MOSBY'S TEXTBOOK FOR

LONG TERM CARE

assistants

SECOND EDITION

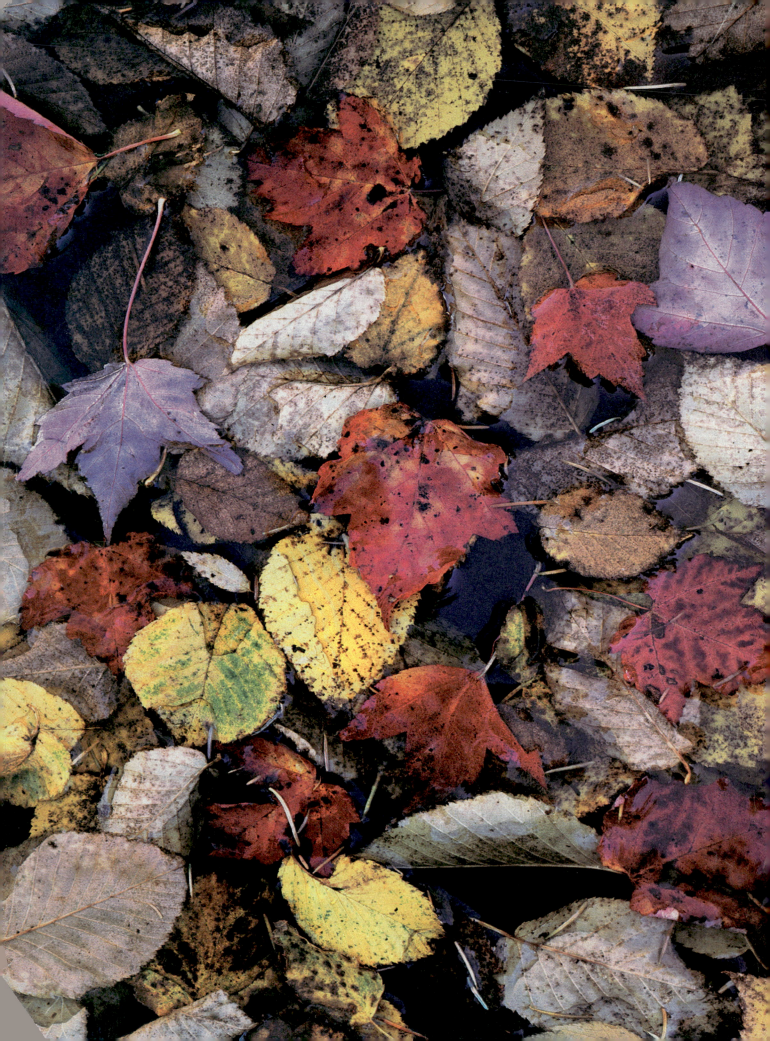

Mosby's Textbook for

LONG TERM CARE

assistants

SECOND EDITION

Sheila A. Sorrentino, RN, BSN, MA, PhD
DIRECTOR OF CAREER EDUCATION AND TRAINING
HEARTLAND COMMUNITY COLLEGE • BLOOMINGTON, IL

Jean Hogan, RN, MSN
CLINICAL NURSE SPECIALIST, GERONTOLOGY
VA MEDICAL CENTER • LIVERMORE, CA

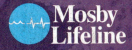
Mosby
Lifeline

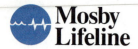
**Mosby
Lifeline**

Publisher: David T. Culverwell
Executive Editor: Richard A. Weimer
Managing Editor: Doris E. Smith
Editorial Staff: Mary Beth Ryan Warthen, Christine Ambrose, and Christi Mangold,
Production Editor: Kathleen L. Teal
Photography: Rick Brady
Design: Studio Montage, St. Louis, MO
Cover Photo: FPG International
Preface Illustration: Jim Branscum

Second Edition
Copyright © 1994 by Mosby-Year Book, Inc.
A Mosby Lifeline imprint of Mosby-Year Book, Inc.

Previous edition, copyrighted 1988

Printed in the United States of America

Mosby-Year Book, Inc.
11830 Westline Industrial Drive
St. Louis, Missouri 63146

International Standard Book Number:
0–8016–7021–7

94 95 96 97 98 CL/CL 9 8 7 6 5 4 3 2 1

The following illustrations were originally used in Sorrentino, SA: Mosby's Textbook for Nursing Assistants, ed. 3, St. Louis, 1992, Mosby.

PREFACE

An adaptation of the third edition of *Mosby's Textbook for Nursing Assistants* by Sheila A. Sorrentino, the second edition of *Mosby's Textbook for Long-Term Care Assistants* emphasizes the needs of the elderly and other persons requiring the services of nursing facilities. The second edition continues to focus on nursing assistant skills and functions, safety, and the psychosocial approach to resident care. In every chapter, caring, understanding, and respect for residents as individuals are important attitudes conveyed to the nursing assistant.

As with the previous edition, the accepted functions of nursing assistants and those functions that they may be asked to perform, if given the necessary education, training, and supervision, are presented. Because facilities vary in their use of nursing assistants, the responsibilities and limitations of nursing assistants are emphasized throughout the book and specifically in Chapter 2 *(The Nursing Assistant)* which deals with the legal and ethical aspects of their role.

Since the first edition of *Mosby's Textbook for Long-Term Care Assistants* was released, four major policies have affected health care delivery in the United States:

- Universal precautions issued by the Centers for Disease Control (CDC)

- The Omnibus Budget Reconciliation Act of 1987 (OBRA)

- The Food Guide Pyramid issued by the United States Department of Agriculture (USDA)

- The bloodborne pathogen standard issued by the Occupational Safety and Health Administration (OSHA)

These policies are explained in the second edition of *Mosby's Textbook for Nursing Assistants.* Universal precautions and the bloodborne pathogen standard are described in Chapter 8 *(Infection Control)* and are integrated throughout the text as they relate to the provision of care and the performance of nursing skills. The Food Guide Pyramid is highlighted in Chapter 15 *(Food and Fluids)* as the focus of good nutrition, replacing the long-standing four basic food groups.

Resident rights identified by OBRA are a major focus of Chapter 1. OBRA implications are highlighted in Chapter 2 *(The Nursing Assistant)* in relation to the legal role of the nursing assistant and Chapter 6 *(The Elderly Resident)* as the law pertains to the quality of life, health, and safety of residents in nursing facilities.

Major features of this new edition are the integration of OBRA throughout the text and the addition of a Quality of Life section to each chapter beginning with Chapter 7. While quality of life and resident rights are integrated throughout Chapters 7 to 28, the Quality of Life section bridges the focus of the chapter with how to protect the resident's rights and enhance the person's quality of life when giving care.

Considerable attention has been given to increasing the awareness and sensitivity of nursing assistants to the psychosocial needs of the elderly. Content related to these qualities has been integrated throughout the text. The Quality of Life sections and resident quotes at the beginning of each chapter are other features that help nursing assistants understand the feelings and needs of residents.

The textbook is intended for use in community colleges, technical colleges, high schools, vocational-career centers, nursing facilities, and other agencies providing nursing assistant education. The organization allows for variations in curricular structure and program length. The order of chapter or chapter section presentation can be determined by the instructor. For example, a course begins with infection control, body mechanics, bedmaking, and bed bath. The appropriate chapters and sections can be assigned for studying in the above order without jeopardizing content or learning.

Organization of the second edition, like *Mosby's Textbook for Nursing Assistants*, was influenced by basic nursing concepts and learning strategies:

- Nursing assistants must be aware of and understand their work environment and the individuals in that environment.

- An understanding of body structure and function promotes safe and competent performance of psychomotor skills.

- Learning proceeds from the simple to the complex. Concepts and procedures integral to other activities and functions (safety, body mechanics, and medical asepsis) are presented early. Psychomotor skills that are easy to learn and basic to the role of nursing assistants are then presented, such as bedmaking, personal care, certain urinary and bowel elimination procedures, measuring intake and output, serving food trays, and feeding residents. More complex content follows. Vital signs and heat and cold applications are more complex in regard to learning and safe practice and may not be nursing assistant functions in all facilities.

- The basic needs according to Abraham Maslow are emphasized.
- The resident is presented as a person with physical, psychological, social, and spiritual needs.
- The influence and importance of cultural heritage to a person's activities of daily living and responses to illness are presented where appropriate.

Mosby's Textbook for Long-Term Care Assistants is comprehensive and is intended to serve as a reference for nursing assistants as they expand their skills and knowledge. A new chapter titled *Confusion and Dementia* (Chapter 24) and chapters focusing on safety, rehabilitation, care of the elderly, common health problems, human sexuality, and

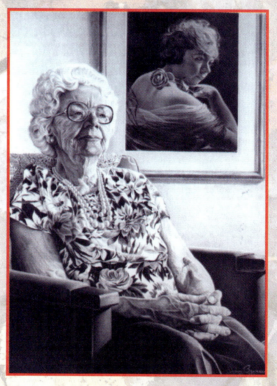

From a series of drawings entitled "Aging in America" by Jim Branscum, Phoenix, Arizona.

basic emergency care are part of the book's comprehensiveness. Chapter 23 *(Common Health Problems)* describes the basic causes, signs and symptoms, and care of residents with common health problems. Chapter 25 *(Human Sexuality)* addresses the sensitive issue of sexuality, including sexuality in nursing facilities, sexuality in the elderly, sexually transmitted diseases, and the sexually aggressive resident.

The reading level for *Mosby's Textbook for Long-Term Care Assistants* should appeal to a broad range of students with various reading abilities. Except for medical terms which are defined throughout the text, the vocabulary is basic, using common terms. The readability of the text does not compromise professionalism, caring, and sensitivity.

Mosby's Textbook for Long-Term Care Assistants includes a full-color format with illustrations and photographs that enhance the student's understanding of the material presented. Other important features include learning objectives and key terms with definitions at the beginning of each chapter and review questions and answers to facilitate and evaluate learning at the end of each chapter.

Sheila A. Sorrentino

Publisher's note:

*W*e hope you enjoy this new edition of *Mosby's Textbook for Long-Term Care Assistants*. Considerable thought has been put into creating an interesting tone and design of this text. We have chosen vintage photographs for the chapter openers. Building this text around these photographs has taught us much about compassion, caring, and the journey of life. We hope that as you see these photographs you, too, will have a similar empathic experience that will not only touch you, but will also affect the relationship you have with the people to whom you give care.

David T. Culverwell,
Doris E. Smith, Mary Beth R. Warthen
Mosby Lifeline

AKNOWLEDGEMENTS

*A*s with any textbook, there are many people who contribute in some way to its completion. Those deserving thanks and appreciation include:

Connie March, Vice President of Geriatric Services at ServantCor (Kankakee, Illinois), for her advice, suggestions, and provision of reference materials.

Tammy Taylor and Jane DeBlois, nursing assistant instructors at Heartland Community College in Bloomington, Illinois, and Helen Chigaros, nursing assistant instructor at Kankakee Community College in Kankakee, Illinois, for providing ideas, insight, reference materials, and support for this work.

Relda Kelly, for writing the second edition of the workbook to accompany this textbook.

Cheryl Owoc, for writing the instructor's manual and the instructor's resource kit.

The many who reviewed the manuscript and provided invaluable ideas and suggestions.

The editorial staff at Mosby Lifeline in Hanover, Maryland: Rick Weimer, Dave Culverwell, Doris Smith, Mary Beth Warthen, Christi Mangold, Eric Duchinsky, and Christine Ambrose for their expertise, interest, and dedication to this book and my other works; and to Kathleen Teal for her production efforts.

And finally to Don Ladig, Editor-in-Chief for Allied Health at Mosby in St. Louis, who conceived the idea of *Mosby's Textbook for Nursing Assistants* first published in 1984. That first book and those that followed have served to educate thousands of nursing assistants who, in turn, gave quality to the care and lives of even more patients and residents. ❧

Sheila A. Sorrentino

TABLE of CONTENTS

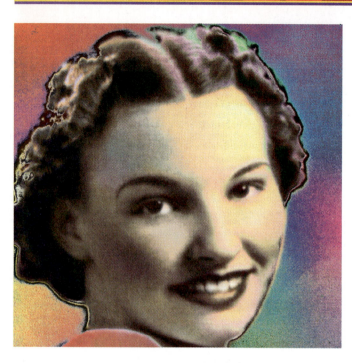

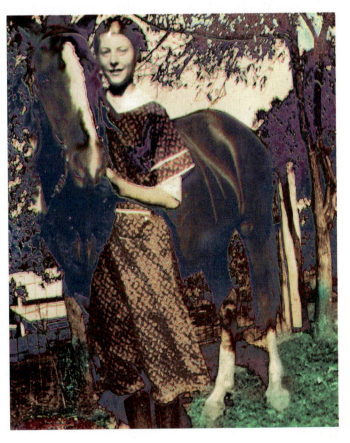

1

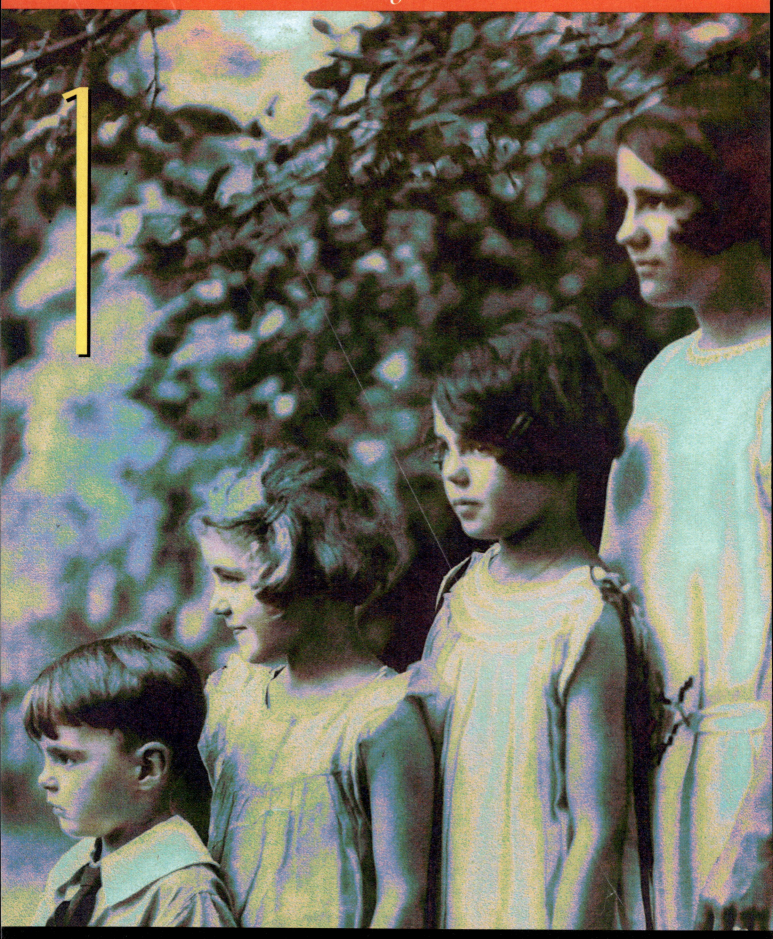

Key TERMS

acute illness
A sudden illness from which the person is expected to recover

Alzheimer's disease
A disease that affects brain tissue; victims suffer increasing memory loss and confusion until they cannot meet their simplest personal needs; some even forget their own names

board and care facility
A facility which provides custodial care to a few independent residents, often in a home setting; no licensed nurse is required

chronic illness
An illness, slow or gradual in onset, for which there is no known cure; the illness can be controlled and complications prevented

communicable disease
A disease that can be spread from one person to another

custodial care
Care provided on a 24-hour basis that meets a person's basic physical needs

deconditioning
The process of becoming weak from illness or lack of exercise

functional nursing
A method of organizing nursing care; nursing staff members perform specific tasks for all assigned residents

health care team
A variety of health care workers who work together in providing health care for residents; interdisciplinary health care team

hospice
A health care facility or program for individuals dying of terminal illnesses

interdisciplinary health care team
The health care team

licensed practical nurse (LPN)
An individual who has completed a 1-year nursing program and who has passed the licensing examination for practical nurses; called licensed vocational nurse (LVN) in some states

Medicaid
A health insurance program sponsored by state and federal governments

Medicare
A health insurance plan administered by the Social Security Administration of the federal government

nursing assistant
An individual who gives basic nursing care under the supervision of an RN or an LPN; also called nurse's aide, nursing attendant, health care assistant, and orderly

nursing facility (NF)
A facility that provides nursing care for many residents; a licensed nursing staff is required; commonly called a nursing home or convalescent hospital

nurse practitioner (NP)
A registered nurse who has received advanced training in physical examination and assessment; in some states the NP can diagnose and prescribe under a doctor's supervision

nursing team
The individuals involved in providing nursing care: registered nurses, LPNs, and nursing assistants

OBRA
The Omnibus Budget Reconciliation Act of 1987; concerned with the quality of life, health, and safety of residents

orderly
A male nursing assistant

primary nursing
A method of organizing nursing care; a nurse is responsible for the total care of specific residents on a 24-hour basis

registered nurse (RN)
A person who has studied nursing for 2, 3, or 4 years and who has passed a licensing examination

restorative aide
A nursing assistant who has special training in rehabilitation skills

skilled nursing facility (SNF)
A facility that provides nursing care for residents who need complex care but do not require hospital services; may be part of a nursing facility or a hospital

team nursing
A method of organizing nursing care in which a nurse serves as a team leader; the team leader assigns other nurses and nursing assistants to care for certain residents

My family is gone and there was no one to help me after my surgery. So I came here. I have help and new friends. That makes me happy.

This chapter describes the purposes, goals, and services of long-term care. Emphasis is given to nursing facilities that employ nursing assistants. The chapter also describes the organization of nursing facilities, the nursing team, insurance programs, and some of the federal laws regarding resident care.

LONG-TERM CARE FACILITIES

Long-term care facilities provide health care services to persons unable to care for themselves at home but who do not need hospital care. Services range from very simple custodial care to more complex care. Medical, nursing, food, recreational, rehabilitative, and social services usually are provided.

Persons living in long-term care facilities are called *residents,* not patients. The facility is their permanent or temporary home. Long-term care facilities are designed and constructed to meet the special needs of elderly or disabled residents (Fig. 1-1). Some residents return home when well enough. Others require nursing care until death occurs.

Board and Care Facilities

A **board and care facility** (custodial or residential facility) often is in a home setting. The facility provides simple custodial care to a few residents. **Custodial care** is care that is provided on a 24-hour basis and that meets the person's basic physical needs. A safe environment is provided for individuals who need supervision but not nursing care. Residents need very little assistance with their personal care. They usually can dress themselves and tend to their grooming and bathroom needs with little assistance. A caregiver always is present to help with their needs and to see that they are fed, clean, and in good health. This caregiver may be a nursing assistant. Licensed nurses may or may not be employed by the facility.

Nursing Facilities

A **nursing facility** (nursing home or convalescent hospital) provides nursing care to many residents. A licensed nursing staff is required. Residents usually have more severe health problems than do persons in board and care facilities. Services range from very simple custodial care to more complex care. Medical, nursing, food, recreational, rehabilitative, and social services usually are provided. Licensed nurses, nursing assistants, physical therapists, dietary personnel, and other health care workers are needed to provide such services. These employees have specific skills and knowledge. The focus of their care, however, is always on the residents.

Some nursing facilities also provide more complex care and are called **skilled nursing facilities (SNFs).** A part of the facility (skilled nursing unit) is reserved for residents with more severe health problems. These residents have many health problems but do not require hospital services. Many residents are admitted to SNFs directly from hospitals. They stay for a short time to recover from an illness or surgery or to be rehabilitated. Others do not recover enough to return home. These residents transfer to other types of facilities or become permanent residents of the nursing facility.

Hospital-based skilled nursing facilities provide more skilled nursing care than is available in most SNFs. Persons in a hospital-based SNF may be called *patients* because, as in a hospital, they stay for a short time. Patients may receive intravenous therapy, special nutritional therapy, special treatments, or other specialized nursing care or rehabilitation. They usually are transferred to another SNF or nursing facility after a few weeks.

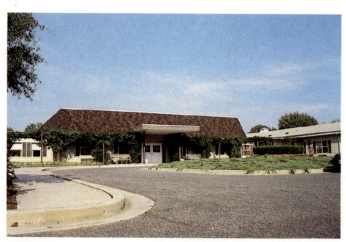

A

FIGURE 1-1 *A, A one-story long-term care facility.*

2

Purposes and goals of nursing facilities. Nursing facilities have several purposes. Most residents suffer from one or more chronic illnesses. One goal is to *promote good physical and mental health* by helping residents accept the limits of their chronic diseases and to function within those limits. The goal is accomplished through teaching, counseling, and caring by concerned health care providers. Residents are helped to change habits that can make their illnesses worse. They are encouraged to eat proper diets and to get the proper amount and type of exercise. They also are encouraged to focus on their abilities rather than their disabilities and to do as much for themselves as possible.

Families are given help in accepting the physical and mental changes that they see in their loved ones. They are helped to understand the reasons for these physical and mental changes. They are taught how to assist their loved ones to maintain the highest possible level of functioning and to accept the limits of the chronic illnesses.

Prevention of communicable disease is another goal. A **communicable disease** can be spread from one person to another (see Chapter 8). Communicable diseases—for example, colds and influenza (flu)—can create major health problems for elderly persons. You will be closely involved in the care of residents. Therefore you may be the first person to detect the signs and symptoms of a communicable disease.

The *treatment of chronic illness* is another major purpose. A **chronic illness** is slow or gradual in onset. There is no cure. The illness can be controlled and complications can be prevented with proper treatment. Chronic illness is different from acute illness. An **acute illness** is one that begins suddenly and from which the person is expected to recover. Persons with acute illnesses may need hospital care.

A nurse observes residents for signs and symptoms of worsening illness. The nurse is involved in the treatment of illness by giving care and carrying out therapeutic measures ordered by the doctor. You will be assisting the nurse. Therefore you will be involved in the observation and care of residents (Fig. 1-2, p. 4).

Rehabilitation or *restorative care* also is a purpose of nursing facilities. It is aimed at helping residents return to their highest possible level of physical and mental functioning. This does not necessarily mean that the resident can be discharged from the facility. In the past, rehabilitation focused primarily on individuals who could return home. Now all residents are helped to remain as independent as possible. This includes those residents who will be in nursing facilities for the rest of their lives.

Restorative care begins when an individual is admitted to the facility. Often residents have become **deconditioned** after an acute illness. This means that they have become weak from bed rest or lack of exercise while ill. Other residents may have suffered a disability as a result of a stroke, fracture, or surgery. Many health care workers may be involved in helping the resident become as independent as possible. These include physical therapists, occupational therapists, language therapists, and restorative aides. **Restorative aides** are nursing assistants with special rehabilitation training. They assist other health care workers in the restorative program. The entire staff, whether specially trained or not, helps residents reach and maintain their highest level of functioning.

Some nursing facilities provide educational experiences for students. The students may be studying to become nurses, nursing assistants, or nurse practitioners. In some areas medical students study in nursing facilities. All students are concerned with the same purposes and goals as those of the facility. They assist in the promotion of health, the treatment of illness, and the prevention of communicable disease, as well as in restorative care.

Nursing facilities provide services in addition to rehabilitation and nursing. They may provide laboratory, dietary, and portable x-ray services, respiratory therapy, and recreational therapy. Many facilities also may have special units for different types of care. These include hospice and Alzheimer's disease units.

Hospice units. A **hospice** is a unit especially designed for those who are dying. The physical, emotional, social, and spiritual needs of the resident and family are provided for in a setting that allows much freedom. Children and pets may be allowed to visit at any time. Family and friends are encouraged to help in giving care. Hospice care also may be provided in hospitals or home care agencies.

B
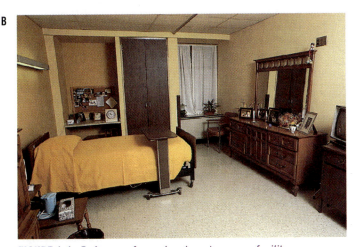

FIGURE 1-1 *B, A room of a modern long-term care facility.*

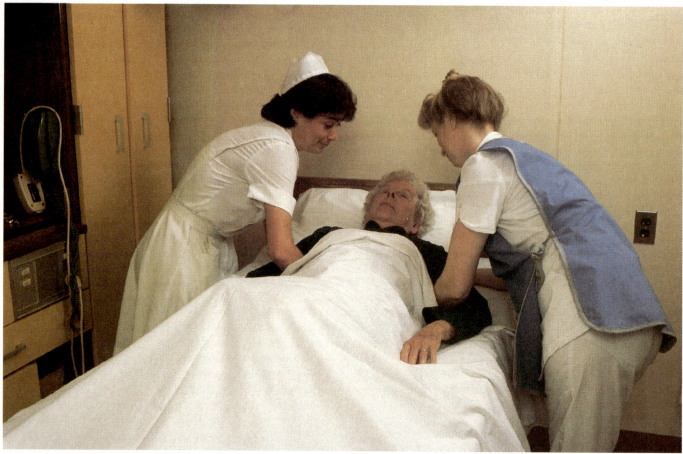

FIGURE 1-2 *A nursing assistant helping an RN give care to a resident.*

Alzheimer's units. An Alzheimer's unit is designed for residents with **Alzheimer's disease.** Alzheimer's disease affects brain tissue (see Chapter 24). Victims suffer increasing memory loss and confusion until they cannot take care of their own simplest personal needs. Eventually, they may forget their own names. They often wander about and may become agitated or even combative. The Alzheimer's unit usually is closed off from the rest of the facility. Keeping the unit closed provides a safe environment where these special residents can wander freely. They are cared for by a specially trained staff.

HOW A NURSING FACILITY IS ORGANIZED

Nursing facilities usually are owned by an individual or by a corporation. The owner is responsible for making sure that the facility provides adequate and safe care at the lowest possible cost. The owner must make sure that local, state, and OBRA (see pp. 8-10) regulations are followed. The owner makes facility policies and hires others to manage the facility. In corporate-owned facilities there usually is a regional manager. The regional manager hires an administrator for the facility. In privately owned facilities the owner also may be the administrator.

In larger facilities, department heads report to the administrator. An office manager is responsible for resident billing, admissions, and personnel records. There may be housekeeping, maintenance, and laundry supervisors. Activities directors or recreational therapists plan and organize resident activities. A director of staff development is responsible for staff training and in-service programs. OBRA requires that all nursing facilities have a medical director. The medical director is a doctor who is a consultant to the staff for all medical problems not handled by a resident's personal doctor. The medical director also helps guide resident care policies and programs. The director of nurses is in charge of the entire nursing staff and the activities involved in providing safe nursing care to residents. The nursing service department is discussed later in this chapter.

The Health Care Team

The **health care team** involves a variety of workers whose skills and knowledge are directed to the total care of the resident. Members of the health care team provide supportive services for the overall goal of quality resident care. The team works together to meet the needs of each resident. Because many health care workers are involved in the care of each resident, coordination of care is needed. The nursing staff usually is responsible for the coordination of care. An RN serves in the key leadership position. Fig. 1-3 shows the members of the health care team, with the resident as the focus of all health care workers. Because the health care team involves individuals from many disciplines, it also is called the **interdisciplinary health care team.**

Nursing Service

Nursing service is a major department in nursing facilities. A director of nurses (DON) is found in most nursing facilities. A DON is an RN. The DON is assisted in managing the responsibilities of the department of nursing by nursing supervisors. Nursing supervisors usually are RNs. Some are LPNs. There usually is one supervisor per shift. This person supervises and coordinates resident care for that shift.

Licensed nurses are assigned to each nursing station or unit. They provide nursing care and assign and supervise the work of nursing assistants. The nursing assistant reports to the nurse who is supervising his or her work. The nurse reports to the nursing supervisor. The nursing supervisor reports to the DON.

Nursing education is a part of nursing service. There may be a director of staff development (DSD) who reports to the DON. The DSD usually is an RN. The DON, however, may have this responsibility. The DSD plans and presents educational sessions to nursing personnel so that up-to-date and safe resident care can be provided. The DSD also may conduct a nursing assistant training program.

Methods of Organizing Nursing Care

Nursing care can be organized in several ways to provide safe and effective care. The number of residents needing care, available staff members, and cost are factors in or-

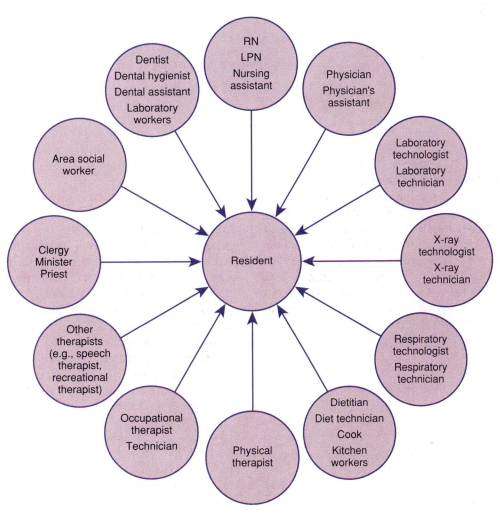

FIGURE 1-3 *Members of the health care team, with the resident as the focus of care.*

ganizing nursing care. Common methods of organizing care in nursing facilities are functional nursing, team nursing, and primary nursing.

Functional nursing is perhaps the oldest and least effective method. Each member of the nursing team is given certain functions or tasks to do for all residents. One nurse may give all medications. Another may change all dressings and give all treatments. Some nursing assistants give all the baths, take all vital signs, and weigh all residents. Others may make all beds, pass all drinking water, and feed residents who cannot feed themselves. Functional nursing care is uncoordinated and fragmented. There are many disadvantages to the resident. These include interrupted rest, having to learn several names and titles of nursing staff members, waiting to have total care completed, and frequent interruptions. Having to deal with so many different individuals can cause confusion and disorientation in elderly persons.

Team nursing is a popular and efficient method of organizing nursing care. The team is led by a nurse who determines the amount and kind of care required by each resident. The team leader assigns nursing assistants or other nurses to care for specific residents. Assignments are made according to the resident's needs and the skills of the team members. Team members report to the team leader about any observations made and the care given.

Primary nursing involves total and comprehensive resident care. Each resident is assigned to a primary nurse. The primary nurse is responsible for the resident's care on a 24-hour basis. Other nurses and nursing assistants assist the primary nurse. The primary nurse is involved in the resident's care and gives necessary teaching and guidance. Home care or hospital transfers are arranged as needed. The primary nurse also is responsible for communicating with the family. Both the resident and family know which nurse to ask for and to whom questions about care and treatment should be directed.

THE NURSING TEAM

The **nursing team** involves RNs, LPNs, and nursing assistants. Each member has different roles and responsibilities, depending on the amount and kind of education received. All are concerned with the basic needs and quality of life of each resident.

Registered Nurses

A **registered nurse (RN)** studies for 2 years at a community college, 2 or 3 years in a hospital-based diploma program, or 4 years at a college or university. The person studies nursing, as well as the biological, social, and physical sciences. The graduate takes a licensing examination offered by a state board of nursing. The examination must be passed for the nurse to become *registered*

and to receive a license to practice. RNs must be licensed by the state in which they practice.

RNs assess, plan, implement, and evaluate nursing care. The RN identifies the resident's needs and develops a plan of care for the resident. The RN then carries out the plan of care and evaluates its effectiveness on the person's condition. RNs are concerned with the physical, social, emotional, and spiritual needs of residents and their quality of life. Residents are helped to become more independent and are taught ways to stay healthy. Residents, families, and other nursing staff members are instructed by RNs at the bedside or in classrooms.

RNs also carry out the doctor's orders. They may delegate doctor's orders to LPNs or nursing assistants. RNs cannot diagnose diseases or illnesses and do not have the right to prescribe treatments or medications.

Nurse Practitioners

A **nurse practitioner (NP)** is an RN who has had additional education in physical examination and assessment. In some states a nurse practitioner, in addition to being licensed as an RN, must be certified by the state board of nursing. Nurse practitioners may specialize in many different areas. Most NPs who work in nursing facilities, however, are either family nurse practitioners (FNPs) or gerontological nurse practitioners (GNPs). GNPs specialize in the care of the elderly. NPs work for doctors or under the direction of the facility's medical director. The NP assists the nursing staff in assessing residents. The NP may be permitted to write orders for medications and treatments for uncomplicated illnesses or other problems.

Licensed Practical Nurses

A **licensed practical nurse (LPN)** completes 1 year of study in a hospital-based nursing program, community college, vocational school, or technical school. Some public high schools offer 2-year practical nursing programs. In classroom and clinical settings the study of nursing is emphasized. Students also study body structure and function, basic psychology, arithmetic, and communication skills. Graduates take the licensing examination for practical nursing. After passing the test, the individual receives a license to practice and the title of *licensed practical nurse*. In some states the title is *licensed vocational nurse (LVN)*. Like RNs, practical nurses must be licensed to practice nursing.

LPNs work under the supervision of RNs, licensed physicians, and licensed dentists. Their responsibilities and functions are more limited than those of an RN because the LPN has less education in the biological, physical, and social sciences. An LPN can function with a limited amount of supervision when the resident's needs are simple and condition is stable.

Nursing Assistants

Nursing assistants are employed in nursing facilities to assist nurses in providing care to residents. Nurse's aide, nursing attendant, and health-care assistant are other titles. A male nursing assistant may be called an **orderly.** Under the direct supervision of RNs and LPNs, nursing assistants give simple, basic nursing care. Some nursing assistants have taken formal courses in community colleges or high school vocational programs. Others may have taken a course through the nursing education department of a health facility. Some nursing assistants have received on-the-job training instead of a formal course. However, the **Omnibus Budget Reconciliation Act (OBRA) of 1987** requires that nursing assistants have formal training and pass a competency evaluation. Nursing assistant training and competency evaluation are discussed in Chapter 2.

You may wish to continue your education to become an RN or LPN. Community colleges and 4-year colleges and universities in your area can help you select the best program to meet your needs, abilities, and financial situation.

PAYING FOR HEALTH CARE

Hospital care and long-term care are very costly and can financially ruin individuals and their families. Even after a person returns home, bills may continue for doctor's visits, medicines, medical supplies, and home care services.

Most elderly and disabled persons cannot afford large medical bills. Some avoid medical care because they cannot pay. To pay their medical bills, others may go without food. These people and their families often experience worry, fear, and emotional upset over paying for health care. For those with insurance, part of or all of their hospital costs usually are covered. Rarely is the total cost of long-term care covered.

Insurance Programs

Private and government insurance programs pay part or all of a person's health care costs. The basic programs that affect long-term care include the following.

1. *Private insurance* and *group insurance plans* are bought by individuals or by groups for individuals. These plans rarely pay for long-term care. If long-term care is covered, there usually are strict limitations regarding eligibility for coverage, amount paid, and length of stay. Long-term care insurance also can be purchased. However, there are limitations on coverage. Individual policies should be reviewed before purchase.

2. **Medicare** is a health insurance plan administered by the Social Security Administration of the federal government. Benefits are for persons 65 years of age and older. Younger, disabled people also may be covered. Monthly premiums are paid by those insured. Medicare has two parts. Part A pays for some hospital costs up to certain amounts during a specified time period (see discussion of diagnostic-related groups in the next section). Long-term care and home care costs are included if certain regulations are met. Part B pays for some medical expenses, such as doctor visits, diagnostic tests, and treatments. Part B also may cover such things as physical therapy, language therapy, and hospital equipment for home use if ordered by a doctor. Medicare benefits and regulations are complex and change often. Your local Social Security office can provide information and answer questions.

3. **Medicaid** is a health insurance program sponsored by the state and federal governments. Benefits, regulations, and eligibility requirements vary from state to state. Persons older than 65 may qualify. The blind, the disabled, and low-income families usually are eligible. Medicaid usually pays for hospital services, doctors' fees, x-ray and laboratory tests, home care, family planning, dental and eye care, immunizations, and rehabilitation. There is no insurance premium. However, the amount paid for each covered service is limited.

Diagnostic-Related Groups

Diagnostic-related groups (DRGs) were legislated by Congress in 1983 to reduce Medicare and Medicaid costs. Before DRGs, Medicare and Medicaid paid for a certain percentage of actual hospital costs. The amount was determined *after* the hospital stay. Under the DRG system, Medicare and Medicaid payments are determined *before* hospitalization.

A DRG consists of specific diagnoses. The government has determined the length of stay and the cost of treating illnesses in the specific category. The hospital is paid the predetermined amount for Medicare and Medicaid patients. If the hospital's costs for treating the patient are less than the DRG amount, the hospital keeps the extra money. If costs are greater than the DRG amount, the hospital takes the loss.

DRGs have had a great impact on health care. Hospitals want to avoid financial loss from lengthy patient stays. Therefore patients sometimes are discharged earlier than in the past. These patients often are still quite ill. Additional care in nursing facilities frequently is needed until they are well enough and strong enough to return home.

Most nursing facilities receive Medicare or Medicaid funds. These facilities must meet OBRA requirements. Otherwise funding will not occur. Unannounced surveys are conducted to determine if nursing facilities are meeting OBRA requirements.

REQUIREMENTS OF THE OMNIBUS BUDGET RECONCILIATION ACT OF 1987

OBRA is concerned with the quality of life, health, and safety of residents. Nursing facilities must provide care in a manner and in an environment that maintains or improves each resident's quality of life, health, and safety. Training and competency evaluation of nursing assistants are OBRA requirements (see Chapter 2). Many other requirements must be met as well.

Resident Rights

Residents of nursing facilities have certain rights under federal and state laws. Residents have rights as citizens of the United States. They also have rights relating to their everyday lives and care in a nursing facility. Nursing facilities must protect and promote resident rights. Residents must be able to exercise their rights without interference from the facility. Some residents are incompetent (not able) and cannot exercise their rights. Legal guardians exercise rights for them.

Nursing facilities must inform residents of their rights. They must be informed orally and in writing.

Such information is given before or during admission to the facility. It must be given in the language used and understood by the resident.

Privacy and confidentiality. Residents have the right to personal privacy. The resident's body must not be exposed unnecessarily. Only those workers directly involved in care, treatments, or examinations should be present. The resident must give consent for others to be present. For example, a student may want to observe a procedure or treatment. The resident's consent is necessary for the student to be an observer. A resident also has the right to use the bathroom in private. Privacy must be maintained for personal care activities as well.

Residents also have the right to visit with others in private. They have the right to visit in an area where they cannot be seen or heard by others. The facility must try to provide private space when it is requested. Offices, chapels, dining rooms, meeting rooms, and conferences rooms can be used if available.

The right to visit in privacy also involves telephone conversations (Fig. 1-4). In addition, residents have the right to send and receive mail without interference by others. Letters sent and received by the resident must not

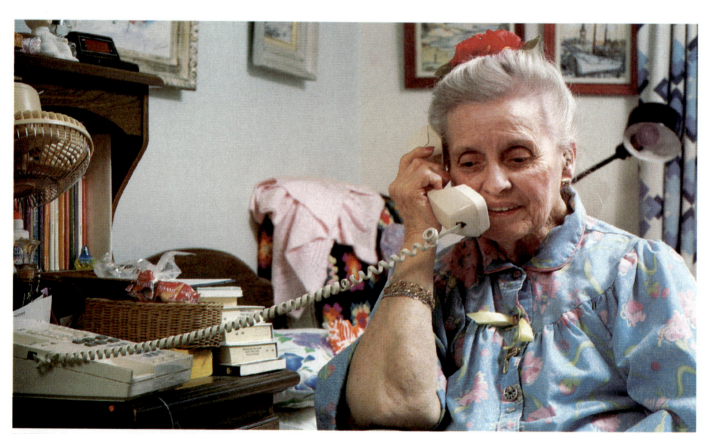

FIGURE 1-4 *A resident talking privately on a telephone.*

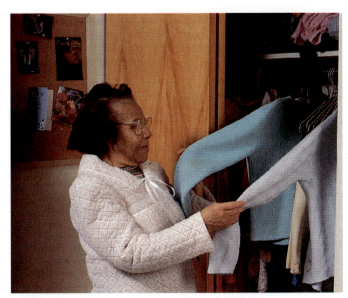

FIGURE 1-5 *A resident choosing what clothing to wear.*

be opened by others without the resident's permission.

Information about the resident's care, treatment, and condition must be kept confidential. Medical and financial records also are confidential. The resident must give consent for them to be released to other facilities or individuals. Consent is not needed, however, for the release of medical records when the resident is being transferred to another facility. Records also can be released without the resident's consent when they are required by law or for insurance purposes.

Throughout this textbook you will be reminded to keep information about the person confidential. Providing for privacy and keeping medical and personal information confidential show respect for the individual. They also protect the person's dignity. The right to privacy and confidentiality are discussed in Chapter 2.

Personal choice. OBRA requires that residents be free to choose their own doctors. They also have the right to participate in planning their own care and treatment. This means that residents have the right to choose activities, schedules, and care based on their personal preferences. For example, residents have the right to choose when to get up and go to bed, what to wear, how to spend their time, and what to eat (Fig. 1-5). They also can choose companions and visitors inside and outside of the facility.

Personal choice is important for quality of life, dignity, and self-respect. You will be reminded throughout this book to allow the person's preferences whenever it is safely possible.

Disputes and grievances. Residents have the right to voice concerns, questions, and complaints about care or treatment. The dispute or grievance may involve another resident. It may be about treatment or care that was not given. The facility must promptly try to correct the situation. The resident must not be punished in any way for voicing the dispute or grievance.

Participation in resident and family groups. Residents have the right to participate in resident and family groups. This means that residents have the right to form groups (Fig. 1-6). In addition, a resident's family has the right to meet with the families of other residents. These groups can discuss concerns and suggest ways to improve quality of life in the facility. They also can plan activities for residents and families. The group can provide support and reassurance for group members. Residents also have the right to participate in social, religious, and community activities. They also have the right to assistance in getting to and from activities of their choice.

Care and security of personal possessions. Residents have the right to keep and use personal possessions. Available space and the health and safety of other residents can affect the type and amount of personal possessions allowed. A person's property must be treated with care and respect. Although the items may not have value to you, they are important to the resident. They also relate to personal choice, dignity, and quality of life.

The facility must take reasonable measures to protect the person's property. Items should be labeled with the resident's name. The facility must investigate reports of lost, stolen, or damaged items. Police assistance sometimes is necessary. The resident and family probably will be advised not to keep jewelry and other expensive items in the facility.

You must protect yourself and the facility from being accused of stealing a resident's property. Do not go through a resident's closet, drawers, purse, or other space without the person's knowledge and consent. Have an-

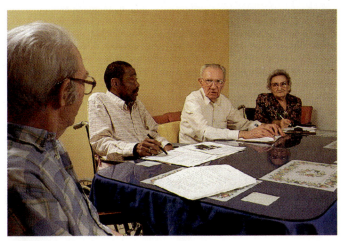

FIGURE 1-6 *Residents at a group meeting.*

other worker with you and the resident or legal guardian present if it is necessary to inspect closets and drawers. The worker serves as a witness to your activities.

Freedom from abuse, mistreatment, and neglect. OBRA states that residents have the right to be free from verbal, sexual, physical, or mental abuse. Elder abuse is discussed in Chapter 6.

Residents also have the right to be free from involuntary seclusion. Involuntary seclusion is separating the resident from others against his or her will. It also can mean keeping the person confined to a certain area or away from his or her room without consent. If the person is incompetent, involuntary seclusion occurs against the legal guardian's consent.

No one can abuse, neglect, or mistreat the resident. This includes facility staff members, volunteers, staff members from other agencies or groups, other residents, family, visitors, and legal guardians. Nursing facilities must have policies and procedures for investigating suspected or reported cases of resident abuse. Also, nursing facilities cannot employ persons who have been convicted of abusing, neglecting, or mistreating individuals.

Freedom from restraint. Residents have the right not to have body movements restricted. Body movements can be restricted by the application of restraints or the administration of certain drugs. Some drugs can restrain the person because they affect mood, behavior, and mental function. Sometimes residents need to be restrained to protect them from harming themselves or others. A doctors's order is necessary for restraints to be used. Restraints cannot be used for the convenience of the staff. Restraints are discussed in Chapter 7.

Quality of life. OBRA requires that nursing facilities care for residents in a manner that promotes dignity, self-esteem, and physical, psychological, and emotional well-being. Protecting the rights of residents is one way to promote quality of life. Personal choice, privacy, participation in group activities, having personal property, and freedom from restraint show respect for the person.

The resident should be spoken to in a polite and courteous manner (see Chapter 4). Giving good, honest, and thoughtful care will enhance the resident's quality of life.

Activities. Activities are important to a resident's quality of life. OBRA requires that nursing facilities provide activity programs that meet the interests and physical, mental, and psychosocial needs of each resident. Such activities must allow personal choice and promote physical, intellectual, social, and emotional well-being. Many facilities also provide religious services for spiritual health. You will be responsible for assisting residents to and from activity programs. You also may be assigned to help residents with activities.

Environment. The environment of the facility must promote quality of life. The environment must be clean, safe, and as homelike as possible. Letting the resident have personal possessions enhances quality of life by acknowledging personal choice and promoting a homelike environment. The safe environment is discussed in Chapter 7. The furniture and equipment in a resident's room are discussed in Chapter 10. Information relating to temperature and sound levels also is presented.

SUMMARY

In this chapter you have been introduced to nursing facilities, their general goals and purposes, and the health care workers involved in resident care. You also were introduced to insurance programs that pay for health care. Finally, you were introduced to OBRA and its effect on the residents' quality of life.

Facility size and services offered influence the organization and the number of workers employed by the facility. Whatever the size of the facility, the focus of care is always the resident. Under the supervision of RNs and LPNs, you have an important place in the organization of the facility and on the health care team.

Review QUESTIONS

Circle the *best* answer.

1. Helping individuals return to their highest physical and psychological functioning is known as
   a. Detection and treatment of disease
   b. Promotion of health
   c. Rehabilitation
   d. Disease prevention

2. Who controls policy in a nursing facility?
   a. The director of nurses
   b. The administrator
   c. The owner
   d. The health care team

3. A health care unit for dying residents is called
   a. A hospice
   b. A board and care facility
   c. An intermediate care facility
   d. A hospital

4. The nursing team includes all of the following *except*
   a. Registered nurses
   b. Physicians
   c. Nursing assistants and orderlies
   d. Licensed practical nurses

5. Which statement is *false?*
   a. Medicare is for those 65 years of age and older and for some disabled persons.
   b. DRGs affect Medicare and Medicaid payments.
   c. Most insurance programs pay all costs of long-term care.
   d. Persons older than 65 may be eligible for Medicaid.

Circle *T* if the answer is true and *F* if it is false.

T F 6. Rehabilitation begins when the resident is ready to be discharged from the nursing facility.

T F 7. The DON is responsible for the entire nursing staff and the activities involved in providing safe nursing care.

T F 8. Nursing supervisors are RNs or LPNs.

T F 9. The nursing assistant is a member of both the health care team and the nursing team.

T F 10. Functional nursing involves giving each member of the nursing team certain tasks to perform.

T F 11. An LPN functions under the supervision of an RN, a licensed doctor, or a licensed dentist.

T F 12. A nursing assistant assists RNs and LPNs in providing nursing care to residents.

T F 13. You have the right to open a resident's mail.

T F 14. The resident has the right to decide what he or she will wear.

T F 15. You can search the resident's closets and drawers to look for lost items.

T F 16. Residents can offer suggestions to improve the facility.

T F 17. Residents can be restrained to prevent them from leaving the facility.

T F 18. Residents must be free from abuse, neglect, and mistreatment.

T F 19. Allowing personal choice is important for the resident's quality of life.

T F 20. Participation in activities is important for the resident's quality of life.

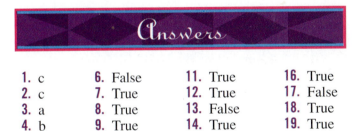

Answers

1. c	6. False	11. True	16. True
2. c	7. True	12. True	17. False
3. a	8. True	13. False	18. True
4. b	9. True	14. True	19. True
5. c	10. True	15. False	20. True

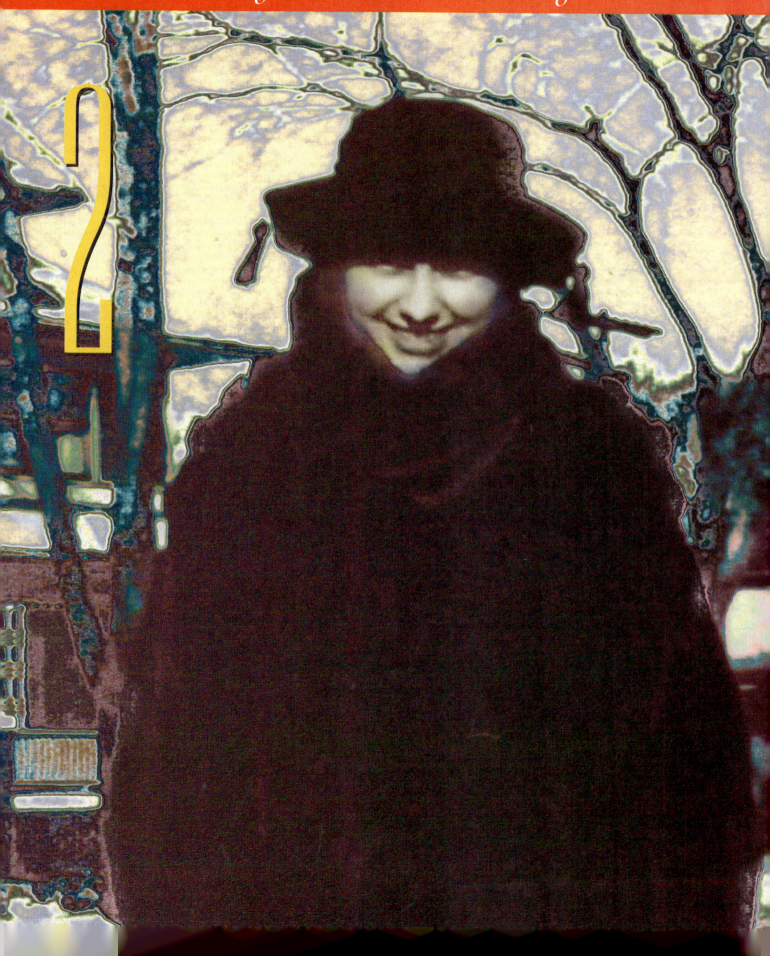

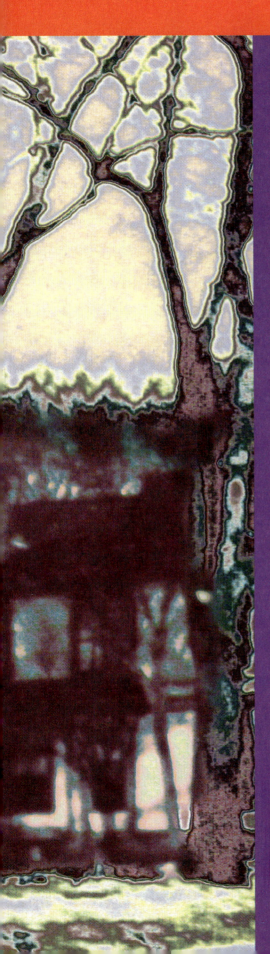

What You Will LEARN

- The key terms listed in this chapter

- The role of nursing assistants and the functions they can and cannot perform

- Why nursing assistants need a job description

- The qualities and characteristics of a successful nursing assistant

- Good health and hygiene practices

- How the nursing assistant should dress for work

- The nursing assistant training and competency evaluation programs required by OBRA

- The information contained in the nursing assistant registry and other OBRA requirements

- How nursing assistants should behave ethically

- How to prevent negligent acts

- The differences among false imprisonment, defamation, assault, and battery

- How to protect the right to privacy

- The nursing assistant's role in relation to wills

- How to work with others and to plan and organize work

assault
Intentionally attempting or threatening to touch the body of another person without the person's consent

battery
The actual unauthorized touching of another person's body without the person's consent

civil law
Laws concerned with the relationships among people; private law

crime
An act that is a violation of criminal law

criminal law
Laws concerned with offenses against the public and society in general; public law

defamation
Injuring the name and reputation of another person by making false statements to a third person

empathy
The ability to see things from another person's point of view

ethics
What is right and wrong conduct

false imprisonment
The unlawful restraint or restriction of another person's movement

invasion of privacy
A violation of a person's right not to have his or her name, photograph, or private affairs exposed or made public without giving consent

law
A rule of conduct made by a government body

libel
Defamation through written statements

malpractice
Negligence by a professional person

negligence
An unintentional wrong in which a person fails to act in a reasonable and careful manner and thereby causes harm to another person or to the person's property

slander
Defamation through oral statements

tort
A wrong committed against another person or the person's property

will
A legal statement of how an individual wishes to have property distributed after death

I like when Betty is here. She's very nice and doesn't rush me. She always looks nice. ✄

Studying to become a nursing assistant in long-term care should be interesting and exciting. You will discover answers to questions you may have wondered about. How can a bed be made with a person lying in it? How can a person receive a complete bath in bed? What sounds are heard through a stethoscope when a blood pressure is taken?

You will learn that many beliefs about aging and the elderly are untrue: all older people become "senile"; people over 65 have no interest in sex; aging is a disease process. You will learn the facts about these issues as they concern aging. But first you must understand the role and responsibilities of nursing assistants. There may be times when you are told to do something that is not within your role. Therefore you need to know the functions you can and cannot perform in your position. To perform your job safely, you also must be aware of what is right and wrong behavior, as well as your legal limitations. Equally important is an understanding of the qualities and characteristics of a good nursing assistant and an understanding of how to work effectively with others.

THE ROLE OF A NURSING ASSISTANT

You will perform simple and basic nursing functions under the supervision of a nurse. Your work will be supervised by an RN or an LPN. To help nurses provide safe and effective care, you must understand that nursing is a scientific and personal service given to the residents. You will be concerned mainly with assisting nurses in giving care to the residents. You often will perform simple functions without a nurse being physically present. At other times you will actually help the nurse give bedside nursing care. The following rules should help you understand your role.

1. You are an assistant to the nurse.
2. A nurse assigns and supervises your work.
3. You report any changes in a resident's physical or mental status to the nurse.
4. You do not make decisions about what should or should not be done for a resident.
5. If you do not understand directions or instructions, ask the nurse for clarification before going to the resident.
6. Perform no function or task that you have not been prepared to do or that you do not feel comfortable performing without the supervision of a nurse.

FUNCTIONS AND RESPONSIBILITIES

The functions and responsibilities of a nursing assistant vary among nursing facilities. *Responsibility* is a duty or obligation to perform some act or function and being able to answer for one's actions. The procedures in this book have been performed by nursing assistants. Some are more advanced than others. You will find that the functions and responsibilities of nursing assistants often are greater in nursing facilities than in hospitals.

You will perform functions and procedures relating to the personal hygiene, safety, comfort, nutrition, exercise, and elimination needs of residents (Fig. 2-1). You also will perform related functions such as lifting and moving residents, making observations, and collecting specimens. Also, because you provide care daily over many months, you will play an important role in the residents' psychological comfort. In addition, you may assist with the admission and discharge of residents and measure temperatures, pulses, respirations, and blood pressures.

Your training may prepare you to perform certain procedures. Your employer, however, may not allow nursing assistants to perform those procedures. Other facilities may ask that you perform procedures you may not have learned.

There are certain functions, procedures, and tasks that you should never perform. It is extremely important that you understand what you *cannot* do as a nursing assistant.

Never give medications. This includes medication given orally, rectally, by injection, directly into the bloodstream, through an intravenous line, or applied to the skin. There have been times when a nurse has brought a medication to a resident's room while the resident was in the bathroom or busy with some other activity. The nurse then instructed the nursing assistant to give the medication to the resident later. In this (and other similar situations) you should respectfully, but firmly, refuse to follow the nurse's direction. If you give a medication, you are performing a function and a responsibility beyond the scope of nursing assistants.

Never insert tubes or objects into a resident's body openings or remove them from the body. You must not insert tubes into the resident's bladder, esophagus, trachea, nose, ears, bloodstream, or body openings that have been surgically created. Exceptions to the rule are those procedures in this textbook that you will study and practice with your instructor's supervision.

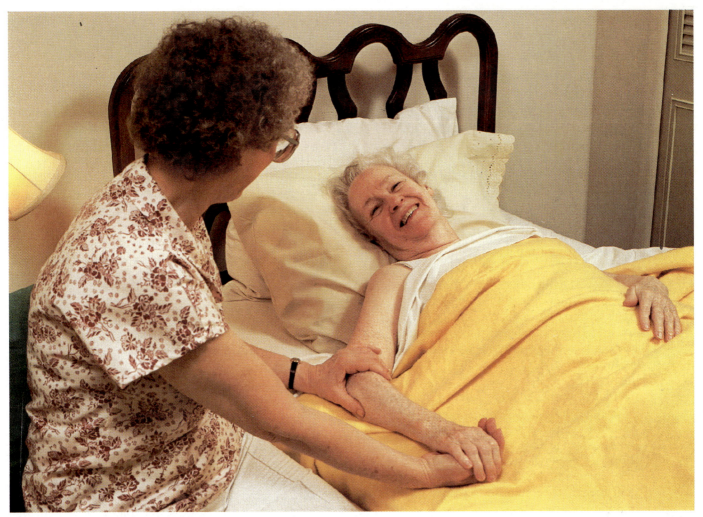

FIGURE 2-1 *A nursing assistant helping an RN make the resident comfortable.*

Never take verbal or telephone orders from doctors. You might answer the telephone or be near a doctor who wants to give you an order. You should politely give your name and title, ask the doctor to wait, and promptly find a nurse to speak with the doctor.

Never perform procedures that require sterile technique. With sterile technique, all objects that will be in contact with the resident's body are free of all microorganisms. Sterile technique and procedures require skills, knowledge, and judgment beyond the training you will receive. You can assist a nurse during a sterile procedure. However, you must never perform the procedure yourself.

Never tell the resident or family the resident's diagnosis or medical or surgical treatment plans. The doctor is responsible for informing the resident and family about the diagnosis and treatment. Nurses may provide further explanations about what the doctor has already told the resident and family if they seem confused.

Never diagnose or prescribe treatments or medications for residents. Only doctors can diagnose and prescribe.

Never supervise other nursing assistants. Nurses are responsible for supervising nursing assistants. You will not be trained to supervise the work of others. Supervising other nursing assistants can have serious legal consequences.

Never just ignore an order or request to do something that you cannot do or that is beyond your scope of practice as a nursing assistant. Promptly explain to the nurse why you cannot carry out the order or request. The nurse will assume you are doing what you were told unless you explain otherwise. Resident care cannot be neglected.

Always request a written job description from an employer. A job description lists the responsibilities and functions you will perform. Before taking a job, inform your employer of any functions you do not know how to do. Also advise the employer of functions you are op-

Job Description

Job Title: Nursing Assistant
Department: Nursing
Job Summary: The nursing assistant provides resident care under the direction of a nurse and assists the nursing team in maintaining nursing and resident units.
Supervisor: Charge nurse

Qualifications:

1. High school education preferred but must have at least a grade school education.
2. Documentation of a formal nursing assistant course and the passing of a competency evaluation.
3. Willingness to learn and work under close supervision.
4. Ability to work with others.
5. Ability to communicate with residents.
6. Genuine interest in residents and co-workers as demonstrated by timeliness and working when scheduled, including weekends and holidays.

Responsibilities:

1. Resident care
   a. Demonstrates a genuine interest in working with the elderly.
   b. Protects residents' rights and treats residents with respect at all times.
   c. Provides personal care such as baths, showers, oral hygiene, skin care, hair care, fingernail and toenail care, monitoring fluid intake and output, toileting, etc.
   d. Assists residents to shave daily.
   e. Assists in serving and feeding residents.
   f. Passes fresh drinking water each shift.
   g. Uses safety measures for residents and self when using body mechanics, side rails, mechanical or electric lifts, collapsible tubs, etc.
   h. Assists with restorative and reconditioning nursing procedures: good body alignment, bed positioning, range-of-motion exercises, transferring residents using a gait belt, provides opportunities for self-care, ambulation, etc.
   i. Follows the bowel or bladder training program established for a resident.
   j. Assists the resident to the bathroom as necessary.
   k. Attends scheduled therapy sessions for a better understanding of a resident's needs and progress.
   l. Encourages and assists the resident to attend all therapies and programs ordered by the doctor (e.g., physical therapy).
   m. Assists the resident to practice activities or exercises learned in therapy programs.
   n. Assists in mental rehabilitation programs.
   o. Organizes care so residents can attend activities or therapies as scheduled.
   p. Assists in transferring residents to activity programs.
   q. Answers call lights promptly and provides or obtains the necessary care.
   r. Observes and reports unusual symptoms, changes, accidents, and injuries to the charge nurse.
   s. Participates in resident care conferences.
   t. Reports to the charge nurse before going off duty.
   u. Performs other duties as directed by the supervisor.

2. Departmental
   a. Makes beds and cleans units on a daily basis as assigned by the charge nurse.
   b. Cares for soiled and clean linen and personal resident laundry according to procedure.
   c. Follows established cleaning schedule for drawers, closets, clean and dirty utility rooms, and nurses' station.
   d. Cleans and cares for equipment and utensils as assigned by the charge nurse.

3. Personal
   a. Wears the official uniform.
   b. Is clean and well groomed.
   c. Completes the nursing assistant orientation program and successfully passes the examination.
   d. Attends staff meetings and staff development programs as required.
   e. Is able to interpret the "Resident's Rights" to the resident and family.

4. Physical demands
   Must have good physical health and be willing and able to be on his or her feet and active during the entire work shift.

I HAVE READ AND UNDERSTAND THE JOB DESCRIPTION AS STATED. THE JOB DESCRIPTION IS SATISFACTORY AS STATED. I AGREE TO ACCEPT THE POSITION OF NURSING ASSISTANT AS DESCRIBED.

Signature _____ Date _____

*Adapted from "Nursing Assistant Job Description" courtesy of Americana Health Care Center, Kankakee, Illinois.

posed to performing for moral or religious reasons. Clearly understand what will be expected of you before taking a job. Do not take a job if you will have to function beyond your educational limitations or against your moral or religious principles. A sample job description for nursing assistants is detailed on p. 16.

No one can force you to perform a function, task, or procedure that is beyond the scope of a nursing assistant. Many times a nursing assistant's job will be threatened for refusing to follow a nurse's orders. Often a nursing assistant will obey an order out of fear. That is why you must understand the role and responsibilities of nursing assistants. You also need to know which functions you can safely perform, the things you should never do, and your job description. Understanding the ethical and legal aspects of your roles is equally important.

QUALITIES AND CHARACTERISTICS

Caring about elderly and disabled residents is an important trait for health care team members in long-term care. It is essential that you *want* to help the elderly and disabled residents be as happy and independent as possible. It is equally important that you *believe* that each person has value as a human being no matter how old, ill, or disabled that person may be. There are certain traits, atti-

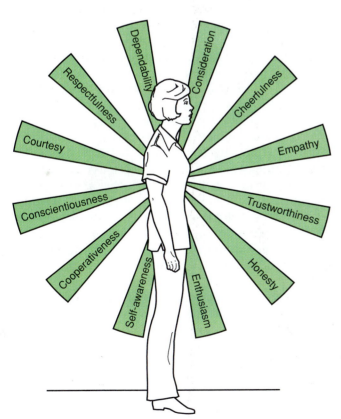

FIGURE 2-2 *The qualities and characteristics of a successful nursing assistant.*

tudes, and manners that help one perform a job well. These are called "qualities and characteristics."

In addition to caring, the following qualities and characteristics are necessary for you to function effectively (Fig. 2-2).

1. *Dependability.* Residents and the nursing team rely on you to report to work when scheduled and on time. They also expect you to perform duties and tasks as assigned and to keep your obligations and promises.

2. *Consideration.* You must be considerate of your residents' physical and personal feelings. Residents rely on you for care. They deserve respect and kindness.

3. *Cheerfulness.* You need to greet and talk with residents and others in a pleasant manner. You must not be moody, bad tempered, or sarcastic when caring for residents. If you are unhappy, you must not show or share your feelings.

4. *Empathy.* **Empathy** is the ability to see things from the resident's point of view—to put yourself in the resident's position. How would you feel if you had the resident's problems?

5. *Patience.* Patience is very important in caring for the elderly and disabled. These people often move slowly, talk slowly, or have difficulty understanding or remembering directions. You must be patient. Let them do tasks at their own pace.

6. *Trustworthiness.* Residents and co-workers place their confidence in you. They believe that you will keep resident information confidential. They also believe that you will not gossip about residents, co-workers, doctors, or other members of the health care team.

7. *Respectfulness.* A resident has certain rights, values, beliefs, and feelings. Although these may differ from yours, you must not criticize or condemn the resident. Treat the resident with respect and dignity at all times. You should show the same respect for your supervisors and co-workers.

8. *Courtesy.* You must be polite and courteous to residents, families, visitors, and co-workers. Address people by title and name, such as "Mrs. Johnson" or "Dr. Wilson," unless they request otherwise. Other courteous acts are explaining a procedure to a resident before you do it; saying "please" and "thank you"; and not interrupting others unnecessarily.

9. *Conscientiousness.* You must be careful, alert, and exact in following orders and instructions. Give thorough care with knowledge and skill. Imagine that you are caring for your parent, grandparent, or someone else that you love. How would you want that person to be cared for? Always perform to the best of your ability.

10. *Honesty.* You must be truthful, sincere, and genuine and show a true interest in residents. The amount and kind of care you give, your observations, and your errors must be reported truthfully and accurately.

11. *Cooperation.* You must be willing to help and work with others. You can show your cooperation by getting along well with others and by being willing to take that "extra step" during busy and stressful times.

• **12.** *Self-awareness.* Being self-aware means that you know your own feelings, strengths, and weaknesses. You need to understand yourself before you can understand others.

Personal Health, Hygiene, and Appearance

The health care team serves as an example to others. Residents, families, and visitors expect you to set a healthy example. A resident may wonder about health care workers who smoke, especially when the resident is told to stop smoking. Therefore your personal health, appearance, and hygiene deserve careful attention.

Your Health

Feeling and looking healthy are important to you as a person, to your residents, and to your employer. Your residents and employer trust you to provide conscientious and effective care. To fulfill this trust you must be physically and mentally healthy. Otherwise you cannot function at your best.

Diet. Good nutrition means eating a balanced diet. A balanced diet includes dairy products, fish and meats, fruits and vegetables, and breads and cereals. Start your day with a good breakfast. To maintain your weight, the number of calories taken in must balance your daily energy needs. To lose weight, caloric intake must be less than energy needs. Avoid excess sweets, salty foods, high-fat foods, and crash diets.

Sleep and rest. Sufficient sleep and rest are needed to do your job well and to stay healthy. Most people need 7 to 8 hours of sleep daily. However, the amount varies with each person. Fatigue, lack of energy, and irritability may mean you need more rest and sleep.

Body mechanics. You will bend, carry heavy objects, and lift, move, and reposition residents. These activities cause stress and strain on your body. You need to have good posture and learn to use your muscles effectively (see Chapter 9).

Exercise. Exercise is important for muscle tone, circulation, and weight control. There also are psychological benefits from exercise. Walking, running, swimming, and biking are excellent forms of exercise. You will feel better physically and be more alert mentally if you exercise regularly. Do not begin a vigorous exercise program until you have consulted your doctor.

Your eyes. Just wonder for a moment what it would be like if you could not see. Losing your sight would require major changes in all your activities, such as the way you live, work, and travel. Your eyes deserve special care and respect. Have your eyes examined and wear glasses or contact lenses as prescribed. Make sure you have good lighting when you read or do fine work.

Good vision is necessary in your work. In addition to reading instructions, you will measure blood pressures and temperatures. The procedures require the ability to read fine measurements. Inaccurate readings can place your residents in danger.

Smoking. Smoking has been linked to lung cancer, chronic lung diseases, and many heart and circulatory disorders. If you smoke, remember that cigarette smoke can be offensive to others. Smoke only where it is allowed and never smoke in or near a resident's room. Many facilities do not allow employees to smoke in the building. Smoke odors stay on your hands, clothing, and hair. Therefore handwashing and good personal hygiene are essential. Wash your hands immediately after smoking and before giving care.

Drugs. Drug abuse is a major problem in today's society. People can become physically and psychologically dependent on drugs. Drugs affect thinking, feeling, behavior, and functioning. Accidents, suicides, divorce, crime, and other tragic and violent events have been linked to drug abuse. Aquired immunodeficiency syndrome (AIDS) (see Chapter 23) has been linked to intravenous drug use. Individuals who are dependent on drugs may go to any length to get them.

Drugs that have an undesirable effect on your mind and body affect your ability to work effectively. Working under the influence of drugs places your residents in danger. You should take only drugs that have been prescribed by a doctor and only in the prescribed way.

Alcohol. At first, alcohol may produce a feeling of well-being and stimulation. Alcohol, however, is a drug that has a depressing effect on the brain. Thinking, balance, coordination, and mental alertness are affected. Some people are physically or psychologically dependent on alcohol. They suffer from alcoholism, an illness that can be treated and controlled with the person's desire and cooperation.

The moderate use of alcohol is socially accepted by many people and religious groups. However, it affects your mind and body. Therefore you must never report to work under the influence of alcohol or drink alcohol on the job. You must consider the safety of your residents, co-workers, and yourself.

Your Hygiene

You must pay careful attention to personal cleanliness. Preventing offensive body and breath odors is important. You should bathe daily, use a deodorant or antiperspirant, and brush your teeth after meals. You also should use mouthwash regularly. Your hair should be clean and styled in an attractive and simple way. Your fingernails should be clean, short, and neatly shaped.

For women special hygiene measures are necessary during menstrual periods. Change tampons or sanitary napkins frequently, especially if flow is heavy. The genital area should be washed with soap and water at least twice a day. Handwashing is necessary after using the bathroom, changing tampons or napkins, and washing the genital area.

Foot care prevents odors and infection. Your feet should be bathed daily and dried thoroughly between the toes. Cut toenails straight across after bathing or soaking them in water.

Your Appearance

Good health and personal hygiene practices will help you to look and feel well. The following practices and suggestions will help you to look neat, clean, and professional (Fig. 2-3).

1. Uniforms should fit well and be modest in length and style.
2. Be sure your uniforms are clean, pressed, and mended. Wear a clean uniform daily.
3. Underclothes should be clean, fit properly, and be changed daily. Because of perspiration, you may want to change underclothing more often during hot, humid weather and after vigorous exercise.
4. Jewelry should not be worn while you are on duty. Most facilities allow employees to wear a wedding ring; some allow an engagement ring. Large rings and bracelets can scratch and tear the skin of elderly residents. Necklaces, bracelets, and earrings can be pulled off by confused or combative residents, causing you injury.
5. Stockings and socks should be clean, well-fitting, and changed daily. Do not roll stockings down or wear round garters. These practices interfere with the circulation in your legs.
6. Shoes should be comfortable, give support, and fit properly. Clean and polish shoes often to keep them white and neat in appearance. Wash and replace shoelaces as necessary.
7. Nail polish should not be worn. Chipped nail polish provides a place for microbes to grow and multiply.
8. Hair should be worn simply and attractively. Keep hair off your collar and out of your face. Use simple pins, combs, barrettes, and bands to keep long hair up and in place.
9. Makeup should be modest in amount and moderate in color. Avoid a painted and severe look when you wear makeup.
10. Do not wear perfumes, colognes, or aftershave lotion. They may offend and nauseate residents. Some facilities allow lightly scented colognes or aftershave lotion.

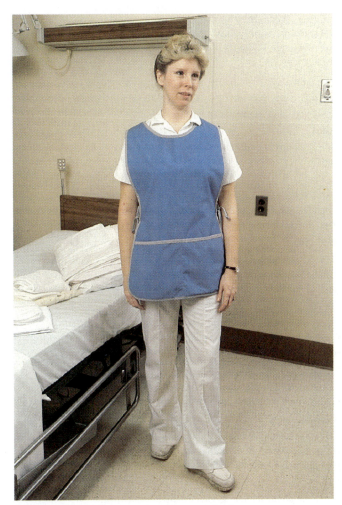

FIGURE 2-3 *A well-groomed nursing assistant.*

NURSING ASSISTANT TRAINING AND COMPETENCY EVALUATION

The care you give is very important to the health and welfare of your residents. Safe, effective, quality care is essential to protect residents from harm. Until recently, nursing assistant training was required by law only in some states. The law required that individuals learn basic nursing knowledge and skills for employment as nursing assistants. The purpose of such training was to protect residents from unsafe and poor nursing care.

In 1987 the Congress of the United States passed the Omnibus Budget Reconciliation Act (OBRA) (see Chapter 1). This law applies to all 50 states. A major purpose of OBRA is to improve the quality of care given to residents of nursing facilities. OBRA requires education and competency evaluation for all nursing assistants employed in nursing facilities. The purpose is to ensure that nursing assistants have the necessary knowledge and skills to give safe care.

The Training Program

Now every state has a nursing assistant training and competency evaluation program. Training must be at least 75 hours long and include supervised practical experience. Such training occurs in a laboratory or clinical setting. The student actually performs nursing care and procedures on other persons. This practical training (also called a *clinical practicum* or *clinical experience*) is supervised by a nurse. Usually the nurse is the course instructor.

The training program includes the knowledge and skills needed by nursing assistants to perform their roles and responsibilities. Areas of study include communication, infection control, safety and emergency procedures, residents' rights, basic nursing skills, personal care skills, feeding techniques, and skin care. Students also learn how to transfer, position, dress, and ambulate residents, and how to perform range-of-motion exercises. They also learn the signs and symptoms of common diseases and conditions and how to care for cognitively impaired residents (those who have problems with thinking and memory).

Competency Evaluation

The competency evaluation program includes a written test and a skills test. The *written test* involves multiple-choice questions. Each question has 4 possible answers. Only 1 answer is correct. The test is made up of about 75 questions. The *skills evaluation* involves the demonstration of nursing skills. You will have to perform certain skills learned in your training program.

The written and skills competency evaluations are taken after you complete your training program. Your instructor or supervisor can help you find where to take the tests and how to complete the required application form. There is a fee for the competency evaluation. This fee must be sent with your application. You will be notified about the location and time of the tests after your application has been processed.

Your training program will prepare you for the competency evaluation. If the first attempt was unsuccessful, you can retest. OBRA requires that individuals be allowed three attempts to complete the evaluation successfully.

Nursing Assistant Registry

OBRA requires each state to have a nursing assistant registry. The registry is an official record or listing of persons who have successfully completed a nursing assistant training and competency evaluation program. The registry contains the following information about each nursing assistant:

1. Full name, including maiden name and any married names

2. Last known home address
3. Social Security number
4. Date of birth
5. Last known employer, date hired, and date employment was terminated
6. Date the competency evaluation was passed
7. Information about findings of abuse, neglect, or dishonest use of property. Such information includes the nature of the offense and evidence supporting the finding. If a hearing was held, the date and its outcome are included. The person has the right to include a statement disputing the finding. All this information must remain in the registry for at least 5 years.

Registry information can be requested by any nursing facility or agency needing the information. The nursing assistant also receives a copy of all information in her or his registry file. The copy is provided when the entry is first included in the registry and again when information is changed or added. The nursing assistant can correct inaccurate information.

Other OBRA Requirements

OBRA also requires retraining and a new competency evaluation program for nursing assistants who have not worked for 2 consecutive years (24 months). Say, for example, that you completed a training and competency evaluation. After working as a nursing assistant, you quit your job. You were either not working or you worked in some other field for 2 or more years. Now you want to work as a nursing assistant again. OBRA requires that you take another training and competency evaluation program. This is to ensure that your knowledge and skills are current for safe care. It does not matter how long you worked as a nursing assistant, but how long you did *not* work.

Regular in-service education and performance reviews are other OBRA requirements. Nursing facilities must provide 12 hours of in-service training per year to nursing assistants. A nursing assistant's work also will be evaluated regularly. These are ways to help ensure that nursing assistants have the knowledge and skills to give safe, effective care.

ETHICAL AND LEGAL CONSIDERATIONS

You often will face situations in which you must decide what you should or should not do or what you can or cannot do. These circumstances may involve ethical or legal questions. What would you do in the following situations?

1. A resident asks you to be a witness to the signing of a will.
2. A nurse tells you to "tie down" Mr. Elliott because he keeps trying to get out of bed.

3. A friend's neighbor is one of your residents. The friend asks you what is wrong with the neighbor and what is being done for her.

4. The nurse tells you to give Mrs. Andrews an enema. Mrs. Andrews refuses to let you.

5. You are helping Susan Jones, RN, give a resident a treatment. She tells you to leave the privacy curtains open so she can see when Dr. James arrives to make rounds.

The following discussion will help you to decide what to do in these and other situations.

Ethics

Ethics is the discipline concerned with right and wrong conduct. It involves morals and making choices or judgments about what should or should not be done. An ethical person behaves and acts in the right way.

Every professional group has a code of ethics. The code consists of rules, or standards of conduct, that members of the group are to follow. The American Nurses Association (ANA) has a code of ethics for RNs. The National Federation of Licensed Practical Nurses (NFLPN) has one for LPNs. You should develop your own personal code of ethics. Consider the following rules of conduct for nursing assistants.

1. Respect each resident as an individual.
2. Perform no act that is not within the legal scope of a nursing assistant.
3. Perform no act for which you have not been adequately prepared.
4. Take no drug without the prescription and supervision of a doctor.
5. Carry out the nurse's directions and instructions to your best possible ability.
6. Be loyal to your employer and to those with whom you work.
7. Act as a responsible citizen at all times.
8. Know the limits of your role and knowledge.
9. Keep resident information confidential.
10. Consider the resident's needs to be more important than your own.

Legal Considerations

Legal considerations relate to laws. **Laws** are rules of conduct made and passed by a governmental body such as Congress or a state legislature. Laws to protect the public welfare are enforced by the government.

Criminal laws are concerned with offenses against the public and against society in general. A violation of a criminal law is called a **crime.** A person found guilty of a crime will be fined or sent to prison. Murder, robbery, rape, and kidnapping are examples of crimes.

Civil laws are concerned with relationships between people. Examples of civil laws are those that pertain to contracts and nursing practice. A person found guilty of breaking a civil law usually will have to pay a sum of money to the injured person.

Torts. **Tort** comes from a French word meaning *wrong*. Torts are part of civil law. A tort is committed by an individual against another person or the person's property. Torts may be intentional or unintentional. The following torts are common to health care.

Negligence is an unintentional wrong. The person fails to act in a reasonable and careful manner and thereby causes harm to the person or property of another. The negligent person failed to do what a reasonable and careful person would have done. Or he or she did what a reasonable and careful person would not have done. The negligent person may have to pay damages (i.e., a sum of money) to the injured party.

Malpractice refers to negligence on the part of professionals. A person is considered to be a professional because of the training and education received and the type of service provided. Nurses, doctors, lawyers, and pharmacists, for example, are considered professional persons.

Common negligent acts committed by nursing assistants include the following.

1. Side rails have been ordered for a confused resident. The nursing assistant leaves the side rails down. The resident falls out of bed and breaks a hip.
2. A resident is burned because a nursing assistant applied a warm water bottle that was too hot.
3. A resident's dentures break after being dropped by a nursing assistant.
4. A resident complains to the nursing assistant of difficulty breathing and chest pain. The nursing assistant does not report the complaints to the nurse. The resident dies of a heart attack.
5. A resident puts on the signal light, and the nursing assistant does not answer the light for several minutes. The resident goes into shock because of sudden, severe bleeding.

As a nursing assistant you are legally responsible *(liable)* for your own actions. What you do or do not do can lead to a lawsuit if harm results to the person or property of another. At times a nurse may direct you to do something that is beyond the legal scope of your role or for which you have not been prepared. Giving medications is an example. You may be told not to worry—that the nurse will take full responsibility if anything happens. The nurse may indeed be held liable as your supervisor, but you are not relieved of personal liability. *You are responsible for your own actions.*

You function under the direction and supervision of a nurse. However, at times you have a right and a duty to refuse to follow the nurse's directions. You should refuse to carry out the nurse's order if one of the following occurs.

1. You are asked to do something that is beyond the legal scope of your role.
2. You have not been prepared to perform the function safely.
3. You know that the act or procedure may harm the resident.
4. The nurse's directions or orders are unethical, illegal, or against facility policy.
5. Directions are unclear or incomplete.

You can protect residents and yourself from negligent acts by using common sense. Ask yourself if what you are about to do is safe for the resident.

Defamation is injuring the name and reputation of another person by making false statements to a third person. **Libel** involves making false statements in writing or through drawings. **Slander** is false statements made orally. Protect yourself from committing defamation by never making false statements about a resident, coworker, or any other person. The following remarks are examples of defamation:

1. Implying or suggesting that an individual has AIDS
2. Stating that a resident is insane
3. Implying or suggesting that a person is corrupt or dishonest in dealing with others

Assault and **battery** are two separate intentional torts. They may result in both civil and criminal charges. **Assault** is intentionally attempting or threatening to touch the body of another person without the person's consent. The individual is placed in fear of bodily harm. Threatening to "tie down" or restrain an uncooperative resident is an example of assault.

Battery is the actual unauthorized touching of another person's body without the person's consent. Consent is the important factor in assault and battery. The resident or the resident's responsible party must give consent for any procedure, treatment, or other act that involves touching the body. The consenting person can withdraw consent at any time.

Consent is more than a person's verbal okay or signature on a form. For the consent to be valid, it must be *informed* consent. Informed consent recognizes a resident's or responsible party's right to decide what will be done to the resident's body and who can touch that body. Consent is considered to be informed when the individual giving consent clearly understands the reason for a treatment, what will be done, how it will be done, who will do it, and the expected outcomes and risks. The person also must understand the treatment alternatives and the consequences of not having the treatment. The doctor is responsible for informing the individual.

You can protect yourself from being accused of bat-

tery. Explain to your residents what you are planning to do for them and get their consent. The consent may be verbal. It may be a gesture (such as a nod), turning over for a backrub, or holding out an arm so the pulse can be taken. Some residents are confused or mentally incompetent. For these individuals, written consent for care usually is given by their responsible party or legal guardian when they are admitted.

False imprisonment is the unlawful restraint or restriction of a person's freedom of movement. Threat of restraint or actual physical restraint constitutes false imprisonment. It is considered an intentional tort. The most common examples of false imprisonment are these:

1. Preventing a person who wants to leave the health care facility from doing so
2. Restraining a resident unnecessarily

Invasion of privacy is another tort. Each person has the right not to have his or her name, photograph, or private affairs exposed or made public without having

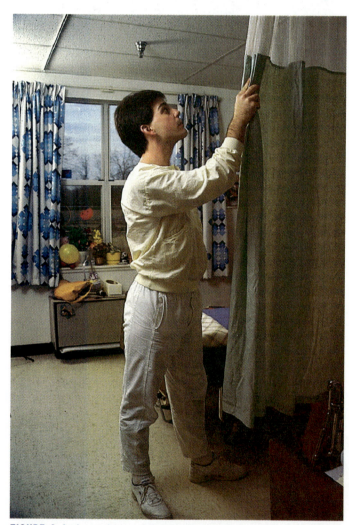

FIGURE 2-4 *A nursing assistant protecting the resident's privacy by pulling the curtain around the resident's bed.*

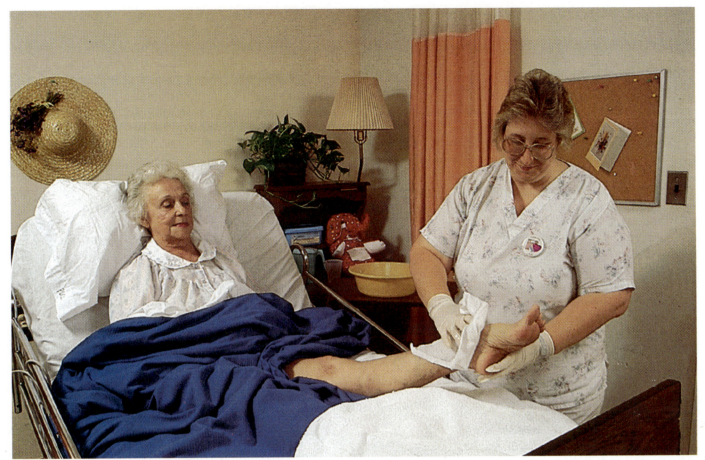

FIGURE 2-5 *Only the body part involved in the procedure is exposed.*

given consent. A violation of this right is an invasion of privacy. You must treat residents with respect and ensure their privacy. Only health care workers involved in the resident's care should see, handle, or examine the resident's body. You can ensure the resident's right to privacy by doing the following.

1. Make sure residents are covered when you move them through the corridors.
2. Screen residents as in Fig. 2-4; use privacy curtains, or close the door when giving care. Also close drapes, blinds, or window shades.
3. Expose only the body part involved in a treatment or procedure (Fig. 2-5).
4. Do not discuss the resident or the resident's treatment with anyone except the nurse supervising your work. "Shop talk" is one of the most common causes of invasion of privacy.

Wills. A **will** is a legal statement of how a person wishes to have property distributed after death. There is no ethical or legal reason why you cannot witness the signing of a will if you are asked to do so. You also may refuse to witness the signing of a will without fear of legal liability.

A resident or family member may ask you to help prepare a will. You should politely refuse. Explain that you do not have the necessary knowledge or legal ability to prepare a will. Ask a nurse to speak to the resident or family member about contacting a lawyer.

Do not witness a resident's will if you are named in the will. To do so would prevent you from receiving that which had been left to you. As a witness, you may have to testify that the resident was of sound mind when the will was signed. You also should be prepared to testify that the resident stated that the document being signed was his or her last will. Be sure to tell your supervisor that you were a witness to a resident's will.

WORKING WITH OTHERS

You are a member of both the nursing and health care teams. You will work closely with RNs, LPNs, and other nursing assistants. Your ability to work well with others will affect how well you function as a nursing assistant and the quality of care received by your residents. In addition to the ethical and legal considerations just discussed, the following guidelines will help you work well with others.

1. Understand the roles, functions, and responsibilities in your job description.
2. Develop the desired qualities and characteristics of a nursing assistant working in long-term care.
3. Report to work on time.
4. Call the facility if you cannot report to work. Call as soon as possible and give the reason for your absence.
5. Practice good personal health and hygiene measures.
6. Take pride in your appearance, and follow the facility dress code.
7. Act in an ethical and a legal manner at all times.
8. Follow the directions and instructions of your supervisor.
9. Question unclear instructions and things you do not understand.
10. Report resident or family complaints and your observations to the nurse promptly.
11. Help others willingly when asked.
12. Do not waste supplies and equipment.
13. Do not use the telephone, supplies, or equipment for your personal use.
14. Do not use the resident's telephone or personal belongings for your personal use.
15. Follow the rules and regulations of the facility in which you are employed.
16. Measure, report, and record accurately.
17. Tell the nurse when you are leaving and when you have returned to your work area.
18. Do not discuss your personal problems with residents.
19. Protect the resident's rights at all times.

Planning and Organizing Your Work

Working well with others includes working in an organized and efficient way. You will be assigned to give nursing care to residents and to perform routine tasks in your assigned area. Some assignments must be completed by a certain time. Others must be done by the end of the shift. You must plan and organize your work to give safe, thorough care and to make good use of your time. The following guidelines will help you to plan and organize your work.

1. Discuss priorities with the RN or LPN when you receive your assignment.
2. Know the routine of your shift and your assigned work area.
3. List care or procedures that must be performed on a schedule. Some residents must be positioned or toileted every 2 hours.
4. Estimate how much time is needed for each resident, procedure, and task.
5. Identify the tasks and procedures that can be done while residents are eating, visiting, or involved in activities or therapies.
6. Plan care around meal times, visiting hours, therapies, and daily recreation and social activities.
7. Identify situations in which you will need help from a co-worker. Ask a co-worker to help you when needed. Tell the person the approximate time when you will need help.
8. Schedule any equipment or rooms if necessary. Some facilities have only one shower or bathtub. You will need to schedule the tub or shower for your resident's use.
9. Review the procedures to be performed and gather the necessary supplies beforehand.

SUMMARY

This chapter has presented many important considerations about your role as a nursing assistant. You have learned what you can and cannot do both legally and ethically. The important qualities and characteristics of nursing assistants and health, hygiene, and personal appearance have been presented. The nursing assistant training and competency evaluation program, registry, and other OBRA requirements were explained. Working well with others also was discussed.

What you do and how you do it affects you, your residents, and your co-workers. All are affected personally and legally. You have an important role, and you are a very special person for wanting to be a nursing assistant in long-term care. Use common sense, and act in a reasonable and careful manner. Respect your residents, protect their rights, and enjoy your work!

Review QUESTIONS

Circle *T* if the answer is true and *F* if it is false.

 1. You perform simple and complex procedures under the supervision of a nurse.

 2. You must perform all tasks and procedures as directed by the nurse.

 3. You make decisions about what should be done for residents.

 4. All health care facilities let nursing assistants perform the same procedures and tasks.

 5. You should have a written job description before employment.

 6. You should never give a resident medication unless told to do so by an RN.

 7. You do not take verbal or telephone orders from doctors.

 8. You are responsible for informing the resident or family about the diagnosis and treatment.

 9. You can show empathy by feeling sorry for the residents.

 10. You must respect the values, beliefs, and feelings of residents.

 11. You should take drugs only under the advice and supervision of a doctor.

 12. Alcohol must never be consumed on duty.

 13. Vision problems of a nursing assistant can affect the resident's safety.

 14. Bathing is not necessary during menstrual periods.

 15. Jewelry is part of your uniform.

 16. You can wear pastel nail polish while on duty.

 17. OBRA requires a training program and a competency evaluation for nursing assistants.

 18. The nursing assistant registry is private and confidential.

 19. OBRA requires retraining if you have not worked for 2 consecutive years.

20. Laws are ethical standards of right and wrong conduct.

21. You are always responsible for your own actions.

22. Defamation is the unauthorized touching of another person.

 23. Assault is attempting or threatening to touch another person without that person's consent.

 24. False imprisonment is the illegal restraint of another person's movement.

 25. A resident has the right to have information about treatment and care kept private and confidential.

26. You cannot witness the signing of a will.

27. If unable to report to work, you should call and give the employer a reason for the absence.

Answers

1. False	**8.** False	**15.** False	**22.** False
2. False	**9.** False	**16.** False	**23.** True
3. False	**10.** True	**17.** True	**24.** True
4. False	**11.** True	**18.** False	**25.** True
5. True	**12.** True	**19.** True	**26.** False
6. False	**13.** True	**20.** False	**27.** True
7. True	**14.** False	**21.** True	

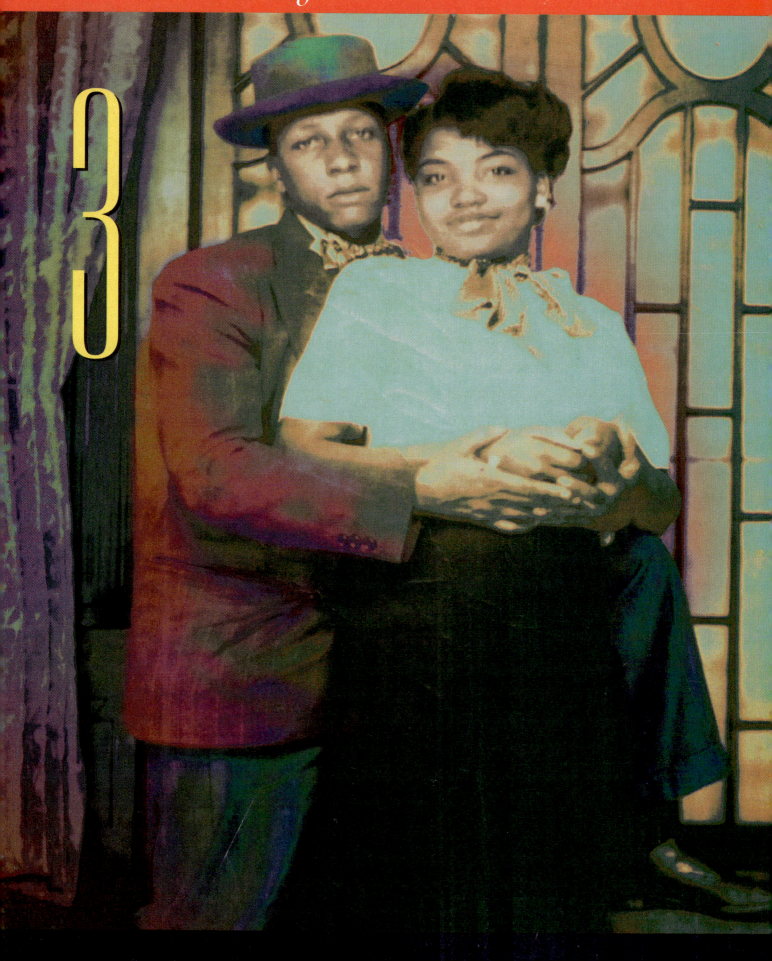

3

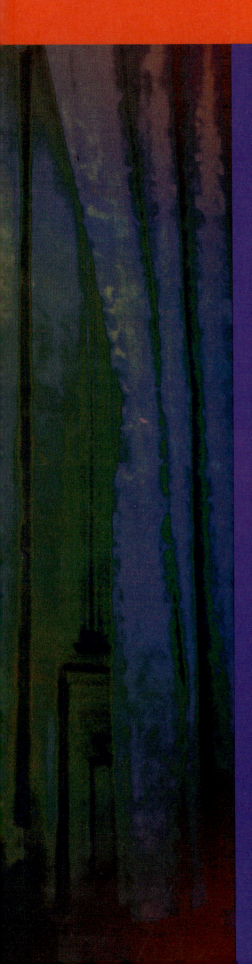

What You Will LEARN

- The key terms listed in this chapter

- The purpose of communication among members of the health care team

- Five rules for communicating effectively

- The purpose, parts, and information contained in the resident's record

- Legal and ethical responsibilities of nursing assistants who have access to resident records

- Information you can collect about a resident by use of sight, hearing, touch, and smell

- Information that you always should include when reporting to the nurse

- The difference between end-of-shift reports and resident care conferences

- Fifteen basic rules for recording

- The purpose of the comprehensive care plan and Kardex

- How care plans are developed according to OBRA regulations

- How computers are used in long-term care

chart
The resident's record

communication
The exchange of information; a message sent is received and interpreted by the intended person

comprehensive care plan
A written guide that gives direction about the care a resident should receive from the health care team

Kardex
Card file that summarizes information in the resident's record; it includes treatments, diagnosis, routine care measures, and special equipment used by the resident

minimum data set (MDS)
A form used by nurses to assess a resident's mental, physical, and psychosocial function

objective data
Information about a resident that can be seen, heard, felt, or smelled by another person; signs

observation
Using the senses of sight, hearing, touch, and smell to collect information about the resident

recording
Writing or charting resident care and observations

reporting
An oral account of the resident's care and observations

resident assessment protocol summary (RAPS)
Guidelines used in developing the comprehensive care plan

resident's record
A written account of the resident's physical or mental status and his or her response to the treatment and care given by members of the health care team; the chart

signs
Objective data

subjective data
Information communicated by the resident that the health care worker cannot observe by using the senses; symptoms

symptoms
Subjective data

triggers
Clues that direct the caregiver to the appropriate resident assessment protocol (RAPS)

There's a lot of personal information in my chart. Sometimes I wonder about what the staff has written and who reads my chart. But I know they need the information to give me good care.

Members of the health care team must communicate with one another to provide coordinated and effective resident care. Information must be shared about what has been done and what needs to be done for the resident. The health care team also must share information about the resident's response to care and treatment.

Consider the following example of communication by the health care team. The doctor has ordered a blood test for Mrs. Carter. Eating would affect the test results. Mrs. Carter cannot have breakfast until a blood sample has been taken by the laboratory technician. The nurse asks the dietary department not to send Mrs. Carter's breakfast until notified. She explains to Mrs. Carter why breakfast will be delayed. The nurse also tells you about the breakfast delay. The laboratory technician draws the blood sample and tells the nurse that the resident may have breakfast. The nurse orders the meal. A dietary worker brings the tray to the nursing station. You are asked to serve Mrs. Carter's tray. When she has finished eating, you remove the tray and observe how much she has eaten of each food. You report your observations to the nurse. The nurse records them in Mrs. Carter's record. Because the team members communicated with one another and the resident, Mrs. Carter's care was coordinated and effective. She understood that she was not being neglected or forgotten.

You will communicate with the health care team. However, you will have more direct and frequent communication with the nursing team. You need to understand the basic elements and rules of communication. Then you can learn ways to communicate resident information to the health care team. Communication with residents and families is discussed in Chapter 4.

COMMUNICATION

Communication is the exchange of information—a message sent is received and interpreted by the intended person. For communication to be effective, the words must have the same meaning for the sender and the receiver of the message. The words "small," "moderate," and "large" often are used in health care. The words, however, mean different things to different people. Is

small the size of a dime or the size of a half dollar? In health care the difference in meaning can affect resident safety. Try to avoid words that have more than one meaning.

Using words familiar to people you communicate with is important. You will learn medical terminology as you study and gain experience as a nursing assistant. If a member of the health care team uses an unfamiliar term, ask for an explanation. If you do not understand the message, communication will not occur. Likewise, avoid using terms that are unfamiliar to the residents.

Try to be brief and concise when communicating. Do not add unrelated or unnecessary information. You must stay on the subject, avoid wandering in thought, and not get wordy. Being brief and concise reduces the chance of omitting important details.

Information should be presented in a logical and orderly manner. Organize your thoughts so that you can present them logically and in the right order. Think about what happened step-by-step, and give the information to the nurse in that way.

You need to present facts and be specific. The receiver should have a clear picture of what you are communicating. Asking for clarification or for more information should not be necessary. Reporting that a resident's tem-

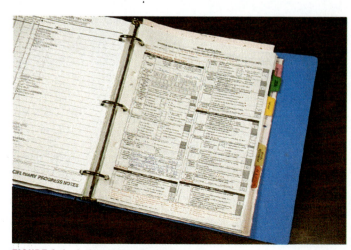

FIGURE 3-1 *A, A traditional chart.*

perature is 100.2° is more specific and factual than saying the "temperature is up."

THE RESIDENT'S RECORD

The **resident's record (chart)** is a written account of the resident's condition and response to care and treatment given by the health care team. The record may be in traditional written form in a chart cover or on computer (Fig. 3-1). The main purpose of the chart is to provide a way for the health care team to communicate information about the resident. The record is permanent and can be used many years later if a resident's health history is needed. The record is a legal document. It can be used in court as evidence of the resident's problems, treatment, and care.

The record has many forms organized into sections for easy use. Chart organization may vary among facilities. It usually includes the results of the resident's history and physical examination, doctors' orders, and progress notes. Some facilities have separate sections for the progress notes of each service (e.g., nursing, social service, and physical therapy). In other facilities, members of the health care team use the same progress notes. There also are laboratory and x-ray reports and the intake and output record, intravenous (IV) therapy record, and graphic records. Also included are the admission sheet and admitting assessments from nursing, social service, dietary service, and recreational therapy. Each page must have the resident's name, room number, and other identifying information. This reduces the chance of errors and the improper placement of records.

Members of the health care team record data on the progress notes and on forms for their department or service. The information is then available to other health care team members who need to know what care has been given and the resident's response (Fig. 3-2).

Nursing facilities have policies about the contents of

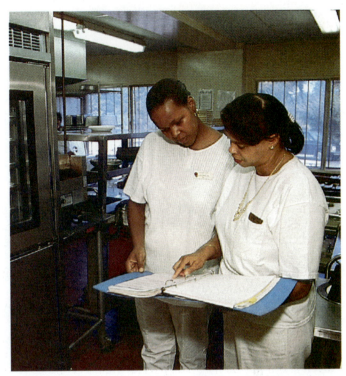

FIGURE 3-2 *The nurse and dietitian review the resident's record.*

resident records and about who may see them. There are policies about how often recordings need to be made and who records information on the specific forms. There also are policies about acceptable abbreviations, correcting errors, the color of ink to be used, and how to sign entries. You need to know your facility's policies as they relate to resident records.

Some facilities do not let nursing assistants write in the chart. They feel that this is the nurse's responsibility. Others allow and rely on nursing assistants to record observations and care. General guidelines for recording are presented on pp. 35 and 37.

Usually all professional health care workers involved in a resident's care have access to the chart. Those not directly involved in the resident's care are not allowed to review the record. Cooks, laundry and housekeeping staff members, and office clerks have no need to see resident records. Some facilities do not let nursing assistants read charts. The nurse shares necessary resident information with them.

Remember that you have an ethical and a legal responsibility to keep resident information confidential. Also remember that only those members of the health care team involved in the resident's care need to read the chart. You may have a friend or relative in the facility. If you are not involved in that resident's care, you have no right to review that person's chart. To review the chart would be an invasion of privacy.

B

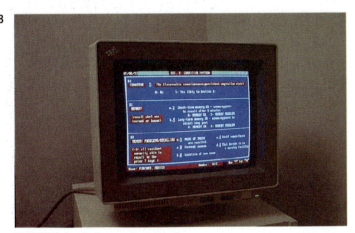

FIGURE 3-1 *B, A computer record.*

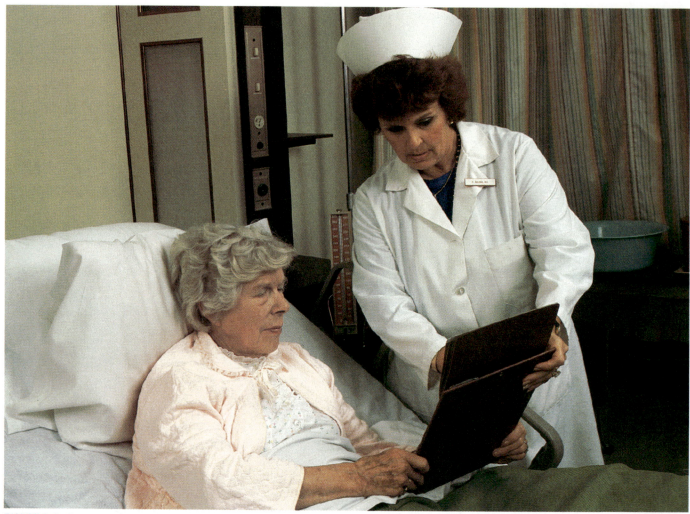

FIGURE 3-3 *A nurse reviews a resident's record with the resident.*

Many facilities allow residents to see their records if they ask to do so. In some states it is their legal right. You should know your employer's policy regarding residents or their guardians seeing a resident's chart. If a resident or guardian asks you for the chart, report the request to your supervisor. The nurse is responsible for dealing with the request (Fig. 3-3).

The following section details parts of the record that relate to your work as a nursing assistant.

The Admission Sheet

The admission sheet is completed when the person is admitted to the facility. It contains identifying information. The identifying information is the resident's legal name, birth date, age, sex, current address, marital status, religion, and Medicare or Social Security number. The name of the resident's responsible party or guardian also is in-

cluded. Some facilities add the resident's diagnosis, date and time of admission, and the doctor's name. An identification (ID) number is given to each resident and included on the admission sheet.

You might use the admission sheet to learn background information about a resident. You also might use it to fill out other forms that require some of the same information. In that way the resident or guardian does not have to answer the same questions several times.

Activities of Daily Living Flow Sheet

The activities of daily living (ADL) flow sheet (Fig. 3-4) is used to record a resident's ability to perform ADLs. This flow sheet may have places to record the resident's intake at each meal, bowel and bladder elimination, hygiene, and mental status. The resident's activity level also is included.

Activities of Daily Living Flow Sheet

MONTH:				YEAR:										
				DATE:										

HYGIENE: BSS = Bath/Shave/Shampoo   L = Linen Change
OF = Oral/Face
0 = Not one of the above

N
D
E

FOOD: G = Good (80–100%)   FT = Feeding Tube (Nasogastric/Gastrostomy)
F = Fair   (60–80%)   N = NPO
P = Poor   (0–60%)   0 = No monitoring

N
D
E

FLUIDS: E = Encourage   I = IV   QS = Quantity Sufficient
R = Restrict   T = TPN   QI = Quantity Insufficient
M = Monitor Intake

N
D
E

ELIMINATION: BOWEL   S = Suppository   L = Large BM   C = Colostomy
E = Enema   M = Mod. BM   0 = No BM
I = Incontinent   S = Small BM

N
D
E

ELIMINATION: F = Foley Catheter   M = Monitor Output   QS = Quantity Sufficient
BLADDER   S = Suprapubic   I = Incontinent   QI = Quantity Insufficient
E = External Catheter   C = Continent

N
D
E

AIR: O = Oxygen   S = Suctioning
0 = No intervention
SS = Supervised Smoking

N
D
E

ENTER IN SPACE BELOW • RESIDENT IDENTIFICATION • TREATING FACILITY • WARD NO. • *Continue on Reverse*

Record code and self-care level
in each shift.
Levels: I = Independent
II = Supervision, assist
III = Partial assist
IV = Complete assist
If self-care category omitted,
circle & explain on back of sheet.
If res. on pass—write pass in
time slot.

FIGURE 3-4 *An ADL flow sheet*   Continued

	REST (R)/SLEEP (S):		RW = Rested Well				SW = Slept Well														
			RF = Rested Fair				SF = Slept Fair														
			RP = Rested Poorly				SP = Slept Poorly														

FIGURE 3-4, cont'd *An ADL flow sheet*

Nurses' Progress Notes

The nurses' progress notes are a written description of the nursing care given and the resident's response (Fig. 3-5). They also include the signs and symptoms the nurse observes about the resident. Nurses use the progress notes to record information about special treatments and medications that are given. Resident teaching and counseling, procedures performed by the doctor, and visits by other health care team members are recorded in the nurses' progress notes.

Nurses in long-term care do not chart daily in the progress notes unless there has been a change in the resident's condition, an unusual occurrence, or a problem. Summaries of care are written. These summaries reflect the resident's progress toward the goals established in the resident care plan and the resident's response to care. Facility policy states how often summaries are written.

Other Types of Flow Sheets

Other flow sheets are used to record any series of measurements or observations made at frequent intervals. For example, pulse, respirations, and blood pressure may be measured frequently. Or a resident with a heart condition may be weighed daily (Fig. 3-6, p. 34). These measurements will be recorded on flow sheets. The intake and output record is another type of flow sheet (see Chapter 15).

REPORTING AND RECORDING OBSERVATIONS

Reporting and recording are ways to communicate with the health care team. Each method is an account of what has been done for and observed about the resident. **Reporting** is the oral account of the resident's care and observations. **Recording (charting)** is the written account.

NURSE'S NOTES

(Reference tags: F311 - F351)

(Cross reference tags: F157, F158, F164, F174, F221, F222, F253, F289, F301, F517 - F527, F531)

DATE/ TIME	PROB. NO.	NOTES MUST BE SIGNED WITH NAME AND TITLE

NAME—Last	First	Middle	Attending Physician	Chart No.

CFS 6-32HH © 1992 Briggs Corporation, Des Moines, IA 50306 (800) 247-2343
Printed in U.S.A.

FIGURE 3-5 Nurses' progress notes. (Reprinted with permission. Copyright 1993, Briggs Corporation, Des Moines, IA 50306.)

VITAL SIGNS AND WEIGHT RECORD

(Reference tags: F327, F328 and F331-F333; Cross reference tags: F164, F274, F277 and F441)

ADMISSION INFORMATION

Admission Date _____ / _____ / _____   Admission Weight _____ lbs   Usual Weight _____ lbs

Admission Height _____   Ideal Body Weight (IBW) Range_____ —

(Obtain from Initial Nutritional History/Assessment CFS 5-5)

Date of Birth _____ / _____ / _____   Age _____

INSTRUCTIONS: Date each entry. Record blood pressure (BP), temperature, pulse, respirations and weight in the appropriate columns. Indicate by checking (✓) the actual route of measuring temperature and pulse based on the following—**TEMPERATURE:** O-Oral, R-Rectal, A-Axillary; **PULSE:** R-Radial, A-Apical. Identify weight gain or loss in the appropriate **WT CHANGE** column by specifying the difference (in pounds) between "new" weight and previous weight. The **DATE NOTIFIED** columns need only be completed when it is necessary to notify the individuals listed. Refer to the bottom of this form for undesired weight loss parameters. Each entry must be signed by the nurse.

DATE	BP	TEMPERATURE				PULSE			RESPIR-ATIONS	WEIGHT (lbs)	WT CHANGE		DATE NOTIFIED			COMMENTS	NURSE'S SIGNATURE
		Temp.	O	R	A	Pulse	R	A			Gain	Loss	Family	Doctor	Dietary		

SUGGESTED PARAMETERS FOR EVALUATING SIGNIFICANCE OF UNPLANNED AND/OR UNDESIRED WEIGHT LOSS

Interval	Significant Loss	Severe Loss	Formula for Determining % of Body Wt Loss
1 month	5%	> 5%	
3 months	7.5%	> 7.5%	$\dfrac{\text{Usual Wt - Actual Wt}}{\text{Usual Wt}} \times 100$
6 months	10%	>10%	

NAME—Last	First	Middle	Attending Physician	Chart No.

CFS 6-21HH © 1992 Briggs Corporation, Des Moines, IA 50306 (800) 247-2343
Printed in U.S.A.

FIGURE 3-6 *Vital signs and daily-weight flow sheet. (Reprinted with permission. Copyright 1993, Briggs Corporation, Des Moines, IA 50306.)*

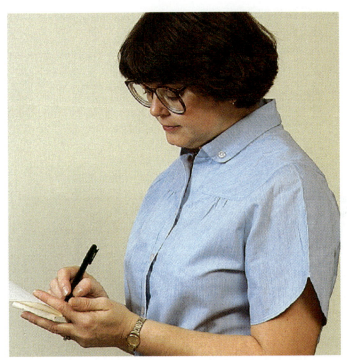

FIGURE 3-7 *A nursing assistant making notes of observations on a note pad.*

You need to make notes of your observations. They will be valuable later when you report to the nurse. Carry a note pad and pen in your pocket. Then you can note your observations at the time they are made (Fig. 3-7).

Reporting

You report resident care and observations to the nurse. Reports must be prompt, thorough, and accurate. Always give the nurse the resident's name, room and bed number, and the time observations were made or care was given. Only report what you observed or did yourself. Give reports as often as the resident's condition requires or as often as requested by the nurse. Be sure to give the nurse a final report at the end of your shift. Use your notes to give a specific, concise, and descriptive report (Fig. 3-8).

The nurse gives a report at the end of the shift to nursing personnel of the oncoming shift (end-of-shift report). Information is shared about care that has been given and the care that needs to be given to the residents. Information about the resident's condition also is included. Some facilities require that the entire nursing team hear the end-of-shift report when coming on duty. Others have nursing assistants perform routine tasks while RNs and LPNs hear the report. If this is the case, your supervisor will give you a report on the residents assigned to you.

Observations

Observation involves using the senses of sight, hearing, touch, and smell to collect information about the resident. When you look at the resident, you will observe such things as the way the resident is lying, sitting, or walking. You also will observe if the skin is flushed or pale, or if there are reddened or swollen areas. You will listen to the resident breathe, talk, and cough. A stethoscope is used to listen to the heartbeat. Touching gives you information about skin temperature. Touch also lets you feel if the skin is moist or dry. You also will use touch to take the resident's pulse. The sense of smell detects body, wound, and breath odors and unusual odors from urine and bowel movements.

Information or data observed about a resident is called **objective data.** Objective data **(signs)** are those things you can see, hear, feel, or smell yourself. You can feel a pulse, and you can see what a resident has vomited. However, you cannot feel or see pain or nausea. The things a resident tells you about but that you cannot observe through your senses are **subjective data (symptoms).**

You will observe many things about your residents. More specific observations are discussed as they relate to procedures and resident care presented throughout this book. The basic observations you need to make and report to the nurse are found in List 3-1 on p. 36.

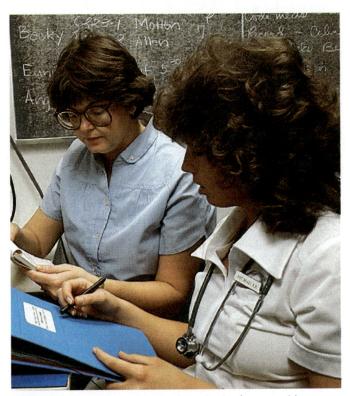

FIGURE 3-8 *A nursing assistant using notes to give a report to a nurse.*

List 3 -1

Basic Observations of the Resident

A. Ability to respond
   1. Is the resident easy or difficult to arouse?
   2. Is the resident able to give his or her name, the time, and the location when asked?
   3. Can the resident identify others accurately?
   4. Can the resident answer questions appropriately?
   5. Can the resident speak clearly?
   6. Are instructions followed appropriately?
   7. Is the resident calm, restless, or excited?
   8. Is the resident conversing, quiet, or talking a lot?
B. Movement
   1. Can the resident squeeze your fingers with each hand?
   2. Can the resident move his or her arms and legs?
   3. Are the resident's movements shaky or jerky?
C. Pain or discomfort
   1. Where is the pain located? (Ask the resident to point to the pain.)
   2. Is the resident able to tell you if he or she has pain, or does the resident simply appear to be in pain—moaning or restless, an expression of pain on the face
   3. Does the pain go anywhere else?
   4. What is the duration of the pain?
   5. What is the resident's description of the pain?
      a. Sharp
      b. Severe
      c. Knifelike; stabbing
      d. Dull
      e. Burning
      f. Aching
      g. Comes and goes
      h. Depends upon position
   6. Has medication been given?
   7. Did medication help relieve the pain? Is pain still present?
   8. Is the resident able to sleep and rest?
   9. What is the position of comfort?

D. Skin
   1. Is the skin pale or flushed?
   2. Is the skin cool, warm, or hot?
   3. Is the skin moist or dry?
   4. What color are the lips and nails?
   5. Are there any sores or reddened areas?
E. Eyes, ears, nose, and mouth
   1. Is there drainage from the eyes?
   2. Are the eyelids closed?
   3. Are the eyes reddened?
   4. Does the resident complain of spots, flashes, or blurring?
   5. Is the resident sensitive to bright lights?
   6. Is there drainage from the eyes?
   7. Is the resident able to hear? Does the resident need to have things repeated?
   8. Is there drainage from the nose?
   9. Is the resident able to breathe through the nose?
   10. Is there breath odor?
   11. Does the resident complain of a bad taste in the mouth?
F. Respirations
   1. Do both sides of the resident's chest rise and fall with respirations?
   2 Is there noisy breathing?
   3. Is there difficulty breathing?
   4. Does the resident breathe easier sitting up or on one side or the other?
   5. Is there a cough? What is the frequency? is it dry or productive?
   6 What is the amount and color of the resident's sputum?
G. Bowels and bladder
   1. Is the abdomen firm or soft?
   2. Does the resident complain of gas?
   3. What is the amount, color, and consistency of the resident's bowel movement? Is the odor unusual?
   4. Does the resident have pain (burning) or difficulty urinating?
   5. What is the amount of urine?
   6. What is the frequency of urination?

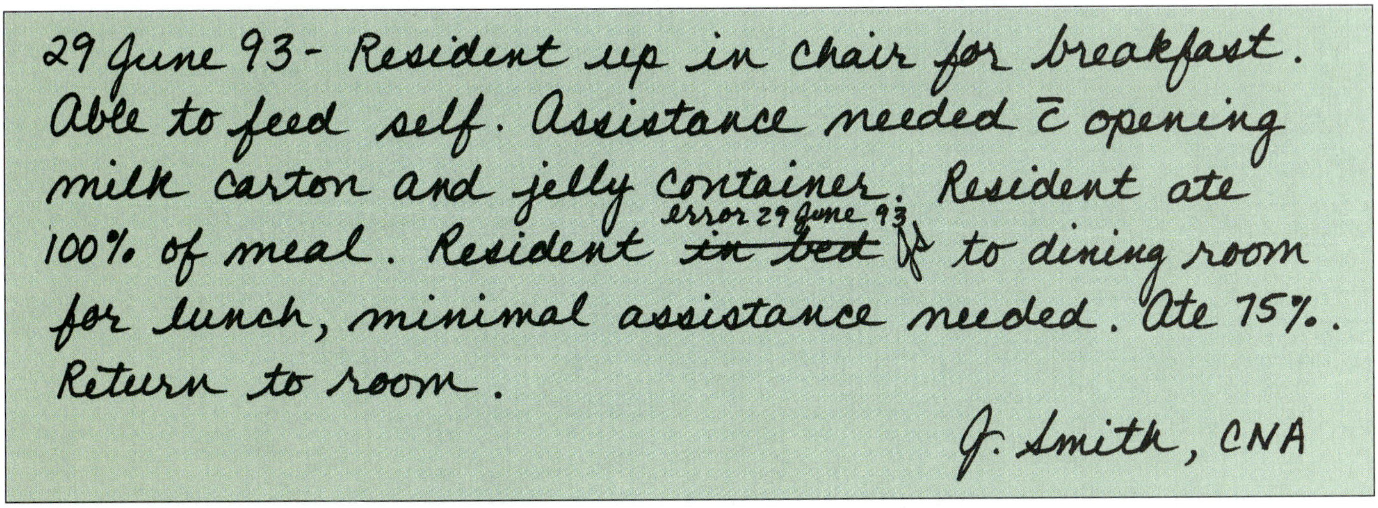

29 June 93 - Resident up in chair for breakfast. Able to feed self. Assistance needed c̄ opening milk carton and jelly container. Resident ate 100% of meal. Resident ~~in bed~~ *error 29 June 93* to dining room for lunch, minimal assistance needed. Ate 75%. Return to room.

J. Smith, CNA

FIGURE 3-9 *Charting by a nursing assistant.*

Recording

If you are allowed to record on the resident's chart, you have an even greater responsibility to communicate clearly and thoroughly. Fig. 3-9 is an example of charting by a nursing assistant. You should follow these basic rules when recording.

1. Always use ink.
2. Include the date and the time whenever a recording is made.
3. Make sure writing is legible and neat.
4. Use only the abbreviations approved by your facility (see Chapter 28).
5. Use correct spelling, grammar, and punctuation.
6. Never erase if you make an error. Draw a line through the incorrect part. Then write "error" and your initials over it. Rewrite the part. Some facilities use "mistaken entry" rather then "error." Follow facility policy for correcting errors.
7. Sign all entries with your name and title according to facility policy (e.g., Jane Gates, CNA).
8. Do not skip lines. Draw a line through the blank space of a partially completed line. This prevents others from recording in a space with your signature.
9. Make sure each form on which you are writing contains the resident's name and other identifying information.
10. Never chart a procedure or treatment until it has been completed.
11. Be accurate, concise, and factual. Do not record judgments, interpretations, or opinions.
12. Record in a logical and sequential manner.
13. Be descriptive. Avoid terms with more than one meaning.
14. Use the resident's exact words whenever possible. Use quotation marks to show that the statement is a direct quote.

COMPREHENSIVE CARE PLANS

The **comprehensive care plan** is a written guide that gives direction about the care a resident should receive. The plan consists of resident problems, goals for care, and actions to be taken to help the resident solve the problems. The health care team (see p. 4) develops the resident's care plan. The team includes the RN responsible for the resident's care, the doctor, and team members from other disciplines that are involved in meeting the resident's needs. The resident, resident's family, or legal representative also are included in the care planning process.

OBRA requires that the physical, mental, and psychosocial status of all residents be assessed and a comprehensive care plan developed. The minimum data set (MDS) is used for these assessments (Fig. 3-10, pp. 38-42). The nurse is responsible for completing the MDS. The observations you make and report to the nurse are used in completing the MDS.

The problems identified on the MDS give **triggers** (clues) for the resident assessment protocols (RAPs). RAPs are guidelines that help the health care team develop the resident's care plan (Fig. 3-11, p. 44 and

Text continued on p. 43.

MINIMUM DATA SET
FOR NURSING FACILITY RESIDENT ASSESSMENT AND CARE SCREENING (MDS)
(Status in last 7 days, unless other time frame indicated)

Code "NA" or (—) = Information unavailable or untrustworthy

[ ] = Write in the appropriate alpha or numeric response

[ ] = Check (✓) if response is applicable

UPON COMPLETION OF THIS FORM, GO TO RAP TRIGGER LEGEND.

SECTION A. IDENTIFICATION AND BACKGROUND INFORMATION

1. ASSESSMENT DATE
Month — Day — Year

2. RESIDENT NAME
(First) (Middle Initial) (Last)

3. SOCIAL SECURITY NO.

4. MEDICAID NO. (If applicable)

5. MEDICAL RECORD NO.

6. REASON FOR ASSESSMENT
1. Initial admission assess.
2. Hosp/Medicare reassess.
3. Readmission assessment
4. Annual assessment
5. Significant change in status
6. Other (e.g., UR)

7. CURRENT PAYMENT SOURCE(S) FOR N.H. STAY
(Billing Office to indicate; **check all that apply**)
a. Medicaid
b. Medicare
c. CHAMPUS
d. VA
e. Self pay/Private insurance
f. Other

8. RESPONSIBILITY/ LEGAL GUARDIAN
(Check all that apply)
a. Legal guardian
b. Other legal oversight
c. Durable power attrny./ health care proxy
d. Family member responsible
e. Resident responsible
f. NONE OF ABOVE

9. ADVANCED DIRECTIVES
(For those items with supporting documentation in the medical record, **check all that apply**)
a. Living will
b. Do not resuscitate
c. Do not hospitalize
d. Organ donation
e. Autopsy request
f. Feeding restrictions
g. Medication restrictions
h. Other treatment restrictions
i. NONE OF ABOVE

10. DISCHARGE PLANNED WITHIN 3 MOS.
(Does not include discharge due to death)
0. No   1. Yes   2. Unknown/uncertain

11. PARTICIPATE IN ASSESSMENT
a. Resident
0. No
1. Yes
b. Family
0. No
1. Yes
2. No family

12. SIGNATURES (Indicate section(s) completed next to name)
Signature & Date of RN Assessment Coordinator

Signatures, Titles & Dates of Others Who Completed Part of the Assessment

SECTION B. COGNITIVE PATTERNS

1. COMATOSE
(Persistent vegetative state/no discernible consciousness)
0. No   1. Yes (Skip to SECTION E)

2. MEMORY
(Recall of what was learned or known)
a. Short-term memory OK—seems/appears to recall after 5 minutes
0. Memory OK   1. Memory problem ▲²
b. Long-term memory OK—seems/appears to recall long past
0. Memory OK   1. Memory problem ▲²

3. MEMORY/ RECALL ABILITY
(Check all that resident normally able to recall during last 7 days) Fewer than 3 ✓ = ▲²
a. Current season
b. Location of own room
c. Staff names/faces
d. That he/she is in a nursing home
e. NONE OF ABOVE are recalled

4. COGNITIVE SKILLS FOR DAILY DECISION-MAKING
(Made decisions regarding tasks of daily life)
0. Independent—decisions consistent/reasonable ▲⁴
1. Modified independence—some difficulty in new situations only ▲⁴ ▲²
2. Moderately impaired—decisions poor; cues/ supervision required ▲⁴ ▲²
3. Severely impaired—never/rarely made decisions ▲²

5. INDICATORS OF DELIRIUM —PERIODIC DISORDERED THINKING/ AWARENESS
(Check if condition over last 7 days appears different from usual functioning)
a. Less alert, easily distracted ●¹
b. Changing awareness of environment ●¹
c. Episodes of incoherent speech ●¹
d. Periods of motor restlessness or lethargy ●¹
e. Cognitive ability varies over course of day ●¹
f. NONE OF ABOVE

6. CHANGE IN COGNITIVE STATUS
Change in resident's cognitive status, skills, or abilities in last 90 days
0. No change   1. Improved   2. Deteriorated ●¹ ▲¹⁴

SECTION C. COMMUNICATION/HEARING PATTERNS

1. HEARING
(With hearing appliance, if used)
0. Hears adequately—normal talk, TV, phone
1. Minimal difficulty when not in quiet setting
2. Hears in special situation only—speaker has to adjust tonal quality and speak distinctly
3. Highly impaired/absence of useful hearing

2. COMMUNICATION DEVICES/ TECHNIQUES
(Check all that apply during last 7 days)
a. Hearing aid, present and used
b. Hearing aid, present and not used
c. Other receptive comm. technique used (e.g., lip read)
d. NONE OF ABOVE

3. MODES OF EXPRESSION
(Check all used by resident to make needs known)
a. Speech
b. Writing messages to express or clarify needs
c. Signs/gestures/sounds
d. Communication board
e. Other
f. NONE OF ABOVE

4. MAKING SELF UNDERSTOOD
(Express information content—however able)
0. Understood
1. Usually Understood-difficulty finding words or finishing thoughts
2. Sometimes Understood-ability is limited to making concrete requests ▲⁴
3. Rarely/Never Understood ▲⁴

5. ABILITY TO UNDERSTAND OTHERS
(Understanding verbal information content-however able)
0. Understands
1. Usually Understands-may miss some part/intent of message ▲²
2. Sometimes Understands-responds adequately to simple, direct communication ▲² ▲⁴ ▲⁵
3. Rarely/Never Understands ▲² ▲⁴ ▲⁵

6. CHANGE IN COMMUNI-CATION/ HEARING
Resident's ability to express, understand or hear information has changed over last 90 days
0. No change   1. Improved   2. Deteriorated ●¹

SECTION D. VISION PATTERNS

1. VISION
(Ability to see in adequate light and with glasses if used)
0. Adequate—sees fine detail, including regular print in newspapers/books
1. Impaired—sees large print, but not regular print in newspapers/books ●³
2. Highly Impaired—limited vision, not able to see newspaper headlines, appears to follow objects with eyes ●³
3. Severely Impaired—no vision or appears to see only light, colors, or shapes ●³

●= Automatic Trigger   ▲ = Potential Trigger

1 - Delirium	5 - ADL Functional/Rehabilitation Potential	9 - Behavior Problems
2 - Cognitive Loss/Dementia	6 - Urinary Incontinence and Indwelling Catheter	10 - Activities
3 - Visual Function	7 - Psychosocial Well-Being	11 - Falls
4 - Communication	8 - Mood State	12 - Nutritional Status

13 - Feeding Tubes	17 - Psychotropic Drug Use
14 - Dehydration/Fluid Maintenance	18 - Physical Restraints
15 - Dental Care	
16 - Pressure Ulcers	

Form 1828HH   © 1990 Briggs Corporation, Des Moines, IA 50306 (800) 247-2343   PRINTED IN U.S.A.   1 of 4   Rev. 3/91
Copyright limited to addition of trigger system.

FIGURE 3-10 *Minimum data set (MDS). (Reprinted with permission of Briggs Corporation, Des Moines, IA. 50306)*

2.	VISUAL LIMITATIONS/ DIFFICULTIES	a. Side vision problems—decreased peripheral vision; (e.g., leaves food on one side of tray, difficulty traveling, bumps into people and objects, misjudges placement of chair when seating self) ●3	a.
		b. Experiences any of the following: sees halos or rings around lights, sees flashes of light; sees "curtains" over eyes	b.
		c. NONE OF ABOVE	c.
3.	VISUAL APPLIANCES	Glasses; contact lenses; lens implant; magnifying glass 0. No 1. Yes	

SECTION E. PHYSICAL FUNCTIONING AND STRUCTURAL PROBLEMS

1. ADL SELF-PERFORMANCE *(Code for resident's PERFORMANCE OVER ALL SHIFTS during last 7 days—Not including setup)*

0. INDEPENDENT—No help or oversight—OR—Help/oversight provided only 1 or 2 times during last 7 days.

1. SUPERVISION—Oversight encouragement or cueing provided 3+ times during last 7 days—OR—Supervision plus physical assistance provided only 1 or 2 times during last 7 days.

2. LIMITED ASSISTANCE—Resident highly involved in activity, received physical help in guided maneuvering of limbs, or other nonweight bearing assistance 3+ times—OR—More help provided only 1 or 2 times during last 7 days.

3. EXTENSIVE ASSISTANCE—While resident performed part of activity, over last 7-day period, help of following type(s) provided 3 or more times:
  — Weight-bearing support
  — Full staff performance during part (but not all) of last 7 days.

4. TOTAL DEPENDENCE—Full staff performance of activity during entire 7 days.

2. ADL SUPPORT PROVIDED—*(Code for MOST SUPPORT PROVIDED OVER ALL SHIFTS during last 7 days; code regardless of resident's self-performance classification)*

			1 SELF-PERFORMANCE	2 SUPPORT
	0. No setup or physical help from staff 2. One-person physical assist 1. Setup help only 3. Two+ person physical assist			
a.	BED MOBILITY	How resident moves to and from lying position, turns side to side, and positions body while in bed 3 or 4 for self-perf = ▲5		
b.	TRANSFER	How resident moves between surfaces—to/from: bed, chair, wheelchair, standing position (EXCLUDE to/from bath/toilet) 3 or 4 for self-perf = ▲5		
c.	LOCO-MOTION	How resident moves between locations in his/her room and adjacent corridor on same floor. If in wheelchair, self-sufficiency once in chair 3 or 4 for self-perf = ▲5		
d.	DRESSING	How resident puts on, fastens, and takes off all items of street clothing, including donning/removing prosthesis 3 or 4 for self-perf = ▲5		
e.	EATING	How resident eats and drinks (regardless of skill) 3 or 4 for self-perf = ▲5		
f.	TOILET USE	How resident uses the toilet room (or commode, bedpan, urinal); transfers on/off toilet, cleanses, changes pad, manages ostomy or catheter, adjusts clothes 3 or 4 for self-perf = ▲5		
g.	PERSONAL HYGIENE	How resident maintains personal hygiene, including combing hair, brushing teeth, shaving, applying makeup, washing/drying face, hands, and perineum (EXCLUDE baths and showers)		

| 3. | BATHING | How resident takes full-body bath, sponge bath, and transfers in/out of tub/shower (EXCLUDE washing of back and hair. Code for most dependent in self-performance and support. Bathing Self-Performance codes appear below.) 3 or 4 for (a) = ▲5
0. Independent—No help provided
1. Supervision—Oversight help only
2. Physical help limited to transfer only
3. Physical help in part of bathing activity
4. Total dependence | a. | b. |

4.	BODY CONTROL PROBLEMS	*(Check all that apply during last 7 days)*		
		a. Balance—partial or total loss of ability to balance self while standing ▲11	a.	
		b. Bedfast all or most of the time ▲11	b.	
		c. Contracture to arms, legs, shoulders, or hands	c.	
		d. Hemiplegia/hemiparesis ▲11	d.	
		e. Quadriplegia ▲11	e.	
		f. Arm—partial or total loss of voluntary movement	f.	
		g. Hand—lack of dexterity (e.g., problem using toothbrush or adjusting hearing aid)	g.	
		h. Leg—partial or total loss of voluntary movement ▲11	h.	
		i. Leg—unsteady gait	i.	
		j. Trunk—partial or total loss of ability to position, balance, or turn body ▲11	j.	
		k. Amputation	k.	
		l. NONE OF ABOVE	l.	

5.	MOBILITY APPLIANCES/ DEVICES	*(Check all that apply during last 7 days)*		
		a. Cane/walker	a.	
		b. Brace/prosthesis	b.	
		c. Wheeled self	c.	
		d. Other person wheeled		d.
		e. Lifted (manually/mechanically)		e.
		f. NONE OF ABOVE		f.

| 6. | TASK SEG-MENTATION | Resident requires that some or all of ADL activities be broken into a series of subtasks so that resident can perform them.
0. No   1. Yes | |

7.	ADL FUNC-TIONAL REHAB. POTENTIAL	a. Resident believes he/she capable of increased independence in at least some ADLs ▲5	a.
		b. Direct care staff believe resident capable of increased independence in at least some ADLs ▲5	b.
		c. Resident able to perform tasks/activity but is very slow	c.
		d. Major difference in ADL Self-Performance or ADL Support in mornings and evenings (at least a one category change in Self-Performance or Support in any ADL)	d.
		e. NONE OF ABOVE	e.

| 8. | CHANGE IN ADL FUNCTION | Change in ADL self-performance in last 90 days
0. No change   1. Improved   2. Deteriorated | |

SECTION F. CONTINENCE IN LAST 14 DAYS

1. CONTINENCE SELF-CONTROL CATEGORIES
(Code for resident performance over all shifts.)

0. CONTINENT—Complete control

1. USUALLY CONTINENT—BLADDER, incontinent episodes once a week or less; BOWEL, less than weekly;

2. OCCASIONALLY INCONTINENT—BLADDER, 2+ times a week but not daily; BOWEL, once a week

3. FREQUENTLY INCONTINENT—BLADDER, tended to be incontinent daily, but some control present (e.g., on day shift); BOWEL, 2-3 times a week

4. INCONTINENT—Had inadequate control. BLADDER, multiple daily episodes; BOWEL, all (or almost all) of the time.

| a. | BOWEL CON-TINENCE | Control of bowel movement, with appliance or bowel continence programs if employed | |
| b. | BLADDER CONTI-NENCE | Control of urinary bladder function (if dribbles, volume insufficient to soak through underpants), with appliances (e.g., foley) or continence programs, if employed 2, 3 or 4 = ▲6 | |

2.	INCONTI-NENCE RELATED TESTING	*(Skip if resident's bladder continence code equals 0 or 1 AND no catheter is used)*	
		a. Resident has been tested for a urinary tract infection	a.
		b. Resident has been checked for presence of a fecal impaction, or there is adequate bowel elimination	b.
		c. NONE OF ABOVE	c.

3.	APPLIANCES AND PROGRAMS	a. Any scheduled toileting plan	a.	e. Did not use toilet room/commode/urinal	e.
		b. External (condom) catheter ▲6	b.	f. Pads/briefs used ▲6	f.
		c. Indwelling catheter ▲6	c.	g. Enemas/irrigation	g.
		d. Intermittent catheter ▲6	d.	h. Ostomy	h.
				i. NONE OF ABOVE	i.

| 4. | CHANGE IN URINARY CONTINENCE | Change in urinary continence or programs in last 90 days
0. No change   1. Improved   2. Deteriorated | |

SKIP TO SECTION J IF COMATOSE

SECTION G. PSYCHOSOCIAL WELL-BEING

1.	SENSE OF INITIATIVE/ INVOLVE-MENT	a. At ease interacting with others	a.
		b. At ease doing planned or structured activities	b.
		c. At ease doing self-initiated activities	c.
		d. Establishes own goals	d.
		e. Pursues involvement in life of facility (i.e., makes/keeps friends; involved in group activities; responds positively to new activities; assists at religious services)	e.
		f. Accepts invitations into most group activities	f.
		g. NONE OF ABOVE	g.

2.	UNSETTLED RELATION-SHIPS	a. Covert/open conflict with and/or repeated criticism of staff ●7	a.
		b. Unhappy with roommate ●7	b.
		c. Unhappy with residents other than roommate ●7	c.
		d. Openly expresses conflict/anger with family or friends ●7	d.
		e. Absence of personal contact with family/friends	e.
		f. Recent loss of close family member/friend	f.
		g. NONE OF ABOVE	g.

●= Automatic Trigger   ▲ = Potential Trigger

1 - Delirium	5 - ADL Functional/Rehabilitation Potential	9 - Behavior Problems	13 - Feeding Tubes	17 - Psychotropic Drug Use
2 - Cognitive Loss/Dementia	6 - Urinary incontinence and indwelling Catheter	10 - Activities	14 - Dehydration/Fluid Maintenance	18 - Physical Restraints
3 - Visual Function	7 - Psychosocial Well-Being	11 - Falls	15 - Dental Care	
4 - Communication	8 - Mood State	12 - Nutritional Status	16 - Pressure Ulcers	

2 of 4   Rev. 3/91

FIGURE 3-10, cont'd *For legend see opposite page.*   *Continued.*

3.	PAST ROLES	a. Strong identification with past roles and life status	a.
		b. Expresses sadness/anger/empty feeling over lost roles/status ●7	b.
		c. *NONE OF ABOVE*	c.

SECTION H. MOOD AND BEHAVIOR PATTERNS

1.	SAD OR ANXIOUS MOOD	*(Check all that apply during last 30 days)*	
		a. VERBAL EXPRESSIONS of DISTRESS by resident (sadness, sense that nothing matters, hopelessness, worthlessness, unrealistic fears, vocal expressions of anxiety or grief) ●8	a.
		DEMONSTRATED (OBSERVABLE) SIGNS of mental DISTRESS	
		b. Tearfulness, emotional groaning, sighing, breathlessness ●8	b.
		c. Motor agitation such as pacing, handwringing or picking ●8	c.
		d. Failure to eat or take medications, withdrawal from self-care or leisure activities ●8 ▲14	d.
		e. Pervasive concern with health ●8	e.
		f. Recurrent thoughts of death—e.g., believes he/she is about to die, have a heart attack ●8	f.
		g. Suicidal thoughts/actions ●8	g.
		h. *NONE OF ABOVE*	h.
2.	MOOD PERSISTENCE	Sad or anxious mood intrudes on daily life over last 7 days—not easily altered, doesn't "cheer up" 0. No 1. Yes ●8	
3.	PROBLEM BEHAVIOR	*(Code for behavior in last 7 days)* 0. Behavior **not exhibited** in last 7 days 1. Behavior of this type occurred **less than daily** 2. Behavior of this type occurred **daily or more frequently**	
		a. WANDERING (moved with no rational purpose; seemingly oblivious to needs or safety) 1 or 2 = ●9	a.
		b. VERBALLY ABUSIVE (others were threatened, screamed at, cursed at) 1 or 2 = ●9	b.
		c. PHYSICALLY ABUSIVE (others were hit, shoved, scratched, sexually abused) 1 or 2 = ●9	c.
		d. SOCIALLY INAPPROPRIATE/DISRUPTIVE BEHAVIOR (made disrupting sounds, noisy, screams, self-abusive acts, sexual behavior or disrobing in public, smeared/threw food/feces, hoarding, rummaged through others' belongings) 1 or 2 = ●9	d.
4.	RESIDENT RESISTS CARE	*(Check all types of resistance that occurred in the last 7 days)*	
		a. Resisted taking medications/injection	a.
		b. Resisted ADL assistance	b.
		c. *NONE OF ABOVE*	c.
5.	BEHAVIOR MANAGEMENT PROGRAM	Behavior problem has been addressed by clinically developed behavior management program. (Note: Do not include programs that involve only physical restraints or psychotropic medications in this category.) 0. No behavior problem 1. Yes, addressed 2. No, not addressed	
6.	CHANGE IN MOOD	Change in mood in last 90 days 0. No change 1. Improved 2. Deteriorated ▲1	
7.	CHANGE IN PROBLEM BEHAVIOR	Change in problem behavioral signs in last 90 days 0. No change 1. Improved 2. Deteriorated ●1	

SECTION I. ACTIVITY PURSUIT PATTERNS

1.	TIME AWAKE	*(Check appropriate time periods—last 7 days)* Resident awake all or most of time (i.e., naps no more than one hour per time period) in the:	
		a. Morning 7a.m.–Noon (or when resident wakes up) a.	c. Evening 5p.m.–10p.m. (or bedtime) c.
		b. Afternoon Noon–5p.m. b.	d. *NONE OF ABOVE* d.
2.	AVERAGE TIME INVOLVED IN ACTIVITIES	0. Most—(more than 2/3 of time) ▲10 2. Little—(less than 1/3 of time) ▲10 1. Some—(1/3 to 2/3 time) ▲10 3. None ▲10	
3.	PREFERRED ACTIVITY SETTINGS	*(Check all settings in which activities are preferred)*	
		a. Own room a.	d. Outside facility d.
		b. Day/activity room b.	e. *NONE OF ABOVE* e.
		c. Inside NH/off unit c.	

4.	GENERAL ACTIVITIES PREFERENCES (adapted to resident's current abilities)	*(Check all specific preferences whether or not activity is currently available to resident)*	
		a. Cards/other games a.	f. Spiritual/religious activ. f.
		b. Crafts/arts b.	g. Trips/shopping g.
		c. Exercise/sports c.	h. Walking/wheeling outdoors h.
		d. Music d.	i. Watch TV i.
		e. Read/write e.	j. *NONE OF ABOVE* j.
5.	PREFERS MORE OR DIFFERENT ACTIVITIES	Resident expresses/indicates preference for other activities/choices. 0. No 1. Yes ●10	

SECTION J. DISEASE DIAGNOSES

Check only those diseases present that have a relationship to current ADL status, cognitive status, behavior status, medical treatments, or risk of death. (Do not list old/inactive diagnoses.) (If none apply, check the NONE OF ABOVE box)

1.	DISEASES	**HEART/CIRCULATION**		r. Manic depressive (bipolar disease)	r.
		a. Arteriosclerotic heart disease (ASHD)	a.	**SENSORY**	
		b. Cardiac dysrhythmias	b.	s. Cataracts	s.
		c. Congestive heart failure	c.	t. Glaucoma	t.
		d. Hypertension	d.	**OTHER**	
		e. Hypotension	e.	u. Allergies	u.
		f. Peripheral vascular disease	f.	v. Anemia	v.
		g. Other cardiovascular disease	g.	w. Arthritis	w.
		NEUROLOGICAL		x. Cancer	x.
		h. Alzheimer's	h.	y. Diabetes mellitus	y.
		i. Dementia other than Alzheimer's	i.	z. Explicit terminal prognosis	z.
		j. Aphasia	j.	aa. Hypothyroidism	aa.
		k. Cerebrovascular accident (stroke)	k.	bb. Osteoporosis	bb.
		l. Multiple sclerosis	l.	cc. Seizure disorder	cc.
		m. Parkinson's disease	m.	dd. Septicemia	dd.
		PULMONARY		ee. Urinary tract infection—in last 30 days ▲14	ee.
		n. Emphysema/asthma/COPD	n.	ff. *NONE OF ABOVE*	ff.
		o. Pneumonia	o.		
		PSYCHIATRIC/MOOD			
		p. Anxiety disorder	p.		
		q. Depression	q.		
2.	OTHER CURRENT DIAGNOSES AND ICD-9 CODES	260–263.9=●12 276.5=▲14 291.0–293.1=●1 a. b. c. d. e. f.			

SECTION K. HEALTH CONDITIONS

1.	PROBLEM CONDITIONS	*(Check all problems that are present in last 7 days unless other time frame indicated)*	
		a. Constipation	a.
		b. Diarrhea ▲14	b.
		c. Dizziness/vertigo ▲14	c.
		d. Edema	d.
		e. Fecal impaction	e.
		f. Fever ▲14	f.
		g. Hallucinations/delusions	g.
		h. Internal bleeding ▲14	h.
		i. Joint pain	i.
		j. Pain—resident complains or shows evidence of pain daily or almost daily	j.
		k. Recurrent lung aspirations in last 90 days	k.
		l. Shortness of breath	l.
		m. Syncope (fainting)	m.
		n. Vomiting ▲14	n.
		o. *NONE OF ABOVE*	o.
2.	ACCIDENTS	a. Fell—past 30 days ●11	a.
		b. Fell—past 31-180 days ●11	b.
		c. Hip fracture in **last 180 days**	c.
		d. *NONE OF ABOVE*	d.

FIGURE 3-10, cont'd *Minimum data set (MDS). (Reprinted with permission of Briggs Corporation, Des Moines, IA. 50306.)*

Resident Name _____ I.D. Number _____

3.	STABILITY OF CONDITIONS	a. Conditions/diseases make resident's cognitive, ADL, or behavior status unstable—fluctuating, precarious, or deteriorating.	a.
		b. Resident experiencing an acute episode or a flare-up of a recurrent/chronic problem.	b.
		c. *NONE OF THE ABOVE*	c.

SECTION L. ORAL/NUTRITIONAL STATUS

| 1. | ORAL PROBLEMS | a. Chewing problem | a. | c. Mouth pain ●15 | c. |
| | | b. Swallowing problem | b. | d. *NONE OF ABOVE* | d. |

| 2. | HEIGHT AND WEIGHT | *Record height (a) in inches and weight (b) in pounds.* *Weight based on most recent status in* **last 30 days;** *measure weight consistently* **in accord with standard facility** *practice— e.g., in a.m. after voiding, before meal, with shoes off, and in nightclothes.* HT (in.) [a.] WT (lb.) [b.] |
| | | c. **Weight loss** (i.e., **5% +** in **last 30 days;** or **10%** in **last 180 days**) 0. No 1. Yes ●12 ▲14 | c. |

3.	NUTRITIONAL PROBLEMS	a. Complains about the taste of many foods ●12	a.	d. Regular complaint of hunger ●12	d.
		b. Insufficient fluid; dehydrated ●14	b.	e. Leaves 25%+ food uneaten at most meals ●12 ▲14	e.
		c. Did **NOT** consume all/almost all liquids provided **during last 3 days** ▲14	c.	f. *NONE OF ABOVE*	f.

4.	NUTRITIONAL APPROACHES	a. Parenteral/IV ▲14 ●12	a.	e. Therapeutic diet ●12	e.
		b. Feeding tube ▲14 ●13	b.	f. Dietary supplement between meals	f.
		c. Mechanically altered diet ●12	c.	g. Plate guard, stabilized built-up utensil, etc.	g.
		d. Syringe (oral feeding) ●12	d.	h. *NONE OF ABOVE*	h.

SECTION M. ORAL/DENTAL STATUS

1.	ORAL STATUS AND DISEASE PREVENTION	a. Debris (soft, easily movable substances) present in mouth prior to going to bed at night ●15	a.
		b. Has dentures and/or removable bridge	b.
		c. Some/all natural teeth lost—does not have or does not use dentures (or partial plates) ●15	c.
		d. Broken, loose, or carious teeth ●15	d.
		e. Inflamed gums (gingiva), oral abscesses, swollen or bleeding gums, ulcers, or rashes ●15	e.
		f. Daily cleaning of teeth/dentures If not checked = ●15	f.
		g. *NONE OF ABOVE*	g.

SECTION N. SKIN CONDITION

1.	STASIS ULCER	(i.e., open lesion caused by poor venous circulation to lower extremities) 0. No 1. Yes	
2.	PRESSURE ULCERS	(Code for highest stage of pressure ulcer) 0. No pressure ulcers 1. Stage 1 A persistent area of skin redness (without a break in the skin) that does not disappear when pressure is relieved ●12 ●16 2. Stage 2 A partial thickness loss of skin layers that presents clinically as an abrasion, blister, or shallow crater ●12 ●16 3. Stage 3 A full thickness of skin is lost, exposing the subcutaneous tissues—presents as a deep crater with or without undermining adjacent tissue ●12 ●16 4. Stage 4 A full thickness of skin and subcutaneous tissue is lost, exposing muscle and/or bone ●12 ●16	
3.	HISTORY OF RESOLVED/ CURED PRESSURE ULCERS	Resident has had a pressure ulcer that was resolved/cured in **last 90 days** 0. No 1. Yes	

4.	SKIN PROBLEMS/ CARE *If None Checked From C Thru G = ▲16*	a. Open lesions other than stasis or pressure ulcers (e.g., cuts)	a.
		b. Skin desensitized to pain/pressure/discomfort	b.
		c. Protective/preventive skin care	c.
		d. Turning/repositioning program	d.
		e. Pressure-relieving beds, bed/chair pads (e.g., egg crate pads)	e.
		f. Wound care/treatment (e.g., pressure ulcer care, surgical wound)	f.
		g. Other skin care/treatment	g.
		h. *NONE OF ABOVE*	h.

SECTION O. MEDICATION USE

1.	NUMBER OF MEDI-CATIONS	(Record the number of *different* medications used in *the last 7 days;* enter "0" if none used.)	
2.	NEW MEDI-CATIONS	Resident has received new medications during the **last 90 days** 0. No 1. Yes	
3.	INJECTIONS	*(Record the number of days injections of any type received during the last 7 days.)*	
4.	DAYS RECEIVED THE FOLLOWING MEDICATION	*(Record the number of days during last 7 days; Enter "0" if not used; enter "1" if long-acting meds. used less than weekly)*	
		a. Antipsychotics 1-7 = ▲9 ▲11 ▲17	a.
		b. Antianxiety/hypnotics 1-7 = ▲9 ▲11 ▲17	b.
		c. Antidepressants 1-7 = ▲9 ▲11 ▲17	c.
5.	PREVIOUS MEDICATION RESULTS	*(SKIP this question if resident currently receiving anti-psychotics, antidepressants, or antianxiety/hypnotics— otherwise code correct response for last 90 days)* Resident has previously received psychoactive medications for a mood or behavior problem, and these medications were effective (without undue adverse consequences). 0. No, drugs not used 1. Drugs were effective 2. Drugs were not effective 3. Drug effectiveness unknown	

SECTION P. SPECIAL TREATMENTS AND PROCEDURES

1.	SPECIAL TREAT-MENTS AND PROCE-DURES	SPECIAL CARE—*Check treatments received during the last 14 days.*	
		a. Chemotherapy	a.	f. IV meds	f.
		b. Radiation	b.	g. Transfusions	g.
		c. Dialysis	c.	h. O2	h.
		d. Suctioning	d.	i. Other _____	i.
		e. Trach. care	e.	j. *NONE OF ABOVE*	j.
		THERAPIES—*Record the number of days each of the following therapies was administered (for at least 10 minutes during a day) in the last 7 days:*	
		k. Speech—language pathology and audiology services	k.
		l. Occupational therapy	l.
		m. Physical therapy	m.
		n. Psychological therapy (any licensed professional)	n.
		o. Respiratory Therapy	o.
2.	ABNORMAL LAB VALUES	Has the resident had any **abnormal lab values** during the last 90-day period? 0. No 1. Yes 2. No tests performed	
3.	DEVICES AND RESTRAINTS	*Use the following code for last 7 days:* 0 Not used 1 Used less than daily 2 Used daily	
		a. Bed rails	a.
		b. Trunk restraint 1 or 2 = ▲9 ●18	b.
		c. Limb restraint 1 or 2 = ▲9 ●18	c.
		d. Chair prevents rising 1 or 2 = ▲9 ●18	d.

● = Automatic Trigger   ▲ = Potential Trigger

1 - Delirium	5 - ADL Functional/Rehabilitation Potential	9 - Behavior Problems	13 - Feeding Tubes	17 - Psychotropic Drug Use
2 - Cognitive Loss/Dementia	6 - Urinary Incontinence and Indwelling Catheter	10 - Activities	14 - Dehydration/Fluid Maintenance	18 - Physical Restraints
3 - Visual Function	7 - Psychosocial Well-Being	11 - Falls	15 - Dental Care	
4 - Communication	8 - Mood State	12 - Nutritional Status	16 - Pressure Ulcers	

4 of 4   Rev. 3/91

FIGURE 3-10, cont'd *For legend see opposite page.*

Continued.

FACE SHEET FOR NURSING FACILITY RESIDENT ASSESSMENT AND CARE SCREENING (MDS)
BACKGROUND INFORMATION/INTAKE AT ADMISSION

I. IDENTIFICATION INFORMATION

1. RESIDENT NAME _____
(First)   (Middle Initial)   (Last)

ID# _____

2. DATE OF CURRENT ADMISSION
Month — Day — Year

3. MEDICARE No. (SOC. SEC. or Comparable No. if no Medicare No.)

4. FACILITY PROVIDER NO.

Federal No.

5. GENDER — 1. Male   2. Female

6. RACE/ETHNICITY
1. American Indian/Alaskan Native
2. Asian/Pacific Islander
3. Black, not of Hispanic origin
4. Hispanic
5. White, not of Hispanic origin

7. BIRTHDATE
Month — Day — Year

8. LIFETIME OCCUPATION _____

9. PRIMARY LANGUAGE
Resident's primary language is a language other than English.   0. No   1. Yes _____
(Specify)

10. RESIDENTIAL HISTORY PAST 5 YEARS
(Check all settings resident lived in during 5 years prior to admission)
a. Prior stay at this nursing home — a.
b. Other nursing home/residential facility — b.
c. MH/psychiatric setting — c.
d. MR/DD setting — d.
e. *NONE OF ABOVE* — e.

11. MENTAL HEALTH HISTORY
Does resident's RECORD indicate any history of mental retardation, mental illness, or any other mental health problem?   0. No   1. Yes

12. CONDITIONS RELATED TO MR/DD STATUS
Check all conditions that are related to MR/DD Status, that were manifested before age 22, and are likely to continue indefinitely.
a. Not Applicable—no MR/DD (Skip to Item 13) — a.
MR/DD with Organic Condition
b. Cerebral palsy — b.
c. Down's syndrome — c.
d. Autism — d.
e. Epilepsy — e.
f. Other organic condition related to MR/DD — f.
g. MR/DD with no organic condition — g.
h. Unknown — h.

13. MARITAL STATUS
1. Never Married   3. Widowed   5. Divorced
2. Married   4. Separated

14. ADMITTED FROM
1. Private home or apt.   3. Acute care hospital
2. Nursing facility   4. Other

15. LIVED ALONE — 0. No   1. Yes   2. In other facility

☐ = Code the appropriate response   b. = Check (✓) if response is applicable

16. ADMISSION INFORMATION AMENDED   *(Check all that apply)*
a. Accurate information unavailable earlier — a.
b. Observation revealed additional information — b.
c. Resident unstable at admission — c.

II. BACKGROUND INFORMATION AT RETURN/READMISSION

1. DATE OF CURRENT READMISSION
Month — Day — Year

2. MARITAL STATUS
1. Never Married   3. Widowed   5. Divorced
2. Married   4. Separated

3. ADMITTED FROM
1. Private home or apt.   3. Acute care hospital
2. Nursing facility   4. Other

4. LIVED ALONE — 0. No   1. Yes   2. In other facility

5. ADMISSION INFORMATION AMENDED   *(Check all that apply)*
a. Accurate information unavailable earlier — a.
b. Observation revealed additional information — b.
c. Resident unstable at admission — c.

III. CUSTOMARY ROUTINE (ONLY AT FIRST ADMISSION)

1. CUSTOMARY ROUTINE (Year prior to first admission to a nursing home)
(Check all that apply. If all information UNKNOWN, check last box only.)

CYCLE OF DAILY EVENTS
a. Stays up late at night (e.g., after 9 pm) — a.
b. Naps regularly during day (at least 1 hour) — b.
c. Goes out 1+ days a week — c.
d. Stays busy with hobbies, reading, or fixed daily routine — d.
e. Spends most time alone or watching TV — e.
f. Moves independently indoors (with appliances, if used) — f.
g. *NONE OF ABOVE* — g.

EATING PATTERNS
h. Distinct food preferences — h.
i. Eats between meals all or most days — i.
j. Use of alcoholic beverage(s) at least weekly — j.
k. *NONE OF ABOVE* — k.

ADL PATTERNS
l. In bedclothes much of day — l.
m. Wakens to toilet all or most nights — m.
n. Has irregular bowel movement pattern — n.
o. Prefers showers for bathing — o.
p. *NONE OF ABOVE* — p.

INVOLVEMENT PATTERNS
q. Daily contact with relatives/close friends — q.
r. Usually attends church, temple, synagogue (etc.) — r.
s. Finds strength in faith — s.
t. Daily animal companion/presence — t.
u. Involved in group activities — u.
v. *NONE OF ABOVE* — v.
w. UNKNOWN—Resident/family unable to provide information — w.

Signature and Date of RN Assessment Coordinator: _____

Signatures and Dates of Others Who Completed Part of the Assessment:

_____ _____ _____

_____ _____ _____

END

Form 1827HH   BRIGGS, Des Moines, IA 50306 (800) 247-2343   PRINTED IN U.S.A.   (9-90)

FIGURE 3-10, cont'd *Minimum data set (MDS). (Reprinted with permission of Briggs Corporation, Des Moines, IA. 50306.)*

Fig. 3-12, p. 45). For example, Mr. Smith is *deconditioned*. **Deconditioning** is the process of becoming weak from illness or lack of exercise. The MDS shows that Mr. Smith cannot do his activities of daily living (ADLs). This *triggers* the *RAPs,* which provides guidelines for actions to solve the problem. The *goal* is for Mr. Smith to be independent in all ADLs. The actions to help Mr. Smith reach the goal are as follows:

◆ Occupational therapy to work with the resident on ADLs daily
◆ Physical therapy to work with the resident on strengthening exercises daily
◆ Nursing staff member to walk the resident 20 feet twice daily

Health care team members from the three disciplines (occupational therapy, physical therapy, and nursing) work to solve one problem. Care plan suggestions are welcomed from all health care team members, including nursing assistants. A comprehensive care plan is developed for each resident. You can use the care plan as a guide to individualized resident care.

Care plan forms vary in each facility. Often the care plan is included in the resident's record or in a Kardex.

THE KARDEX

The **Kardex** is a type of card file used in some health facilities. There is a card for each resident. It contains some of the information found in the resident's record. The Kardex in long-term care is basically a summary of the resident's care plan, current diagnosis, routine care measures, special equipment used, and any special needs (Fig. 3-13, p. 45). The Kardex card is a quick and easy source of resident information.

RESIDENT CARE CONFERENCE

There are two types of resident care conferences. One is the interdisciplinary care planning (IDCP) conference, and the other is a problem-focused conference. The IDCP conference is held regularly to review and update resident care plans or to develop care plans for new residents. This conference includes the RN in charge of the resident's care, the doctor, and health care team members from other disciplines. Dietary, recreation, rehabilitation therapies, and social work are examples of other disciplines that may be included. The resident and a family member also are included.

Problem-focused conferences are held whenever there is a single problem affecting a resident's care. Only health care team members directly involved in the problem attend. The resident or the resident's family may be asked to attend.

Nursing assistants often are included in both types of conferences. They are encouraged to share their suggestions and observations.

COMPUTERS IN HEALTH CARE

The use of computers is a growing trend in health care. Information systems are available that collect, send, record, and store information. The information can be retrieved when needed. Resident records and care plans are kept on computers in more and more nursing facilities. Instead of recording on the resident's chart, it is easier, faster, and more efficient to enter information into a computer (Fig. 3-13, p. 46).

Computers also are being used to monitor certain measurements such as blood pressures, temperatures, and heart rates. The computer recognizes normal and abnormal measurements. When the abnormal is sensed, an alarm alerts the nursing staff. Computerized monitoring is common in hospitals. It also may be used in skilled nursing units.

Computers help save time. The quality and safety of resident care are increased. Less information is omitted from the residents' records, and fewer errors are made in recording. Records are more complete, and personnel are more efficient.

Computers are easy to use and vast amounts of information can be stored in them. Therefore the resident's right to privacy must be protected. Only certain individuals may use the computer. They have their personal codes (passwords) that are used to access the computer. Nursing assistants usually are not allowed to use the computer. If allowed access, you must follow the ethical and legal considerations related to privacy, confidentiality, and defamation (see Chapter 2).

Learning to use a computer is easy and fun. If you have the opportunity to use the computer where your work, you should do so. Eventually all health care facilities will be computerized. If you know how to use computers, you have an additional skill that makes you a good person to employ.

TELEPHONE COMMUNICATIONS

In some facilities clerical staff members answer the telephones on the nursing units. Others do not have a clerical staff on the nursing units. In any case there are times when you must answer the telephone. Good telephone communication skills are essential. The caller cannot see you. Your tone of voice, how clearly you speak, and your attitude give much information. You must be as professional speaking on the telephone as you would be speaking to the person face-to-face.

Most facilities have policies about answering the telephone. Know your facility's policy. The guidelines here and on p. 46 can help you be professional and courteous.

1. Answer the telephone as quickly as possible. This avoids excessive ringing of phones, which can disturb residents. It also tells the caller that the staff is efficient.

Resident's Name:			Medical Record No.:

RESIDENT ASSESSMENT PROTOCOL SUMMARY

1. For each RAP area triggered, show whether you are proceeding with a care plan intervention.

2. Document problems, complications, and risk factors; the need for referral to appropriate health professionals; and the reasons for deciding to proceed or not to proceed to care planning. Documentation may appear anywhere the facility routinely keeps such information, such as problem sheets or nurses' progress notes.

3. Show location of this information.

RAP PROBLEM AREA	CARE PLANNING DECISION (✓)		LOCATION OF INFORMATION
	PROCEED	NOT PROCEED	
1 DELIRIUM			
2 COGNITIVE LOSS/DEMENTIA			
3 VISUAL FUNCTION			
4 COMMUNICATION			
5 ADL FUNCTIONAL/ REHABILITATION POTENTIAL			
6 URINARY INCONTINENCE & INDWELLING CATHETER			
7 PSYCHOSOCIAL WELL-BEING			
8 MOOD STATE			
9 BEHAVIOR PROBLEMS			
10 ACTIVITIES			
11 FALLS			
12 NUTRITIONAL STATUS			
13 FEEDING TUBES			
14 DEHYDRATION/FLUID MAINTENANCE			
15 DENTAL CARE			
16 PRESSURE ULCERS			
17 PSYCHOTROPIC DRUG USE			
18 PHYSICAL RESTRAINTS			

Signature of RN Assessment Coordinator:	Date:

Form 1833HH   BRIGGS, Des Moines, IA 50306 (800) 247-2343 PRINTED IN U.S.A.

RESIDENT ASSESSMENT PROTOCOL SUMMARY

FIGURE 3-11 *Resident assessment protocols (RAPS). (Reprinted with permission of Briggs Corporation, Des Moines, IA. 50306)*

Diet: **Bland**

Activities:	Bath:	Travel:	Position:
___ Complete bed rest	___ Bed bath	___ Wheelchair	
___ Bed rest	✓ Partial	___ Stretcher	
___ Bathroom privileges	___ Bathe self	✓ Ambulatory	
✓ Up ad lib	___ Tub	✓ Walker	
	___ Shower	___ Cane	
		___ Crutches	

Side rails:	Oxygen:	Special equipment:
___ Constantly	___ Liters per minute	
✓ Nights only	___ PRN ___ Constantly	
___ Side rail release	___ Tent ___ Catheter	
	___ Mask ___ Cannula	

Prosthesis:	Special privileges:	
✓ Dentures	shampoo hair as	
✓ Eye glasses	desired	
___ Contact lenses		
✓ Hearing aid		**Allergies:**
___ Limb		None known
___ Other		

Date	Medications	Date	Treatments
8/21	Tagamet 300 mg qid — 9-1-5-9 — po	8/21	Vital signs — qid
8/21	Mylanta 10 ml po 90 min pc + HS		Fluids
		8/21	Intake and output
		8/21	Hematest stools for occult blood
8/22	HS Med Dalmane 30 mg po		
PRN 8/22	Tylenol tabs 2 po q4h — headache		IVs
		8/21	D5W 1000 ml q8h

Room	Name	Age	Diagnosis	Doctor
33-1	Bailey, Laura	96	Duodenal ulcer	J. Wilson

FIGURE 3-12 *A sample Kardex.*

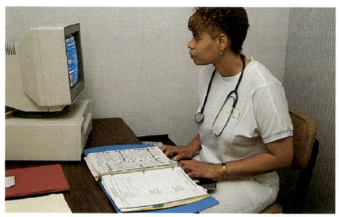

FIGURE 3-13 *A nurse enters resident information into a computer.*

2. Do not answer the phone in a rushed manner. Take a deep breath before answering to avoid sounding breathless to the caller.

3. Identify the facility and the area. Identify yourself, and give a courteous greeting. For example: "Rock Hill Nursing Facility, 2B, Wendy Storm; may I help you?"

4. Have a pencil and paper ready when you answer the phone. This allows you take a message for other health care workers or for a resident.

5. Write down the caller's name. This way, you will not have to ask the caller to repeat his or her name later during the call.

6. Get the correct spelling of the caller's name. This allows you to address the caller correctly and give correct messages.

7. Write the following information when taking a message: the caller's name, date and time of the call, telephone number, and the message.

8. Repeat the message and telephone number back to the caller. This makes sure you have the correct information.

9. Ask a caller to "please hold" if necessary. You may place a caller on hold if another line is ringing. Find out who is calling before placing the call on hold. Do not put a caller with an emergency on hold.

10. Do not lay the phone down or cover the receiver with your hand when you are not speaking to the caller. The caller may overhear confidential conversations.

11. Return to a caller on hold within 30 seconds. It is impolite to keep a caller on hold. Ask if the caller can wait longer or if the call can be returned.

12. Do not give confidential information to any caller. Remember that resident information is confidential. Refer such calls to a nurse.

13. Transfer the call if appropriate. Tell the caller you are going to transfer the call. Give the caller the phone number in case the call gets disconnected or the line is busy.

14. End the conversation politely. Thank the person for calling and say good-bye.

15. Give the message to the appropriate person.

SUMMARY

Communication among members of the health care team is essential for effective and coordinated resident care. Whether oral or written, communication should be factual, concise, understandable, and presented in a logical order. Reports, the comprehensive care plan, the Kardex, resident records, and resident care conferences are ways health team members communicate with one another.

The traditional resident record presented in this chapter is being replaced in some facilities with computerized records. Regardless of the type of resident record used, you must remember that the resident's chart is a legal document. It contains highly personal and confidential information. Confidential information is shared only with the health care members involved in a resident's care. It is never shared with the resident's friends or family without the resident's permission.

The resident has the right to participate in his or her care planning. OBRA requires that the resident be included in this process. The resident may refuse actions suggested by the health care team.

Review QUESTIONS

Circle *T* if the answer is true and *F* if it is false.

 1. The health care team members communicate with each other to provide effective and coordinated resident care.

 2. The resident's chart is destroyed after the resident leaves the facility to protect his or her privacy.

 3. The resident's chart cannot be used in a lawsuit because of the right to privacy.

 4. You generally can read the charts of all residents in the facility.

 5. Information is collected about the resident by using sight, hearing, touch, and smell.

 6. Subjective data can be observed with the senses.

 7. The resident's care plan is a card that contains a summary of the medications and treatments ordered by the doctor.

 8. The end-of-shift report and the resident care conference have the same purpose.

 9. You can let the telephone ring until you have time to answer it.

 10. You can place a caller on hold if necessary.

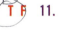 **11.** Never give confidential information to any caller.

Circle the *best* answer.

12. When communicating, you should do all of the following *except*
  a. Use terms with more than one meaning
  b. Be brief and concise
  c. Present information logically and in sequence
  d. Give facts and be specific

13. These statements are about resident records. Which is *false*?
  a. The record is used to communicate information about the resident.
  b. The record is a written account of the resident's condition and response to treatment.
  c. The record is a written account of care given by the health care team.
  d. Anyone working in the facility can read the resident's record.

14. Where does the nurse describe the nursing care given?
  a. Comprehensive care plan
  b. Nurses' notes
  c. Flow sheet
  d. Kardex

15. When recording information, you should do the following *except*
  a. Use ink
  b. Include the date and time
  c. Erase if you make an error
  d. Sign all entries with your name and title

16. The following statements are about recording. Which is *false*?
  a. Use the resident's exact words whenever possible.
  b. Record only what you have observed and done yourself.
  c. Do not skip lines.
  d. To save time, chart a procedure before it is completed.

17. The comprehensive plan
  a. Is written by the doctor
  b. Consists of actions taken to help a resident
  c. Is the same for all residents
  d. Is also called the Kardex

18. The following statements are about computers in health care. Which is *false*?
  a. Computers are used to collect, send, record, and store information.
  b. The resident's privacy must be protected.
  c. Residents' care plans can be computerized.
  d. All employees will be able to use the computer.

Answers

1. True	**6.** False	**11.** True	**16.** d
2. False	**7.** False	**12.** a	**17.** b
3. False	**8.** False	**13.** d	**18.** d
4. False	**9.** False	**14.** b	
5. True	**10.** True	**15.** c	

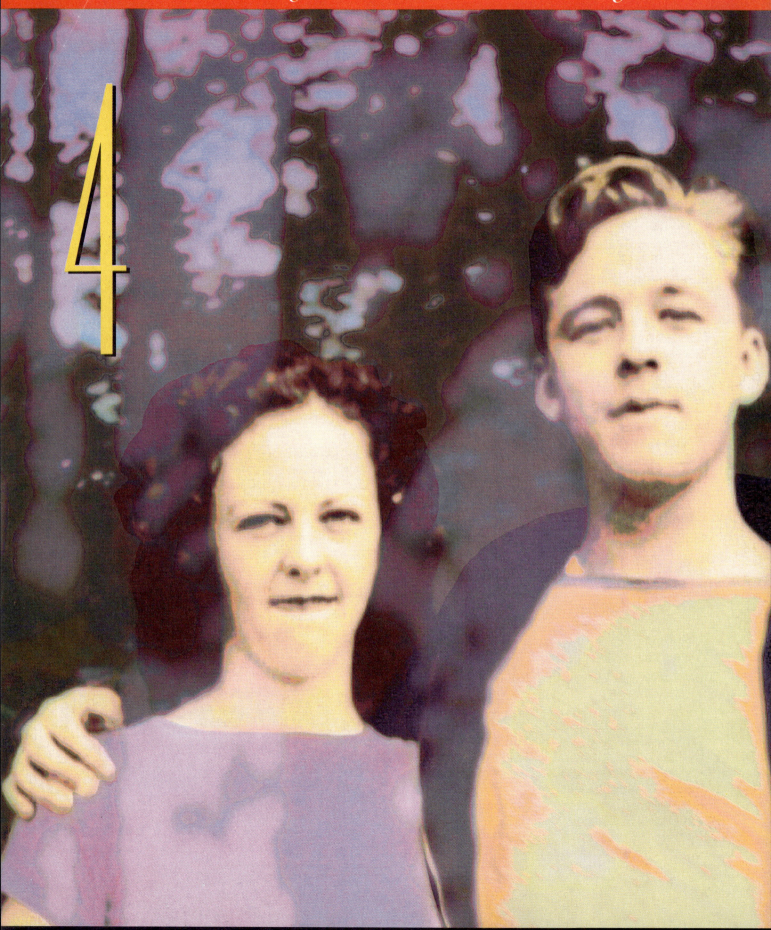

4

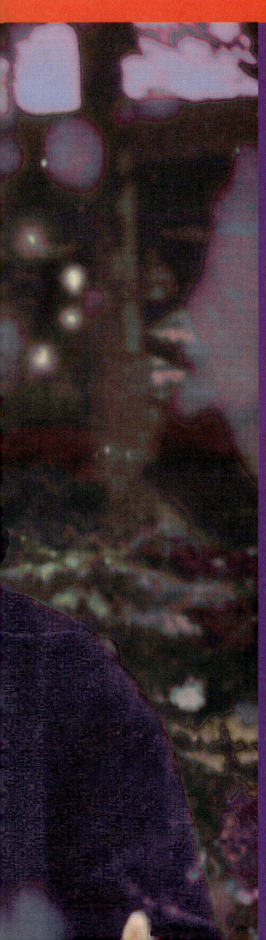

What You Will LEARN

- The key terms listed in this chapter

- The parts that make up the whole person

- The basic needs for life as identified by Abraham Maslow

- How culture and religion influence health and illness

- The psychological and social effects of illness

- The types of residents cared for in nursing facilities

- How to promote a resident's quality of life

- How verbal and nonverbal communication are used

- Six communication barriers

- Why family and visitors are important to residents

- The courtesies you should give to residents and visitors

body language
Facial expressions, gestures, posture, and other body movements that send messages to others

comatose
The inability to respond to verbal stimuli

culture
The values, beliefs, habits, likes, dislikes, customs, and characteristics of a group that are passed from one generation to the next

esteem
The worth, value, or opinion one has of a person

need
That which is necessary or desirable for maintaining life and mental well-being

nonverbal communication
Communication that does not involve the use of words

optimal level of function
A person's highest potential for mental and physical performance

religion
Spiritual beliefs, needs, and practices

self-actualization
Experiencing one's potential

verbal communication
Communication that uses the written or spoken word

Cheryl usually spends a little time with me every day. Sometimes we talk a lot and sometimes we don't say much at all. Its just good knowing someone cares.

The resident is the most important person in the nursing facility. Age, religion, nationality, education, occupation, and life-style are some factors that make each resident unique. Each resident is an important, special, valuable human being. The resident must be treated as a person who can think, act, and make decisions.

You will care for many residents, most of them elderly. Keep in mind that each resident is a person. You need to understand the fears, needs, and rights of that person. Also, you need to understand the losses that the person may have suffered. This is especially true of elderly residents. They may have lost homes, family members, friends, and body functions. They also may have lost their roles in families or communities. This chapter will help you understand and communicate with the residents you will serve, help, and care for.

THE RESIDENT AS A PERSON

Too often a resident is referred to as a room number, such as "12A needs a pain pill," rather than "Mrs. Brown in 12A needs a pain pill." This strips the person of his or her identity and reduces the individual to a thing. Residents often are denied the dignity and respect of being called by their titles, such as Mrs. Jones, Mr. Smith, or Miss Turner. Instead, they are called Jane, Tom, or Mary. Some have been called Grandma, Papa, or Sweetheart. Never call residents by their first name or any other name unless you have been asked to do so. Residents are not things, your relatives, or children. They are complex, adult human beings. To give effective care, you must be aware of the whole person.

The whole person has physical, social, psychological, and spiritual parts. These parts are woven together and cannot be separated (Fig. 4-1). Each part relates to and depends on the others. As a social being, a person speaks and communicates with others. Physically, the brain, mouth, tongue, lips, and throat structures must function for speech. Communication also is highly psychological because it involves the thinking and reasoning abilities of the mind. To consider only the physical part is to ignore the resident's ability to think, make decisions, and interact with others. You also ignore the fact that the resident is a living person with a life history of experiences, joys, sorrows, and needs.

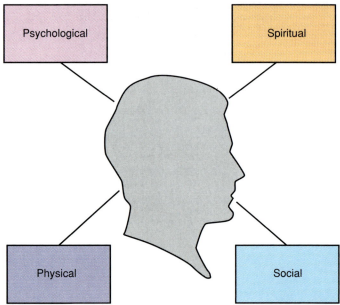

FIGURE 4-1 *A person is a physical, psychological, social, and spiritual being. The parts overlap and cannot be separated.*

NEEDS

A **need** is that which is necessary or desirable for maintaining life and mental well-being. According to Abraham Maslow, a famous psychologist, certain basic needs must be met if a person is to survive and function. These needs are arranged in order of importance. Lower-level needs must be met before higher-level needs. These basic needs, from the lowest level to the highest, are physiological or physical needs, the need for safety and security, the need for love and belonging, esteem needs, and the need for self-actualization (Fig. 4-2). People normally meet their own needs. Inability to meet basic needs usually results because of disease, illness, injury, or advanced age. Those who are ill or injured usually seek help from doctors, nurses, and other health care team members.

Physiological Needs

Human beings share certain physical needs with other forms of life such as animals, fish, and plants. The physical needs required for life are oxygen, food, water, elimination, and rest. They must be met before higher-level needs.

A person will die within minutes without oxygen. People can survive longer without food or water, but they begin to feel weak and ill within a few hours. If the kidneys or intestines do not function normally, poisonous wastes build up in the blood stream. If the problem is not corrected, the person will die. Without enough rest and sleep, an person becomes exhausted.

You will assist the other health care team members in helping residents meet their physical needs. You need to develop a true appreciation of these physical needs. Most people take them for granted until a problem develops. How do you feel when you have difficulty breathing or feel as if you are choking? How do you react when you are thirsty, hungry, or do not get enough sleep?

The Need for Safety and Security

Safety and security needs include shelter, clothing, and protection from harm or danger. Health problems often occur from inadequate shelter, heat, or clothing. Frostbite, for example, is a common problem during the

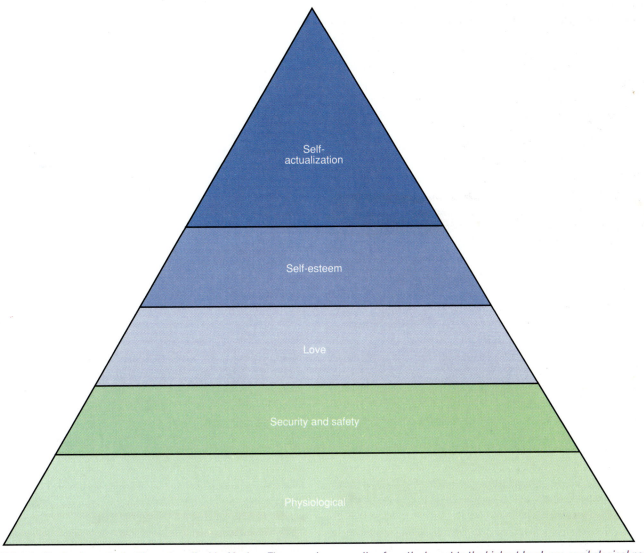

FIGURE 4-2 *The basic needs for life as described by Maslow. These needs, proceeding from the lowest to the highest level, are psychological needs, the need for safety and security, the need for love and belonging, the need for esteem, and the need for self-actualization.*

winter because of inadequate clothing, shelter, or heat in the home.

Many elderly persons feel a loss of security and safety when they are admitted to a nursing facility. They are not in the familiar, secure surroundings of their homes. They are in a strange place, with strange routines, and strangers to care for them. Often they become frightened and confused. You can help them feel secure by being kind, understanding, and patient. Show them their new surroundings, listen to their concerns, and explain all routines and procedures. You may have to repeat explanations and directions many times for several days or weeks until the resident feels safe and unafraid. Be patient.

The Need for Love and Belonging

The need for love and belonging relates to love, closeness, affection, belonging, and meaningful relationships with others. There have been cases where people have slowly become weaker and unable to care for themselves, or have died, because of the lack of love and belonging. This is particularly true of elderly persons, especially those who have outlived families and friends. Belonging needs usually can be met by family and friends. If none exist or care about the resident, then these needs must be met by you and other health care workers. Help the resident become acquainted with other residents and staff members. Remind the resident that you are there to care for him or her.

The Need for Esteem

Esteem means the worth, value, or opinion one has of a person or oneself. Esteem needs relate to thinking well of oneself, seeing oneself as useful, and being well thought of by others. Residents of nursing facilities often lack self-esteem because they are elderly, disabled, or chronically ill. An elderly man may once have built his own home, worked a farm, and supported and raised a family. How might he feel about himself now that he cannot dress or feed himself because of crippling arthritis? A woman who has lost her hair because of cancer treatments may feel unattractive and less than whole. Persons with slow, crippling diseases or those who have lost a limb also may feel less than whole. Treat residents with respect and encourage them to do as much for themselves as possible (even though it takes more time). This helps increase self-esteem.

The Need for Self-Actualization

Self-actualization means experiencing one's potential. It involves learning, understanding, and creating to the limit of a person's capacity. This is the highest need. Rarely, if ever, is it totally met. Most people constantly try to learn and understand more. The need for self-actualization can be postponed, and life will continue.

CULTURE AND RELIGION

Culture is defined as the values, beliefs, habits, likes, dislikes, customs, and characteristics of a group of people that are passed from one generation to the next. The resident's culture influences health beliefs and practices. Culture also influences the resident's behavior in a nursing facility.

You will care for persons of different cultural backgrounds. People in the United States come from various cultures, races, and nationalities. Therefore you may care for residents from cultures that differ from your own. They may have family practices, food preferences, hygiene habits, and clothing styles that are different from yours. The resident also may speak and understand a foreign language. Some cultural groups have beliefs about the causes and cures of illnesses. They may perform certain rituals aimed at ridding the body of disease. Learn as much as you can about a resident's cultural beliefs and health care practices. This will help you provide care that meets the resident's needs.

Religion relates to spiritual beliefs, needs, and practices. Like culture, a person's religion influences health and illness practices. Religions may have beliefs and practices about diet, healing, days of worship, birth, and death.

Most Americans are Jewish, Protestant, or Roman Catholic. There also are many Moslems, Buddhists, and Hindus. Many residents find religion to be a source of comfort and strength during illness. They may wish to observe religious practices. If religious services are held in your facility, assist residents to attend the services if they wish. A resident may want to leave the facility to attend services or have a visit from a spiritual leader or adviser. You need to report the request to the nurse. A resident may want the pastor to visit in the room. If so, make sure the room is neat and orderly and that there is a chair for the cleric to use. Be sure the resident and pastor have privacy during the visit.

You need to respect and accept the resident's culture and religion. When you meet people from other cultures or religions, take time to learn about their beliefs and practices. This will help you understand your resident and give better care.

Individuals may not follow all the beliefs and practices of their culture or religion. Some people may not practice a religion. Remember that each person is unique. Avoid judging residents by your standards.

BEING CHRONICALLY ILL OR DISABLED

If people had a choice between staying healthy and active or becoming ill or disabled, surely they would choose a healthy, active life. Unfortunately, people do become ill and disabled. They suffer not only physical problems but psychological and social problems as well.

Residents of nursing facilities can no longer live in their own homes. They can no longer take care of their own personal needs. They can no longer go to work, prepare meals, do housework or yard work. They cannot go to the store or participate in social activities as they did before. Being involved in these activities brings personal satisfaction, feelings of self-worth, and contact with others. Residents may feel alone and isolated if they have outlived friends or lost spouses. It is not unusual for residents to feel frustrated, useless, or angry. The anger may be directed at you. Try to remember that they are angry with their situation and really not angry at you.

Chronically ill and disabled residents may have many fears and anxieties about living in a nursing facility. They may feel lonely and believe families and friends have abandoned them. They may fear being dependent on strangers. Many may fear increasing loss of function. Some will express their fears. Others will not or cannot. You will work closely with these residents. You can anticipate these concerns and help the resident feel safe, secure, and loved. You can take an extra minute to "visit," to quietly hold a hand, or to give a hug.

Show your willingness to take care of their personal needs. Respond promptly and treat each person with respect and dignity. You may not be able to prevent increasing loss of function. You can, however, help the resident maintain his or her **optimal level of functioning.** This refers to a person's highest potential for mental and physical performance. Encourage the person to be as independent as possible. Always focus on the person's abilities, not on the disabilities.

Hospitalized patients often are treated as sick, dependent people. Encouraging this "sick role" in a nursing facility reduces the resident's quality of life. Your job, and that of all health care workers, is to improve the resident's quality of life. You can do this by helping each person regain or maintain as much physical and mental function as possible.

Residents You Will Care For

You will care for different types of residents. Most will be elderly. Some are mentally alert and oriented but have chronic illnesses or disabilities that keep them from living alone or with family (Fig. 4-3). Others are too confused and disoriented to care for themselves. Still others may be recovering from a fracture, an acute illness, or surgery. You may care for terminally ill residents. These residents need frequent care to maintain comfort and make their last days as peaceful as possible.

Alert, Oriented Residents

Many residents are alert and oriented. They know who they are, where they are, the year, and the time of day. These residents have physical problems that require

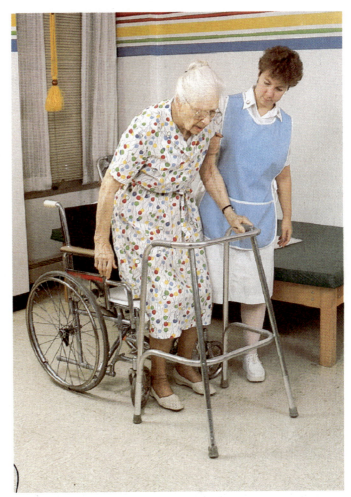

FIGURE 4-3 *An elderly person who requires the services of a long-term care facility.*

them to live in a nursing facility. They may be paralyzed as a result of stroke, injury, or birth defects. They may have crippling diseases such as arthritis or multiple sclerosis. Or they may be suffering from a chronic heart, liver, kidney, or respiratory disease. The amount of care required depends on how disabled they are. Because these residents are alert and oriented, they may have problems adjusting to a nursing facility. Remember, you need to help these residents accept the nursing facility as home.

Confused and Disoriented Residents

Many residents are mildly to severely confused and disoriented. Some simply have trouble remembering where the dining room is or the month and year. Others are more confused and disoriented—thinking that they are in another city waiting for a train. The most severely disoriented do not even know who they are. Sometimes the confusion and disorientation are temporary. This is especially true of the newly admitted resident. For other resi-

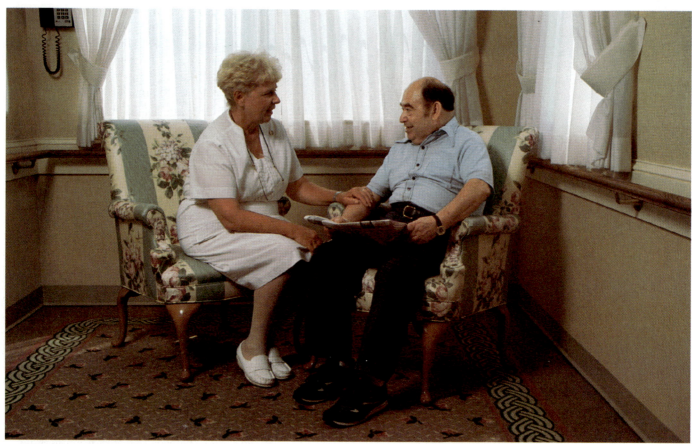

FIGURE 4-4 *A nursing assistant talking with a resident.*

dents, such as those with Alzheimer's disease, the confusion and disorientation are permanent and become worse. You will learn how to work with all types of confused residents in Chapter 24.

Short-Term Residents

Some residents will stay in a facility for a short time. They may be recovering from fractures, acute illness, or surgery. The goal is to help these residents increase their strength and mobility so they can return home or to their former living situation. Some residents may be so ill that they need skilled care. They may need IV therapy, feeding through special tubes, special wound care, or other treatments. Others may need special therapy programs: physical, occupational, or language therapy or special restorative nursing care. You will assist other health care workers in helping these residents return to their optimal level of functioning.

Some people are cared for at home and are admitted to nursing facilities for short stays. This is *respite care*. The caregiver is given time to take a vacation, take care of business, or simply to rest. Respite care may last from a few days to several weeks.

Terminally Ill Residents

Terminally ill residents require a lot of care. They may have advanced cancer, liver, kidney, or respiratory or heart disease. Some may have AIDS. Some are alert and oriented; others are **comatose.** Comatose residents cannot respond to verbal stimuli, but may still feel pain.

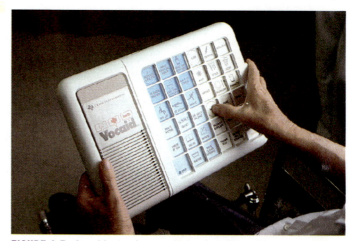

FIGURE 4-5 *A resident using an electronic talking aid.*

They may show pain by grimacing or groaning. Some residents have a great deal of pain and need frequent care to maintain comfort. Pain medication can help. You should promptly report any sign of discomfort to the nurse. Pain medication is important, but so is the care you give. Turning and positioning, gentle back rubs, touch, and holding a hand can be very effective in promoting comfort and peace.

COMMUNICATING WITH THE RESIDENT

Several elements are necessary for effective communication between you and the resident. *First,* you must understand and respect the resident as a person. If the resident is elderly, remember that this is a mature, adult person. Often elders are spoken to as if they are children. *Second,* you must view the resident as more than an illness, disability, or room number. The resident is a physical, psychological, social, and spiritual human being. *Third,* you need to appreciate the problems and frustrations that result from being ill, disabled, or very old. *Fourth,* you must speak to the resident as if he or she understands you even if the person is confused and disoriented. *Fifth,* you must recognize and respect the resident's rights. *Finally,* you must accept and respect the resident's culture and religion.

The rules for communication discussed in Chapter 3 apply when you are communicating with residents. Remember these guidelines.

1. Use words that mean the same to you and the resident.
2. Speak in short sentences.
3. Avoid medical terminology and unfamiliar words.
4. Communicate in a logical and orderly manner.
5. Be specific and factual when presenting information.
6. Give the resident time to process (understand) the information that you give.
7. Ask questions to be sure you have been understood. Repeat information as often as necessary. Repeat exactly what you said so the person does not have to process a new message. This is especially important for residents with hearing problems.
8. Be patient. Residents with memory problems may ask the same question several times a day. Do not remind them that you are repeating information. Accept their memory loss as you would any other disability.

You will use both verbal and nonverbal communication when relating to your residents. Understanding how to use both methods will help you communicate effectively.

Verbal Communication

Words are used in **verbal communication.** They may be spoken or written. Verbal communication is used to talk with residents to find out how they are feeling, what their needs are, and to share information with them (Fig. 4-4).

Most verbal communication involves the spoken word. When speaking, control the volume and tone of your voice. Speak clearly and distinctly. Avoid using slang or vulgar words. Face the resident whenever possible, and keep your hands away from your mouth. Residents understand better if they can see your face and lips. This is important for persons with hearing problems. Also avoid shouting, whispering, and mumbling. They interfere with effective communication.

Written communication is used when a resident cannot speak or hear but can read. Magic slates, paper and pencil, communication boards, or electronic talking aids (Fig. 4-5) can be used. If a resident cannot speak or read, you need to provide a way for the resident to communicate needs. The nurse will tell you how to communicate with the resident. If the resident can hear but cannot speak or read, ask questions that can be answered yes or no with nods, blinks, or other gestures. A picture board also may be helpful (Fig. 4-6). You will write messages to communicate with residents who are deaf or who have severe hearing problems (Fig. 4-7). When writing mes-

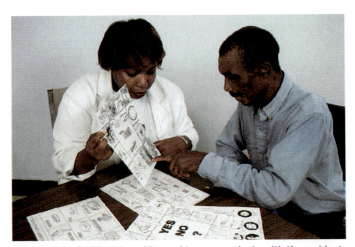

FIGURE 4-6 *A picture board is used to communicate with the resident.*

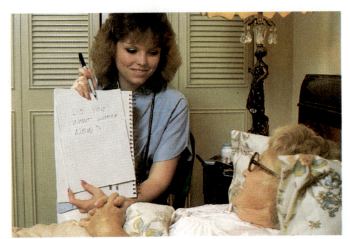

FIGURE 4-7 *A nursing assistant writing a note to a resident with hearing and vision difficulties.*

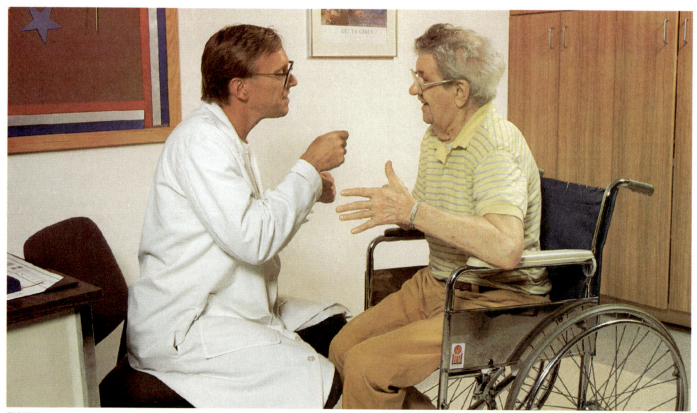

FIGURE 4-8 *A resident using sign language to communicate.*

sages for those with poor vision, use a black felt pen on white paper. Print the message in large letters. Deaf residents may use sign language and written messages to communicate (Fig. 4-8).

Your communication with residents should be kind, courteous, and friendly. This may be hard when residents are not courteous in return. Remember, residents who are the hardest to deal with probably need your kindness the most.

Nonverbal Communication

Nonverbal communication (body language) does not rely on words. Gestures, facial expressions, posture, body movements, touch, and smell are examples of how messages are sent and received without the use of words. Nonverbal messages are considered a truer reflection of a person's feelings. They usually are involuntary and hard to control. A resident may say one thing but act in a different way. Therefore you need to watch the person's eyes and the way hands are held or moved. Gestures, posture, and other actions can tell you more than the spoken word. For example, a resident who normally stands straight has slumped posture. This person probably is not feeling well or happy. Another resident denies having pain. However, the resident stands, sits, or lies down in an unusual way to protect an affected body part.

Residents send messages to you nonverbally. You also send messages to them by the way you act and move. You communicate with residents through facial expressions and how you stand, sit, walk, and look at them. Your body language should show interest and enthusiasm about your work. It also should convey love, caring, and respect for residents. Be sure to control your body language in relation to odors from a resident's body or excretions. Many odors are beyond the resident's control. You will increase the person's embarrassment and humiliation if you react to the odor.

Touch. Touch is a very important form of nonverbal communication. It can convey comfort, caring, love, affection, and reassurance. Touch means different things to different people. The meaning depends on the person's age, culture, sex, and life experiences. Although some people do not like to be touched, do not be afraid to try touch to convey caring and warmth. Often it is easier to comfort residents by holding their hands or touching their forearms than it is to use words. You soon will learn which residents do not want to be touched. Be sure to respect their wishes.

Barriers to Effective Communication

Communication may fail for many reasons. You and the resident must use and understand the same language. Otherwise, messages sent will not be accurately interpreted.

Changing the subject is another barrier to communication. The subject often is changed when it causes discomfort. Residents, health care workers, family members, and visitors have all been known to change the subject when it becomes uncomfortable. Avoid changing the subject. If the resident changes the subject, allow it to happen. Forcing the resident to return to the subject will only increase that person's discomfort.

Never offer your opinion to a resident. Giving your opinion usually shows the resident that you are making a judgment about the resident's values, behavior, or feelings. Let residents express their feelings and concerns without adding your opinion, making a judgment, or jumping to conclusions.

Be sure that you understand what the resident is saying. Residents may use unfamiliar terms or expressions. A resident may ask to "go out" when he or she needs to have a bowel movement. A resident may ask for a "vase" instead of a urinal. Ask questions to make sure you understand what the resident is trying to tell or ask you.

You may find that you talk a lot when residents are silent or speak infrequently. Excessive talking usually is due to nervousness and uncomfortable feelings about the silence. Silences have meaning. Acceptance, rejection, fear, or the need for quiet and time to think may be conveyed by silence. Elderly persons may need time to process (think through) what they have heard. Allow silences to happen. You will learn to be comfortable with them.

Listening is very important for effective communication. Communication will be blocked if you fail to listen with interest and sincerity. Do not pretend to be listening. This results in inappropriate responses to the resident. It conveys a lack of interest and caring. Also, you may miss important information about physical or emotional changes that must be reported to the nurse.

Pat answers such as "Don't worry," "Everything will be okay," and "Your doctor knows best" block communication. These make residents feel that their concerns, feelings, and fears are not being taken seriously and are not important to you or the health care team.

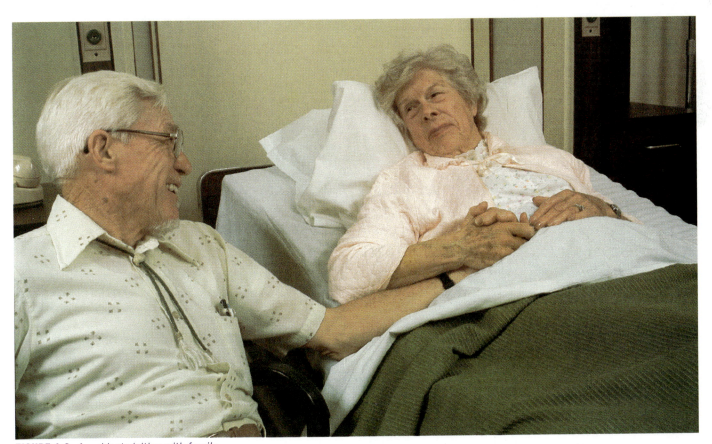

FIGURE 4-9 *A resident visiting with family.*

THE RESIDENT'S FAMILY AND VISITORS

Family, relatives, and friends can help meet the resident's needs for safety and security, love and belonging, and esteem. They can offer support and comfort and lessen feelings of loneliness. Some also want to help give care. This helps both the family and resident. The family knows they are doing something to help the resident, and the resident's physical and emotional needs are met. Often recovery is influenced by the presence or absence of significant family members or friends.

The resident has the right to visit with family and friends in private and without unnecessary interruptions (Fig. 4-9, p. 57). Sometimes care must be given while visitors are present. Remember the resident's right to privacy. The resident's body should not be exposed in the presence of visitors. Politely ask visitors to leave the room, and show them where they can wait. Promptly notify the visitors when they can return. If a spouse or close family member wants to help you and the resident gives consent, allow that person to stay.

Family and visitors need to be treated with courtesy and respect. They may be very concerned and frightened about the resident's condition and care. They also need the support and understanding of the nursing team. However, you should not discuss the resident's condition with them. Refer any questions to the nurse responsible for the resident's care.

Visitors often have questions about visiting rules. The number of visitors allowed and the visiting hours vary among facilities. Often they depend on the resident's age or condition. Dying residents usually can have family members present constantly. This always is true in hospice units. You need to know your facility's visiting policies and the special considerations allowed for an individual resident.

Sometimes a family member or friend can have a negative effect on the resident. If the resident becomes upset or is becoming tired from a visit, report your observations to the nurse. The nurse can then speak with the visitor about the resident's needs.

SUMMARY

People are physical, psychological, spiritual, and social beings. They have basic needs necessary for life: physical needs, the need for safety and security, love and belonging, esteem, and self-actualization. When unable to meet their own needs, people usually seek help from a doctor or other health care workers.

Culture and religion influence the lives of most people. Beliefs, values, habits, diet, and health and illness practices may relate to a person's culture or religion. Try to become aware of the beliefs and practices of the major cultural and religious groups in your area. Being ill or disabled will affect a person physically, psychologically, and socially. How a person handles illness or disability is influenced by religion, culture, family, the resident's basic personality, the seriousness of the illness or disability, and the speed and degree of recovery. The resident may have many fears and anxieties about illness, basic needs, and being able to function normally again. You need to have empathy for your residents if you are to provide effective care.

Residents may be grouped in a nursing facility according to their ability to function and the seriousness of their illness or disability. These residents may have different types of problems, but all have the same basic needs and rights.

Verbal and nonverbal communication is used by residents and health care workers. Remember the strongest and truest messages usually are nonverbal. You need to observe facial expressions, gestures, and other body language for clues about a resident's physical and emotional condition. Control your own nonverbal messages so that you do not send negative feelings. Use touch to communicate understanding, comfort, and caring. Avoid blocking communication by being aware of the common barriers to effective communication.

Remember, family and visitors are important individuals to the resident. They can help meet the resident's basic needs and influence recovery. Treat them with respect and courtesy.

Review QUESTIONS

Circle *T* if the answer is true and *F* if the answer is false.

T F 1. A person is a physical, psychological, social, and spiritual being.

T F 2. Physical needs are the most essential for survival.

T F 3. Clothing and shelter are physiological needs.

T F 4. The need for love and belonging is not important to the sick person.

T F 5. Esteem means love, closeness, affection, and meaningful relationships with others.

T F 6. Self-actualization is the need to learn, create, and understand to the limit of a person's capacity.

T F 7. The resident's cultural background will probably influence health and illness practices.

T F 8. Diet may be influenced by culture and religion.

T F 9. The resident's religious and cultural practices should not be allowed in the nursing facility.

T F 10. Fears and anxieties about being sick or disabled are normal reactions.

T F 11. Verbal communication is the truest reflection of a person's feelings.

T F 12. Messages can be sent by facial expressions, gestures, posture, and touch.

T F 13. Changing the subject promotes communication. More interests and concerns can be discussed.

T F 14. You should talk when the resident is silent.

T F 15. Listening is essential for effective communication.

T F 16. Pat answers such as "Don't worry" encourage the resident to express feelings and concerns.

T F 17. Family and friends can help meet the resident's basic needs.

T F 18. Residents and visitors should be allowed privacy.

T F 19. Visitors should be politely asked to leave the room when care needs to be given to the resident.

T F 20. Nursing facilities are not allowed to have visiting hours or regulations.

Answers

1. True	6. True	11. False	16. False
2. True	7. True	12. True	17. True
3. False	8. True	13. False	18. True
4. False	9. False	14. False	19. True
5. False	10. True	15. True	20. False

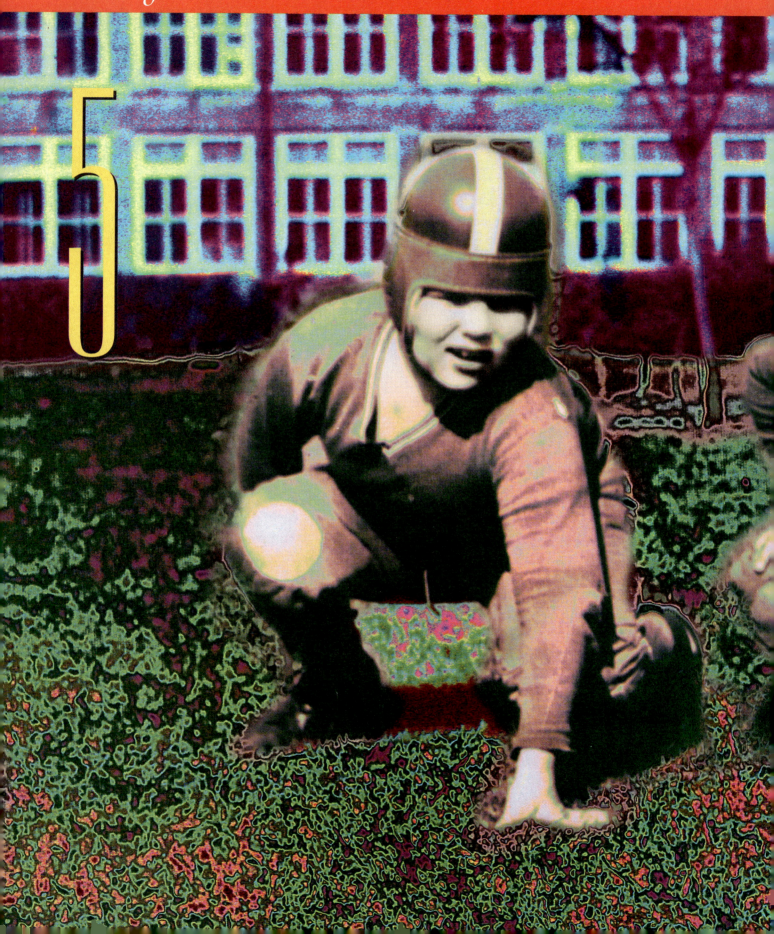

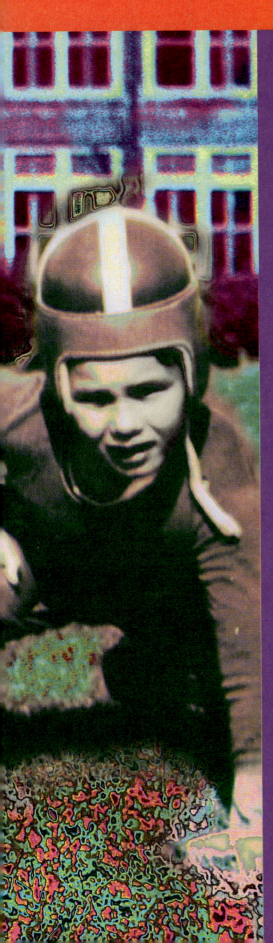

What You Will LEARN

- The key terms listed in this chapter

- The basic structures of the cell and a knowledge of how the cells divide

- Four types of tissue

- The structures of each body system

- The functions of each body system

Note: Students are responsible for only those terms mentioned in the text. Additional terms used in illustrations and legends throughout this chapter are for illustrative purposes only.

artery
A blood vessel that carries blood away from the heart

capillary
A tiny blood vessel; food, oxygen, and other substances pass from the capillaries to the cells

cell
The basic unit of body structure

digestion
The process of physically and chemically breaking down food so that it can be absorbed for use by the cells of the body

hemoglobin
The substance in red blood cells that gives blood its color and carries oxygen in the blood

hormone
A chemical substance secreted by the glands into the blood stream

menstruation
The process in which the endometrium of the uterus breaks up and is discharged from the body through the vagina

metabolism
The burning of food by the cells for heat and energy

organ
Groups of tissues with the same function

peristalsis
Involuntary muscle contractions in the digestive system that move food through the alimentary canal

respiration
The process of supplying the cells with oxygen and removing carbon dioxide from them

system
Organs that work together to perform special functions

tissue
Groups of cells with the same function

vein
A blood vessel that carries blood back to the heart

I was a ballerina when I was young. My husband was a football player. The human body is very powerful.

You will care for persons who need help in meeting their basic needs. Their bodies are unable to work at peak efficiency because of illness, disease, injury, or advanced age. As a result, residents often need medical and nursing care. You will be directed to provide care and perform procedures to promote physical and emotional comfort, physical and spiritual healing, and a return to the highest possible level of functioning. A basic knowledge of the body's normal structure and function will help you understand certain signs, symptoms and behaviors, reasons for care, and purposes of procedures. This knowledge should result in safer, more efficient, and understanding resident care. The changes in body structure and function that occur with aging will be discussed in Chapter 6.

CELLS, TISSUES, AND ORGANS

The basic unit of body structure is the **cell.** Each cell of the body has the same basic structure. However, the functions, size, and shape may be different (Fig. 5-1). Cells are so small that a microscope is needed to see them. They need food, water, and oxygen to live and perform their functions.

The cell and its basic structures are shown in Fig. 5-2. The *cell membrane,* the outer covering that encloses the cell, helps it hold its shape. The *nucleus* is the control center of the cell; it directs the cell's activities. The nucleus is located in the center of the cell. The *cytoplasm* is the portion of the cell that surrounds the nucleus. The cytoplasm contains many smaller structures that perform the functions of the cell. The *protoplasm,* which means "living substance," refers to all the structures, substances, and water within the cell. Protoplasm is a semiliquid substance much like the white of an egg.

Within the nucleus are threadlike structures called *chromosomes.* Each cell has 46 chromosomes. The chromosomes contain *genes.* Genes control the physical and chemical traits inherited by children from their parents. Inherited traits include eye color, height, sex, and skin color.

In addition to controlling the activities of the cell, the nucleus is responsible for cell reproduction. Cells reproduce by dividing in half. The process of cell division is called *mitosis.* Cell division is necessary for the growth and repair of body tissues. During mitosis the 46 chromosomes arrange themselves in 23 pairs. As the cell di-

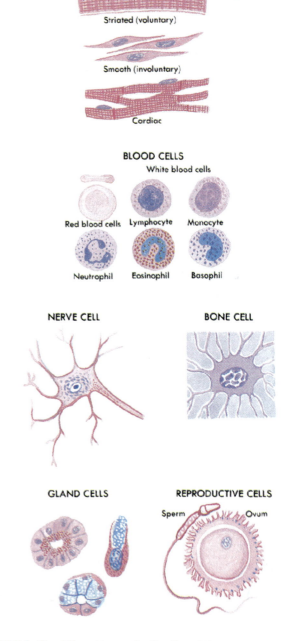

FIGURE 5-1 *The different types of cells. (From Thibodeau GA,* Anthony's textbook of anatomy and physiology, *ed 13, St Louis, 1990, Mosby–Year Book.)*

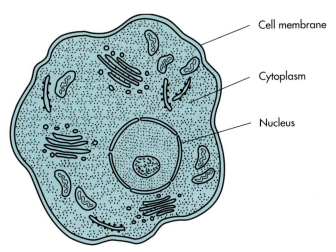

FIGURE 5-2 *The parts of a cell.*

Cell membrane

Cytoplasm

Nucleus

vides, the 23 pairs of chromosomes are pulled in half. The two new cells are identical and each contains 46 chromosomes (Fig. 5-3).

Cells are the building blocks of the body. Groups of cells with similar functions combine to form **tissues.** The body has four basic types of tissue.

1. *Epithelial tissue* covers the internal and external surface of the body. The tissue that lines the nose, mouth, respiratory tract, stomach, and intestines is epithelial tissue. Skin, hair, nails, and glands are included in this category.
2. *Connective tissue* anchors, connects, and supports other body tissues. Connective tissue is found in every part of the body. Bones, tendons, ligaments, and cartilage are connective tissue. Blood is a form of connective tissue.
3. *Muscle tissue* allows the body to move by stretching and contracting. There are three types of muscle tissue (see pp. 67 and 71).
4. *Nerve tissue* receives and carries impulses to the brain and back to the parts of the body.

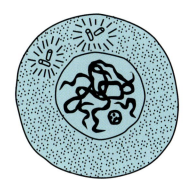

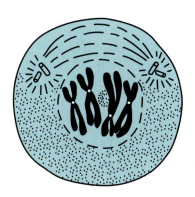

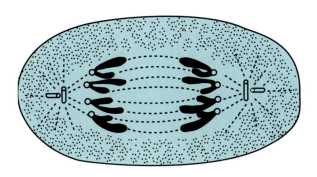

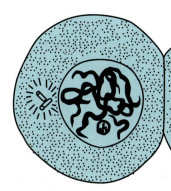

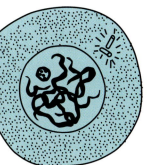

FIGURE 5-3 *Cell division.*

Groups of tissues form **organs.** An organ performs one or more functions. Examples of organs include the heart, brain, liver, lungs, and kidneys. **Systems** are formed by organs that work together to perform special functions (Fig. 5-4).

THE INTEGUMENTARY SYSTEM

The *integumentary system,* or skin, is the largest system of the body. *Integument* means covering, and the skin is the natural covering of the body. The skin is made up of epithelial, connective, and nerve tissue, as well as oil and sweat glands. There are two skin layers, the epidermis and the dermis (Fig. 5-5). The *epidermis,* or outer layer, contains living and dead cells. The dead cells were once deeper in the epidermis and were pushed upward as other cells divided. The dead cells constantly flake off and are replaced with living cells. The living cells also eventually die and flake off. The living cells of the epidermis contain pigment. The pigment is responsible for the color of the skin. There are no blood vessels and few nerve endings in the epidermis. The *dermis* is the inner layer of the skin and is composed of connective tissue. Blood vessels, nerves, sweat and oil glands, and hair roots are contained in the dermis.

Oil and *sweat glands, hair,* and *nails* are considered appendages of the skin. The entire body is covered with hair except for the palms of the hands and soles of the feet. The hair of the nose, eyes, and ears protects these organs from dust, insects, and other foreign objects. Nails protect the tips of the fingers and toes. Nails help the fingers pick up and handle small objects. Sweat glands help the body regulate temperature. Sweat consists of water, salt, and a small amount of waste. Sweat is secreted through the pores. The body is cooled as sweat evaporates. The oil glands lie near the hair shafts. They secrete an oily substance into the space near the hair shaft. The oil travels to the surface of the skin, helping to keep the hair and skin soft and shiny.

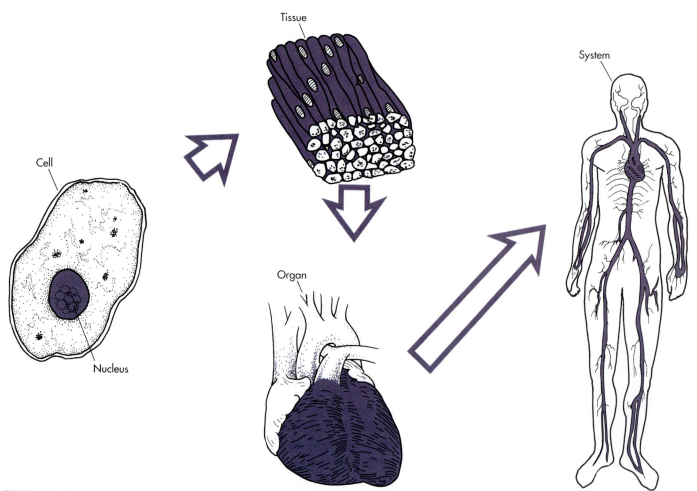

FIGURE 5-4 *The organization of the body. (Modified from Lafleur-Brooks M:* Exploring medical language: a student-directed approach, *ed 3, St Louis, 1994, Mosby–Year Book.)*

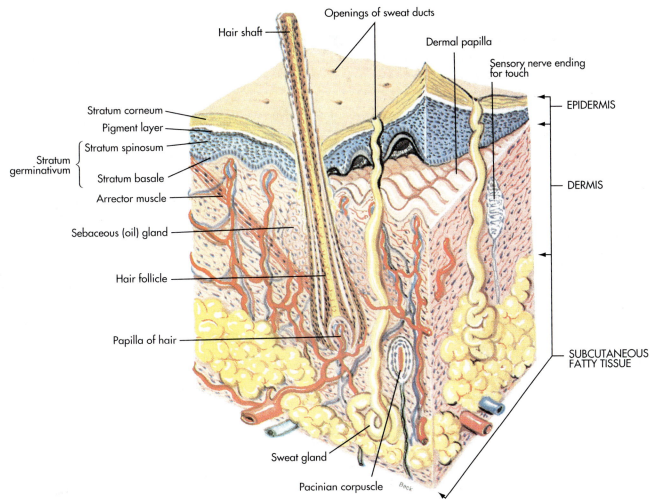

Hair shaft

Openings of sweat ducts

Dermal papilla

Sensory nerve ending for touch

Stratum corneum

Pigment layer

Stratum germinativum { Stratum spinosum / Stratum basale

Arrector muscle

Sebaceous (oil) gland

Hair follicle

Papilla of hair

EPIDERMIS

DERMIS

SUBCUTANEOUS FATTY TISSUE

Sweat gland

Pacinian corpuscle

FIGURE 5-5 *The layers of the skin. (From Thibodeau GA: Anthony's textbook of anatomy and physiology, ed 13, St Louis, 1990, Mosby–Year Book.)*

The skin performs many important functions. It serves as a protective covering for the body. Bacteria and other substances are prevented from entering the body. The skin prevents excessive amounts of water from leaving the body and protects the organs from injury. Nerve endings in the skin sense both pleasant and unpleasant stimulation. There are nerve endings over the entire body. The body is protected because cold, pain, touch, and pressure can be sensed. The skin helps regulate body temperature. Blood vessels dilate (widen) when temperature outside of the body is high. More blood is brought to the body surface to be cooled during evaporation. When blood vessels constrict (narrow), heat is retained by the body because less blood reaches the skin.

THE MUSCULOSKELETAL SYSTEM

The musculoskeletal system provides the framework for the body, allowing the body to move. This system also protects and gives the body shape. In addition to bones and muscles, the system includes ligaments, tendons, and cartilage.

Bones

The bony framework of the body consists of 206 bones (Fig. 5-6, p. 66). There are four types.

1. *Long bones* bear the weight of the body. The bones of the legs are long bones.
2. *Short bones* allow skill and ease in movement. The bones in the wrists, fingers, ankles, and toes are short bones.
3. *Flat bones* protect the organs of the body. These bones include the ribs, skull, pelvic bones, and shoulder blades.
4. *Irregular bones,* such as the vertebrae in the spinal column, allow various degrees of movement and flexibility.

Bones are hard, rigid structures made up of living cells. They are covered by a membrane called the *periosteum.* The periosteum contains blood vessels that supply bone cells with oxygen and food. Inside the hollow centers of the bones is a substance called *bone marrow.* Blood cells are manufactured in the bone marrow.

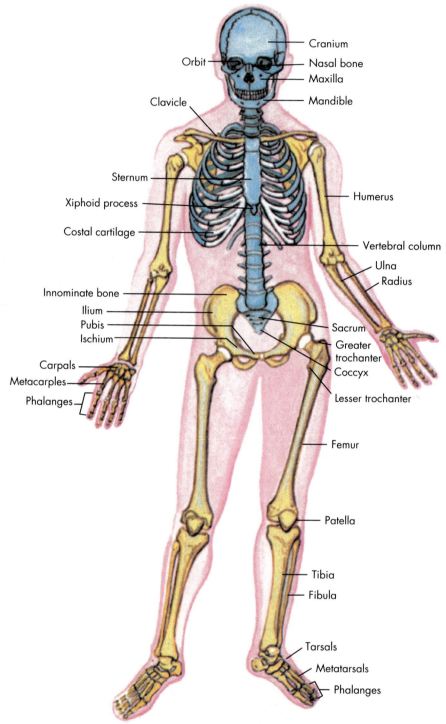

FIGURE 5-6 *The bones of the body. (From Anderson KN, Anderson LE, Glanze WD:* Mosby's medical, nursing, and allied health dictionary, *ed 4, St Louis, 1994, Mosby–Year Book.)*

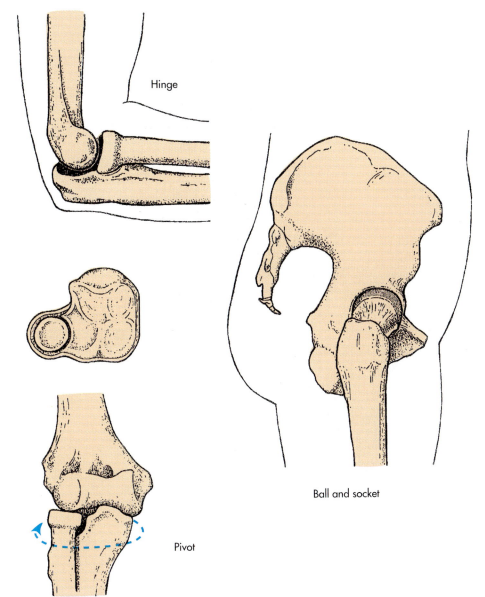

Hinge

Pivot

Ball and socket

FIGURE 5-7 *The types of joints. (Modified from Austrin MG:* Young's learning medical terminology step by step, *ed 7, St Louis, 1991, Mosby–Year Book.)*

Joints

The point at which two or more bones meet is called a *joint*. Joints allow movement. The connective tissue at the end of long bones is called *cartilage*. The cartilage cushions the joint so that the ends of the bones do not rub together. The *synovial membrane* lines the joints. The membrane secretes *synovial fluid*. The synovial fluid acts as a lubricant to allow the joint to move smoothly. Bones are held together at the joint by strong bands of connective tissue called *ligaments*.

There are three types of joints in the human body (Fig. 5-7). The *ball-and-socket joint* is made up of the rounded end of one bone and the hollow end of another bone. The rounded end of one fits into the hollow end of the other. Movement is possible in all directions. The joints of the hips and shoulders are ball-and-socket joints. The elbow is an example of the *hinge joint*, which allows movement in one direction. The *pivot joint* allows turning from side to side. The skull is connected to the spine by a pivot joint. Joint movement is discussed further in Chapter 17.

Muscles

The human body contains more than 500 muscles (Figs. 5-8 and 5-9, pp. 68-69). Some muscles are voluntary and others are involuntary. *Voluntary muscles* can be con-

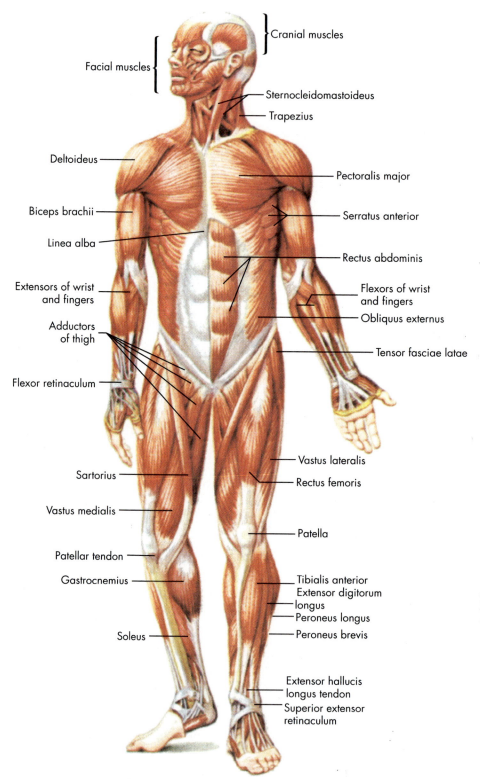

FIGURE 5-8 *Anterior view of the muscles of the body. (From Anderson KN, Anderson LE, Glanze WD:* Mosby's medical, nursing, and allied health dictionary, *ed 4, St Louis, 1994, Mosby–Year Book.)*

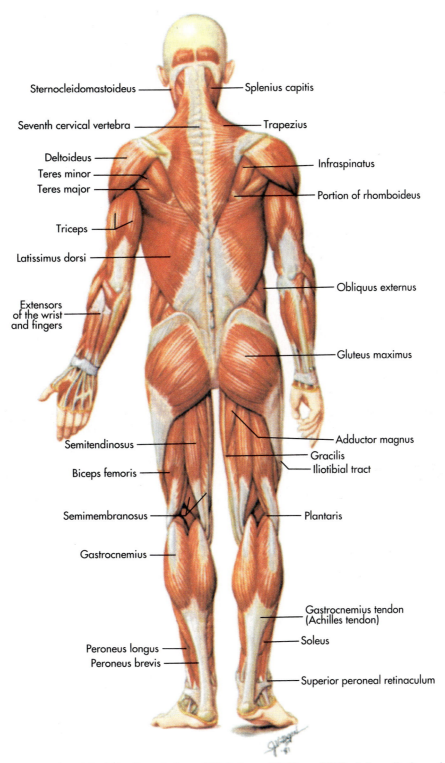

Sternocleidomastoideus — Splenius capitis

Seventh cervical vertebra — Trapezius

Deltoideus — Infraspinatus

Teres minor —

Teres major — Portion of rhomboideus

Triceps —

Latissimus dorsi —

Obliquus externus

Extensors
of the wrist
and fingers —

Gluteus maximus

Adductor magnus

Semitendinosus — Gracilis

Iliotibial tract

Biceps femoris —

Semimembranosus — Plantaris

Gastrocnemius —

Gastrocnemius tendon
(Achilles tendon)

Soleus

Peroneus longus —
Peroneus brevis —

Superior peroneal retinaculum

FIGURE 5-9 *Posterior view of the muscles of the body. (From Anderson KN, Anderson LE, Glanze WD:* Mosby's medical, nursing, and allied health dictionary, *ed 4, St Louis, 1994, Mosby–Year Book.)*

sciously controlled. Muscles that are attached to bones, the *skeletal muscles,* are voluntary. The muscles of your arm do not work unless you move your arm; likewise for the muscles of your legs. Skeletal muscles are *striated;* that is, the muscles appear striped or streaked. *Involuntary muscles* work automatically and cannot be consciously controlled. Involuntary muscles control the action of the stomach, intestines, blood vessels, and other body organs. Involuntary muscles also are called *smooth muscles.* They are smooth in appearance, not streaked or striped. Another type of muscle tissue, *cardiac muscle,* is found in the heart. An involuntary muscle, it has the striated appearance of skeletal muscle.

Muscles perform three important body functions: the movement of body parts, the maintenance of posture, and the production of body heat. Strong, tough connective tissue called *tendons* connects muscles to bones. When muscles contract (shorten), the tendons at each end of the muscle cause the bone to move. There are many tendons in the body; the Achilles tendon is shown in Fig. 5-9, p. 69. Some muscles remain constantly contracted to maintain the body's posture. When muscles contract, they burn food for energy, resulting in the production of heat. The greater the muscular activity, the greater the amount of heat produced in the body. Shivering is a way in which the body produces heat during exposure to cold. The shivering sensation is the result of rapid, general muscle contractions.

THE NERVOUS SYSTEM

The nervous system controls, directs, and coordinates body functions. There are two main divisions of the nervous system: the *central nervous system* (CNS) and the *peripheral nervous system.* The central nervous system consists of the *brain* and *spinal cord* (Fig. 5-10). The peripheral nervous system involves the *nerves* throughout the body (Fig. 5-11, p. 72). Nerves carry messages or impulses to and from the brain. The nerves are connected to the spinal cord. The nerve cell, called a *neuron,* is the basic unit of the nervous system (Fig. 5-12, p. 73). Threadlike projections from the cytoplasm of the neuron are called *nerve fibers.* The nerve fibers that bring impulses to the cell are called *dendrites.* The fibers that carry impulses away from the neurons are called *axons.* A neuron usually has only one axon. Dendrites may be short or as long as 3 feet.

Receptors or *end-organs* are found inside and outside of the body. Each receptor is attached to a neuron by a dendrite. A stimulus is received by the receptor and travels to the brain. Such stimuli include heat, cold, touch, smell, hearing, vision, balance, hunger, and thirst. If the body or body part must respond to the stimulus, the brain sends an impulse through the neurons to the proper muscles and glands.

Nerves are easily damaged and take a long time to heal. Some nerve fibers have a protective covering called a *myelin sheath.* The myelin sheath also insulates the nerve fiber. Nerve fibers covered with myelin are able to conduct impulses faster than fibers without the protective covering.

The Central Nervous System

The central nervous system consists of the brain and spinal cord. The brain is covered by the skull. The three main parts of the brain are the *cerebrum,* the *cerebellum,* and the *brainstem* (Fig. 5-13, p. 74).

The cerebrum is the largest part of the brain and is the center of thought and intelligence. The cerebrum is divided into two halves called the right and left *hemispheres.* The right hemisphere controls the movement and activities of the left side of the body. The left hemisphere controls the body's right side. The outside of the cerebrum is called the *cerebral cortex.* The cerebral cortex controls the highest functions of the brain. Reasoning, memory, the conscience, speech, voluntary muscle movement, vision, hearing, sensation, and other activities are controlled by the cerebral cortex.

The cerebellum regulates and coordinates body movements. The smooth movements of voluntary muscles and balance are made possible because of control by the cerebellum. Injury to the cerebellum results in jerky movements, loss of coordination, and muscle weakness.

The brainstem connects the cerebrum to the spinal cord. There are three important structures within the brainstem: the *midbrain, pons,* and *medulla.* The midbrain and pons relay messages between the medulla and the cerebrum. The medulla is located directly below the pons. Heart rate, breathing, the size of blood vessels, swallowing, coughing, and vomiting are some of the bodily functions controlled by the medulla. The brain is connected to the spinal cord at the lower end of the medulla.

The spinal cord lies within the spinal column. The cord is approximately 18 inches long. The pathways that conduct messages to and from the brain are contained within the cord.

The brain and spinal cord are covered and protected by three layers of connective tissue called *meninges.* The outer layer, which lies next to the skull, is a tough covering called the *dura mater.* The middle layer is called the *arachnoid,* and the inner layer is the *pia mater* (see Fig. 5-10). The space between the middle and inner layers is called the *arachnoid space.* The space is filled with fluid. This fluid, called *cerebrospinal fluid,* circulates around the brain and spinal cord. The cerebrospinal fluid protects the central nervous system by cushioning shocks that could easily injure the structures of the brain and spinal cord.

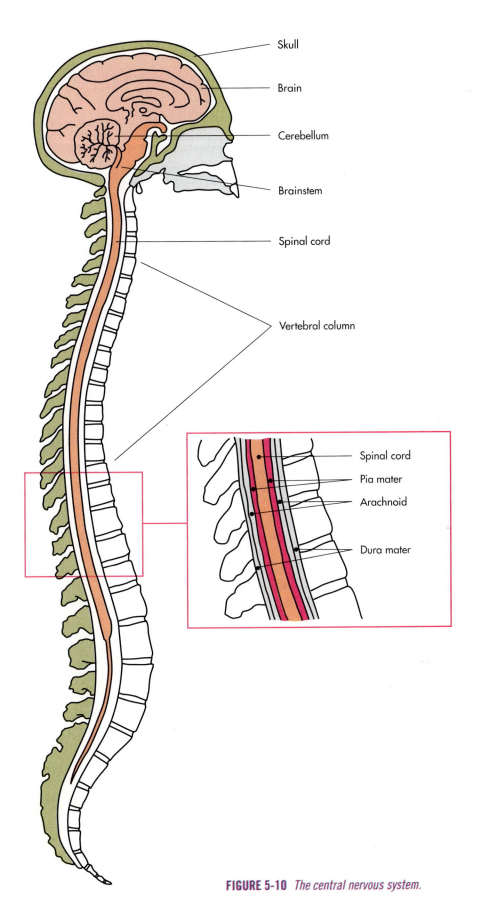

Skull

Brain

Cerebellum

Brainstem

Spinal cord

Vertebral column

Spinal cord

Pia mater

Arachnoid

Dura mater

FIGURE 5-10 *The central nervous system.*

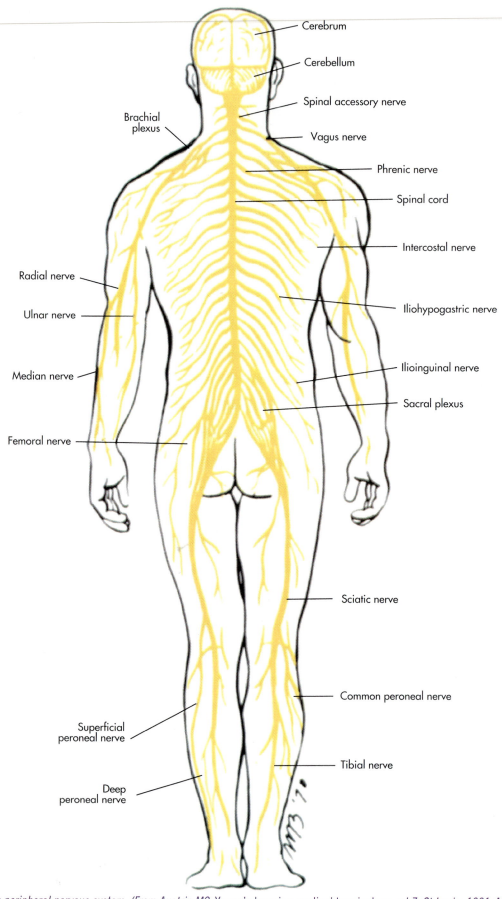

Cerebrum

Cerebellum

Spinal accessory nerve

Vagus nerve

Brachial plexus

Phrenic nerve

Spinal cord

Intercostal nerve

Radial nerve

Ulnar nerve

Iliohypogastric nerve

Median nerve

Ilioinguinal nerve

Sacral plexus

Femoral nerve

Sciatic nerve

Common peroneal nerve

Superficial peroneal nerve

Tibial nerve

Deep peroneal nerve

FIGURE 5-11 *The peripheral nervous system. (From Austrin MG:* Young's learning medical terminology, *ed 7, St Louis, 1991, Mosby–Year Book.)*

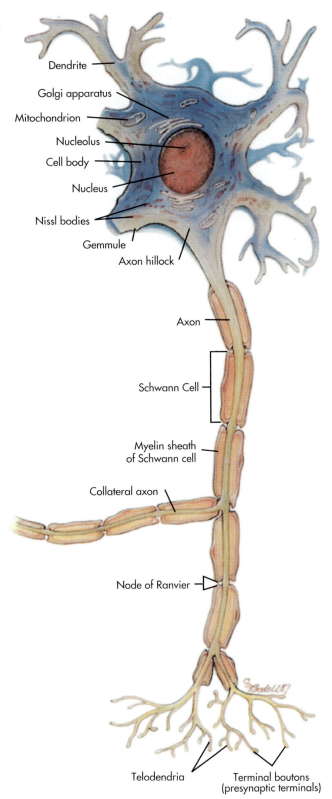

Dendrite

Golgi apparatus

Mitochondrion

Nucleolus

Cell body

Nucleus

Nissl bodies

Gemmule

Axon hillock

Axon

Schwann Cell

Myelin sheath
of Schwann cell

Collateral axon

Node of Ranvier

Telodendria

Terminal boutons
(presynaptic terminals)

FIGURE 5-12 *A neuron. (From Seeley RR, Stephens TD, Tate P:* Anatomy and physiology, *ed 2, St Louis, 1992, Mosby–Year Book.)*

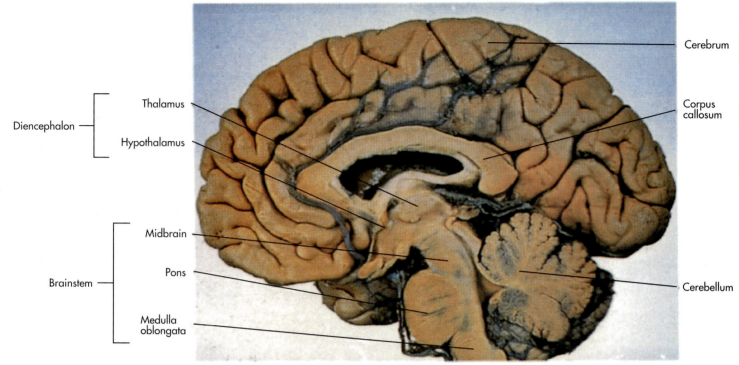

FIGURE 5-13 *The brain. (From Seeley RR, Stephens TD, Tate P:* Anatomy and physiology, *ed 2, St Louis, 1992, Mosby–Year Book.)*

The Peripheral Nervous System

The peripheral nervous system involves 12 pairs of *cranial nerves* and 31 pairs of *spinal nerves.* The cranial nerves conduct impulses between the brain and the head, neck, chest, and abdomen. Impulses for smell, vision, hearing, pain, touch, temperature, pressure, voluntary muscle control, and involuntary muscle control are conducted through the cranial nerves. The spinal nerves carry impulses from the skin, extremities, and the internal body structures not supplied by the cranial nerves.

Some peripheral nerves with special functions are grouped together to form the *autonomic nervous system.* This system has control over involuntary muscles and certain body functions. The functions include the heartbeat, blood pressure, intestinal contractions, and glandular secretions. The functions occur automatically without conscious effort. The autonomic nervous system is divided into the *sympathetic nervous system* and the *parasympathetic nervous system.* These divisions balance each other. The sympathetic nervous system tends to speed up functions whereas the parasympathetic nervous system slows them down. When you are angry, frightened, excited, or exercising, the sympathetic nervous system is stimulated. The parasympathetic system is activated when you relax or when the sympathetic system has been under stimulation for too long.

The Sense Organs

The five major senses are sight, hearing, taste, smell, and touch. Receptors for taste are in the tongue and are called *taste buds.* The receptors for smell are located in the nose. Touch receptors are found in the dermis, especially in the toes and fingertips.

The eye. Receptors for vision are located in the eyes. The eye is a delicate organ that can be easily injured. The bones of the skull, the eyelids and eyelashes, and tears protect the eyes from injury. The structures of the eye are shown in Fig. 5-14. The eye has three separate layers. The *sclera,* which is the white of the eye, is the outer layer. The sclera is made of tough connective tissue. The second layer is the *choroid.* Blood vessels, a muscle called the *ciliary muscle,* and the *iris* make up the choroid. The iris gives the eye its color. The opening in the middle of the iris is the *pupil.* The size of the pupil varies with the amount of light entering the eye. The pupil constricts (narrows) in bright light and dilates (widens) in dim or dark places. The inner layer of the eye is called the *retina.* The receptors for vision and the nerve fibers of the optic nerve are contained in the retina.

Light enters the eye through the *cornea.* The cornea is the transparent part of the outer layer that lies over the eye. Light rays pass to the *lens,* which lies behind the pupil. The light is then reflected to the retina and carried to the brain by the optic nerve.

The *aqueous chamber* separates the cornea from the lens. The chamber is filled with a fluid called *aqueous humor*. The fluid helps the cornea keep its shape and position. The *vitreous body* is located behind the lens. The vitreous body is a gelatin-like substance that supports the retina and maintains the shape of the eye.

The ear. The ear is a sense organ that functions in hearing and balance. The ear is divided into three parts: the *external ear*, the *middle ear*, and the *inner ear*. The structures of the ear are shown in Fig. 5-15 on p. 76.

The external ear (outer part) is called the *pinna* or *auricle*. Sound waves are guided through the external ear into the *auditory canal*. There are many glands in the auditory canal that secrete a waxy substance. The waxy substance is called *cerumen*. The auditory canal extends about 1 inch to the *eardrum*. The eardrum, also called the *tympanic membrane*, separates the external and middle ear.

The middle ear is a small space that contains the *eu-stachian tube* and three small bones called *ossicles*. The eustachian tube connects the middle ear and the throat. Air enters the eustachian tube so that there is equal pressure on both sides of the eardrum. The ossicles amplify sound received from the eardrum and transmit the sound to the inner ear. The three ossicles are called the *malleus*, which looks like a hammer; the *incus*, which resembles an anvil; and the *stapes*, which is shaped like a stirrup.

The inner ear consists of the *semicircular canals* and the *cochlea*. The cochlea, which looks like a snail shell, contains fluid. The fluid carries the sound waves received from the middle ear to the *auditory nerve*. The auditory nerve then carries the message to the brain.

The three semicircular canals are bony loops filled with fluid. They are involved with balance. They sense the position of the head and changes in position, and they send messages to the brain.

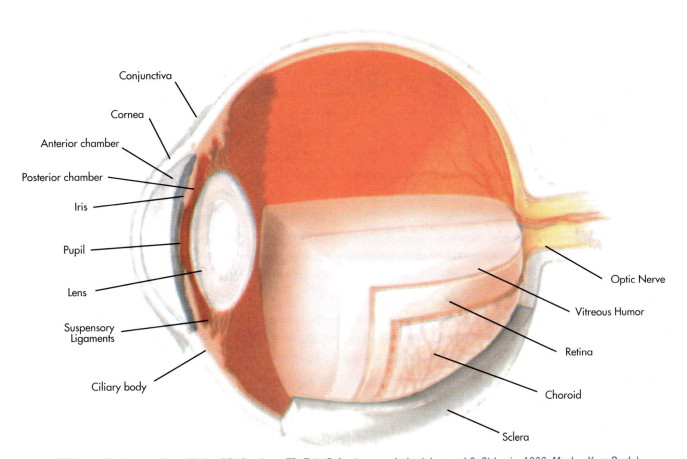

Conjunctiva
Cornea
Anterior chamber
Posterior chamber
Iris
Pupil
Lens
Suspensory Ligaments
Ciliary body
Optic Nerve
Vitreous Humor
Retina
Choroid
Sclera

FIGURE 5-14 *The eye. (From Seeley RR, Stephens TD, Tate P:* Anatomy and physiology, *ed 2, St Louis, 1992, Mosby–Year Book.)*

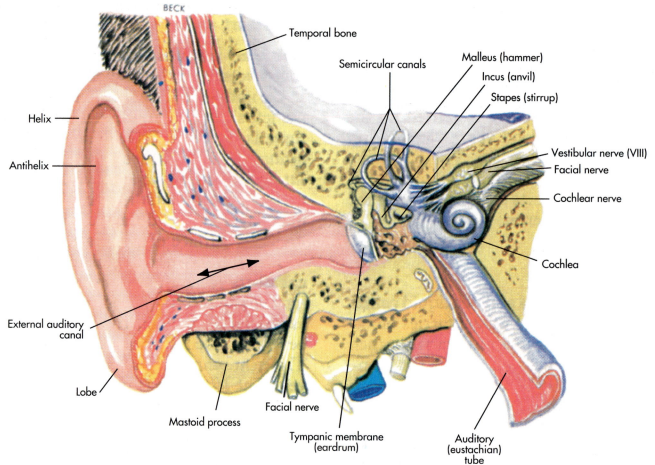

BECK

Temporal bone

Semicircular canals

Malleus (hammer)

Incus (anvil)

Stapes (stirrup)

Helix

Antihelix

Vestibular nerve (VIII)

Facial nerve

Cochlear nerve

Cochlea

External auditory canal

Lobe

Facial nerve

Mastoid process

Tympanic membrane (eardrum)

Auditory (eustachian) tube

FIGURE 5-15 *The ear. (Modified from Thibodeau GA: Anthony's textbook of anatomy and physiology, ed 13, St Louis, 1990, Mosby–Year Book.)*

THE CIRCULATORY SYSTEM

The circulatory system consists of the blood, heart, and blood vessels. The heart pumps blood through the blood vessels. The circulatory system performs many important functions. The blood carries food, oxygen, and other substances to the cells. Blood also removes waste products from the cells. Regulation of body temperature is aided by the blood and blood vessels. Heat from muscle activity is carried by the blood to other parts of the body. Blood vessels in the skin dilate if the body needs to be cooled. They constrict if heat needs to be kept in the body. The circulatory system also produces and carries cells that defend the body from harmful disease-causing germs.

The Blood

The blood consists of the blood cells and of a liquid called *plasma*. Plasma, which is mostly water, carries blood cells to the other cells of the body. The plasma also carries other substances needed by body cells for proper functioning. Food (proteins, fats, and carbohydrates),

hormones (see the section on the endocrine system), and chemicals are among the many substances carried in the plasma. Waste products also are carried in the plasma.

Red blood cells are called *erythrocytes.* They give the blood its red color because of a substance in the cell called **hemoglobin.** As the red blood cells circulate through the lungs, the hemoglobin picks up oxygen. The hemoglobin carries oxygen to the body cells. When the blood appears bright red, the hemoglobin in the red blood cells is saturated with oxygen. As the blood circulates through the body, oxygen is given to the cells. The cells release carbon dioxide (a waste product), which is picked up by the hemoglobin. Red blood cells saturated with carbon dioxide make the blood appear dark red.

There are approximately 25 trillion red blood cells in the body. About 4½ to 5 million are found in a cubic milliliter of blood. (A cubic milliliter is equivalent to a tiny drop of blood.) These cells live for 3 or 4 months. They are destroyed by the liver and spleen as they wear out. The bone marrow produces new red blood cells.

About 1 million new red blood cells are produced every second.

The *white blood cells* are called *leukocytes* and are colorless. These cells protect the body against infection. There are 5,000 to 10,000 white blood cells in a cubic milliliter of blood. At the first sign of infection, the white blood cells rush to the site of the infection and begin to multiply rapidly. The number of white blood cells increases when there is an infection in the body. White blood cells also are produced by the bone marrow. They live about 9 days.

Platelets, also called *thrombocytes*, are necessary for the clotting of blood. They also are produced by the bone marrow. There are about 200,000 to 400,000 platelets in a cubic milliliter of blood. A platelet will survive for about 4 days.

The Heart

The heart is a muscle that pumps blood through the blood vessels to the tissues and cells of the body. The heart lies in the mid to lower part of the chest cavity toward the left side (Fig. 5-16). The heart is hollow and is

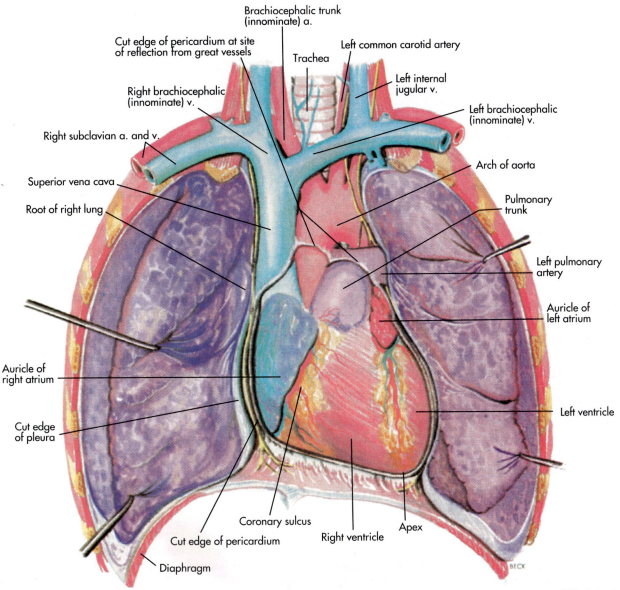

Brachiocephalic trunk (innominate) a.

Cut edge of pericardium at site of reflection from great vessels

Trachea

Left common carotid artery

Right brachiocephalic (innominate) v.

Left internal jugular v.

Left brachiocephalic (innominate) v.

Right subclavian a. and v.

Arch of aorta

Superior vena cava

Pulmonary trunk

Root of right lung

Left pulmonary artery

Auricle of left atrium

Auricle of right atrium

Left ventricle

Cut edge of pleura

Coronary sulcus

Cut edge of pericardium

Right ventricle

Apex

Diaphragm

BECK

FIGURE 5-16 *The location of the heart in the chest cavity. (From Thibodeau GA: Anthony's textbook of anatomy and physiology, ed 13, St Louis, 1990, Mosby–Year Book.)*

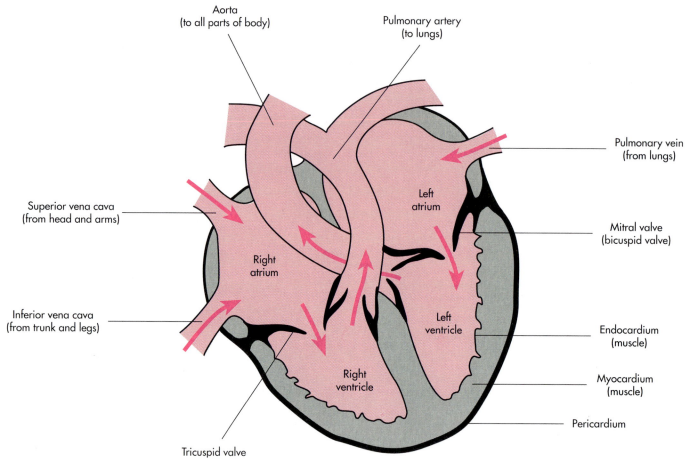

Aorta
(to all parts of body)

Pulmonary artery
(to lungs)

Pulmonary vein
(from lungs)

Superior vena cava
(from head and arms)

Left
atrium

Mitral valve
(bicuspid valve)

Right
atrium

Inferior vena cava
(from trunk and legs)

Left
ventricle

Endocardium
(muscle)

Right
ventricle

Myocardium
(muscle)

Pericardium

Tricuspid valve

FIGURE 5-17 *The structures of the heart.*

made up of three layers (Fig. 5-17). The outer layer is called the *pericardium;* it is a thin sac that covers the heart. The *myocardium* is the second layer. This layer is the thick muscular portion of the heart. The *endocardium* is the inner layer of the heart. The endocardium is the membrane that lines the inner surface of the heart.

The heart has four chambers (see Fig. 5-17). The upper chambers receive blood and are called *atria*. The *right atrium* receives blood from the body tissues. The *left atrium* receives blood from the lungs. The lower chambers are called *ventricles*. The ventricles pump blood. The *right ventricle* pumps blood to the lungs for oxygen. The *left ventricle* pumps blood to all parts of the body. Valves are located between the atria and the ventricles. The valves allow blood to flow in one direction. They prevent blood from flowing back into the atria from the ventricles. The *tricuspid valve* is located between the right atrium and right ventricle. The *mitral valve*, also called the *bicuspid valve*, is located between the left atrium and left ventricle.

There are two phases of heart action: systole and diastole. During *diastole*, the resting phase, the heart cham-

bers fill with blood. During *systole*, the working phase, the heart contracts. Blood is pumped through the blood vessels when the heart contracts.

The Blood Vessels

Blood flows to body tissues and cells through the blood vessels. There are three groups of blood vessels: arteries, capillaries, and veins. The **arteries** carry blood away from the heart. Arterial blood is rich in oxygen. The *aorta* is the largest artery of the body. The aorta receives blood directly from the left ventricle. The aorta branches off into other arteries that carry blood to all parts of the body (Fig. 5-18, *A*). These arteries branch off into smaller parts within the tissues. The smallest branch of an artery is called an *arteriole*.

Arterioles connect with blood vessels called **capillaries.** Capillaries are very tiny vessels. Food, oxygen, and other substances pass from the capillaries into the cells of the body. Waste products, including carbon dioxide, are picked up from the cells by the capillaries. The waste products are carried back to the heart by the veins.

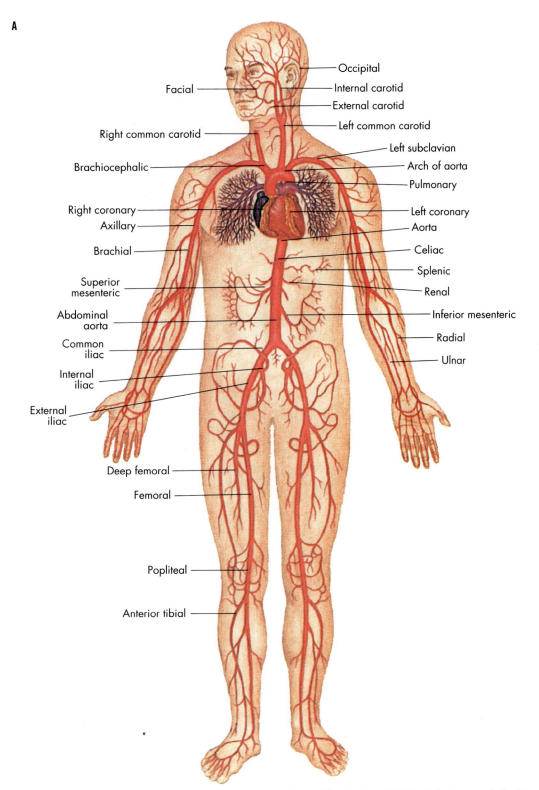

A

Occipital

Facial

Internal carotid

External carotid

Right common carotid

Left common carotid

Left subclavian

Brachiocephalic

Arch of aorta

Pulmonary

Right coronary

Left coronary

Axillary

Aorta

Brachial

Celiac

Superior mesenteric

Splenic

Renal

Abdominal aorta

Inferior mesenteric

Radial

Common iliac

Ulnar

Internal iliac

External iliac

Deep femoral

Femoral

Popliteal

Anterior tibial

FIGURE 5-18 *The arterial and venous systems. A, The arterial system. (From Seeley RR, Stephens TD, Tate P:* Anatomy and physiology, *ed 2, St Louis, 1992, Mosby–Year Book.)*

Continued.

B

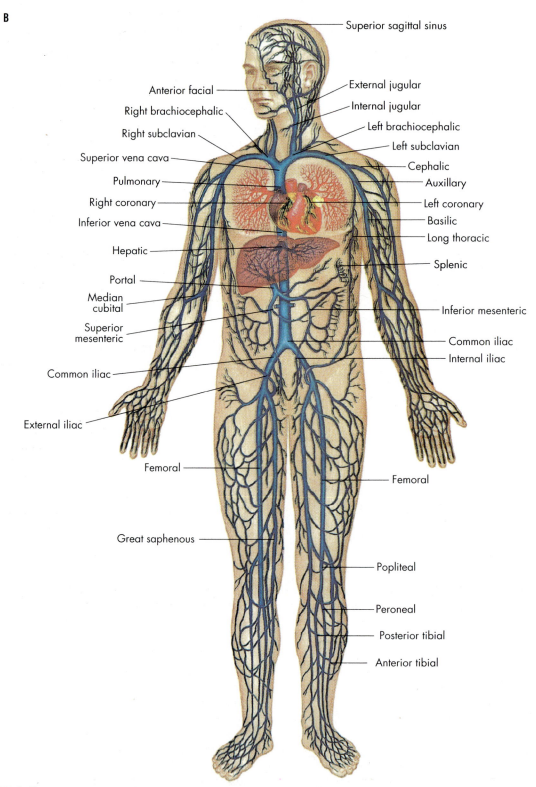

- Superior sagittal sinus
- Anterior facial
- External jugular
- Right brachiocephalic
- Internal jugular
- Right subclavian
- Left brachiocephalic
- Superior vena cava
- Left subclavian
- Pulmonary
- Cephalic
- Right coronary
- Auxillary
- Inferior vena cava
- Left coronary
- Hepatic
- Basilic
- Portal
- Long thoracic
- Median cubital
- Splenic
- Superior mesenteric
- Inferior mesenteric
- Common iliac
- Common iliac
- External iliac
- Internal iliac
- Femoral
- Femoral
- Great saphenous
- Popliteal
- Peroneal
- Posterior tibial
- Anterior tibial

FIGURE 5-18, *B,* *The venous system. (From Seeley RR, Stephens TD, Tate P:* Anatomy and physiology, *ed 2, St Louis, 1992, Mosby–Year Book.)*

The **veins** return blood to the heart. They are connected to the capillaries by *venules*. Venules are small veins. The venules begin branching together to form veins. The many branches of veins also branch together as they near the heart to form two main veins (Fig. 5-18, *B*). The two main veins are the *inferior vena cava* and the *superior vena cava*. Both empty into the right atrium. The inferior vena cava carries blood from the legs and trunk. The superior vena cava carries blood from the head and arms. Venous blood is dark red in color because it contains little oxygen and a great deal of carbon dioxide.

Blood flow through the circulatory system is diagrammed in Fig. 5-17, on p. 78, and can be summarized as follows. Venous blood, poor in oxygen, empties into the right atrium. Blood flows through the tricuspid valve into the right ventricle. The right ventricle pumps blood into the lungs to pick up oxygen. Oxygen-rich blood from the lungs enters the left atrium. Blood from the left atrium passes through the mitral valve into the left ventricle. The left ventricle pumps the blood to the aorta, which branches off to form other arteries. The arterial blood is carried to the tissues by arterioles and to the cells by capillaries. The cells and capillaries exchange oxygen and nutrients for carbon dioxide and waste products. The capillaries connect with venules. The venules carry blood that contains carbon dioxide and waste products. The venules form veins. The veins return blood to the heart.

THE RESPIRATORY SYSTEM

Oxygen is necessary for survival. Every cell of the body requires oxygen. The air contains about 20% oxygen, which is enough to meet the needs of the body under normal conditions. The respiratory system brings oxygen into the lungs and eliminates carbon dioxide. The process of supplying the cells with oxygen and removing the carbon dioxide from them is called **respiration.** Respiration involves *inhalation* (breathing in) and *exhalation* (breathing out). The terms *inspiration* (breathing in) and *expiration* (breathing out) also are used. The respiratory system is shown in Fig 5-19 on p. 82.

Air enters the body through the *nose*. The air then passes into the *pharynx* (throat), a tube-shaped passageway for both air and food. Air passes from the pharynx into the *larynx*. The larynx is commonly called the *voice box*. A piece of cartilage called the *epiglottis* acts like a lid over the larynx. The epiglottis prevents food from entering the airway during swallowing. During inhalation the epiglottis lifts up to let air pass over the larynx. Air passes from the larynx into the *trachea,* commonly called the *windpipe*. The trachea divides at its lower end into the *right bronchus* and the *left bronchus.* Each bronchus enters a lung. On entering the lungs the bronchi

further divide several times into smaller branches called *bronchioles*. Eventually, the bronchioles subdivide and end in tiny one-celled air sacs called *alveoli*. The alveoli look like small clusters of grapes. They are supplied with capillaries. Oxygen and carbon dioxide are exchanged between the alveoli and the capillaries. The blood in the capillaries picks up oxygen from the alveoli. Then the blood is returned to the left side of the heart and pumped to the rest of the body. The alveoli pick up carbon dioxide from the capillaries for exhalation.

The lungs are spongy tissues filled with alveoli, blood vessels, and nerves. Each lung is divided into lobes. The right lung has three lobes and the left lung has two. The lungs are separated from the abdominal cavity by a muscle called the *diaphragm*. Each lung is covered by a two-layered sac called the *pleura*. One layer is attached to the lung and the other to the chest wall. The pleura secretes a very thin fluid that fills the space between the layers. The fluid prevents the layers from rubbing together during inhalation and exhalation. A bony framework consisting of the ribs, sternum, and vertebrae protects the lungs.

THE DIGESTIVE SYSTEM

The digestive system is responsible for breaking down food physically and chemically so that it can be absorbed for use by the cells of the body. This process is called **digestion.** The digestive system also is called the *gastrointestinal (GI) system*. The system eliminates solid wastes from the body. The digestive system consists of the *alimentary canal (GI tract)* and the accessory organs of digestion (Fig. 5-20, p. 83). The alimentary canal is a long tube extending from the mouth to the anus. The mouth, pharynx, esophagus, stomach, small intestine, and large intestine are the major parts of the alimentary canal. The accessory organs of digestion are the teeth, tongue, salivary glands, liver, gallbladder, and pancreas.

Digestion begins in the *mouth*. The mouth also is called the *oral cavity*. The oral cavity receives food and prepares it for digestion. Through chewing motions, the *teeth* cut, chop, and grind food into smaller particles for digestion and swallowing. The *tongue* aids in chewing and swallowing. The *taste buds* on the surface of the tongue contain nerve endings. The taste buds allow sweet, sour, bitter, and salty tastes to be distinguished. *Salivary glands* in the oral cavity secrete *saliva*. The saliva moistens food particles for easier swallowing and begins the digestion of food. During the act of swallowing the tongue pushes food into the *pharynx*.

The pharynx is a muscular tube known as the *throat*. The act of swallowing is continued as the pharynx contracts. Contraction of the pharynx pushes food into the *esophagus*. The esophagus is a muscular tube about 10 inches long. The esophagus extends from the pharynx to

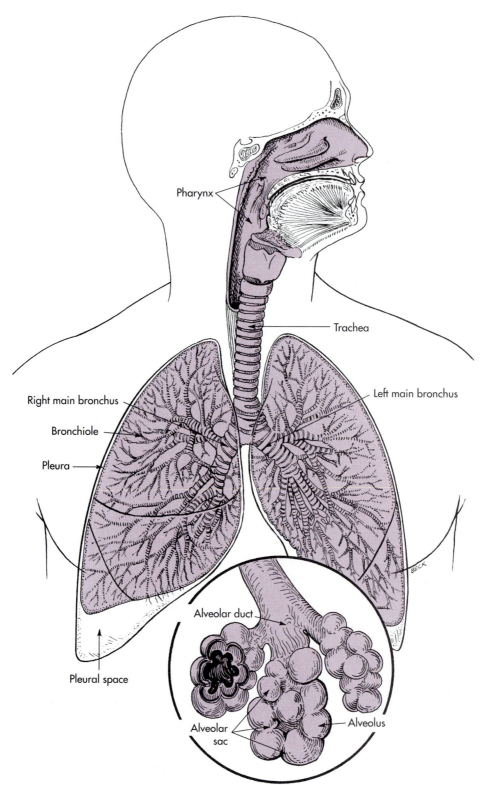

Pharynx

Trachea

Right main bronchus

Left main bronchus

Bronchiole

Pleura

Alveolar duct

Pleural space

Alveolar sac

Alveolus

FIGURE 5-19 *The respiratory system. (From Thibodeau GA:* Anthony's textbook of anatomy and physiology, *ed 13, St Louis, 1990, Mosby–Year Book.)*

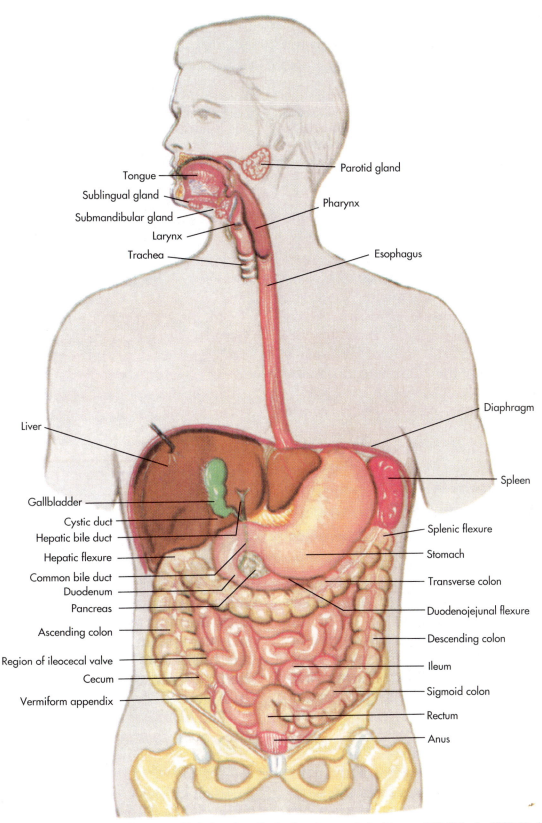

Tongue

Sublingual gland

Submandibular gland

Larynx

Trachea

Parotid gland

Pharynx

Esophagus

Diaphragm

Liver

Spleen

Gallbladder

Cystic duct

Hepatic bile duct

Hepatic flexure

Common bile duct

Duodenum

Pancreas

Ascending colon

Region of ileocecal valve

Cecum

Vermiform appendix

Splenic flexure

Stomach

Transverse colon

Duodenojejunal flexure

Descending colon

Ileum

Sigmoid colon

Rectum

Anus

FIGURE 5-20 *The digestive system. (From Thibodeau GA:* Anthony's textbook of anatomy and physiology, *ed 13, St Louis, 1990, Mosby—Year Book.)*

the stomach. Involuntary muscle contractions called **peristalsis** move the food down the esophagus into the stomach.

The *stomach* is a muscular, pouchlike sac located in the upper left portion of the abdominal cavity. Strong stomach muscles stir and churn food to break it up into even smaller particles. The stomach is lined with a mucous membrane that contains glands that secrete *gastric juices*. Food is mixed and churned with the gastric juices to form a semiliquid substance called *chyme*. Through peristalsis, the chyme is pushed from the stomach into the small intestine.

The *small intestine* is about 20 feet long and is divided into three parts. The first part is called the *duodenum*. In the duodenum, more digestive juices are added to the chyme. One of the juices is called *bile*. Bile is a greenish liquid produced by the *liver* and stored in the *gallbladder*. Juices from the *pancreas* and small intestine also are added to the chyme. The digestive juices chemically break down food so that it can be absorbed.

Peristalsis moves the chyme through the two remaining portions of the small intestine: the *jejunum* and the *ileum*. Tiny projections called *villi* line the small intes-

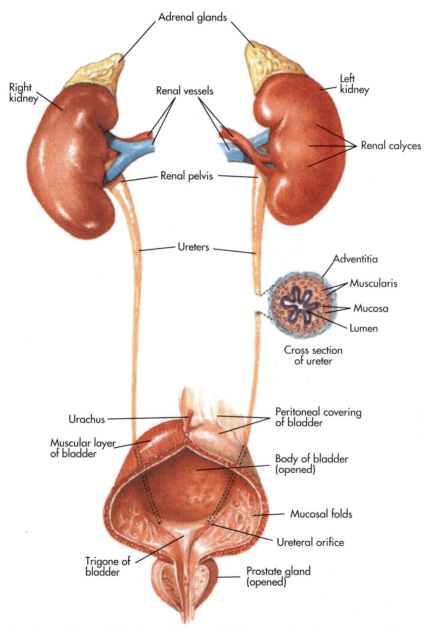

FIGURE 5-21 *The urinary system. (From Anderson KN, Anderson LE, Glanze WD:* Mosby's medical, nursing, and allied health dictionary, *ed 4, St Louis, 1994, Mosby–Year Book.)*

tine. The villi absorb the digested food into the capillaries. Most of the absorption of food takes place in the jejunum and ileum.

Some chyme remains undigested. The undigested chyme passes from the small intestine into the *large intestine*. The large intestine also is called the *large bowel* or the *colon*. The colon absorbs most of the water from the chyme. The remaining semisolid material is called *feces*. The feces consist of a small amount of water and solid wastes and some mucus and germs. These are the

waste products of digestion. The feces pass through the colon into the *rectum* by peristalsis. Feces pass out of the body through the *anus*.

THE URINARY SYSTEM

Wastes are removed from the body through the respiratory system, the digestive system, and the skin. The digestive system rids the body of solid wastes. The lungs rid the body of carbon dioxide. Water and other substances are contained in sweat. There are other waste

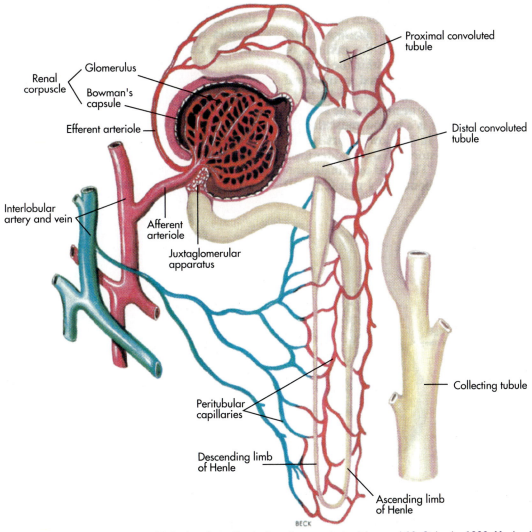

FIGURE 5-22 *A nephron. (From Thibodeau GA:* Anthony's textbook of anatomy and physiology, *ed 13, St Louis, 1990, Mosby–Year Book.)*

85

products in the blood as a result of body cells burning food for energy. The functions of the urinary system are to remove waste products from the blood and to maintain water balance within the body. The structures of the urinary system are shown in Fig. 5-21 on p. 84.

The *kidneys* are two bean-shaped organs located in the upper abdomen. They lie against the muscles of the back on each side of the spine. They are protected by the lower edge of the rib cage. Each kidney consists of over a million tiny *nephrons* (Fig. 5-22, p. 85). The nephron is the basic working unit of the kidney. Each nephron contains a *convoluted tubule,* which is a tiny coiled tubule. Each convoluted tubule has a *Bowman's capsule* at one

end. The capsule partially surrounds a cluster of capillaries called a *glomerulus.* Blood passes through the glomerulus and is filtered by the capillaries. The fluid portion of the blood is squeezed into the Bowman's capsule. The fluid then passes into the tubule. Most of the water and other necessary substances are reabsorbed by the blood and recirculated in the body. The rest of the fluid and the waste products form *urine* in the tubule. Urine flows through the tubule to a *collecting tubule.* All of the collecting tubules within the millions of nephrons drain into the *renal pelvis* within the kidney.

A tube, called the *ureter,* is attached to the renal pelvis of the kidney. Each ureter is about 10 to 12 inches long.

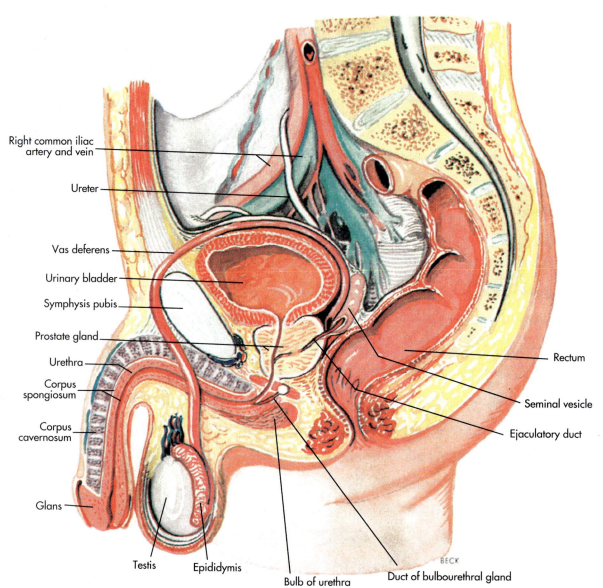

FIGURE 5-23 *The male reproductive system. (From Thibodeau GA: Anthony's textbook of anatomy and physiology, ed 13, St Louis, 1990, Mosby–Year Book.)*

The ureters carry urine from the kidneys to the *bladder.* The bladder is a hollow muscular sac that lies in the lower part of the abdominal cavity toward the front. Urine is stored in the bladder until the desire to urinate is felt. The need to urinate usually occurs when there is about half a pint (250 ml) of urine in the bladder. Urine passes from the bladder through the *urethra.* The opening at the end of the urethra is the *meatus.* Urine passes from the body through the meatus. Urine is a clear yellowish fluid.

THE REPRODUCTIVE SYSTEM

Human reproduction is the result of the union of a sex cell from the female and a sex cell from the male. The structures of the male reproductive system and the female reproductive system are different. The differences allow for the process of reproduction.

The Male Reproductive System

The structures of the male reproductive system are shown in Fig. 5-23. The *testes,* also called *testicles,* are the sex glands of the male. Sex glands also are called *gonads.* The two testes are glands of oval or almond shape. The male sex cells are produced in the testes. Sex cells of the male are called *sperm* cells. *Testosterone,* the male hormone, also is produced in the testes. This hormone is necessary for the functioning of the reproductive organs and for the development of secondary sex characteristics in the male. Male secondary sex characteristics include facial hair and growth of a beard; pubic and axillary hair; hair on the arms, chest, and legs; deepening of the voice; and increases in neck and shoulder size. The testes are suspended between the thighs in a sac called the *scrotum.* The scrotum consists of skin and muscle

The sperm travel from the testis to the *epididymis.* The epididymis is a coiled tube located on top and to the side of the testis. From the epididymis the sperm travel through a tube called the *vas deferens.* Eventually each vas deferens joins a *seminal vesicle.* The two seminal vesicles store sperm and produce *semen.* Semen is a fluid that carries sperm from the male reproductive tract. The ducts of the seminal vesicles unite to form the *ejaculatory duct.* The ejaculatory duct passes through the prostate gland.

The *prostate gland,* shaped like a doughnut, lies just below the bladder. The gland secretes a fluid into the semen. As the ejaculatory ducts leave the prostate, they join the *urethra,* which also runs through the prostate. The urethra is the outlet for both urine and semen. The urethra is contained within the penis.

The *penis* is located outside of the body and is composed of *erectile* tissue. When the man becomes sexually excited, blood fills the erectile tissue, causing the penis to become enlarged, hard, and erect. The erect penis is then able to enter the vagina of the female reproductive tract. The semen containing sperm is then released into the vagina of the female.

The Female Reproductive System

The structures of the female reproductive system are shown in Fig. 5-24 on p. 88. The female gonads are two almond-shaped glands called the *ovaries.* Each ovary is located on either side of the uterus in the abdominal cavity. The ovaries produce and contain the *ova,* or eggs. The ova are the female sex cells. One ovum (egg) is released monthly during a woman's reproductive years. The release of an ovum from an ovary is called *ovulation.* The ovaries also secrete the female hormones *estrogen* and *progesterone.* These hormones are responsible for the functioning of the female reproductive system and the development of secondary sex characteristics in the female. These include increase in breast size; pubic and axillary hair; slight deepening of the voice; and widening and rounding of the hips.

When an ovum is released from an ovary, it is picked up by one of the *fallopian tubes.* There are two fallopian tubes, one on each side. The tubes are attached at one end to the uterus. The ovum then travels through the fallopian tube to the *uterus.* The uterus is a hollow muscular organ shaped like a pear. The uterus is located in the center of the pelvic cavity behind the bladder and in front of the rectum. The main part of the uterus is called the *fundus.* The neck or narrow section of the uterus is called the *cervix.* The tissue lining the uterus is known as the *endometrium.* Many blood vessels are contained in the endometrium. If sex cells from the male and female unite into one cell, the cell will implant into the endometrium where it will grow into a baby. The uterus serves as a place for the unborn baby to grow and receive nourishment.

The cervix of the uterus projects into a muscular canal called the *vagina.* The vagina opens to the outside of the body and is located just behind the urethra. The vagina receives the penis during sexual intercourse and serves as part of the birth canal. Glands in the walls of the vagina keep it moistened with secretions. The external opening of the vagina is partially closed by a thin piece of membrane called the *hymen.*

The external genitalia of the female are referred to as the *vulva* (Fig. 5-25, p. 88). The *mons pubis* is a rounded fatty pad over a bone called the *symphysis pubis.* The mons pubis is covered with hair in the adult female. The *labia majora* and *labia minora* are two folds of tissue on each side of the vaginal opening. The *clitoris* is a small organ composed of erectile tissue. The clitoris becomes hard when sexually stimulated.

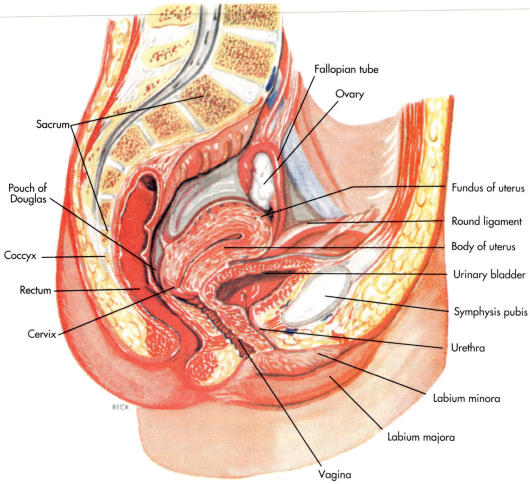

Sacrum

Pouch of
Douglas

Coccyx

Rectum

Cervix

Fallopian tube

Ovary

Fundus of uterus

Round ligament

Body of uterus

Urinary bladder

Symphysis pubis

Urethra

Labium minora

Labium majora

Vagina

BECK

FIGURE 5-24 *The female reproductive system. (From Thibodeau GA:* Anthony's textbook of anatomy and physiology, *ed 13, St Louis, 1990, Mosby–Year Book.)*

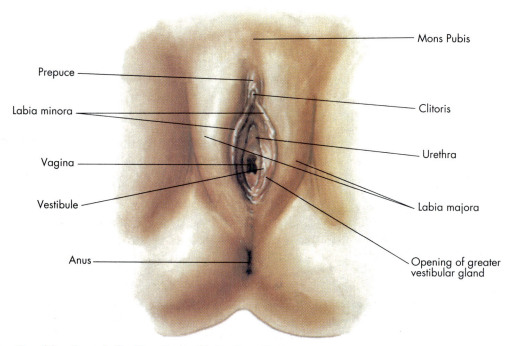

Prepuce

Labia minora

Vagina

Vestibule

Anus

Mons Pubis

Clitoris

Urethra

Labia majora

Opening of greater
vestibular gland

FIGURE 5-25 *The external female genitalia. (From Seeley RR, Stephens TD, Tate P:* Anatomy and physiology, *ed 2, St Louis, 1992, Mosby–Year Book.)*

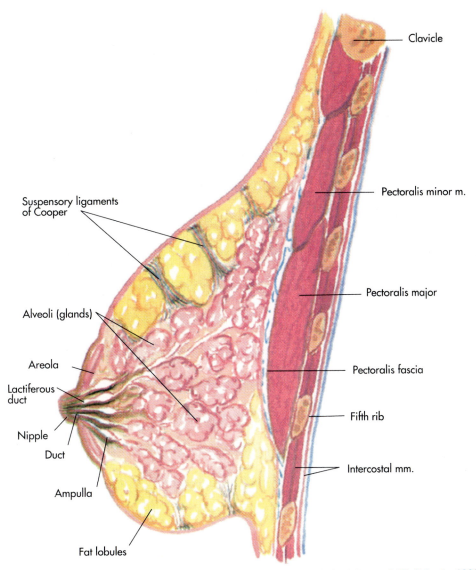

Clavicle

Pectoralis minor m.

Pectoralis major

Pectoralis fascia

Fifth rib

Intercostal mm.

Suspensory ligaments of Cooper

Alveoli (glands)

Areola

Lactiferous duct

Nipple

Duct

Ampulla

Fat lobules

FIGURE 5-26 *The female breast. (From Thibodeau GA:* Anthony's textbook of anatomy and physiology, *ed 13, St Louis, 1990, Mosby–Year Book.)*

The *mammary glands,* or *breasts,* are considered organs of reproduction because they secrete milk after childbirth. The glands are located on the outside of the chest. They are made up of glandular tissue and fat (Fig. 5-26). The milk drains into ducts that open onto the nipple.

Menstruation. The endometrium is rich in blood to nourish the cell that grows into an unborn baby *(fetus).* If a woman does not become pregnant, the endometrium breaks up and is discharged through the vagina to the outside of the body. This process is called **menstruation.** Menstruation occurs about every 28 days. Therefore, it also is called the *menstrual cycle.*

The first day of the cycle begins with menstruation. Blood flows from the uterus through the vaginal opening. The menstrual flow usually lasts between 3 to 7 days. Ovulation occurs during the next phase of the cycle. An ovum matures in an ovary and is released. Ovulation usually occurs on or about the fourteenth day of the cycle. Meanwhile, estrogen and progesterone (the female hormones) are secreted by the ovaries. These hormones cause the endometrium to thicken for a possible pregnancy. If pregnancy does not occur, the hormones decrease in amount. The blood supply to the endometrium decreases because of the decrease in hormones. The endometrium breaks up and is discharged through the vagina. Another menstrual cycle begins.

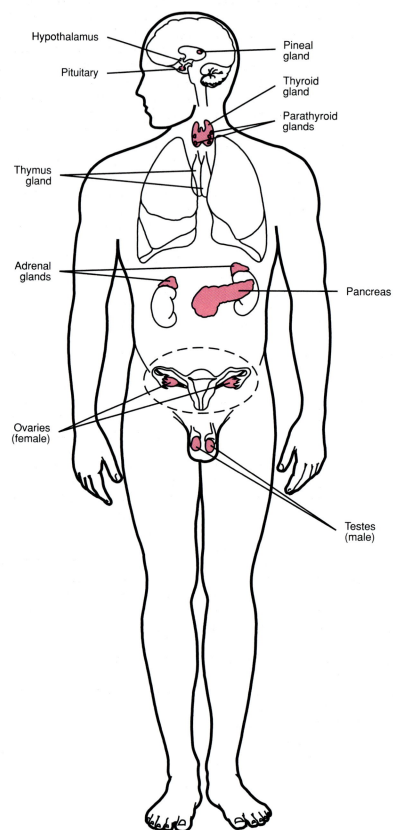

FIGURE 5-27 *The endocrine system. (From Seeley RR, Stephens TD, Tate P:* Anatomy and physiology, *ed 2, St Louis, 1992, Mosby–Year Book.)*

Fertilization. For human reproduction to occur, a sex cell from the male (sperm) must unite with a sex cell from the female (ovum). The uniting of the sperm and ovum into one cell is called *fertilization.* A sperm contains 23 chromosomes, and an ovum contains 23 chromosomes. When the two cells unite, the fertilized cell contains 46 chromosomes.

During intercourse millions of sperm are deposited in the vagina. The sperm travel up the cervix, through the uterus, and into the fallopian tubes. If a sperm and an ovum unite in the fallopian tube, fertilization occurs and results in pregnancy. The fertilized cell travels down the fallopian tube to the uterus. After a short time the fertilized cell will implant in the thick endometrium and grow during pregnancy.

THE ENDOCRINE SYSTEM

The endocrine system consists of glands called the *endocrine glands* (Fig. 5-27, p. 90). The endocrine glands secrete chemical substances called **hormones** into the blood stream. The hormones regulate the activities of other organs and glands in the body.

The *pituitary gland* is called the *master gland.* About the size of a cherry, the pituitary gland is located at the base of the brain behind the eyes. The pituitary gland is divided into lobes: the anterior pituitary lobe and the posterior pituitary lobe. The *anterior pituitary lobe* secretes important hormones. *Growth hormone* is needed for the growth of muscles, bones, and other organs. An adequate amount of growth hormone is needed throughout life to maintain normal-sized bones and muscles. Growth will be stunted if a baby is born with deficient amounts of the growth hormone. Too much of the hormone causes excessive growth.

Thyroid-stimulating hormone (TSH) also is secreted by the anterior pituitary lobe. The thyroid gland requires thyroid-stimulating hormone to function properly. *Adrenocorticotropic hormone (ACTH)* is another hormone secreted by the anterior lobe. This hormone stimulates the adrenal gland. The anterior lobe also secretes hormones that regulate the growth, development, and function of the male and female reproductive systems.

The *posterior pituitary lobe* secretes two hormones: *antidiuretic hormone (ADH)* and *oxytocin.* Antidiuretic hormone prevents the kidneys from excreting excessive amounts of water. Oxytocin causes the smooth muscles of the uterus to contract during childbirth.

The *thyroid gland,* shaped like a butterfly, is located in the neck in front of the larynx. Thyroid hormone (TH) is secreted by the thyroid gland. *Thyroxine* is another term for thyroid hormone. Thyroid hormone regulates **metabolism.** Metabolism is the burning of food for heat and energy by the cells. Too little thyroid hormone results in slowed body processes, slowed movements, and weight gain. Too much of the hormone causes increased metabolism, excess energy, and weight loss. If a baby is born with deficient amounts of thyroid hormone, physical and mental growth will be stunted.

The *parathyroid glands* secrete *parathyroid hormone.* There are four parathyroid glands. Two are located on each side of the thyroid gland. Parathormone regulates the body's use of calcium. Calcium is needed for the proper functioning of nerves and muscles. Insufficient amounts of calcium cause *tetany.* Tetany is a state of severe muscle contraction and spasm. If untreated, tetany can cause death.

There are two *adrenal glands.* An adrenal gland is located on the top of each kidney. The adrenal gland is divided into two parts: the *adrenal medulla* and the *adrenal cortex.* The adrenal medulla secretes *epinephrine* and *norepinephrine.* These hormones stimulate the body to produce energy quickly during emergencies. Heart rate, blood pressure, muscle power, and energy all increase. The adrenal cortex secretes three groups of hormones that are essential for life. The *glucocorticoids* regulate metabolism of carbohydrates. They also control the body's response to stress and inflammation. The *mineralocorticoids* regulate the amount of salt and water that is absorbed and lost by the kidneys. The adrenal cortex also secretes small amounts of the male and female sex hormones.

The *pancreas* secretes *insulin.* Insulin regulates the amount of sugar in the blood available for use by the cells. Insulin is needed for sugar to enter the cells. If there is too little insulin, sugar cannot enter the cells. If sugar cannot enter the cells, excess amounts of sugar build up in the blood. This condition is called *diabetes mellitus.*

The *gonads* are the glands of human reproduction. Male sex glands, the testes, secrete *testosterone.* Female sex glands, the ovaries, secrete *estrogen* and *progesterone.*

SUMMARY

The human body is made up of several systems. Each system has its own structures and functions. The body systems are related to and dependent on each other for proper functioning and survival. Injury or disease of one part of the system affects the entire system and the whole body. You may need to refer to this chapter as you study other chapters in this book and as you learn to perform basic nursing procedures. Each procedure will involve the resident's body and your body. To give safe and effective care, you need to have a basic understanding of the body's structure and function.

Review QUESTIONS

Circle the *best* answer.

1. The basic unit of body structure is the
   a. Cell
   c. Nephron
   b. Neuron
   d. Ovum

2. Organs are formed by groups of
   a. Cells
   c. Systems
   b. Tissues
   d. Chromosomes

3. Which is not a function of the skin?
   a. Providing the protective covering for the body
   b. Regulating body temperature
   c. Sensing cold, pain, touch and pressure
   d. Providing the shape and framework for the body

4. Which part of the musculoskeletal system allows movement?
   a. Bone marrow and periosteum
   b. Synovial membrane
   c. Joints
   d. Ligaments

5. Skeletal muscles
   a. Are under involuntary control
   b. Appear smooth
   c. Are under voluntary control
   d. Appear striped and smooth

6. Muscles are connected to bones by
   a. Cartilage
   c. Nerve fibers
   b. Ligaments
   d. Tendons

7. Which is *not* a main part of the brain?
   a. Cerebrum
   c. Brainstem
   b. Pons
   d. Cerebellum

8. The highest functions of the brain take place in the
   a. Cerebral cortex
   c. Brainstem
   b. Medulla
   d. Spinal nerves

9. In addition to serving as the organ for hearing, the ear is involved with
   a. Regulating body movements
   b. Balance
   c. Smoothness of body movements
   d. Controlling involuntary muscles

10. The liquid part of the blood is the
    a. Hemoglobin
    c. Plasma
    b. Red blood cell
    d. Alveolus

11. Which part of the heart pumps blood to the body?
    a. Right atrium
    c. Left atrium
    b. Right ventricle
    d. Left ventricle

12. Blood vessels that carry blood away from the heart are called
    a. Capillaries
    c. Venules
    b. Veins
    d. Arteries

13. Oxygen and carbon dioxide are exchanged
    a. In the bronchi
    b. Between the alveoli and capillaries
    c. Between the lungs and the pleura
    d. In the trachea

14. Food is made easier to swallow by
    a. Bile
    c. Chyme
    b. Gastric juices
    d. Saliva

15. Most of the absorption of food takes place in the
    a. Stomach
    c. Colon
    b. Small intestine
    d. Large intestine

16. Urine passes from the body through
    a. The ureters
    c. The anus
    b. The urethra
    d. Nephrons

17. The male sex cell is the
    a. Semen
    c. Gonad
    b. Ovum
    d. Sperm

18. The female sex gland is the
    a. Ovary
    c. Uterus
    b. Fallopian tube
    d. Vagina

19. The endocrine glands secrete substances called
    a. Hormones
    c. Semen
    b. Mucus
    d. Insulin

20. The "master gland" of the body is the
    a. Endocrine gland
    b. Pituitary gland
    c. Thyroid gland
    d. Adrenal gland

Answers

1. a	6. d	11. d	16. b
2. b	7. b	12. d	17. d
3. d	8. a	13. b	18. a
4. c	9. b	14. d	19. a
5. c	10. c	15. b	20. b

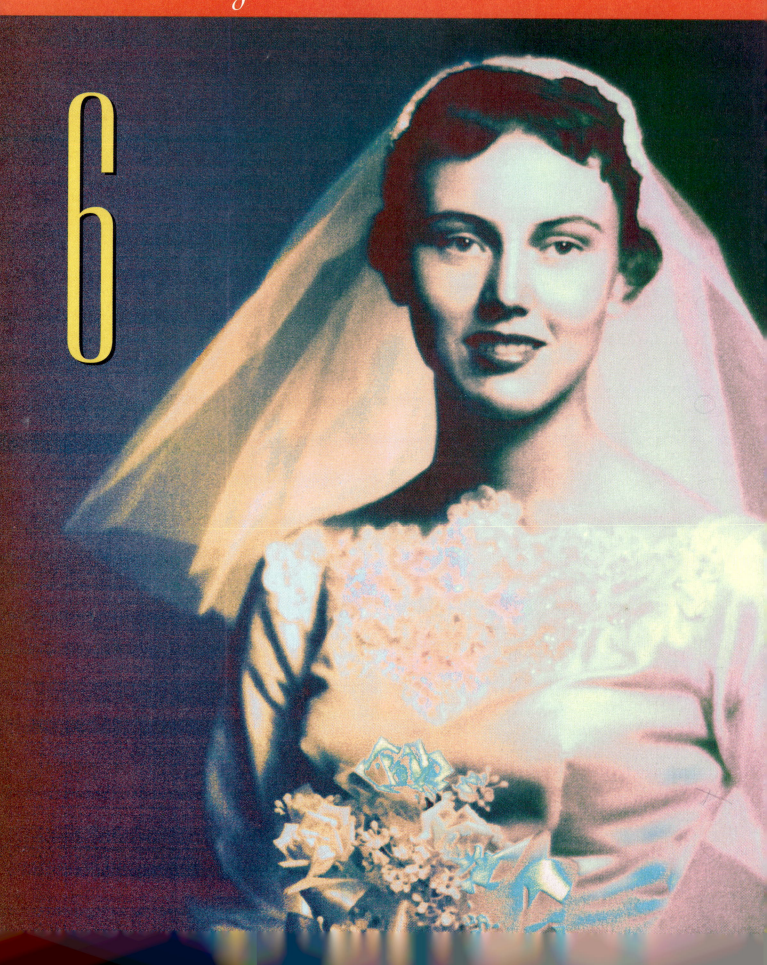

6

What You Will LEARN

- The key terms listed in this chapter

- The effects of retirement

- Common changes in social relationships of elderly persons

- How the death of a spouse affects the survivor

- Changes in body systems as a result of aging and the care that is required

- Housing alternatives for elderly persons

- Why residents of nursing facilities may avoid social relationships

- How to promote the resident's quality of life

- Signs of elderly abuse

- What to do if elderly abuse is suspected

dysphagia
Difficulty *(dys)* swallowing *(phagia)*

dyspnea
Difficulty *(dys)* in breathing *(pnea)*

geriatrics
The care of aging people

gerontology
The study of the aging process

old
Those persons between the ages of 65 and 85

old-old
Those persons over the age of 85

young-old
Those persons between the ages of 55 and 65

This is our wedding picture. Hilda was so lovely. She died a few years back. She was 86. She was as lovely to me the day she died as she was the day we were married. I miss her so. ✍

The number of older persons is increasing every day. People are living longer and are healthier than before. Most people can expect to live into their 70s. Many live into the 80s and 90s. More and more people are living past 100.

But what is old? Age ranges have been given for the young-old, old, and the old-old. The **young-old** are between the ages of 55 and 65. The **old** are between the ages of 65 to 85. The **old-old** are people over 85.

Gerontology is the study of the aging process. **Geriatrics** is the care of the aged. Aging is a normal process. It is not a disease. Normal changes occur in body structure and function. The elderly have special needs because of these changes. They are at greater risk for illnesses, chronic diseases, and injuries. This does not mean that all elderly persons are mentally and physically disabled. Many continue to live healthy and happy lives in their own homes. Fewer than 10% of the elderly live in nursing facilities.

PSYCHOLOGICAL AND SOCIAL EFFECTS OF AGING

Physical, psychological, and social changes occur as a person grows older. Graying hair, wrinkles, and slower movements are physical reminders of growing old. Retirement and death of a spouse, relatives, and friends are social reminders. The person must prepare for his or her own death. Growing old can be a painful process socially, psychologically, and physically.

Retirement

People traditionally retire at the age of 65. Some retire earlier. Others work until the age of 70 or longer. Retirement is a reward for a lifetime of hard work. The person has earned the right not to work and can now relax and enjoy life (Fig. 6-1). Travel, leisure, and doing whatever one wants are "benefits" of retirement (Fig. 6-2). Many people enjoy retirement. Others are not so fortunate. Some must retire because of chronic disease or disability. Poor health and medical expenses can make the enjoyment of retirement very difficult.

Work has social and psychological effects. Work helps meet the basic needs of love, belonging, and esteem. Personal satisfaction and usefulness result from working. Friendships develop and day-to-day events are shared with co-workers. Leisure activities, recreation, and companionship often involve co-workers. Some people need work for psychological and social fulfillment. Retirement can be hard for them. Some retired people have part-time jobs or do volunteer work (Fig. 6-3). Such activities promote feelings of usefulness and well-being.

Retirement usually means reduced income. The monthly Social Security check may be the only source of income. Retirement and aging, however, do not mean fewer expenses. There still may be rent or mortgage payments. Food, clothing, gas and electricity, water bills, and taxes are other expenses. Car expenses, home repairs, medicine, and health care are additional costs. So are entertainment and gifts for children and grandchildren. Retirement can cause severe financial problems. Some people plan for retirement through savings, investments, retirement plans, and insurance.

Social Relationships

Social relationships change throughout life. Children grow up and move away. They have families of their own.

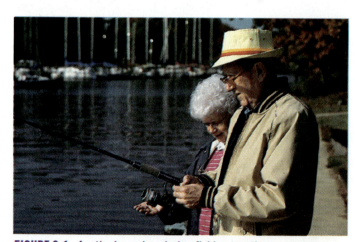

FIGURE 6-1 *A retired couple enjoying fishing together.*

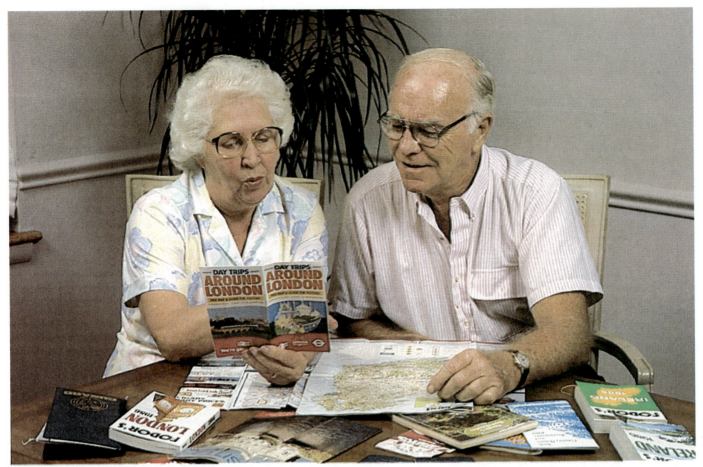

FIGURE 6-2 *An elderly couple planning a vacation.*

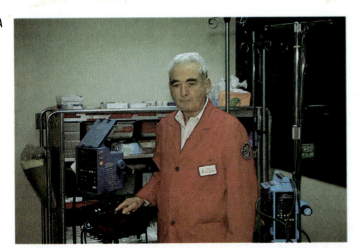

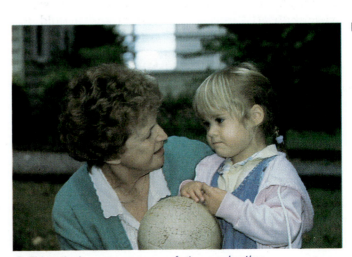

FIGURE 6-3 *A, This retired gentleman does volunteer work at a hospital.*

B, This retired woman serves as a foster grandmother.

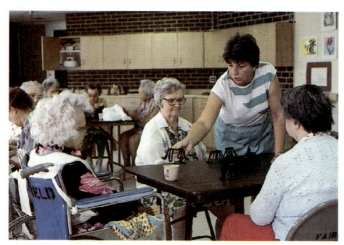

FIGURE 6-4 *Elderly persons enjoying companionship with people their own age.*

Many live far away from their elderly parents. Elderly family members and friends die, move away, or become disabled. These changes can cause feelings of loneliness and isolation. Separation from children and the lack of companionship with people their own age are common causes of loneliness in elderly persons (Fig. 6-4).

Many older people adjust to these changes. Hobbies, church and community activities, and new friends help prevent loneliness. Some communities and organizations sponsor bus trips to ball games, shopping, plays, and concerts. Being a grandparent can bring great love and enjoyment (Fig. 6-5). Being included in family activities helps prevent loneliness. It also allows the elderly person to feel useful and wanted (Fig. 6-6).

Elderly persons who speak and understand a language other than English may have social problems. Their communication occurs with family and friends who speak the same language. These relatives and friends may move away or die. Greater loneliness and isolation for the foreign-speaking individual may result. The person may not have anyone to talk to and may not be understood by others. In addition, the person's cultural values and practices may not be understood or recognized.

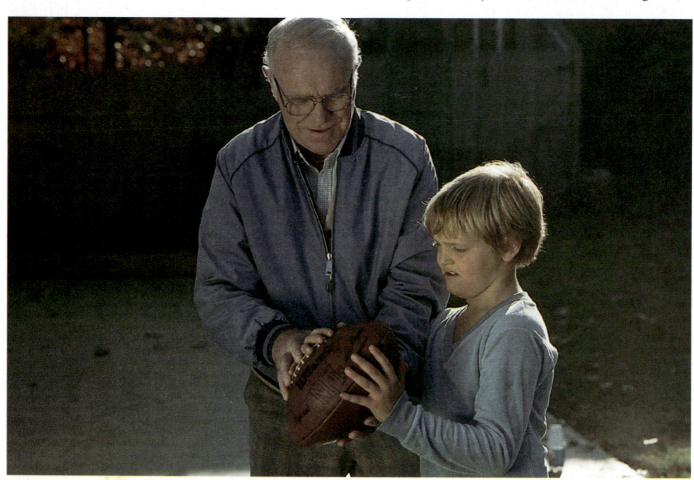

FIGURE 6-5 *An elderly man playing with his grandchild.*

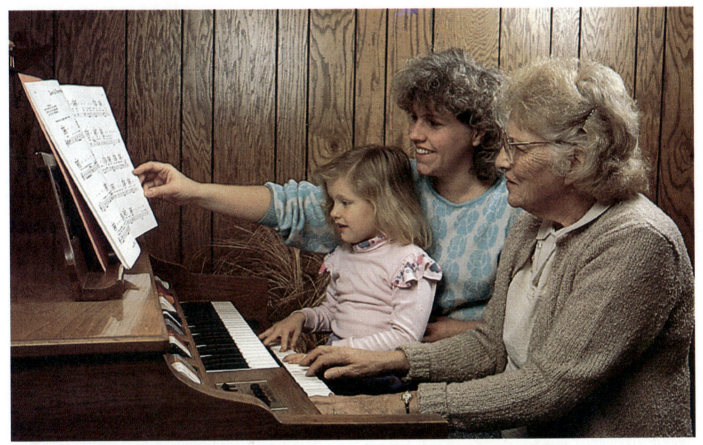

FIGURE 6-6 *An elderly woman is included in family activities.*

A social change some elderly persons experience is being cared for by their children. Parents and children change roles. Instead of the parent caring for the child, the child cares for the parent. This role change and dependency on a child can make some elderly persons feel more secure. Others, however, feel unwanted, in the way, and useless. Some feel a loss of dignity and self-respect. Tensions may develop among the child, parent, and other members in the household. Tension can be caused by the lack of privacy and by disagreements. Criticisms about housekeeping, child rearing, cooking, and friends are common causes of tension.

Death of a Spouse

As couples grow older, the chances increase that one of them will die. Women live longer than men. Therefore becoming a widow is a reality for many women.

A person may try to prepare psychologically for the death of a life partner. When death does occur, however, the loss is devastating. No amount of preparation is ever enough for the emptiness and changes that result. The person loses a lover, friend, companion, and confidant. The grief felt by the survivor can be very great. Serious physical and mental health problems can result. The will to live may be lost or suicide may be attempted.

THE PHYSICAL EFFECTS OF AGING

Certain physical changes are a normal part of aging. The changes occur in everyone (List 6-1, p. 99). The changes are gradual and may go unnoticed as the person adjusts to them. Some people age faster than others. The rate and degree of change vary with each person. Body processes slow down. Energy level and body efficiency decline.

Normal aging is not always accompanied by illness, injury, or disability. Quality of life does not have to decline. The changes in body processes take place over many years. This allows the person to adjust to such things as reduced activity and mobility.

The Integumentary System

The skin loses its elasticity and fatty tissue layer. As a result, the skin thins and sags. Folds, lines, and wrinkles appear. There is decreased secretion from oil and sweat glands. Dry skin develops. The skin is fragile and easily damaged. Skin breakdown and pressure sores are dangers.

List 6-1

Physical Changes During the Aging Process

System	Changes	System	Changes
Integumentary	Skin becomes less elastic		Pupils less responsive to light
	Fatty tissue layer is lost		Decreased vision at night or in dark rooms
	Skin thins and sags		Difficulty seeing green and blue colors
	Skin is fragile and easily injured		Poor vision
	Folds, lines, and wrinkles appear		Changes in auditory nerve
	Decreased secretion of oil and sweat glands		Eardrums atrophy
	Dry skin develops		High-pitched sounds not heard
	Itching		Wax secretion decreases
	Increased sensitivity to cold		Hearing loss
	Nails become thick and tough	Circulatory	Heart pumps with less force
	Whitening or graying hair		Arteries narrow and are less elastic
	Loss or thinning of hair		Less blood flows through narrowed arteries
Musculoskeletal	Muscle atrophy and decreased strength		Weakened heart has to work harder to pump blood through narrowed vessels
	Bone mass decreases	Respiratory	Respiratory muscles weaken
	Decreasing bone strength		Lung tissue becomes less elastic
	Bone becomes brittle; can break easily		Difficulty breathing (dyspnea)
	Vertebrae shorten		Decreased strength for coughing
	Joints become stiff and painful	Digestive	Decreased saliva production
	Hip and knee joints become flexed		Difficulty swallowing
	Gradual loss of height		Decreased appetite
	Loss of strength		Decreased secretion of digestive juices
	Decreased mobility		Difficulty digesting fried and fatty foods
Nervous	Reduction in nerve cells		Indigestion
	Slower nerve conduction		Loss of teeth
	Reflexes slow		Decreased peristalsis, causing flatulence and constipation
	Slower response to stimuli	Urinary	Kidney function decreases
	Reduced blood flow to the brain		Reduced blood flow to the kidneys
	Progressive loss of brain cells		Kidneys atrophy
	Shorter memory		Urine comes concentrated
	Forgetfulness		Bladder muscles weaken
	Confusion		Urinary incontinence may occur
	Dizziness		
	Changes in sleep patterns		
	Reduced sensitivity to touch and pain		
	Decreased senses of smell and taste		
	Eyelids thin and wrinkle		
	Less tear secretion		

Loss of the skin's fatty layer makes the person more sensitive to cold. Sweaters, lap blankets, socks, and extra blankets often are needed for warmth. Elderly persons need to be protected from drafts and extreme cold. Thermostat settings may need to be higher than normal.

Dry skin is easily damaged and causes itching. A complete bed bath, tub bath, or shower twice a week usually is enough for cleanliness. Partial baths are taken at other times. Only mild soaps are used. Some nursing facilities use soap substitutes. Soaps may be used to clean only the underarms, perineum, and under female breasts. Often soap is not used on the arms, legs, back, chest, and abdomen. Lotions, oils, and creams can be used to prevent drying and itching. Deodorants usually are not needed because there is decreased secretion from the sweat glands. Personal hygiene and skin care are discussed in Chapter 12.

Nails become thick and tough. Feet usually have poor circulation. A nick or cut can lead to a serious infection. Amputation of part of the foot or leg may be necessary to fight the infection. Nail and foot care are described in Chapter 12.

An elderly person may complain of cold feet. Socks should be worn. Hot water bottles and heating pads are not used. The risk of burns is very great. Fragile skin, poor circulation, and decreased sensitivity to heat and cold increase the risk of burns.

White or gray hair is a common sign of aging. Men lose a lot of hair. Hair thins on both men and women. Thinning occurs on the head, in the pubic area, and under the arms. Hair tends to be more dry. This is due to the decreased production of scalp oils. Brushing helps stimulate circulation and oil production. Shampooing frequency depends on personal choice. Usually the frequency of shampooing decreases with age. Shampooing should take place as often as necessary to maintain hygiene and comfort. Women and men may wear wigs because of thinning hair. Some choose to color their hair to cover graying.

The Musculoskeletal System

Muscles atrophy (shrink) and decrease in strength. Bone mass decreases. Minerals, especially calcium, are lost from the bones. Bones decrease in strength, become brittle, and break easily. These changes are severe in some elderly persons. For them, simply turning in bed can cause fractures (broken bones). Vertebrae shorten. Joints become stiff and painful. Hip and knee joints become slightly flexed (bent). These changes result in gradual loss of height, loss of strength, and decrease in mobility.

Elderly persons should be encouraged to be as active as possible. Activity, exercise, and diet can help prevent loss of bone and muscle strength. Walking is one of the best exercises. Participation in exercise groups and range-of-motion exercises are helpful. The diet should be high in protein, calcium, and vitamins. Remember, bones can break easily. The person must be protected from injury. Falls must be prevented (see Chapter 7). The person is turned and moved gently and carefully. A resident may need support and assistance in getting out of bed and in walking.

The Nervous System

Aging causes a reduction in nerve cells. Nerve conduction is slower. Reflexes are slower. Therefore responses to stimuli are slower. For example, if an elderly person slips, he or she is more likely to fall than is a younger person. The message telling the brain the person has slipped travels slowly. The message from the brain needed to prevent the fall also travels slowly. Thus the persons falls.

Blood flow to the brain is reduced. This may cause dizziness, which increases the risk for falls. Measures to prevent falls must be practiced. Residents are reminded to get up slowly from the bed or chair to prevent dizziness.

There also is a progressive loss of brain cells. Reduced blood flow and loss of brain cells affect personality and mental function. Memory is shorter and forgetfulness increases. The ability to respond is slowed. Confusion, dizziness, and fatigue may occur. Elderly people often remember events in the distant past better than those in the recent past. Many elderly persons keep mentally active and involved in current events. They show fewer personality and mental changes. Care of the confused person is described in Chapter 24.

Changes in sleep occur. Loss of energy and decreased blood flow cause fatigue. Elderly persons tend to rest or nap during the day. They usually go to bed early and get up early.

The senses. Touch, smell, taste, sight, and hearing are affected by aging. Touch and sensitivity to pain are reduced. The ability to feel heat and cold also is reduced. These changes increase the elderly person's risk for injury. Injuries and diseases that normally cause considerable pain may go unnoticed. The person may feel only minor discomfort. Therefore elderly residents must be protected from injury. Safety measures need to be practiced when heat and cold are applied (see Chapter 20). The skin must be carefully inspected for signs of breakdown. Good skin care and the measures to prevent pressure sores must be practiced.

Smell and taste are important when eating. These senses become dulled, causing a decrease in appetite. The number of taste buds decreases with aging. The tongue senses only sweet, salty, bitter, and sour. Sweet and salty tastes are lost first. This is important to remember when elderly residents complain that food has no taste. This is also why they often ask for more salt or sugar on their food.

The eye. Many changes occur in the eye with aging. Eyelids become thinner and wrinkled. Tear secretion, which protects the eyes, lessens. Therefore the eye is easily irritated by such things as dust and air pollutants. The pupil becomes smaller and less responsive to light. This causes decreased vision at night or in dark rooms. The ability to see clearly is reduced. This creates the need for eyeglasses. The lens of the eye (see Chapter 5, Fig. 5-14, p. 75) yellows. Yellowing of the lens makes it hard to see green and blue colors. Poor vision is a common cause of falls and other accidents. The nursing assistant needs to make sure that residents wear their eyeglasses. Their rooms need to be well lit. Night lights will help them see when they get up during the night.

The ear. Aging causes changes in the auditory nerve. Eardrums atrophy (shrink). The ability to hear high-pitched sounds is lost. Severe hearing loss occurs if these changes progress. A hearing aid may be needed for the affected ear. Hearing aids must be clean and correctly placed in the ear. Wax secretion decreases. Wax becomes harder and thicker with age. This wax is easily impacted (wedged in the ear) and can increase hearing loss. Wax is removed by the doctor or nurse.

The Circulatory System

The heart muscle becomes less efficient. Blood is pumped through the body with less force. These changes may not cause problems when the person is resting. Activity, exercise, excitement, and illness increase the body's need for oxygen and nutrients. If damaged or severely weakened, the heart may be unable to meet these needs.

Arteries loose their elasticity and become narrow. Less blood flows through them. This results in poor circulation in many parts of the body. A weakened heart has to work harder to pump blood through the narrowed vessels.

Exercise is helpful for maintaining health and well-being. Walking is good exercise for the healthy older adult. Many elderly persons exercise daily. They walk, jog, bicycle, hike, ski, play tennis, swim, or are involved in other sports. Residents in nursing facilities should be kept as active as possible.

Although many older adults are able to be quite active, others are less fortunate. Cardiovascular changes may be severe. Affected persons need periods of rest during the day. Daily activities should be planned to avoid overexertion. Such individuals should not walk long distances, climb many stairs, or carry heavy objects. Personal care items, television, telephone, and other frequently used items should be in convenient locations. A moderate amount of daily exercise helps to stimulate circulation. Exercise also helps prevent the formation of thrombi (blood clots) in leg veins. Active or passive range-of-motion exercises are necessary for persons confined to bed. Cardiovascular changes are more severe in some individuals. Doctors may order certain exercises and activity limitations.

The Respiratory System

Respiratory muscles weaken, and lung tissue becomes less elastic. Lung changes may not be obvious at rest. However, difficulty in breathing (dyspnea) may occur with activity. The person may have not have enough strength to cough and clear the upper airway of secretions. Respiratory infections and diseases may develop. These can severely threaten the elderly person's life.

Measures are necessary to promote normal breathing. Heavy bed linens should not cover the chest. They can prevent normal chest expansion. Turning, repositioning, and deep breathing help prevent respiratory complications from bed rest. Breathing usually is easier in the semi-Fowler's position (see Chapter 10). The person should be as active as possible.

The Digestive System

Aging causes many changes in the digestive system. Salivary glands produce less saliva. This can cause difficulty in swallowing (dysphagia). Dull senses of taste and smell cause a decrease in appetite. Secretion of digestive juices decreases. As a result, fried and fatty foods are hard to digest and may cause indigestion. Loss of teeth and ill-fitting dentures make chewing difficult. This results in digestion problems. Certain foods are avoided because they are hard to chew. Usually high-protein foods such as meat are avoided. Decreased peristalsis results in slower emptying of the stomach and colon. Flatulence and constipation are common because of decreased peristalsis (see Chapter 14).

Dry, fried, and fatty foods should be avoided. This helps lessen the problems of difficulty in swallowing and indigestion. Good oral hygiene and denture care improve the ability to taste. Some persons may not have natural teeth or dentures. Their food has to be pureed or ground. Avoiding high-fiber foods may be necessary even though they help prevent constipation. Foods high in fiber are hard to chew and can irritate the intestines. High-fiber foods include apricots, celery, and fruits and vegetables with skins and seeds. Foods that provide soft bulk often are ordered for those with chewing difficulties or constipation. These foods included whole-grain cereals and cooked fruits and vegetables. Bowel elimination is discussed in Chapter 14.

Aging requires certain dietary changes. Elderly people need fewer calories than do younger people. Energy and activity levels are lower. Additional fluids are needed to promote kidney function. Foods that prevent constipation and musculoskeletal changes need to be included in the diet. Foods high in protein are needed for tissue growth and repair. However, protein may be lacking in the diets of elderly persons. Foods high in protein generally are the most expensive.

The Urinary System

Aging decreases kidney function. Blood flow to the kidneys is reduced. This causes the kidneys to atrophy (shrink). Poisonous substances can build up in the blood and cause serious health problems. Urine becomes more concentrated because elderly persons usually do not drink enough fluids. Bladder muscles weaken, and the bladder holds less urine. Many older persons have to go to the bathroom several times during the night. Urinary incontinence may occur.

Adequate fluids are necessary. Too little fluid can damage the kidneys and cause urinary tract infections. Intake should include water, fruit juices, milk, and gelatin. The person should have a choice in the type of fluids served. You need to make sure that water is available to all residents who are permitted to have water. Remind them to drink, and offer fluids often to those who need help. Most fluids should be ingested before 5:00 PM. This reduces the need to urinate during the night. Bladder training programs may be necessary for those with urinary incontinence. Indwelling catheters sometimes are needed. Urinary elimination is discussed in Chapter 13.

HOUSING ALTERNATIVES

Most elderly persons live in their own homes. Some choose to give up their homes whereas others are forced to. Reduced income, taxes, home repairs, and the inability to do yard work are influencing factors. Some elderly people retire to warmer climates. Others find they no longer need the space of a large home when children are gone. Some are no longer able to care for themselves. Housing alternatives are available to meet the needs of elderly persons.

Living with Family Members

Sometimes elderly brothers, sisters, and cousins live together. They provide companionship for each other. They also can share living expenses. They can care for each other during illness or disability. One may have the role of caregiver if the other is ill or disabled.

Some elderly persons live with their adult children. The elderly parent (or parents) moves in with the child, or the child moves into the parent's home. As discussed earlier in this chapter, living with a child can help the elderly person feel safe and secure. The elderly parent may be healthy, may need some supervision, or may be ill or

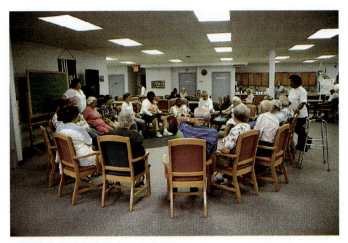

FIGURE 6-7 *An adult day-care center.*

disabled. The adult child can be a caregiver if the elderly parent is ill or disabled. Many children choose to care for a parent so that a nursing home is not required. They first want to try the role of caregiver. A nursing home is an alternative if they find they cannot give the care needed.

As explained on p. 99, living with an adult child is a social change. The parent, adult child, and the child's family all need to adjust. Sleeping arrangements may change if an extra bedroom is not available. If the parent is very ill, a hospital bed may be needed. It may need to go in a living room or dining room.

The adult child's family will still need time alone. Other brothers and sisters may help give care. Respite care (see Chapter 4) may be needed when family vacations are planned. Home care agencies may be used to provide nurses or home health care aides. Community and church groups may have volunteers who can help give care.

Adult day-care centers. Adult children may still need to work even though the elderly parent cannot be left alone. Adult day-care centers provide meals, supervision, and activities for the elderly. Some provide transportation from home to the center.

Eligibility requirements may vary. Some may require that the person be able to walk using a cane or walker if needed. Others allow wheelchairs. Most require that the person be capable of some self-care activities.

Various activities are available at the facility. Cards, board games, movies, crafts, dancing, walks, and lectures are some examples (Fig. 6-7). Some provide bowling and swimming opportunities. All the activities are supervised, and assistance is given as needed.

Intergenerational day-care centers are a new trend. Children and elderly persons are cared for in the same center. Both groups benefit. The elders and the children work together on some of the same activities. They eat

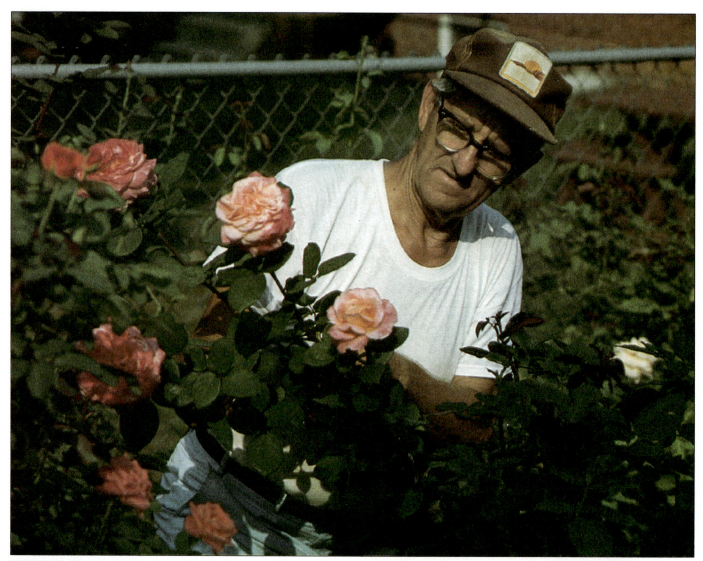

FIGURE 6-8 *This man is enjoying gardening. Apartment living usually does not provide opportunities for gardening or other yard work.*

together and play together. Young children bring out much joy and caring in the elderly whether healthy, ill, or disabled. The children give older persons purpose, love, and affection. In turn, children learn about aging. Intergenerational day-care gives them the opportunity to receive love and affection from elderly persons.

Apartments

Apartments have some advantages for elderly persons. Maintenance, yard work, snow removal, and repair of major appliances are the landlord's responsibility. The elders still can be independent. Personal belongings can be kept. Rent, however, can be costly. Utility bills are another expense. Many elderly persons enjoy gardening and yard work (Fig. 6-8). Apartment living usually does not provide those opportunities.

Residential Hotels

Some cities have residential hotels. Private rooms or efficiency apartments can be rented. Food services may include a dining room, cafeteria, or room service. Recreational activities and emergency medical services may be provided. Most hotels are close to shopping areas, churches, and other civic services. Residential hotels and apartments have similar disadvantages.

Senior Citizen Housing

State and federal funds have helped to build housing for senior citizens. An elderly person or couple can live independently in an apartment near people of the same age. The buildings have wheelchair access, handrails, elevators, and other safety measures. Apartments may be furnished. Appliances are arranged to meet the special needs of the elderly. Many services may be available. There usually is a dining room and a nurse or doctor on call. A daily telephone call is made to check on each tenant. Transportation usually is available to church, the doctor, or shopping areas. The residents pay monthly rent. If government funds are involved, however, rent usually is less than that for a regular apartment.

Nursing Facilities

Nursing facilities are housing alternatives for elderly persons who can no longer care for themselves (see Chapter 1). Nursing facilities offer different levels of care. Some merely provide room, food, and laundry services. Others provide nursing, rehabilitation, dietary, recreational, social, and religious services.

Some people stay in nursing facilities for the rest of their lives. Others stay until they can return to their own homes. The nursing facility is the person's temporary or permanent home. The surroundings are made as homelike as possible (Fig. 6-9).

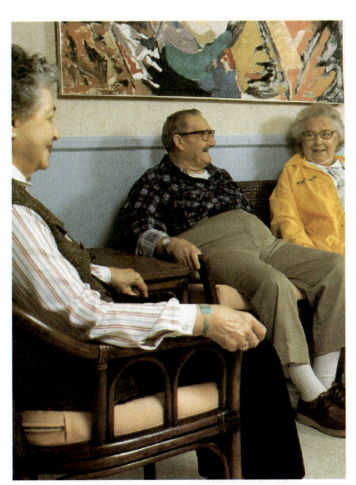

FIGURE 6-9 *The atmosphere of a nursing facility is similar to that of a home.*

Nursing facilities are designed to meet the special needs of elderly persons. Physical changes of aging and the safety needs of the elderly are considered in the design and construction of the facility. The following features are desirable in a nursing facility.

1. Elevators or a one-level building
2. Spacious and uncluttered areas
3. Handrails along hallways
4. Adequate lighting without shadows or glares
5. Floors that are carpeted or not heavily waxed
6. Pleasant landscaping
7. Variations in the use of color
8. Acoustics for noise control
9. Ventilation for control of odors
10. Smoke detectors and a sprinkling system
11. Emergency exits
12. Windows with a pleasant view of the outdoors

Many facilities have independent living units. A wing of the facility has small apartments. Elderly persons living alone or elderly couples live in the units. They perform personal hygiene activities and take their own medications. Food services are available, and help is nearby if needed. Each person, however, takes care of himself or herself. Little supervision or assistance is needed.

Long-term care units in hospitals are common. These units are for persons who still need skilled care but not to the extent previously required. At one time these individuals were transferred to nursing facilities. Now they can receive skilled care on the long-term care unit. Some eventually go home. Others may go to nursing facilities.

Most nursing facilities receive Medicare or Medicaid funds. Such facilities must meet OBRA requirements (see Chapters 1 and 2). OBRA protects the resident's rights and sets standards to promote quality of life. Funding will not occur if the requirements are not met. Unannounced surveys are conducted to determine if nursing facilities are meeting OBRA requirements.

Quality of life. The move to a nursing facility can renew feelings of loneliness and isolation. Developing new friendships will help residents adjust to the facility and improve their quality of life. Most residents develop new social relationships within the facility. Others may avoid social contacts for various reasons. Some people are quiet, private persons who have never been sociable. You need to respect their wishes for privacy. Some residents cannot visit with friends or get to activities without assistance. Offer to take them to visit in a friend's room or to a special activity. Those trying to cope with many losses may find it hard to talk to others. Encourage the person to talk about the losses. He or she may find that other residents have similar losses. Urinary frequency or incontinence may cause elderly persons to avoid social activities. These individuals should be taken to the bathroom before the event or visit or given incontinent briefs (see Chapter 13). People usually need to feel good about their appearance before they feel comfortable with others. Help residents with grooming (shaving, make-up, hair). Help them to dress in clothes of their choosing. Make sure that dentures, eyeglasses, and hearing aids are in place. Chapter 12 discusses personal hygiene and grooming procedures.

ABUSE OF ELDERLY PERSONS

Elderly abuse has become more evident in society. The abuser usually is a family member or a person caring for the elderly person. There are different forms of abuse. The person may be intentionally harmed.

1. *Physical abuse* involves hitting, slapping, kicking, pinching, and beating. Physical injury and pain may result. The person may be deprived of needed medical services or treatment.
2. *Verbal abuse* can be described as the use of oral or written words or statements that speak badly of, sneer at, criticize, or condemn the person. OBRA guidelines also include unkind gestures as a form of verbal abuse.
3. *Involuntary seclusion* is confining the person to a specific area. Elderly people have been locked in closets, basements, attics, and other spaces.
4. *Financial abuse* is the use by another person of the elderly person's money.
5. *Mental abuse* relates to humiliation and threats of being punished or deprived of such things as food, clothing, care, a home, or a place to sleep.
6. *Sexual abuse* is when the person is harassed about sex or is attacked sexually. The person may be forced to perform sexual acts out of fear of punishment or physical harm.

Abuse of elderly persons can occur in their own homes, hospitals, or nursing facilities. Often the abuse is unrecognized. There are many signs of elderly abuse. Any one of the following may indicate abuse.

1. Living conditions are unsafe, unclean, or inadequate.
2. Personal hygiene is lacking. The person is unclean, and clothes are dirty.
3. Weight loss occurs, with signs of poor nutrition and inadequate fluid intake.
4. There are frequent injuries, which occur under strange or seemingly impossible circumstances.
5. Old and new bruises are seen.
6. The person seems very quiet or withdrawn.
7. The person seems fearful, anxious, or agitated.
8. The individual does not seem to want to talk or answer questions.
9. The person is restrained or locked in a certain area for long periods of time. Toilet facilities, food and water, and other needed items cannot be reached.
10. Private conversations are not allowed. The caregiver is present during all conversations.
11. The person seems anxious to please the caregiver.
12. Medications are not taken properly. Medications are not purchased, or too much or too little medication is taken.
13. Emergency room visits may be frequent.
14. The person may go from one doctor to another or may not have a doctor.

OBRA and state laws require the reporting of elderly abuse. If abuse is suspected, it must be reported. Where and how to report suspected abuse varies in each state. If you need to report suspected abuse, you must give as much information as possible. The reporting agency will take action based on the information given. They act immediately if there is a life-threatening situation. Sometimes the help of police or the courts is necessary.

Helping abused elderly persons is not always easy or possible. The abuse may never be reported or recognized. Sometimes the investigating agency cannot gain access to the person. Some elderly persons are abused by their children, and a victim may want to protect the child. Some victims are embarrassed or believe the abuse is deserved. A victim may be afraid of what will happen. He or she may think that the present situation is better than no care at all. Some people fear they will not be believed if they report the abuse themselves.

Elderly abuse is an unfortunate situation. You may suspect that a person is being abused. If so, discuss the situation and your observations with your supervisor. Give the nurse as much information as possible. The nurse will then contact the appropriate members of the health care team. The agency that investigates elderly abuse in your community will be contacted.

SUMMARY

Aging is a normal process. Body functions slow down and become less efficient. Most individuals, however, function independently. They enjoy life with loved ones and friends. For others aging can be difficult. Family and friends may have moved away or died. The physical changes of aging, disease, and illness can make even the most simple, everyday tasks difficult or impossible. Income may not cover monthly living expenses. There may be little or no money for medical bills and medicines. Leaving the home of a lifetime for a nursing facility often is the only alternative.

Many people dread having to live in a nursing facility. OBRA, however, protects those who need to be in nursing facilities. Some of the many OBRA requirements relate to resident rights and quality of life.

Some elderly persons are abused. Their needs and problems present additional concerns. You must be alert to the possibility that a person is being abused. You can help the victim by discussing the situation with the nurse as soon as possible.

You need to understand the physical, psychological, and social changes that accompany aging. Imagine yourself being old. Put yourself in the place of the elderly person. The aged person depends on you for assistance in meeting basic needs. You can more effectively meet these needs if you can appreciate the person's situation. Patience, tolerance, and kindness are needed when working with elders. Their behaviors, habits, and body changes may seem unusual. However, they still need love and the companionship of others. You can help bring happiness and cheer to elders. Above all, treat them with respect and dignity.

Review QUESTIONS

Circle the *best* answer.

1. People between the ages of 65 and 85 are considered to be the
   a. Young-old
   b. Old
   c. Old-old
   d. Elderly

2. The study of the aging process is called
   a. Geriatrics
   b. Dysphagia
   c. Gerontology
   d. Dyspnea

3. Retirement usually results in
   a. Lower income
   b. Physical changes from aging
   c. Less free time
   d. Financial security

4. Elderly persons may experience loneliness because
   a. Children may have moved away
   b. Of difficulties communicating with others
   c. Relatives and friends may have died or moved
   d. All of the above

5. When elderly persons live with their children, they often feel
   a. Independent
   b. Wanted and a part of things
   c. Useless
   d. Dignified

6. Death of a spouse results in the loss of a
   a. Friend
   b. Companion
   c. Lover
   d. All of the above

7. Changes occur in the skin during the aging process. Care should include all of the following *except*
   a. Providing lap robes for warmth
   b. Applying lotion
   c. Using soap daily
   d. Providing good skin care

8. An elderly person has cold feet. You should
   a. Provide socks
   b. Apply a hot water bottle
   c. Soak the feet in hot water
   d. Apply a heating pad

9. Changes occur in the musculoskeletal system. Which is *false?*
   a. Bones become brittle and can break easily.
   b. Bed rest is needed because of loss of strength.
   c. Joints become stiff and painful.
   d. Range-of-motion exercises help to slow down the rate of musculoskeletal changes.

10. Changes occur in the nervous system. Which is *true?*
    a. More sleep is needed than when younger.
    b. Recent events are remembered better than past events.
    c. Sensitivity to pain is reduced.
    d. Confusion occurs in every elderly person.

11. Reduced blood supply to the brain can result in
    a. Confusion
    b. Dizziness
    c. Fatigue
    d. All of the above

12. Changes occur in the eye. Which is *false?*
    a. Night vision is decreased.
    b. Blue and green colors are the easiest colors to see.
    c. The lids become thin and wrinkled.
    d. The eye is easily irritated by dust particles.

13. Hearing loss in the elderly can be caused by
    a. Changes in the auditory nerve
    b. Atrophy of the eardrums
    c. Impacted ear wax
    d. All of the above

14. Arteries lose their elasticity and become narrow. These changes result in
    a. A slower heart rate
    b. Lower blood pressure
    c. A decrease in the amount of blood in the body
    d. Poor circulation to many parts of the body

15. An elderly person has cardiovascular changes. Care should include the following *except*
    a. Placing personal items in a convenient location
    b. A moderate amount of daily exercise
    c. Planning activities to avoid exertion
    d. Walking long distances

Review QUESTIONS

16. Respiratory changes occur with aging. Which is *false?*
    a. Heavy bed linens prevent normal chest expansion.
    b. Frequent turning and repositioning are necessary for the person on bed rest.
    c. The side-lying position is the best for breathing when there are respiratory changes.
    d. The person should be as active as possible.

17. Elderly persons should avoid dry foods because of
    a. Decreases in saliva
    b. Loss of teeth or ill-fitting dentures
    c. Decreased amounts of digestive juices
    d. Decreased peristalsis

18. Changes occur in the digestive system. The elderly person should avoid
    a. Cooked fruits and vegetables
    b. Foods high in protein
    c. Apricots and celery
    d. All of the above

19. Changes occur in the urinary system. Which is *true?*
    a. Kidneys increase in size.
    b. Fluids are important for kidney function.
    c. The bladder becomes larger.
    d. There is increased blood flow to the kidneys.

20. The doctor has ordered an increased fluid intake for an elderly resident. You should
    a. Give most of the fluid before noon.
    b. Give most of the fluid before 5:00 PM.
    c. Offer only water.
    d. Start a bladder training program.

21. Which housing alternative does *not* allow elderly persons to live independently?
    a. Apartments
    b. Residential hotels
    c. Senior citizen housing
    d. A nursing facility

22. Residents may avoid socializing in the nursing facility because
    a. They are normally quiet, private persons.
    b. They need assistance getting to and from activities.
    c. They may be bothered by urinary frequency or incontinence.
    d. All of the above.

23. Which is *not* a sign of elderly abuse?
    a. Stiff joints and joint pain
    b. Old and new bruises
    c. Poor personal hygiene
    d. Frequent injuries

24. You suspect a resident has been abused. What should you do?
    a. Tell the family.
    b. Call a state agency.
    c. Tell the nurse about your suspicion.
    d. Ask the resident if he or she has been abused.

Answers

1. b	7. c	13. d	19. b
2. c	8. a	14. d	20. b
3. a	9. b	15. d	21. d
4. d	10. c	16. c	22. d
5. c	11. d	17. a	23. a
6. d	12. b	18. c	24. d

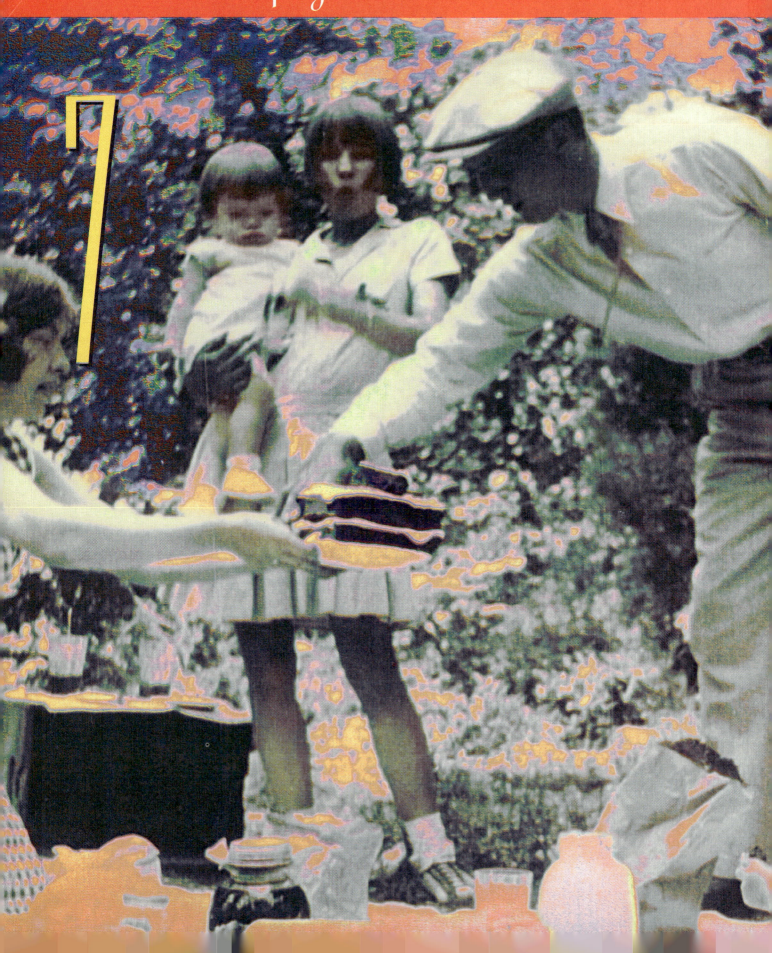

7

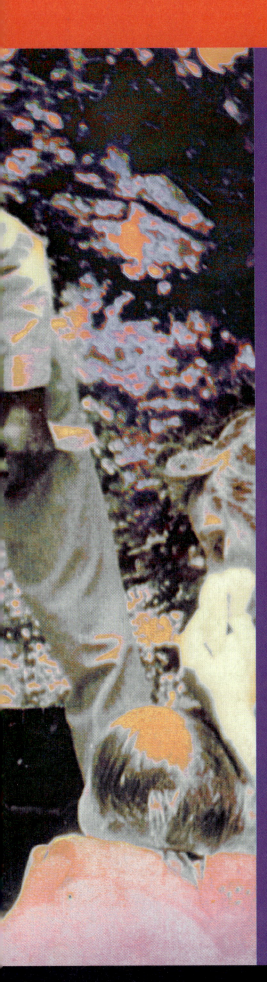

What You Will LEARN

- The key terms listed in this chapter

- Seven reasons why some persons cannot protect themselves

- Common safety hazards in nursing facilities

- Why residents are identified before receiving care and how to accurately identify them

- Safety measures that help to prevent falls

- The purpose of restraints and the required safety rules

- The information that must be reported to the nurse when restraints are used

- How to prevent common equipment-related accidents

- The accidents and errors that need to be reported

- The safety measures for fire prevention and the use of oxygen

- What to do if there is a fire

- The difference between natural disasters and those caused by human beings

- The safety procedures in this chapter

coma
State of being completely unaware of one's surroundings and unable to react or respond

dementia
Set of chronic symptoms in which a person loses memory and the ability to think and reason

disaster
Sudden, catastrophic event in which many people are injured and killed and property is destroyed

ground
That which carries leaking electricity to the earth and away from the electrical appliance

hemiplegia
Paralysis on one side of the body

paraplegia
Paralysis from the waist down

quadriplegia
Paralysis from the neck down

restraint
Devices or chemicals that limit freedom of movement or prevent access to one's body

suffocation
The termination of breathing that results from lack of oxygen

...need to remember to ask for help when getting up. Its just that I want to do things for myself. I don't like needing help.

Safety is a basic need of all people. This is especially true of residents in nursing facilities. These persons have limited physical or mental abilities. They are prone to accident and injury. Many people think that health facilities are free of dangers and hazards. This is not true. Accidental injuries occur in health care facilities. Death has resulted in rare instances.

You and other health care workers are responsible for the safety of residents in nursing facilities. You must practice ordinary and sometimes extraordinary precautions to keep these special persons safe. However, you must not interfere with the resident's rights as outlined by OBRA (see pp. 8-10).

THE SAFE ENVIRONMENT

All health care workers are responsible for ensuring a safe environment. A safe environment is one in which a resident has a very low risk of becoming ill or injured. The resident feels safe and secure, both physically and psychologically. There is little risk of infection, falling, being burned or poisoned, or suffering other injuries. The person is comfortable in relation to temperature, noise, and smells. There is enough lighting and room to move about safely. The person is not afraid and has few worries and concerns.

WHY SOME RESIDENTS CANNOT PROTECT THEMSELVES

There are many reasons why some residents cannot protect themselves. Age, impaired vision or hearing, reduced awareness, and limited mobility are some factors. You need to know the factors that increase a resident's risk of accident so that you can provide for safety.

Age

Most residents are elderly. They are at risk for accidents because of changes in their bodies from aging and chronic illness. They have decreased strength, move slowly, and may be unsteady. Balance may be affected, causing them to fall easily. Because of these physical changes, they cannot move quickly and suddenly to avoid dangers. Other factors make elderly persons prone to accidents and injuries. These include decreased sensitivity to heat and cold, poor vision, hearing problems, and a decreased sense of smell.

Awareness of Surroundings

People need to be aware of their surroundings to protect themselves from injury. Some residents are totally unaware of their surroundings because of illness or injuries. These residents are unconscious or in a **coma.** Coma is defined as a state of being completely unaware of one's surroundings and unable to react or respond. A person in a coma cannot react or respond to people, places, or things. This individual must rely on you and others for protection.

Some persons suffer from **dementia** as a result of certain diseases or injuries. Dementia is a set of chronic symptoms in which a person loses memory and the ability to think and reason. These persons are confused, disoriented, and have a reduced awareness of their surroundings. Demented persons, especially the demented elderly, are very prone to accidents and injury. Some are helpless and totally dependent on others for safety. Others are less helpless. However, they are more dangerous to themselves because of poor judgment. They no longer know what is safe and what is dangerous. They may get into closets, cupboards, or other unsafe and unlocked areas. They may eat or drink cleaning chemicals, medicines, or other poisons.

Impaired Vision

Persons with poor vision have difficulty seeing objects. They often are in danger of falling or tripping over equipment, furniture, or electrical cords. They also may have problems reading labels on containers. This may cause them to mistake such things as perfume, aftershave lotion, hand lotion, or cleaning agents for substances that can be eaten or drunk.

Impaired Hearing

Persons with impaired hearing may have problems hearing warning signals or fire alarms. They may not hear approaching meal carts, medicine carts, or residents in wheelchairs. All workers must make sure that the hearing impaired are out of the way when carts, wheelchairs, or other equipment is being moved through hallways.

Smell and Touch

Smell and touch can be affected by age and illness. If the sense of smell is reduced, a person may be unaware of smoke or gas fumes. People with reduced sense of touch may be burned easily. They may have difficulty sensing the difference between heat and cold. Some residents may have a decreased pain sense and may injure themselves without knowing it. For example, a resident with new shoes may develop a blister without feeling it. If the person has poor circulation to the legs and feet, the blister can become a more serious wound.

Impaired Mobility

Some people have crippling diseases or injuries that make it impossible to move out of danger. Those with arthritis may be unable to walk or propel wheelchairs. Some residents may be paralyzed. **Paraplegia** is paralysis from the waist down. **Quadriplegia** is paralysis from the neck down. Persons with **hemiplegia** are paralyzed on one side of the body. These individuals may be unable to sense pain, heat, or cold. They may be aware of their surroundings and danger but cannot physically move to safety. Part of your job is to keep them safe.

Medications

Medications can affect people in many ways. This is especially true of elderly persons. Side effects include loss of balance, reduced awareness, confusion, disorientation, drowsiness, and lack of coordination. These changes may cause the resident to become fearful and uncooperative. Report these or other unusual behaviors to the nurse.

SAFETY IN THE HEALTH FACILITY

Providing a safe environment for residents is the responsibility of all health care workers. Residents in your care must be properly identified so that they receive the right care and treatment. You must be alert to safety hazards that can cause poisoning, burns, suffocation, the spread of infection, and falls. If you cannot correct a safety hazard, promptly tell the nurse.

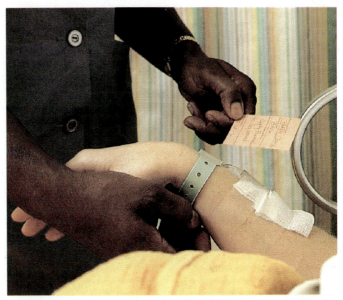

FIGURE 7-2 *A nursing assistant checks the resident's identification bracelet and calls the resident by name before giving care.*

Identifying Your Residents

You will care for several different residents. Each has different treatments, therapies, and activity limitations. Residents must be protected from infections, falls, and equipment-related accidents. Safety also involves giving care to the right person. A resident's life and health can be threatened if the wrong care is given.

Most residents receive identification (ID) bracelets when admitted to the facility. The resident's name, room and bed number, age, religion, doctor, facility name, and other identifying information are shown on the bracelet (Fig 7-1).

The ID bracelet is used to identify the resident before care is given (Fig 7-2). Also call the resident by name while checking the ID bracelet. Calling the resident by name is a courtesy that should be given as the person is being touched and before care is provided. Calling the resident by name, however, is not a reliable way to identify the resident. Confused, disoriented, drowsy, or hearing-impaired residents may respond to any name.

Some nursing facilities have an identification system that uses photographs. The resident's photograph is taken at admission and placed in the person's medical record for identification purposes. If your facility uses such a system, you must to learn to use it safely.

Poisoning

Accidental poisoning as a result of poor vision or mental confusion is a major health hazard in nursing facilities. Be sure that all hazardous materials cannot be reached by vision-impaired or confused residents.

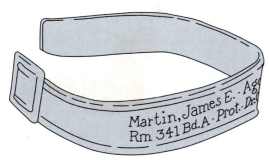

FIGURE 7-1 *Resident identification bracelet.*

Martin, James E. - Age
Rm 341 Bd.A - Prot.- Dr.

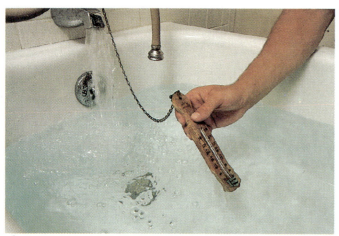

FIGURE 7-3 *A nursing assistant checks the temperature of the bath water.*

Burns

Smoking, spilled hot liquids, electrical appliances, and bath water that is too hot are common causes of burns in nursing facilities.

The following measures can prevent burns.

1. Be sure residents smoke only in smoking areas.
2. Do not leave smoking materials at the bedside unless the resident can be trusted to smoke alone and only in smoking areas.
3. Supervise the smoking of residents who cannot protect themselves.
4. Do not allow smoking in bed.
5. Check equipment for frayed cords and proper operation.
6. Do not allow space heaters in residents' rooms or recreational areas.
7. Do not allow residents to sleep with heating pads.
8. Do not use electric blankets.
9. Check the temperature of the bath water before assisting the resident into the tub (Fig. 7-3).

Suffocation

Suffocation is the termination of breathing that results from lack of oxygen. Death occurs if the person does not start breathing again. Some causes of suffocation include choking on an object, drowning, inhaling gas or smoke, strangulation, and electrical shock. The following safety measures can help prevent suffocation.

1. Cut food into small, bite-sized pieces for residents who cannot do so themselves.
2. Be sure dentures are in place and that the resident can properly chew food being served.
3. Report loose dentures to the nurse.
4. Be sure that a resident has no swallowing problems before giving between-meal snacks or beverages. Some residents may ask you for items that they cannot swallow.

5. If a resident is having difficulty swallowing, promptly tell the nurse.
6. If a resident has a feeding tube in place, do not give food or liquids by mouth unless instructed to do so by the nurse.
7. Never leave a resident unattended in the bathtub.
8. Move all residents from the area if you smell gas or smoke.
9. Be sure that all restraints are used properly (pp. 116-125).
10. Be sure that all electrical cords and appliances are in good repair.

Preventing the Spread of Microorganisms

The spread of infection is a major hazard in health care facilities. Infections are caused by microorganisms that are easily spread from one person to another. The elderly, chronically ill, and disabled are at risk for infections. Infections increase their health problems. Good handwashing helps prevent the spread of infection. Chapter 8 describes how to prevent infections.

Preventing Falls

Falls are the most common accidents in nursing facilities. Falls may result from spills, weakness or dizziness, unfamiliar environment, and medication. Residents may be unable to protect themselves because of confusion, disorientation, or paralysis. Side rails, handrails, and restraints are some safety devices used to prevent falls.

Side rails. Side rails are placed on the sides of hospital beds. They can be raised or lowered. Levers, latches, or buttons lock them in place in the raised position. They protect the resident from falling out of bed. The resident can use the side rails to help move and turn in bed. Side rails can be half the length or the full length of the bed (Fig. 7-4). If the half length side rail is used (see

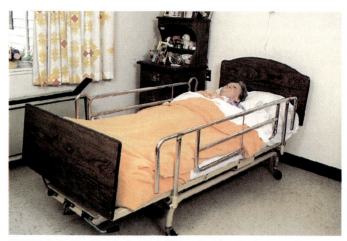

FIGURE 7-4 *Hospital bed with full-length side rails locked in the raised position.*

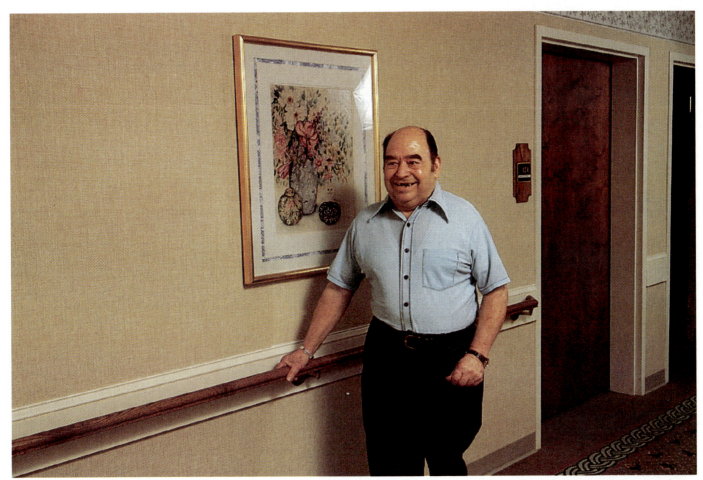

FIGURE 7-5 *An elderly man uses the handrails for support while he is walking.*

Fig. 11-1, p. 210), there usually are two rails on each side. One rail is for the upper part of the bed and the other for the lower part. Side rails are necessary when the bed is raised, as well as for residents who are unconscious or sedated with medication. Side rails must be kept up at all times for these persons except when bedside nursing care is given. Confused or disoriented residents also may need side rails. Ask the nurse which confused residents need the side rails up.

Side rails keep residents from getting out of bed. Therefore they are considered restraints by OBRA. They cannot be used without permission of the resident or the resident's legal guardian. Restraints and OBRA requirements are discussed in this chapter on p. 116.

The procedures in this textbook include the use of side rails. This is done to help you to remember their importance and to use them correctly. If a resident uses his or her right under OBRA not to have side rails, they are not used. You can then omit the steps asking you to lower the side rail at the beginning of the procedure and to raise the side rails at the end of the procedure. *However, whenever the bed is raised to give care or perform a procedure, the side rails must be raised to prevent the resident from falling. The right not to use side rails applies only when the bed is in its lowest position. Be sure to explain to the resident why the side rails are being used.*

Handrails. Handrails are found in hallways (Fig. 7-5) and in the bathrooms of nursing facilities. They provide support for those who are weak or unsteady when walking. They also provide support when residents sit down or get up from a toilet. Handrails also are found along bathtubs and showers for use in getting in and out (Figs. 12-22 and 12-23, pp. 251-252). Handrails are always found in stairways.

Other safety measures. You need to practice other safety measures to prevent residents from falling.

1. Keep the resident's bed in the lowest position except when giving bedside nursing care. The distance from the bed to the floor is reduced if the resident falls or gets out of bed.

2. Have a night light on in the resident's room. The resident who awakens during the night can see. This prevents fear and confusion, and the nursing staff can see in the resident's room.

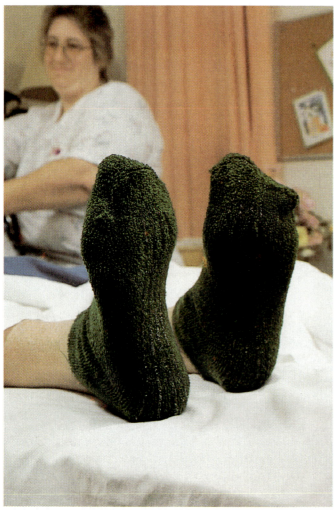

FIGURE 7-6 *Nonskid socks help prevent falls.*

3. Keep floors free of spills and excess furniture.
4. Have residents wear *nonskid* shoes, slippers, or socks when they are up (Fig. 7-6). They should not wear soft bedroom slippers or regular socks.
5. Make sure crutches, canes, and walkers have nonskid tips to prevent slipping and skidding on floors.
6. Keep canes, crutches, and walkers that are not in use out of the way of other residents.
7. Keep the resident's signal light within reach at all times. Explain how to use signal lights, and ask the resident to call for assistance whenever help is needed. The signal light is described in Chapter 10.
8. Lock the wheels of beds, wheelchairs, and stretchers when you transfer residents to or from them.
9. Use a gait belt at all times when you transfer a resident to or from a chair (see Fig. 9-22).
10. Use caution when turning corners, entering corridor intersections, and going through doors. You could bump into and injure another person who may be coming from the other direction.

Restraints

Restraints are devices or chemicals that limit freedom of movement or access to one's body. They are used to protect residents from harming themselves or others. Restraints may be physical or chemical.

OBRA states that residents have the right to be free from restraint (see Chapter 1). However, OBRA does not prevent the use of restraints entirely. Restraints can be used for the physical safety of the resident or other residents. A doctor's order is needed. Restraints cannot be used for staff convenience or to discipline or punish the resident.

A

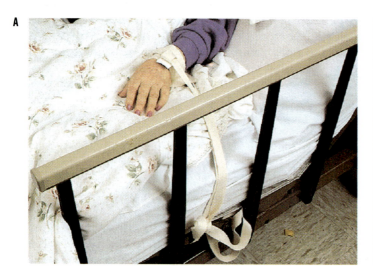

B

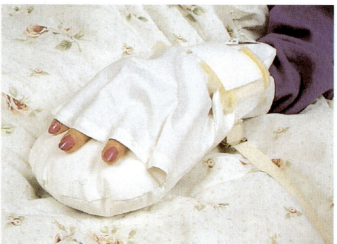

FIGURE 7-7 *Restraints.* **A,** *Limb holder (wrist restraint).* **B,** *Mitt restraint.*

Physical restraints have been defined by law. The definition of physical restraints includes the following key points:

1. May be any manual method, physical or mechanical device, material, or equipment
2. Are attached to or next to the resident's body
3. Cannot easily be removed by the resident
4. Restrict freedom of movement or access to one's body

Restraints can be applied to the wrists, hands, chest, or waist (Fig. 7-7). There also are special types of furniture or barriers that prevent residents from moving about freely. Geriatric chairs or chairs with attached trays that residents cannot remove are other examples (Fig. 7-8). These chairs often are used for residents who cannot sit

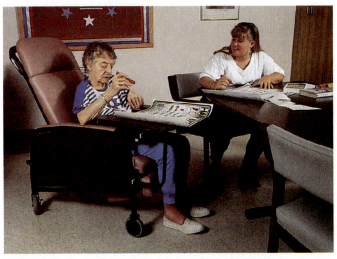

FIGURE 7-8 *The geriatric chair also is a physical restraint.*

C

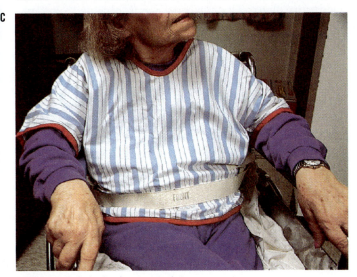

FIGURE 7-7 *C*, *Jacket/vest restraint.*

D

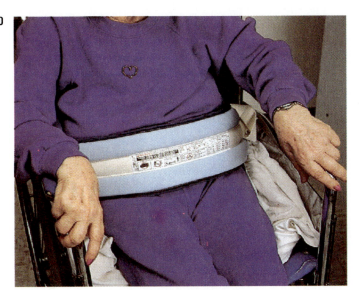

FIGURE 7-7 *D*, *Belt restraint. (Courtesy Posey Co., Arcadia, Calif.)*

up without support. Remember that residents in physical restraints are dependent on you. You must meet their basic needs for food, fluids, and elimination. Physical restraints are used to prevent residents from any of the following:

1. Falling out of bed or from a chair, wheelchair, or stretcher
2. Crawling over side rails or the foot of the bed
3. Interfering with therapies (pulling out tubes, removing dressings, or disconnecting equipment)
4. Harming themselves or others

Chemical restraints are drugs used for discipline or the convenience of the staff and not required for medical treatment. OBRA does not allow the use of chemical restraints. However, drugs may be used to help confused or disoriented residents. These residents may become anxious, agitated, or aggressive. The doctor may order medication to control these behaviors. The goal is to control the behavior without making the resident sleepy and unable to function at the person's highest level. Residents who cannot be controlled usually are transferred to a facility that can meet their special needs.

There are certain considerations you must understand regarding the use of physical restraints.

   1. *Restraints are for protecting residents, not for staff convenience.* Restraining a resident often is easier for the staff than providing necessary supervision, observation, and care. OBRA regulations and professional ethics, however, prevent their use for staff convenience. Restraints are used only as safety precautions for residents. Never use restraints to punish or penalize residents.

   2. *Restraints require a doctor's order.* OBRA and state laws protect residents from unnecessary restraint. There must be a specific medical symptom that requires the use of restraints. In addition, nursing facilities have

policies and procedures about the use of restraints. If a resident needs to be restrained, a doctor's written order must be obtained. The doctor is required by law to give the reason for the restraint. The order and the reason for it will be on the resident's Kardex and care plan. You need to know the laws and facility policies about using restraints.

3. *If restraints are needed, the least restrictive method must be used.* For example, a stroke victim forgets that she cannot stand without assistance. She may be given a removable wheelchair safety belt. The belt reminds her to ask for help before trying to stand. However, it can be removed easily by the resident.

4. *Restraints are used only when other methods of controlling or protecting the resident have been tried.* Many alternatives to restraints are available. The health care team must try other ways of controlling the undesirable behavior first. For example, Mr. Brown often becomes agitated and combative. That is, he hits others when he is upset and disturbed. The health care team needs to determine what things agitate Mr. Brown. His care plan should then list those factors and the measures to help calm him. Restraint alternatives may include television, radio, or music; frequent visits; touch; back rubs; family visits; and a calm approach.

5. *Restraint of a resident unnecessarily constitutes false imprisonment (see Chapter 2).* If you are told to use a restraint, its need must be clearly evident and understood. If not, politely request an explanation. If you apply restraints unnecessarily, you may be charged with false imprisonment.

6. *Restraints require the consent of the resident or the resident's legal guardian.* The resident or the resident's legal guardian must be informed about the need and purpose of the restraint. They also must be told the possible bad effects of restraints: incontinence, weakness, loss of range of motion, reduced social contact, and depression. The doctor or nurse will discuss the need with the family.

7. *Restraints must be used according to the manufacturer's instructions.* The manufacturer will give specific instructions on how the restraint must be applied and secured. Failure to follow such instructions could affect the resident's safety. You could be found negligent for improperly applying the restraint.

8. *The restrained resident's basic needs must be met by the nursing team.* A restraint should be applied so that it is snug and firm, but not tight. A tight restraint may interfere with circulation and breathing. The resident should be comfortable. Movement of the restrained part should be possible to a limited and safe extent. The resident must be checked frequently. Be sure to offer food and fluids and meet the resident's need for elimination.

9. *Restraints may have to be applied rapidly.* They need to be applied with enough help to protect the resident and staff members from injury. Residents in immediate danger of harming themselves or others need to be restrained quickly. Combative and agitated residents can injure themselves and staff members while restraints are being applied. Enough staff members are needed to complete the task safely and efficiently.

10. *A resident may become more confused or agitated after a restraint has been applied.* Whether confused or alert, residents are aware of restricted body movements. They may try to get out of the restraint or struggle or pull at the restraint. These actions often are thought to be confused behaviors. Confused residents may become more confused because they do not understand what is happening to them. The resident needs repeated explanations and reassurance. Spending time with the resident often has a calming effect.

Safety rules. Although used to protect residents, restraints can be dangerous. If it is necessary to restrain a resident, you must observe the resident frequently. The person must be protected from complications that may result from being restrained. These include interferences with breathing and circulation, fractures, burns, and strangulation. Deaths have occurred from the improper use of restraints. You usually will be responsible for applying restraints as ordered. See List 7-1 for the safety measures that need to be practiced in caring for a restrained resident.

Reporting and recording. Certain information about restraints must be included in the resident's record. You may be instructed to apply restraints or be assigned to care for a restrained resident. You must report the following to the nurse:
1. The type of restraint applied
2. The time of application
3. The time of removal
4. The type of care given when the restraint was removed
5. The color and condition of the resident's skin
6. Whether a pulse is felt in the restrained extremity
7. Resident complaints of pain, numbness, or tingling in the restrained part
8. Areas of red or injured skin

Wrist restraints. Wrist restraints also are called hand restraints. They are used to limit the movement of an arm. Commercial wrist restraints usually are used. The procedure for applying wrist restraints is on p. 121.

Safety Measures for Using Restraints

1. Use the type of restraint specified by the nurse and the care plan. Also be sure you have the correct size.

2. Use only commercial restraint products that include manufacturer instructions for use. Do not use sheets, towels, tape, rope, straps, bandages, or other items to restrain a person.

3. Make sure the restraint is intact. There should be no tears, frayed edges, missing loops or straps, or other damage.

4. Never apply any restraint unless you have been instructed in its proper use. You should demonstrate proper application to the nurse before using it on a resident.

5. Do not use restraints to position a resident on a toilet.

6. Follow the facility policies and procedures for the application of restraints.

7. Follow the manufacturer's instructions for safe application. There are many different types of restraints. Some are safe for bed, chair, and wheelchair use. Others can be used only with certain equipment.

8. Make sure the resident is in good body alignment and comfortable before applying the restraint (see Chapter 9).

9. Pad bony areas and skin that may be injured by a restraint. Elderly residents have very fragile skin and may be quite thin. Padding protects body parts from pressure and injury.

10. Apply the restraint securely enough to protect the resident. Allow enough slack so that some movement of the part is possible.

11. Make sure the resident can breathe easily if a restraint has been applied to the chest.

12. Tie restraints according to facility policy. The facility policy should follow the manufacturer's instructions. Quick-release knots or square knots often are used (Fig. 7-9). The knot must be easily released in an emergency. Some restraints have quick-release buckles.

13. Secure the restraint to the movable part of the bed frame or to the bed springs (Fig. 7-10, p. 120). Never secure the restraint to the side rail. Residents may be injured when side rails are raised and lowered. Make sure the resident cannot reach the knot.

14. Make sure full side rails are up when using a vest or belt restraint (Fig. 7-11, p. 120). The side rails should be padded. The resident could accidentally fall off the bed and strangle on the restraint if side rails are not up. If half-length or three-quarter length side rails are used, the resident could get caught between them.

15. Do not criss-cross straps in the back of the resident unless part of manufacturer's instructions.

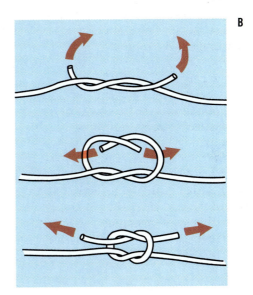

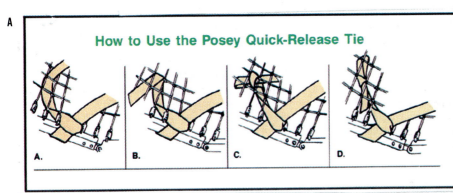

FIGURE 7-9 *A, Posey "quick-release" knot. B, Square knot. (A Courtesy Posey Company, Arcadia, CA.)*

Continued.

16. Check the resident's circulation every 15 minutes if wrist restraints have been applied. You should be able to feel a pulse at a pulse site below the restraint. Fingers or toes should be warm and pink in color.

17. Notify the nurse immediately if:
    a. You are unable to feel a pulse
    b. Fingers are cold, pale, or blue in color
    c. The resident complains of pain, numbness, or tingling in the restrained part
    d. The skin is red or damaged

18. Keep a scissors *in your pocket*. In an emergency, cutting the tie is faster than undoing the knot. Never leave scissors at the bedside or where residents might reach them.

19. Check the resident and the restraint every 15 to 30 minutes to make sure the resident is safe and comfortable. If possible, keep residents where they can be seen by the staff.

20. Remove the restraint and reposition the resident every 2 hours. Give skin care and exercise the part at this time.

21. Make sure the resident receives food and fluids while restrained. Be sure to offer a drink of water often. Toilet the resident or offer the bedpan or urinal every 2 hours.

22. Make sure the signal light always is within the resident's reach.

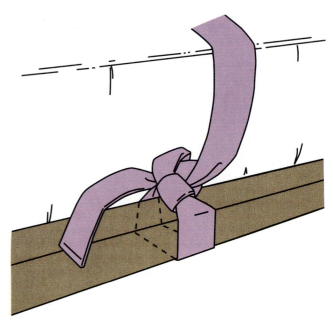

FIGURE 7-10 *The strap of the restraint is tied to the bed frame.*

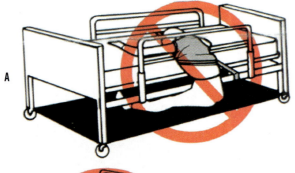

Full siderails should be in the UP position when using any vest or belt in bed. A siderail pad or seizure pad should be used to help prevent the patient from becoming entangled, injured or suffocated.

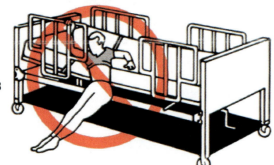

Do not use belts or vests with half- or three-quarter-siderails. The patient may be able to go around the siderail (or between the two half-siderails), fall partially off the bed and suffocate.

FIGURE 7-11 *A,* Full side rails should be used with vest or belt restraints. The side rails should be padded to prevent the resident from getting caught between the rails. *B,* Half-length side rails are dangerous for the restrained resident. (Courtesy Posey Co., Arcadia, Calif.)

PROCEDURE

Applying Wrist Restraints

1. Collect the wrist restraints.

2. Wash your hands.

3. Identify the resident. Check the ID bracelet and call the resident by name.

4. Explain what you are going to do.

5. Provide for privacy.

6. Make sure the resident is in a comfortable position and in good body alignment (see Chapter 9).

7. Apply the restraint. Make sure the soft portion is toward the skin (Fig. 7-12).

8. Check to make sure that the restraint is not too tight. You should be able to place two fingers between the restraint and the skin (Fig. 7-13).

9. Tie the ends to the bed frame or bed springs. Use a knot approved by your facility.

10. Check the pulse, color, and temperature of the restrained part every 15 minutes. Report your observations to the nurse.

11. Place the signal light within the resident's reach.

12. Unscreen the resident.

13. Wash your hands.

14. Remove the restraint every 2 hours, and reposition the resident. Meet the resident's needs for food, fluids, and elimination. Give skin care, perform range-of-motion exercises, and reapply the restraint.

15. Report your observations to the nurse.

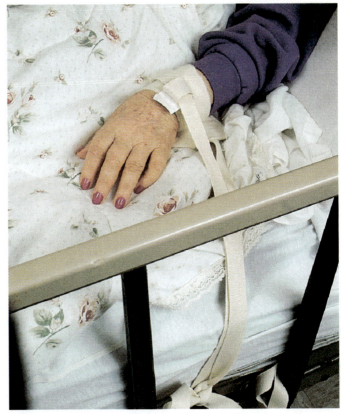

FIGURE 7-12 *The soft portion of the restraint is toward the skin.*

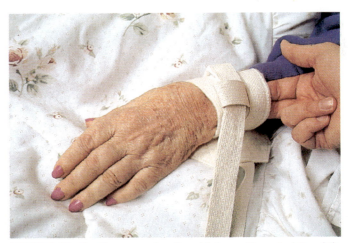

FIGURE 7-13 *Two fingers can be slipped between the restraint and the wrist.*

Mitt restraints. Hands are placed in mitt restraints. They prevent use of the fingers but do not prevent movement of the hands or wrists. The arms also can be immobilized by securing the straps to the bed frame. Mitt restraints are thumbless and prevent the resident from scratching, pulling out tubes, or removing dressings. The resident may be given a hand roll to grasp. The hand roll keeps the fingers in a normal position. A hand roll is not needed with a padded mitt. A padded mitt is made of a thick rounded pad. It is covered on the top with a light net so that tubelike openings are formed for the resident's fingers (Fig. 7-14).

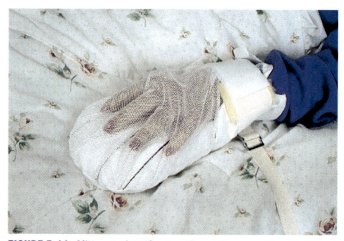

FIGURE 7-14 *Mitt restraint. (Courtesy Posey Company, Arcadia, CA.)*

PROCEDURE

Applying Mitt Restraints

1. Collect
   a. Two mitt restraints
   b. Two washcloths
   c. Tape

2. Make a hand roll (Fig. 7-15), or use a commercial one (Fig. 7-16) if padded mitts are not used.

3. Wash your hands.

4. Identify the resident. Check the ID bracelet and call the resident by name.

5. Explain what you are going to do.

6. Provide for privacy.

7. Make sure the resident's hands are clean and dry.

8. Give the resident a hand roll to grasp if a padded mitt is not used.

9. Apply the mitt restraint (Fig. 7-17).

10. Tie the straps to the bed frame or bed springs if the hand is to be immobilized. Use a knot approved by the facility.

11. Repeat steps 8, 9, and 10 for the other hand.

12. Place the signal light within reach.

13. Unscreen the resident.

14. Wash your hands.

15. Check the resident every 15 to 30 minutes.

16. Remove the restraint every 2 hours, and reposition the resident. Meet the resident's needs for food, fluids, and elimination. Give skin care, perform range-of-motion exercises, and reapply the restraint.

17. Report your observations to the nurse.

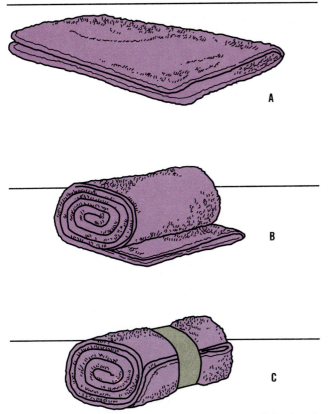

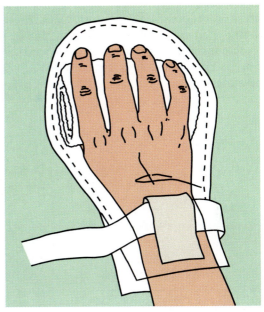

FIGURE 7-15 *Make a hand roll from a washcloth by following these steps.* **A,** *Fold the washcloth in half.* **B,** *Roll up the washcloth.* **C,** *Tape the rolled washcloth.*

FIGURE 7-17 *Mitt restraint applied with the resident grasping a hand roll.*

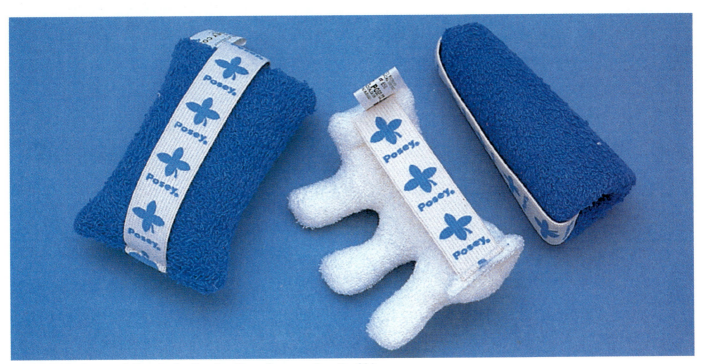

FIGURE 7-16 *Commercial hand rolls. (Courtesy Posey Company, Arcadia, CA.)*

Jacket and vest restraints. Jacket and vest restraints are applied to the chest. They protect the resident from falling out of the bed, a chair, or a wheelchair. The restraint is applied so that the vest crosses in front (Fig. 7-18). The vest must *never* cross in the back. If the straps are in the back, the restraint can slide up around the resident's neck and cause strangulation. (Some brands include this information on warning labels.) The restraint always is applied over clothes, pajamas, or gown. If used for a resident in a chair or wheelchair, the restraint should be tied under the chair, not behind the chair (Fig. 7-19). Remember, padded side rails must be up when jacket or vest restraints are used.

PROCEDURE

Applying a Jacket or Vest Restraint

1. Obtain a jacket or vest restraint in the correct size.

2. Get assistance if needed.

3. Wash your hands.

4. Identify the resident. Check the ID bracelet and call the resident by name.

5. Explain what you are going to do.

6. Provide for privacy.

7. Assist the resident to a sitting position by locking arms with the resident (see p. 163).

8. Slip the resident's arms through the arm holes of the restraint with your free hand. A vest should cross in front.

9. Make sure there are no wrinkles in the front or back of the restraint.

10. Help the resident lie down.

11. Bring the ties through the slots.

12. Make sure the resident is comfortable and in good body alignment (see Chapter 9).

13. Tie the straps to the bed frame or bed springs. Use a knot approved by the facility.

14. Make sure the restraint is not too tight. You should be able to slide your flat hand between the restraint and the resident (Fig. 7-20). Adjust the straps if necessary.

15. Place the signal light within reach.

16. Raise the side rails. Make sure they are padded.

17. Unscreen the resident.

18. Wash your hands.

19. Check the restraint every 15 to 30 minutes.

20. Remove the restraint every 2 hours, and reposition the resident. Meet the resident's needs for food, fluids, and elimination. Give skin care, perform range-of-motion exercises, and reapply the restraint.

21. Report your observations to the nurse.

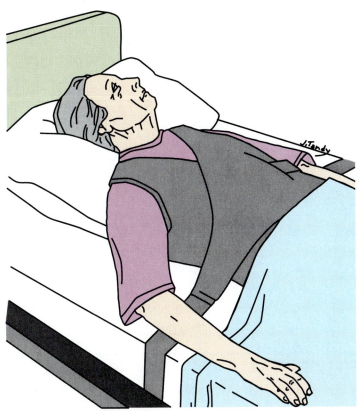

FIGURE 7-18 *Jacket restraint with the ties at the front.*

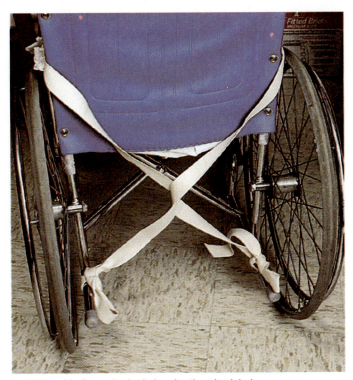

FIGURE 7-19 *Restraint is tied under the wheelchair.*

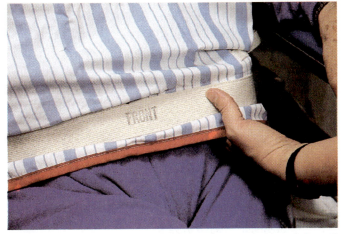

FIGURE 7-20 *A flat hand can slide between the restraint and the resident.*

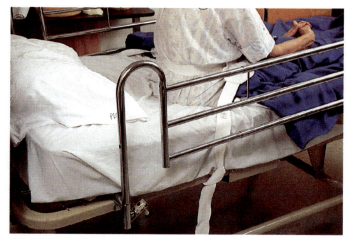

Safety belt. Safety belts (Fig. 7-21) serve the same purpose as jacket and vest restraints. The belt is applied around the resident's waist and secured to the bed or chair. The belt is applied over clothes, a gown, or pajamas. If the resident is sitting in a chair, the belt should be at a 45-degree angle over the hips (Fig. 7-22). Like the vest or jacket restraint, the safety belt is tied under the wheelchair. For residents in bed, padded side rails must be raised.

FIGURE 7-21 *A, Safety belt.*

PROCEDURE

Applying a Safety Belt

1. Obtain a safety restraint in the correct size.

2. Get assistance if needed.

3. Wash your hands.

4. Identify the resident. Check the ID bracelet and call the resident by name.

5. Explain what you are going to do.

6. Provide for privacy.

7. Assist the resident to a sitting position by locking arms with the resident (see p. 163).

8. Place the belt around the front of the resident's waist. Bring the ties to the back with your free hand.

9. Make sure there are no wrinkles in the front or back of the restraint.

10. Bring the ties through the slots.

11. Help the resident lie down.

12. Make sure the resident is comfortable and in good body alignment (see Chapter 9).

13. Tie the straps to the bed frame or bed springs. Use a knot approved by the facility. Lock the straps in place if the restraint locks.

14. Make sure the restraint is not too tight. You should be able to slide your flat hand between the restraint and the resident. Adjust the straps if necessary.

15. Place the signal light within reach.

16. Raise the side rails. Make sure they are padded.

17. Unscreen the resident.

18. Wash your hands.

19. Check the resident every 15 to 30 minutes.

20. Remove the restraint every 2 hours, and reposition the resident. Meet the resident's needs for food, fluids, and elimination. Give skin care, perform range-of-motion exercises, and reapply the restraint.

21. Report your observations to the nurse.

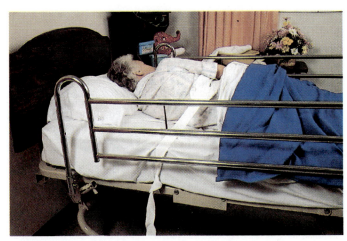

FIGURE 7-21 *B, Safety belt.*

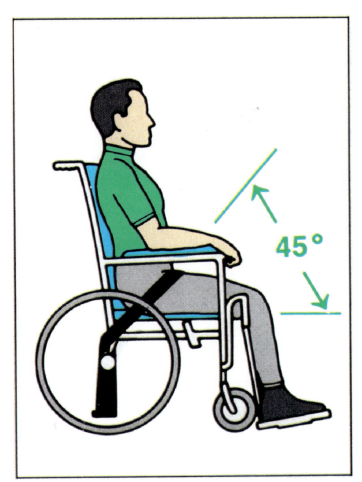

FIGURE 7-22 *The safety belt is at a 45-degree angle over the resident's hips. (Courtesy Posey Company, Arcadia, CA.)*

Quality OF LIFE

Sometimes residents need to be restrained to prevent them from injuring themselves or others. However, restraints should be used for as short a time as possible. A resident's need for restraints must be assessed regularly by the health care team. The resident's care plan should show how the use of restraints will slowly be reduced. The goal is to meet the resident's needs using as little restraint as possible.

Restrained residents depend on you to meet their needs for food, fluids, elimination, and exercise. Remember to provide such care every 2 hours. The care you give can help prevent contractures, incontinence, dehydration, and pressure sores. Psychosocial needs also must be met. You can meet these needs by taking residents to activities and visiting with them when you check on them and give care. Remember to check restrained residents every 15 to 30 minutes to make sure they are safe and comfortable.

Accidents Caused by Equipment

Glass and plastic equipment must be intact and checked before use. Equipment is checked for cracks, chips, and sharp or rough edges, which can easily cut, stab, or scratch residents. Do not use damaged equipment or give it to residents. Instead, take the item to the nurse, point out the defect, and discard the item as instructed.

Electrical equipment must work properly and be in good repair. Frayed cords (Fig. 7-23) and overloaded electrical outlets (Fig. 7-24) can cause electrical shocks that may result in death. The possibility of fires also exists. Frayed cords and equipment that does not function properly must be repaired by an adequately trained person.

Three-pronged plugs (Fig. 7-25) should be used on all equipment. Two prongs carry electrical current. The third prong is the **ground.** A ground carries leaking electricity to the earth, away from the equipment item. Thus leaking electricity cannot be conducted to a person and cause electrical shock and possibly death. Be sure to report the event if you receive a shock while using a piece of equipment. The item should be sent for repair.

Reporting Accidents and Errors

Accidents and errors must be reported immediately to your supervisor. This includes accidents involving residents, visitors, or staff members. You need to report errors in resident care. Errors include giving a wrong treat-

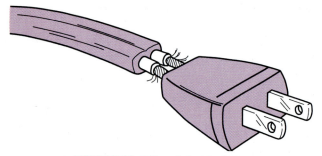

FIGURE 7-23 *A frayed electrical wire.*

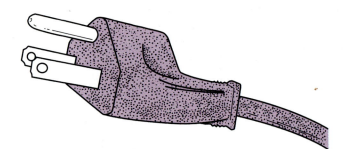

FIGURE 7-24 *A three-pronged plug.*

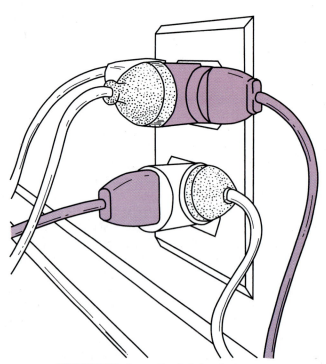

FIGURE 7-25 *An overloaded electrical outlet.*

ment, treating the wrong resident, or forgetting a treatment. Another kind of error is failure to follow special instructions. Examples are allowing a resident on bed rest to sit in a chair or giving too much fluid to a resident on fluid restrictions. Broken items owned by the resident, such as dentures or eyeglasses, must be reported. So should loss of money or clothing belonging to the resident.

When reporting accidents or errors, give the names of the persons involved and the date, time, and location of the accident or error. Also provide a complete description of what happened, names of any witnesses, and any other requested information. Most facilities require written reports about any accident or error. These are commonly called "incident reports."

FIRE SAFETY

Faulty electrical equipment and wiring, overloaded electrical circuits, and smoking are the major causes of fire in the United States. Fire is a constant danger in homes and health care facilities. The entire health care team must prevent fires and act quickly and responsibly in the event of a fire.

Fire and the Use of Oxygen

Three things are needed to start and maintain a fire: a spark or flame, a material that will burn, and oxygen. Air contains a certain amount of oxygen. Some residents, however, need more oxygen than is available in air. Doctors order supplemental oxygen for these residents. Supplemental oxygen is supplied in portable oxygen tanks, through wall outlets, or through air concentrators (see Chapter 21). Because oxygen is needed for fires, special safety precautions are practiced where oxygen is being given and stored.

1. "No smoking" signs are placed on the resident's door and near the bed.
2. Residents and visitors are politely reminded not to smoke in the resident's room.
3. Smoking materials (cigarettes, cigars, and pipes) matches, and lighters are removed from the room.
4. Electrical equipment is turned off *before* being unplugged. Sparks can occur when appliances are unplugged while still turned on.
5. Wool blankets and synthetic fabrics that cause static electricity are removed from the resident's room. The resident should wear a cotton gown or pajamas. Health care workers should wear cotton uniforms.
6. Electrical equipment is removed from the resident's room. This includes electric razors, heating pads, and radios.
7. Materials that ignite easily are removed from the room. This includes oil, grease, alcohol, and nail polish remover.

Fire Prevention

Fire prevention measures have been described for equipment-related accidents and the use of oxygen. These and other fire safety measures are summarized as follows:

1. Follow the fire safety precautions involved in the use of oxygen.
2. Smoke only in areas where smoking is permitted.
3. Be sure all ashes and cigar and cigarette butts are out before emptying ashtrays.
4. Provide ashtrays to residents who are allowed to smoke.
5. Empty ashtrays into a metal container partially filled with sand or water. Do not empty ashtrays into plastic containers or wastebaskets lined with paper or plastic bags.
6. Supervise the smoking of residents who cannot protect themselves. This includes confused, disoriented, and sedated residents.
7. Follow the safety practices necessary when using electrical equipment.
8. Do not leave smoking materials at the bedside of confused or sedated residents.

What to Do If There Is a Fire

Each facility has policies and procedures explaining what to do if there is a fire. You must know the policies and procedures of your facility. You also should know the location of fire alarms, fire extinguishers, and emergency exits. All facilities hold fire drills to practice procedures.

The following practices usually are carried out by the health care team when there is a fire.

1. Sound the nearest fire alarm.
2. Notify the office manager of the exact location of the fire.
3. Move residents in the immediate area of the fire to a safe place.
4. Use a fire extinguisher on a small fire that has not spread to a larger area.
5. Turn off any oxygen or electrical equipment being used in the general area of the fire.
6. Close all doors and windows.
7. Clear all hallways and emergency exits of equipment.
8. Do not use elevators if there is a fire.

You should be able to use a fire extinguisher. Local fire departments often demonstrate to health care workers the use of fire extinguishers. These demonstrations are given once or twice a year. Some facilities require all employees to demonstrate how to use a fire extinguisher.

There are different kinds of extinguishers for different kinds of fires—oil and grease fires, electrical fires, and paper and wood fires—or all-purpose extinguishers for all types of fires. A general procedure for using a fire extinguisher follows.

PROCEDURE

Using a Fire Extinguisher

1.   Pull the fire alarm.

2.   Get the nearest fire extinguisher.

3.   Carry the fire extinguisher upright.

4.   Take the extinguisher to the fire.

5.   Remove the safety pin (Fig. 7-26, *A*).

6.   Push the top handle down (Fig. 7-26, *B*).

7.   Direct the hose at the base of the fire (Fig. 7-26, *C*).

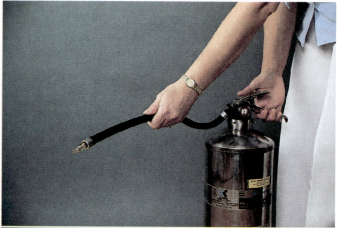

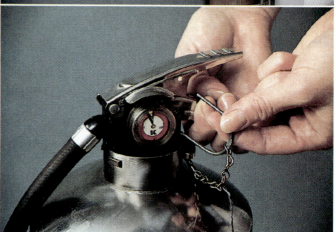

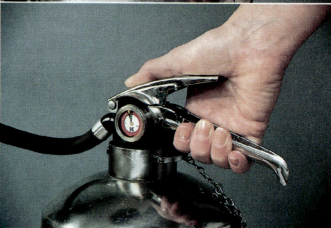

FIGURE 7-26 *A, The safety pin of a fire extinguisher is removed. B, The top handle of the fire extinguisher is pushed down. C, The hose of the fire extinguisher is directed at the base of the fire.*

DISASTERS

A **disaster** is a sudden, catastrophic event in which many people are injured and killed and property is destroyed. Disasters may be natural, such as tornados, hurricanes, blizzards, earthquakes, and floods. Disasters caused by humans include fires, explosions, or auto and air accidents. Local communities and health care facilities have disaster plans. You need to know the disaster plan where you work and the disaster plan of the community where you live and work.

Disaster plans of nursing facilities include policies and procedures to deal with the great numbers of people who will be brought in for treatment. The plan generally provides for the discharge of residents who can go home. Although nursing facilities are not equipped to handle severe injuries, they do have the licensed staff and the beds for the injured. Special equipment can be brought in at a later time. Off-duty staff members may be called in to work.

SUMMARY

Most accidents can be prevented. Knowing the common safety hazards and accidents, knowing who needs protection, and using common sense are all necessary to promote safety. Remember, elderly and disabled persons are more likely to have accidents than are healthy young adults.

Chronic illness, advanced age, physical and mental disability, medications, strange surroundings, and special equipment increase the risk of accidental injury to residents. You need to practice safety precautions and use side rails as appropriate. Encourage residents to use handrails and special equipment, such as walkers and canes, to assist them with walking.

The importance of identifying residents before giving care must be stressed. The resident's life and health can be seriously threatened if the wrong care is given or if care is omitted. Use the ID bracelet to accurately identify the resident. Having two residents on the same nursing unit with the same last name is not uncommon. Some residents may even have the same first and last names.

If restraints are ordered, they must be used for a specific medical symptom. The resident must be checked often to make sure that breathing and circulation are normal. Remember that the restrained resident depends on others for basic needs. Be sure to offer water or other fluids often. Remember, you can be charged with false imprisonment if the resident is restrained unnecessarily.

Fire is a safety hazard. Exercising safety precautions for smoking and electrical equipment helps prevent fires. Extra precautions are needed when oxygen is used. The resident who smokes presents additional fire safety concerns. Check with the nurse to find out which residents may have smoking materials at the bedside. Be sure you know where fire alarms, fire extinguishers, and emergency exits are located and what to do if there is a fire.

Review QUESTIONS

Circle T if the answer is true and F if the answer is false.

T F 1. A safe environment is one in which a person has a very small risk of becoming ill or injured.

T F 2. Cleaning chemicals are kept in locked storage areas that are out of the reach of residents.

T F 3. Aging causes body changes that place an elderly person at risk for accidents.

T F 4. Smell, touch, sight, and hearing can be used to prevent accidents.

T F 5. A paraplegic is paralyzed on one side of the body.

T F 6. Medications are a cause of some accidents.

T F 7. Falls can be prevented by making sure there is enough lighting.

T F 8. Residents should wear bedroom slippers to prevent skidding and slipping on floors.

T F 9. People should not smoke in bed.

T F 10. The spread of infection is not a health hazard in health facilities.

T F 11. Side rails are kept up at all times, even when giving care.

T F 12. Side rails are considered to be restraints by OBRA.

T F 13. Handrails provide support for residents when walking.

T F 14. The resident's ID bracelet should be used to accurately identify the resident before giving care.

T F 15. Restraints are used only for specific medical symptoms.

T F 16. Restraint of a resident unnecessarily is false imprisonment.

T F 17. A resident (or the resident's guardian) must consent to the use of restraints.

T F 18. You can apply restraints any time you think they are needed.

T F 19. Geriatric chairs are not restraints.

T F 20. You can use a jacket restraint to position a resident on the toilet.

T F 21. You should be able to feel a pulse in the wrist if the arm and hand are restrained.

T F 22. Restraints should be removed every 2 hours so that the resident can be repositioned and given skin care.

T F 23. Restrained residents are checked every 15 to 30 minutes to make sure they are safe and comfortable.

T F 24. Restraints are tied to side rails.

T F 25. Jacket restraints are applied so the vest crosses in front.

T F 26. Side rails are left down when jacket restraints are used.

T F 27. Accidents or errors in giving care should be reported to the nurse at the end of the shift.

T F 28. A spark or flame, a material that will burn, and oxygen are needed to start and maintain a fire.

T F 29. Smoking is not allowed where oxygen is used.

T F 30. Wool blankets are used if a resident is receiving oxygen.

T F 31. Oxygen should be turned off if it is being used in the area of a fire.

T F 32. You should close doors and windows when a fire alarm sounds.

Answers

1. True	9. True	17. True	25. True
2. True	10. False	18. False	26. False
3. True	11. False	19. False	27. False
4. True	12. True	20. False	28. True
5. False	13. True	21. True	29. True
6. True	14. True	22. True	30. False
7. True	15. True	23. True	31. True
8. False	16. True	24. False	32. True

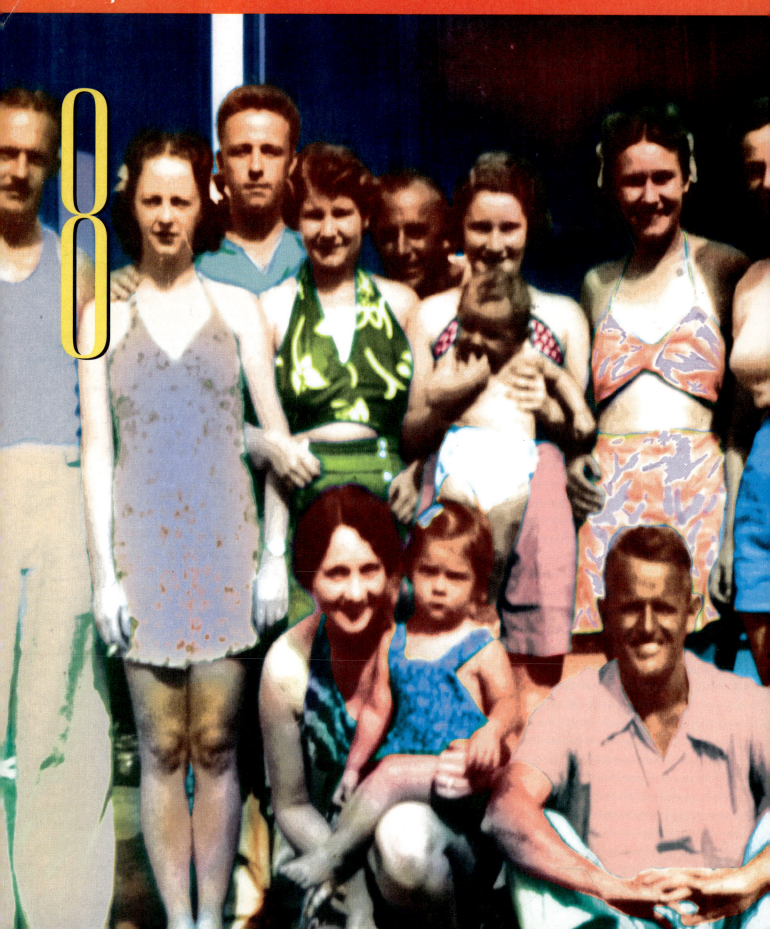

08

Key TERMS

asepsis
The absence of pathogens

autoclave
A pressure steam sterilizer

carrier
A human being or animal that is a reservoir for microorganisms but that does not have the signs and symptoms of an infection

clean technique
Medical asepsis

communicable disease
A disease caused by pathogens that are easily spread; a contagious disease

contagious disease
Communicable disease

contamination
The process by which an object or area becomes unclean

disinfection
The process by which pathogens are destroyed

host
The environment in which microorganisms live and grow; reservoir

infection
A disease state that results from the invasion and growth of microorganisms in the body

infection precautions
Practices that limit the spread of pathogens; barriers are set up that prevent the escape of the pathogen

medical asepsis
The techniques and practices used to prevent the spread of pathogens from one person or place to another person or place; clean technique

microbe
A microorganism

microorganism
A small living plant or animal that cannot be seen without the aid of a microscope; a microbe

nonpathogen
A microorganism that does not usually cause an infection

normal flora
Microorganisms that usually live and grow in a certain location

pathogen
A microorganism that is harmful and capable of causing an infection

personal protective equipment
Specialized clothing or equipment (gloves, goggles, gowns) worn for protection against a hazard

reservoir
The environment in which microorganisms live and grow; the host

spore
A bacterium protected by a hard shell that forms around the microorganism

sterile
The absence of all microorganisms

sterilization
The process by which all microorganisms are destroyed

vaccination
The administration of a vaccine to produce immunity

vaccine
A preparation containing microorganisms

I'm so afraid of getting a cold or some other infection. They weaken me so. I know that's why the staff wears gloves—to help prevent infection.

Infection is a major safety and health hazard. Some infections are minor and cause a short illness. Others are serious and can cause death, particularly in elderly and disabled persons. Healthcare workers need to protect residents and themselves from infection. This is done by preventing the spread of the cause of the infection. In this chapter you will learn the causes of infections and how they spread. You also will learn ways to prevent the spread of infection.

MICROORGANISMS

A **microorganism (microbe)** is a small *(micro)* living plant or animal *(organism)* that cannot be seen without a microscope. Microorganisms are everywhere. They are in the air, food, mouth, nose, respiratory tract, stomach, intestines, and on the skin. They are in the soil and water and on animals, clothing, and furniture. Some microorganisms cause infections and are harmful. They are called **pathogens.** Microorganisms that do not usually cause infection are **nonpathogens.**

Types of Microorganisms

There are five general types of microorganisms.
1. *Bacteria* are microscopic plant life that multiply rapidly. They consist of one cell and often are called *germs.*
2. *Fungi* are plants that live on other plants or animals. Mushrooms, yeasts, and molds are common fungi.
3. *Protozoa* are microscopic one-celled animals.
4. *Rickettsiae* are microscopic forms of life found in the tissues of fleas, lice, ticks, and other insects. They are transmitted to humans by insects bites.
5. *Viruses* are extremely small microscopic organisms that grow in living cells.

Requirements of Microorganisms

Microorganisms require a **reservoir** to live and grow. The reservoir **(host)** is the environment in which the microorganism lives and grows. The reservoir can be a human being, a plant, an animal, the soil, food, water, or other material. The microorganism must receive *water* and *nourishment* from the reservoir. Most microbes require *oxygen* to live. Others cannot live where there is oxygen. A *warm* and *dark* environment is needed. Most microorganisms grow best at body temperature and are destroyed by heat and light.

Normal Flora

Normal flora refers to microorganisms that usually live and grow in a certain location. Certain microorganisms are found in the respiratory tract, the intestines, on the skin, and in other sites outside the body. These microorganisms are nonpathogenic when in or on a natural reservoir. If the nonpathogen is transmitted from its natural location to another site or host, it becomes a pathogen. *Escherichia coli* is a microorganism normally found in the large intestine. If the *E. coli* enters the urinary system, it can cause infection.

INFECTION

An **infection** is a disease state that results from the invasion and growth of microorganisms in the body. It may be localized in a body part or involve the whole body. An infection causes certain signs and symptoms. Some or all of the following may be present: fever, pain or tenderness, fatigue, loss of appetite, nausea, vomiting, diarrhea, rash, sores on mucous membranes, redness, swelling, and discharge or drainage from the infected area. Pathogens can be present without causing an infection. The development of an infection depends on several factors.

The Process of Infection

For an infection to develop there must be a *source*. The source is a pathogen capable of causing disease. The pathogen must have a *reservoir* where it can grow and multiply. Human beings and animals are reservoirs. If they do not have signs and symptoms of infection, they are *carriers*. Carriers can pass the pathogen to others. The pathogen must be able to leave the reservoir. In other words, it must have an *exit*. Body exits are the respiratory, gastrointestinal, urinary, and reproductive tracts, breaks in the skin, and the blood.

The pathogen that has left the reservoir needs to be *transmitted* to another host. Methods of transmission include direct contact, air, food, water, animals, and insects. Microbes also can be transmitted by eating and drinking utensils, dressings, and personal care and hy-

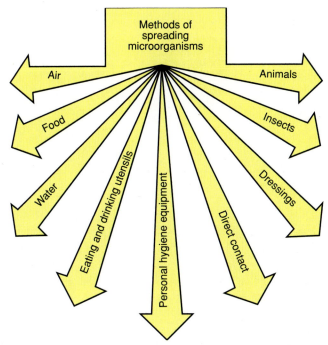

FIGURE 8-1 *Methods by which microorganisms can be spread.*

giene equipment (Fig. 8-1). The pathogen then needs to enter the body through a *portal of entry*. Portals of entry in the body are the same as the exits. Whether or not the pathogen grows and multiplies depends on the *susceptibility of the host*. The human body has the natural ability to protect itself from infection. A person's ability to resist infection is related to age, sex, nutritional status, fatigue, general health, medications, and the presence or absence of other illnesses.

Medical Asepsis

Asepsis means the absence of all disease-producing microorganisms or the absence of pathogens. Because microbes are everywhere, there must be practices to achieve asepsis. These practices are known as **medical asepsis** or **clean technique.** Therefore medical asepsis consists of techniques and practices used to prevent the spread of pathogens from one person or place to another person or place. Medical asepsis is different from disinfection and sterilization. **Disinfection** is the process by which pathogenic microorganisms are destroyed. **Sterilization** is the process in which *all* microorganisms are destroyed. **Sterile** refers to the absence of all pathogenic and nonpathogenic microorganisms.

Contamination is the process by which an object or area becomes unclean. In medical asepsis an object or area is considered clean when it is free of pathogens. Therefore the object or area is contaminated if pathogens are present. Likewise, a sterile object or area is contaminated when pathogens or nonpathogens are present.

Common Aseptic Practices

Aseptic practices are followed in the home, community, and work place. Some common ways to prevent the spread of microbes are as follows:

1. Washing hands after urinating, having a bowel movement, or changing tampons or sanitary napkins
2. Washing hands before handling or preparing food
3. Washing fruits and raw vegetables before eating or serving them
4. Providing individual towels, washcloths, toothbrushes, drinking glasses, and other personal care items for each family member
5. Covering the nose and mouth when coughing, sneezing, or blowing the nose
6. Bathing, washing hair, and brushing teeth regularly
7. Washing cooking and eating utensils with soap and water after they have been used
8. Observing sanitation practices such as the disposal of garbage and the treatment of sewage

Handwashing

Handwashing with soap and water is the easiest and one of the most important ways to prevent the spread of infection. Your hands are used in almost every activity. They are easily contaminated and can spread microbes if you do not practice handwashing before and after giving care. To properly wash your hands, you need to follow these rules.

1. Use warm running water.
2. Hand-operated faucets are considered contaminated. Use a paper towel to turn off the water at the end of the handwashing procedure (Fig. 8-2, p. 138). The paper towel prevents your clean hand from becoming contaminated again. Some facilities consider hand controls to be clean. If hand controls are considered "clean," then you must use a paper towel to turn the faucet both on and off.
3. Bar soap is held during the entire handwashing procedure. When the procedure is completed, rinse the soap under running water. After rinsing, drop it into the soap dish. Avoid touching the soap dish during or after handwashing. Health care facilities have soap dispensers. Bar soap often is used in homes.
4. Your hands and forearms are held lower than your elbows during the procedure. If your hands and forearms are held up, dirty water can run from your hands to your elbows, contaminating those areas.
5. Remember to wash areas that frequently are missed during handwashing: the thumbs, knuckles, sides of the hands, little fingers, and underneath the nails. Use a nail file or orange stick to clean under your fingernails (Fig. 8-3, p. 138).
6. Use a lotion after handwashing to prevent chapping and drying of the skin.

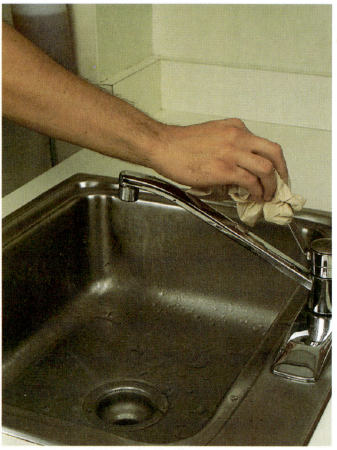

FIGURE 8-2 *A paper towel is used to turn off the faucet.*

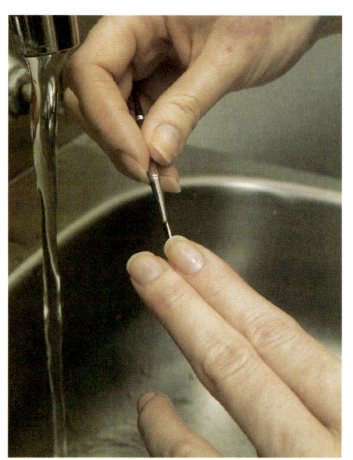

FIGURE 8-3 *An orange stick is used to clean under the fingernails.*

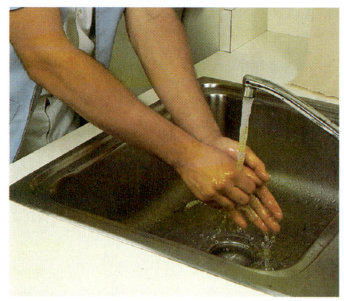

FIGURE 8-4 *The nursing assistant is standing so that his uniform does not touch the sink. He is close enough to reach the soap and water. Hands are lower than elbows.*

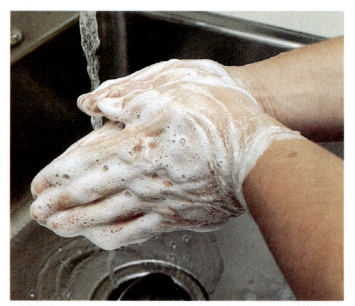

FIGURE 8-5 *The palms are rubbed together to work up a good lather.*

PROCEDURE

Handwashing

1. Make sure that soap, paper towels, orange sticks or nail file, and a wastebasket are available. Collect missing items.

2. Push your watch 4 to 5 inches above your hand.

3. Stand away from the sink so that your clothes do not touch the sink. The soap and faucet must be within reach (Fig. 8-4).

4. Turn on the faucet. Use a paper towel if this is a facility policy.

5. Adjust the water to a warm, comfortable temperature.

6. Throw the paper towel into the wastebasket.

7. Wet your wrists and hands thoroughly under running water. Keep them lower than your elbows during the procedure (see Fig. 8-4).

8. Apply soap to your hands. Rinse bar soap before it is used.

9. Rub your palms together to work up a good lather (Fig. 8-5).

10. Wash each hand and wrist thoroughly, and clean well between the fingers. Clean well under the fingernails by rubbing the tips of your fingers against your palms (Fig. 8-6).

11. Wash for 1 to 2 minutes using friction and rotating motions.

12. Use a nail file or orange stick to clean under your fingernails (see Fig. 8-3).

13. Rinse your wrists and hands well. Water should flow from your arms to your hands.

14. Repeat steps 8 through 13.

15. Return the soap to the soap dish (if bar soap is used).

16. Dry your wrists and hands with paper towels. Pat dry.

17. Turn off the faucet with the paper towels to avoid contaminating your hand.

18. Discard paper towels into the wastebasket.

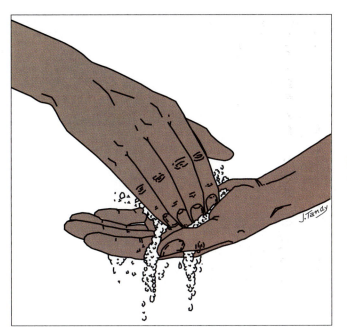

FIGURE 8-6 *The tips of the fingers are rubbed against the palms to clean underneath the fingernails.*

Care of Supplies and Equipment

Most nursing facilities have "clean" and "dirty" utility rooms. Equipment is cleaned in the "dirty" utility room before being disinfected or sterilized in the "clean" utility room. Most health care equipment is disposable. Disposable equipment is used for a resident and then discarded. Some disposable items, however, can be used several times by a resident. Examples include disposable bedpans, urinals, wash basins, thermometers, water pitchers, and drinking cups. Items should be labeled with the resident's name, room, and bed number and never "borrowed" for another resident. When used correctly, disposable equipment helps reduce the spread of infection.

Larger and more expensive equipment usually is not disposable. Nondisposable items have to be disinfected or sterilized before reuse by any resident. Before disinfection or sterilization, equipment is cleaned. Cleaning reduces the number of microbes to be destroyed and removes organic material. Organic material includes blood, pus, drainage from wounds, and body secretions or excretions. You should follow these guidelines when cleaning equipment.

1. Wear disposable gloves when handling or cleaning contaminated equipment.
2. Rinse the item in cold water first to remove organic material. Heat causes organic material to become thick, sticky, and hard to remove.
3. Use soap and hot water to wash the item.
4. Use a brush if necessary.
5. Rinse and dry the item.
6. Disinfect or sterilize the item.
7. Disinfect equipment used for cleaning.

Disinfection. *Disinfection* is the process in which pathogenic microorganisms are destroyed. However, it does not destroy spores. **Spores** are bacteria protected by a hard shell that forms around the microorganism. Spores are killed by extremely high temperatures. Disinfection methods usually do not destroy all spores.

Boiling water is a simple and inexpensive method. Small items are disinfected by placing them in boiling water for at least 15 minutes. *Chemical disinfectants* are used for cleaning instruments and equipment and for housekeeping. They are used to clean commodes, wheelchairs, stretchers, and furniture in the resident unit after a resident has been discharged (Fig. 8-7). There are many types of chemical disinfectants. To prevent skin irritation, you should wear waterproof gloves when using a disinfectant. Specific chemical disinfectants may require special precautions during use or storage. Ask the nurse about procedures for a specific disinfectant.

Sterilization. *Sterilization* procedures destroy all nonpathogens, pathogens, and spores. Extremely high

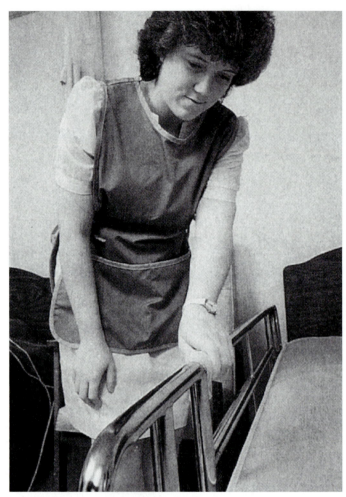

FIGURE 8-7 *The nursing assistant disinfects the bed frame after a resident has been discharged.*

temperatures are used. As stated earlier, microbes grow best at body temperature and are destroyed by heat.

You may learn to sterilize equipment by means of *steam under pressure.* An **autoclave** (Fig. 8-8) is a pressure-steam sterilizer used for metal objects, such as surgical instruments, basins, bedpans, and urinals. Glass and surgical linens also are sterilized in an autoclave. Plastic and rubber items are not placed in an autoclave because they are destroyed by high temperatures. Steam under pressure usually can sterilize objects in 30 to 45 minutes.

Liquid chemicals may be used for sterilizing. Nursing assistants generally are not responsible for using this method.

Other Aseptic Measures

You should practice other aseptic measures to prevent the spread of infection and microorganisms. These measures are essential in the health care facility to protect residents, visitors, and health care workers.

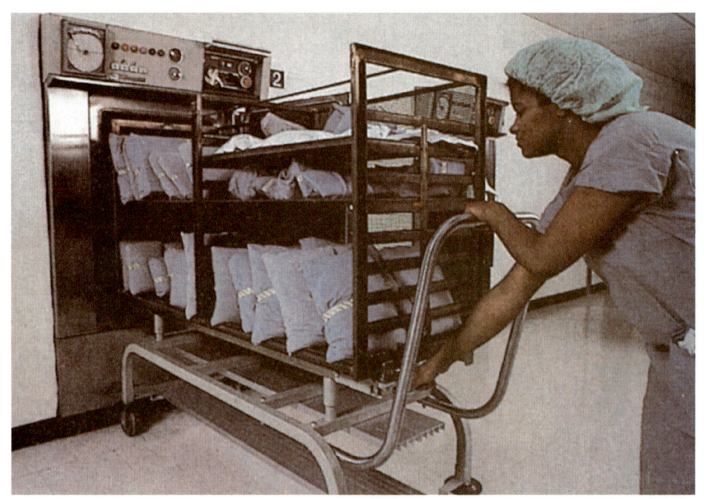

FIGURE 8-8 *An autoclave.*

1. Hold equipment and linens away from your uniform (Fig. 8-9).
2. Avoid shaking linens and other equipment. Use a damp cloth to dust furniture. These actions help prevent the movement of dust.
3. Clean from the cleanest area to the dirtiest. This prevents soiling a clean area.
4. Clean away from your body and uniform. If you dust, brush, or wipe toward yourself, microorganisms are transmitted to your skin, hair, and uniform.
5. Pour contaminated liquids directly into sinks or toilets. Avoid splashing onto other areas.
6. Avoid sitting on a resident's bed. You will pick up microorganisms and transfer them to the next surface that you sit on.
7. Do not take equipment from one resident's room to use for another resident. Even if equipment has not been used, it should not be taken from one room to another.

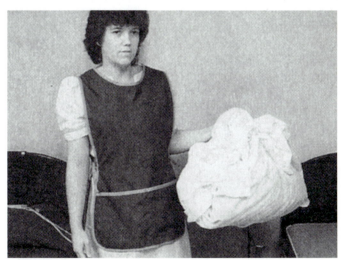

FIGURE 8-9 *The nursing assistant holds soiled linen away from her uniform.*

INFECTION PRECAUTIONS

Sometimes other measures are needed to prevent the spread of microorganisms. **Infection precautions** prevent the spread of pathogens from one area to another. Barriers are set up that prevent the escape of pathogens. The pathogens are kept within a specific area, usually the resident's room. The Centers for Disease Control (CDC) in Atlanta, Georgia, has developed guidelines for infection precautions. Those guidelines are included in this section.

Instead of "infection precautions," you may hear the phrase "isolation techniques." *Isolation* implies separating the resident from others. The pathogen, not the resident, is undesirable. Therefore CDC guidelines now use the phrase "infection precautions." However, the terms *isolation* and *isolation techniques* are still used in describing infection precautions.

Purpose

Infection precautions prevent the spread of **communicable** or **infectious disease.** Communicable diseases are caused by pathogens that are spread easily. Common communicable diseases are tuberculosis (TB), hepatitis B, syphilis, gonorrhea, and acquired immunodeficiency syndrome (AIDS) (see Chapter 23). Residents may have respiratory, skin, wound, gastrointestinal, or blood infections that are highly contagious. The proper use of infection precautions prevents the spread of these and other infectious diseases.

"Clean" Versus "Dirty"

Infection precautions are based on an understanding of clean and dirty. *Clean* refers to those areas or objects that are uncontaminated. Uncontaminated areas are free of pathogens. Areas or objects considered *dirty* are those that are contaminated. If a clean area or object comes in contact with something dirty, the object or area that was clean is now considered dirty. Clean and dirty also depend on the way in which the pathogen is spread.

Types of Infection Precautions

The CDC recognizes three categories of infection precautions. They are *strict precautions, respiratory precautions,* and *universal precautions.* Each category depends on how the pathogen is spread. Special procedures may be required. Gloves, masks, goggles, and gowns may be worn (Fig. 8-10). Linens and equipment may be cared for in special ways.

A 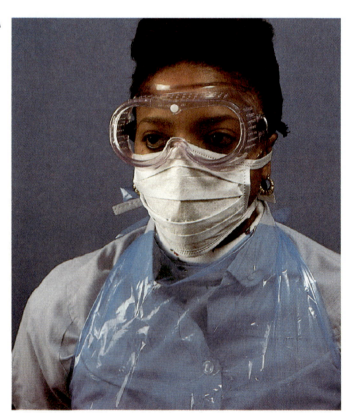 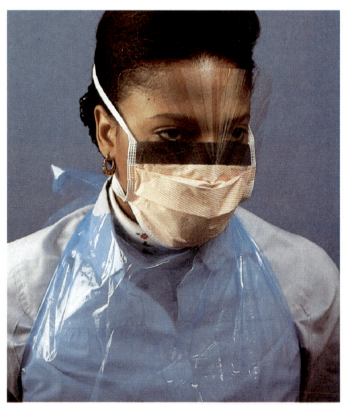 B

FIGURE 8-10 *A, Mask and goggles protect the eyes from splashing body fluids. B, A face shield protects the eyes and mucous membranes of the mouth. Note that a plastic apron is worn to protect the uniform from soil.*

List 8 -1

Universal Precautions

- Gloves are worn when touching blood, body fluids, body substances, and mucous membranes.
- Gloves are worn when there are cuts, breaks, or openings in the skin.
- Gloves are worn when there is possible contact with urine, feces, vomitus, dressings, wound drainage, soiled linen, or soiled clothing.
- Masks, goggles, or face shields are worn when splattering or splashing of blood or body fluids is possible (Fig. 9-10, p. 166). (This protects your eyes and the mucous membranes of your mouth.)
- Gowns or aprons are worn when splashing, splattering, smearing, or soiling from blood or body fluids is possible.
- Hands and other body parts must be washed immediately if contaminated with blood or body fluids.
- Hands are washed immediately after removing gloves.
- Hands are washed after contact with the patient.
- Avoid nicks or cuts when shaving patients.
- Handle razor blades and other sharp objects carefully to avoid injuring the patient or yourself.
- Use resuscitation devices when mouth-to-mouth resuscitation is indicated (see Chapter 29).
- Avoid patient contact when you have open skin wounds or lesions. Discuss the situation with your supervisor.

Strict precautions and respiratory precautions are required for acutely ill patients in hospitals. They may be suffering from illnesses such as smallpox, diphtheria, TB, or mumps. You will not be caring for residents with these diseases in the long-term care setting.

Universal precautions. Universal precautions were issued by the CDC in 1987. They were developed to prevent the spread of AIDS. The AIDS virus is spread through contact with blood. AIDS, hepatitis B, and other infections may be undiagnosed. Universal precautions prevent the spread of AIDS and other infections. Therefore universal precautions are used for *all* residents.

You may care for residents with bleeding or infected wounds. Contact with blood may occur while you give oral care or shave residents. There may be blood or pathogens in urine, feces, or vomitus or in respiratory or vaginal secretions. Many other situations occur in which you could have contact with a resident's blood or body fluids.

Universal precautions involve setting up barriers to prevent contact with the resident's blood, body fluids, or body substances. These precautions are presented in List 8-1. *Remember: the CDC recommends the use of universal precautions for all residents.* Your facility will have policies regarding the use of universal precautions.

General Rules

The following rules are a guide for giving safe care. They will help you to prevent the spread of pathogens to other residents and to yourself.

1. Floors are contaminated. Any object that is on the floor or that falls to the floor is contaminated.
2. Floor dust is contaminated. Mops wetted with a disinfectant solution are used for cleaning. A wet mop keeps dust down.
3. Drafts should be prevented. Pathogens are carried in the air by drafts.
4. Gloves are used to handle contaminated equipment and objects.
5. Contaminated items removed from residents' rooms are bagged.
6. Do not touch your hair, nose, mouth, eyes, or other body part when caring for a resident.
7. If your hands become contaminated, they must not touch any clean area or object.
8. Wash your hands if they become contaminated.
9. Do not shake linen.
10. Use paper towels to turn faucets on and off.
11. Tell the nurse if you have any cuts, open skin areas, a sore throat, vomiting, or diarrhea.

Special Procedures

Universal precautions require special procedures. Gloving, gowning, wearing a mask, and bagging articles removed from the resident's room may be required.

Gloving. Disposable gloves act as a barrier between the resident and you. They protect you from pathogens in the resident's blood, body fluids, and body substances. Residents also are protected from microorganisms that may be on your hands.

Disposable gloves are easy to put on. No special technique is required. You must be careful, however, not to tear the gloves when putting them on. Carelessness, long fingernails, and rings can tear the gloves. Torn gloves must be discarded. Blood, fluids, and other substances can enter the glove through the tear. This contaminates the hand.

The following steps are important in removing gloves. When the gloves are removed, the inside part will be on the outside. The inside of the gloves is considered "clean."

PROCEDURE

Removing Gloves

1. When both hands are still gloved, be sure that only glove touches glove. The gloves should not touch skin on the wrists or arms.

2. Remove one glove by grasping it just below the cuff (Fig. 8-11, *A*).

3. Pull the glove down over your hand so that it is inside out (Fig 8-11, *B*).

4. Hold the removed glove with your gloved hand.

5. Reach inside the other glove with the first two fingers of your ungloved hand (Fig. 8-11, *C*).

6. Pull the glove down (inside out) over your hand and the other glove (Fig. 8-11, *D*).

7. Discard the gloves in the appropriate container.

8. Wash your hands.

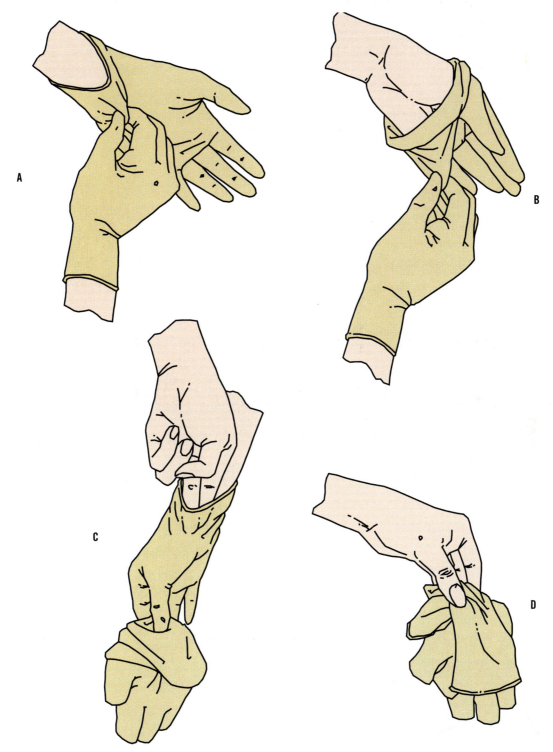

FIGURE 8-11 *Removing gloves.* **A,** *The glove is grasped below the cuff.* **B,** *The glove is pulled down over the hand. The glove is inside out.* **C,** *The fingers of the ungloved hand are inserted inside the other glove.* **D,** *The glove is pulled down and over the hand and glove. The glove is inside out.*

Gowning. Gowns prevent contamination of clothing with blood, body fluids, or body substances when you give care. Gowns are made of paper. They must be long enough and large enough to completely cover clothing. The sleeves are long with tight cuffs. The gown opens at the back, where it is tied at the neck and waist. The inside and the neck of the gown are considered "clean." The outside and waist strings are considered contaminated.

Some facilities use plastic aprons (see Fig. 8-10, p. 142). Gowns are indicated when the arms and wrists must be protected from soiling or contact with blood or body fluids. Possible splashing or splattering indicate the need for gowns. Gowns and aprons are used once and then discarded. A wet gown is considered contaminated. If a gown becomes wet, it is removed and a dry one is put on.

PROCEDURE

Gowning Technique

1. Remove your watch and all jewelry.

2. Roll up long sleeves of your uniform.

3. Wash your hands.

4. Pick up a clean gown. Hold it out in front of you so that it can unfold. Do not shake the gown.

5. Put your hands and arms through the sleeves of the gown as shown in Fig. 8-12, *A*.

6. Make sure the gown completely covers the front of your uniform. The gown should be snug at the neck.

7. Tie the strings at the back of the neck (Fig. 8-12, *B*).

8. Overlap the back of the gown. Your uniform must be completely covered. The gown should be snug (Fig. 8-12, *C*) and should not hang loosely.

9. Tie the waist strings at the back.

10. Provide the necessary resident care.

11. Remove the gown as follows:

    a. Untie the waist strings.

    b. Wash your hands.

    c. Untie the neck strings. Do not touch the outside of the gown.

    d. Pull the gown down from the shoulder.

    e. Turn the gown inside out as it is removed. Hold the gown at the inside shoulder seams and bring your hands together (Fig. 8-12, *D*).

12. Roll up the gown away from you, keeping it inside out.

13. Discard the gown in the wastebasket.

14. Wash your hands.

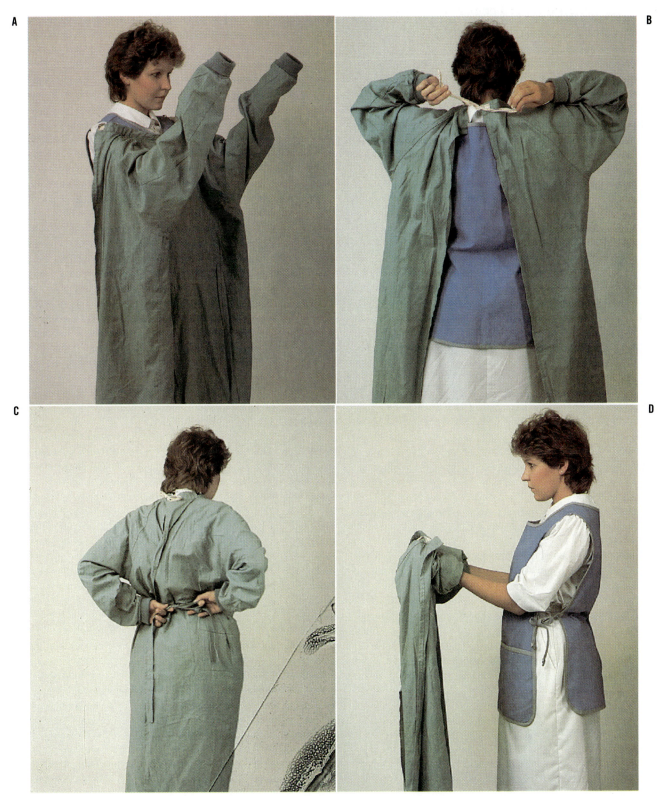

FIGURE 8-12 *Gowning technique.* **A,** *The arms and hands are put through the sleeves.* **B,** *The strings are tied at the back of the neck.* **C,** *The gown is overlapped in the back so that the entire uniform is covered.* **D,** *The gown is turned inside out as it is removed.*

Wearing a face mask and goggles. Face masks and goggles are worn if there is a possibility of splashing or splattering of blood or body fluids while care is given. Disposable masks are used. If a mask becomes wet or moist, it is considered contaminated. A new mask is applied when contamination occurs. Goggles also are disposable and should be discarded after use.

Both the mask and the goggles must fit snugly. Goggles are put on after the face mask (see Fig. 8-10, p. 142). Hands are washed before putting on and before taking off the mask and goggles. Only the ties, elastic, or ear pieces are touched during removal.

PROCEDURE

Wearing a Face Mask

1. Wash your hands.

2. Pick up the mask by its upper ties. Do not touch the part that will cover your face.

3. Position the mask over your nose. Your nose and mouth must be covered (Fig. 8-13, *A*).

4. Place the upper strings over your ears. Tie the strings in the back toward the top of your head (Fig. 8-13, *B*).

5. Tie the lower strings at the back of your neck (Fig. 8-13, *C*). Make sure the lower part of the mask is under your chin. The mask should fit snugly over your nose.

6. Mold the metal strip over the bridge of your nose.

7. Put on the goggles.

8. Wash your hands.

9. Provide necessary care.

10. Change the mask if it becomes contaminated.

11. Remove the mask as follows:

    a. Wash your hands.

    b. Remove your goggles, holding only the ear pieces or elastic. Drop them into the wastebasket.

    c. Wash your hands.

    d. Untie the lower strings.

    e. Untie the upper strings.

    f. Hold the top strings and remove the mask.

    g. Bring the strings together. The inside of the mask will fold together (Fig. 8-13, *D*). Avoid touching the inside of the mask.

12. Discard the mask in the wastebasket.

13. Wash your hands.

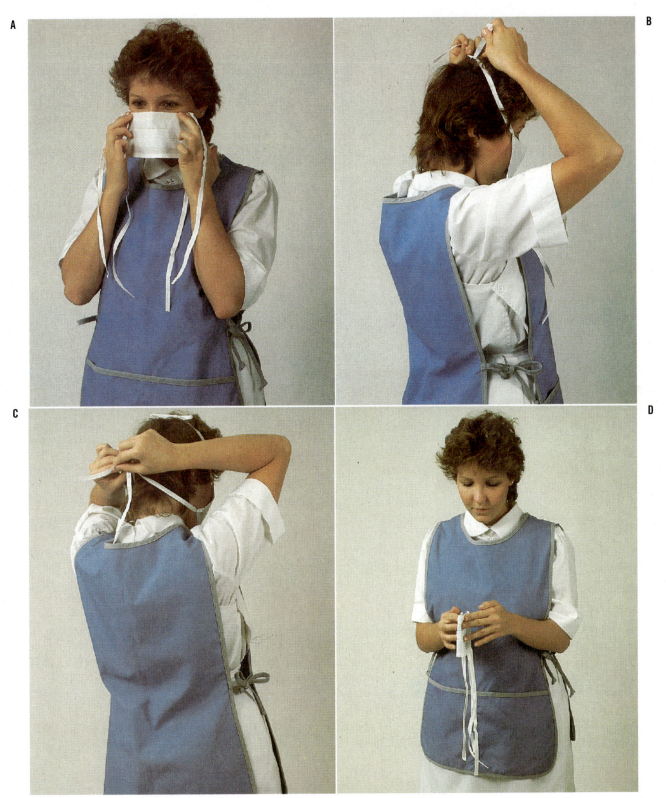

FIGURE 8-13 *A,* *The mask is positioned so that the mouth and nose are covered.* ***B,*** *The upper strings are tied at the back of the head.* ***C,*** *The lower strings are tied at the neck.* ***D,*** *The strings of the face mask are brought together so that the inside of the mask will be folded together after being re-moved.*

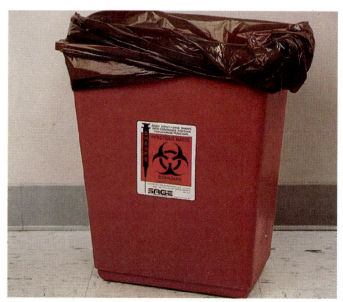

FIGURE 8-14 *Trash is placed in a container with the "biohazard" symbol.*

Bagging articles. Contaminated items are bagged before being removed from the resident's room. Plastic bags are used because they prevent leakage and microorganisms cannot go through them. Trash usually is placed in containers labeled with the "biohazard" symbol (Fig. 8-14). *Biohazardous waste* refers to items that are contaminated with the resident's blood, body fluids, or body substances and may be harmful to others. The prefix *bio* means life and *hazardous* means dangerous or harmful.

Linen is bagged, labeled, and handled according to facility policy. You should know your facility's policy regarding the handling of contaminated waste, linen, and equipment.

BLOODBORNE PATHOGEN STANDARD

The number of people infected with the AIDS virus (HIV) and hepatitis B virus (HBV) is increasing (see Chapter 23). Health care workers care for these people. Therefore health care workers are at risk for exposure. The bloodborne pathogen standard is intended to protect workers from exposure. The standard is a regulation of the Occupational Safety and Health Administration (OSHA). OSHA is part of the U.S. Department of Labor. List 8-2 contains the definitions used by OSHA's bloodborne pathogen standard.

The AIDS and hepatitis B viruses are found in the blood. They are disease-producing pathogens. Therefore they are **bloodborne pathogens.** The viruses exit the body through blood and are transmitted to others by blood. The virus can also be transmitted by other **potentially infectious materials** (see p. 151). Such materials are contaminated with blood or with a body fluid that may contain blood. Potentially infectious materials may also include needles, suction equipment, soiled linens, dressings, and other equipment and items used in the person's care.

Exposure Control Plan

Employers must have a written exposure control plan. The plan identifies those workers who have a risk of occupational exposure. That is, they may be exposed to blood or to other potentially infectious materials. Long-term care workers at risk usually include nurses, nursing assistants, laundry staff, housekeepers, and physical therapists. The plan also includes the actions to take when there is an exposure incident.

Staff at risk for exposure must receive free information and training. Training must be given upon employment. Retraining is done every year. Training is also required for new or changed procedures and tasks that involve exposure to bloodborne pathogens. OSHA requires that training include:

1. An explanation of the bloodborne pathogen standard and where to get a copy
2. The causes, signs, and symptoms of bloodborne diseases
3. How bloodborne pathogens are transmitted
4. An explanation of the facility's exposure control plan and where to get a copy
5. How to know which tasks might cause occupational exposure
6. The use and limitations of safe work practices, **engineering controls,** and **personal protective equipment**
7. Information on the hepatitis B vaccination
8. Who to contact and what to do in an emergency
9. Information on reporting an exposure incident, postexposure evaluation, and follow-up
10. Information on warning labels and color-coding

List 8 -2

Bloodborne Pathogen Standard Definitions

blood Human blood, human blood components, and products made from human blood

bloodborne pathogens Pathogenic microorganisms that are present in human blood and that can cause disease in humans; these pathogens include, but are not limited to, hepatitis B virus (HBV) and human immunodeficiency virus (HIV)

contaminated The presence or the reasonably anticipated presence of blood or other potentially infectious materials on an item or surface

contaminated laundry Laundry that has been soiled with blood or other potentially infectious materials or that may contain sharps

contaminated sharps Any contaminated object that can penetrate the skin, including, but not limited to, needles, scalpels, broken glass, broken capillary tubes, and exposed ends of dental wires

decontamination The use of physical or chemical means to remove, inactivate, or destroy bloodborne pathogens on a surface or item to the point where they can no longer transmit infectious particles and the surface or item is safe for handling, use, or disposal

engineering controls Controls that isolate or remove the bloodborne pathogen hazard from the workplace (sharps disposal containers, self-sheathing needles)

exposure incident A specific eye, mouth, other mucous membrane, nonintact skin, or parenteral contact with blood or other potentially infectious materials that results from the performance of an employee's duties

handwashing facilities A facility providing an adequate supply of running water, soap, single-use towels, or hot-air drying machines

HBV Hepatitis B virus

HIV Human immunodeficiency virus

occupational exposure Reasonably anticipated skin, eye, mucous membrane, or parenteral contact with blood or other potentially infectious materials that may result from the performance of an employee's duties

other potentially infectious materials
1. The following human body fluids: semen, vaginal secretions, cerebrospinal fluid, synovial fluid, pleural fluid, pericardial fluid, peritoneal fluid, amniotic fluid, saliva in dental procedures, any body fluid that is visibly contaminated with blood, and all body fluids in situations where it is difficult or impossible to differentiate between body fluids
2. Any unfixed tissue or organ (other than intact skin) from a human (living or dead)
3. HIV-containing cell or tissue cultures, organ cultures, and HIV- or HBV-containing culture medium or other solutions; blood, organs, or other tissues from experimental animals infected with HIV or HBV

parenteral Piercing mucous membranes or the skin barrier through such events as needlesticks, human bites, cuts, and abrasions

personal protective equipment Specialized clothing or equipment worn by an employee for protection against a hazard

regulated waste
1. Liquid or semiliquid blood or other potentially infectious materials
2. Contaminated items that would release blood or other potentially infectious materials in a liquid or semiliquid state if compressed
3. Items that are caked with dried blood or other potentially infectious materials that are capable of releasing these materials during handling
4. Contaminated sharps; pathological and microbiological wastes containing blood or other potentially infectious materials

source individual Any individual (living or dead) whose blood or other potentially infectious materials may be a source of occupational exposure to employees; examples include, but are not limited to the following:
1. Hospital and clinical patients
2. Clients in institutions for the developmentally disabled
3. Trauma victims
4. Clients of drug and alcohol treatment facilities
5. Residents of hospices and nursing homes
6. Human remains
7. Persons who donate or sell blood or blood components

sterilize The use of a physical or chemical procedure to destroy all microbial life, including highly resistant bacterial endospores

universal precautions An approach to infection control; according to the concept of universal precautions, all human blood and certain human body fluids are treated as if known to be infectious for HIV, HBV, and other bloodborne pathogens

work practice controls Controls that reduce the likelihood of exposure by altering the way the task is performed

Preventive Measures

Preventive measures help reduce the risk of occupational exposure. Such measures include hepatitis B vaccination, universal precautions, engineering and work practice controls, personal protective equipment, and housekeeping measures.

Hepatitis B vaccination. Hepatitis B is an inflammatory disease of the liver. It is caused by the hepatitis B virus (HBV). HBV is usually transmitted by blood and sexual contact. The hepatitis B vaccine is given to produce immunity against hepatitis B. Having **immunity** means that a person has protection against a specific disease and will not get or be affected by the disease. A **vaccination** involves giving a **vaccine** to produce immunity. A vaccine is a preparation containing microorganisms. There are vaccines for many diseases, including measles, mumps, polio, and smallpox. The microorganisms in the vaccine depend on the disease. The polio vaccine contains microorganisms that cause polio. The hepatitis B vaccine contains the virus causing hepatitis B. It provides immunity against hepatitis B.

The hepatitis B vaccination involves three injections (shots). The second injection is given 1 month after the first one. The third injection is given 6 months after the second one. The vaccination can be given before or after exposure to HBV.

Employers must make the hepatitis B vaccination available to employees within 10 working days of being hired. The employee must also receive training about the vaccination. The vaccination is free to the employee. The cost is paid for by the employer.

An employee can refuse the vaccination. If so, the employee must sign a statement saying that the vaccine is being refused. An employee who refuses the vaccine may request and obtain the vaccination at a later date.

Universal precautions. Universal precautions were presented on p. 143. *All* human blood and other potentially infectious materials are treated as if they are infectious for HIV and HBV. OSHA suggests that blood and other infectious materials from all long-term care residents be considered as potentially infectious materials.

Engineering and Work Practice Controls

Engineering and work practice controls are used to control the transmission of HIV and HBV. *Engineering controls* reduce employee exposure in the workplace. The hazard is removed or isolated, or the worker is isolated from the exposure. Special containers for contaminated sharps (needles, broken glass) remove and isolate the hazard from workers. There are also special containers for blood specimens and other body fluid specimens such as urine. All special containers must be puncture-resistant and leakproof. The containers are color-coded in red or labeled with the "biohazard" symbol (see Fig. 8-14).

Work practice controls reduce the risk of exposure. All procedures involving blood or other potentially infectious materials must be done in a way that minimizes spattering, splashing, and spraying. The generation of droplets must also be avoided. OSHA has identified the following work practice controls. The controls address the handling of needles and sharp instruments. Nursing assistant responsibilities do not include the use of needles or sharp instruments. However, such work practice controls are included here so you are aware of how such items should be handled.

1. Do not eat, drink, smoke, apply cosmetics or lip balm, or handle contact lenses in areas of occupational exposure.
2. Do not store food or drink in refrigerators or other locations where blood or potentially infectious materials are kept.
3. Wash hands when gloves are removed and as soon as possible after skin contact with blood or other potentially infectious materials.
4. Never recap, bend, or remove needles by hand unless the employer can demonstrate that no alternative is feasible or that such action is required by a specific medical procedure. When recapping, bending, or removing contaminated needles is required by medical procedure, this must be done by mechanical means (use of forceps) or a one-handed technique.
5. Never shear or break contaminated needles.
6. Discard contaminated needles and sharp instruments in containers that are closable, puncture-resistant, and leakproof. The containers must be color-coded red or labeled with the "biohazard" symbol. Containers must be upright and not allowed to overfill.

Personal Protective Equipment

Personal protective equipment is specialized clothing or equipment worn by an employee for protection against a hazard. Gloves, goggles, and gowns are personal protective equipment. They help prevent occupational exposure to infectious materials. Personal protective equipment meets OSHA's standards if it does not permit blood or other potentially infectious material to pass through the gloves, goggles, or gown. Blood or other potentially infectious materials must not reach the worker's clothes, undergarments, skin, eyes, mouth, or other mucous membranes.

Personal protective equipment must be available at no cost to the worker. Correct sizes must be available. The employer is responsible that equipment is properly cleaned, laundered, repaired, replaced, or discarded.

Personal protective equipment is to be used whenever occupational exposure may occur. OSHA also requires the following precautions for safe handling and use of personal protective equipment.

1. Remove protective equipment before leaving the work area and also after a garment becomes contaminated.
2. Place used protective equipment in designated areas or containers when being stored, washed, decontaminated, or discarded.
3. Wear gloves when it can be expected that there will be contact with blood or other potentially infectious materials. Gloves are also worn when handling or touching contaminated items or surfaces. Gloves are replaced if worn, punctured, or contaminated.
4. Never wash or decontaminate disposable gloves for reuse.
5. Discard utility gloves when they show signs of cracking, peeling, tearing, puncturing, or deteriorating. Utility gloves may be decontaminated for reuse if their integrity is not compromised.

Housekeeping

The bloodborne pathogen standard requires that the facility be kept clean and sanitary. The employer must have a cleaning schedule. The schedule must include the methods of decontamination to be used and the tasks and procedures to be done.

Equipment. Contaminated equipment must be cleaned and decontaminated. So must contaminated work surfaces. Such work surfaces are decontaminated with an appropriate disinfectant:

◆ Upon completion of procedures
◆ Immediately when there is obvious contamination
◆ After any spill of blood or other potentially infectious material
◆ At the end of the work shift when surfaces have become contaminated since the last cleaning

Reusable bins, pails, and cans must be inspected and decontaminated. There must be a schedule for such inspection and decontamination procedures. A brush and dustpan are used to clean up broken glass. Tongs can also be used. You must never pick up broken glass with your hands, not even if wearing gloves.

Waste. Federal, state, and local laws regulate the removal of waste from the facility. The bloodborne pathogen standard requires special measures when discarding contaminated sharps and other *regulated waste*. Regulated waste includes

◆ Liquid or semiliquid blood or other potentially infectious materials
◆ Items contaminated with blood or other potentially infectious materials
◆ Items caked with blood or other potentially infectious materials
◆ Contaminated sharps

Closable, puncture-resistant, and leakproof containers are required for regulated waste. Containers must be color-coded in red or labeled with the "biohazard" symbol.

Laundry

The employer is responsible for laundering contaminated items. Some facilities have their own laundry. Others use a commercial laundry. OSHA requires the following for contaminated laundry:

1. Handle contaminated laundry as little as possible.
2. Wear gloves or other appropriate personal protective equipment when handling contaminated laundry.
3. Bag contaminated laundry at its location of use.
4. Mark laundry bags or containers with the "biohazard" symbol if the laundry is sent off-site.
5. Place wet contaminated laundry in leakproof containers before transporting. The containers should be color-coded in red or labeled with the "biohazard" symbol.

Exposure Incidents

The exposure control plan must include the procedure for evaluating exposure incidents. An *exposure incident* occurs while performing duties of employment. It is a specific eye, mouth, other mucous membrane, nonintact skin, or parenteral contact with blood or other potentially infectious materials. OSHA defines *parenteral* as piercing mucous membranes or the skin barrier. Such piercing can occur through needlesticks, human bites, cuts, and abrasions.

Exposure incidents should be reported at once. Medical evaluation and follow-up are to be made available free to the employee. This includes required laboratory tests. The employee's blood is collected for HBV and HIV testing. The employee may refuse such testing. If so, the blood sample is kept for at least 90 days. Testing can still be done if the employee changes his or her mind.

Confidentiality is very important. The employee must be informed of the results of the evaluation. The employee is also told of any medical conditions resulting from the exposure incident that may need further treatment. The health professional performing the evaluation provides a written opinion to the employer. The employer must give the employee a copy of the opinion within 15 days after the evaluation has been completed.

The source individual's blood is tested for HIV or HBV. The *source individual* is the person whose blood or body fluids are the source of an exposure incident. The results of the testing are to be made available to the exposed employee. State laws vary about releasing such information. The employer must inform the employee about any laws affecting the source's identity and test results.

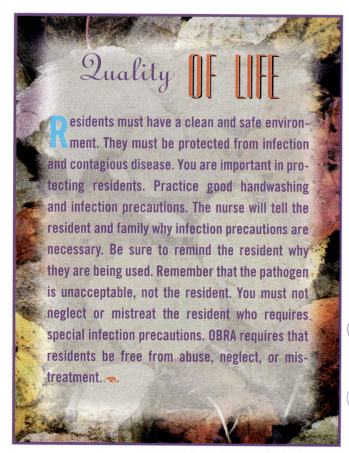

Quality OF LIFE

Residents must have a clean and safe environment. They must be protected from infection and contagious disease. You are important in protecting residents. Practice good handwashing and infection precautions. The nurse will tell the resident and family why infection precautions are necessary. Be sure to remind the resident why they are being used. Remember that the pathogen is unacceptable, not the resident. You must not neglect or mistreat the resident who requires special infection precautions. OBRA requires that residents be free from abuse, neglect, or mistreatment.

SUMMARY

Preventing the spread of infection is the responsibility of every health worker. You must be conscientious about your work. Your employer and your residents assume that you will practice medical asepsis and universal precautions to prevent the spread of microorganisms and infection. Even one act of carelessness can spread microorganisms and endanger resident safety. The reverse is also true. You can develop the same infection that the resident has if you do not practice medical asepsis and universal precautions. The simple procedure of handwashing before and after contact with a resident significantly reduces the spread of microorganisms.

Review QUESTIONS

Circle *T* if the answer is true and *F* if the answer is false.

T F 1. A pathogen is a harmful microorganism capable of causing an infection.

T F 2. Microorganisms are not pathogenic when in their natural environment.

T F 3. The source of an infection is a pathogen.

T F 4. A microorganism must be able to enter the body of a susceptible host for an infection to develop.

T **F** 5. Sterilization is the same as clean technique.

T **F** 6. An object is sterile if nonpathogens are present.

T F 7. Hands and forearms are held up during handwashing.

T F 8. You should clean under your fingernails when washing your hands.

T F 9. The use of disposable equipment helps reduce the spread of infection.

T **F** 10. Unused equipment in a resident's room can be used for another resident.

T F 11. OSHA requires that employees receive free information and training about bloodborne pathogens.

T **F** 12. A person has immunity against hepatitis B. The person will develop the disease.

Circle the *best* answer.

13. A pathogen needs all of the following to grow *except*
    a. Water
    b. Nourishment
    c. Oxygen
    d. Light

14. Microorganisms grow best in an environment that is
    a. Warm and dark
    b. Warm and light
    c. Cool and dark
    d. Cool and light

15. The resident with an infection may have
    a. Fever, nausea, vomiting, rash, and/or sores
    b. Pain or tenderness, redness, and/or swelling
    c. Fatigue, loss of appetite, and/or a discharge
    d. All of the above

154

Review QUESTIONS

16. Microorganisms can enter and leave the body through the
    a. Respiratory tract and/or breaks in the skin
    b. Gastrointestinal system and/or the blood
    c. Reproductive system and/or urinary system
    d. All of the above

17. When cleaning equipment, you should
    a. Rinse the item in cold water before cleaning
    b. Wash the item with soap and hot water
    c. Use a brush if necessary
    d. All of the above

18. Which is used to sterilize equipment?
    a. Handwashing
    b. Boiling water
    c. An autoclave
    d. Chemical disinfectants

19. Infection precautions
    a. Prevent infection
    b. Destroy pathogens
    c. Keep pathogens within a specific area
    d. Destroy pathogens and nonpathogens

20. Universal precautions
    a. Are used for all residents
    b. Prevent the spread of pathogens through the air
    c. Require gowns, masks, goggles, and gloves
    d. All of the above

21. Gloves are worn when the worker is in contact with
    a. Blood
    b. Body fluids
    c. Body substances
    d. All of the above

22. The face mask
    a. Can be reused
    b. Is considered clean on the inside
    c. Is contaminated when it becomes moist
    d. Should fit loosely over the nose and mouth so the person can breathe

23. Goggles are
    a. Always worn when using universal precautions
    b. Worn when there is a risk of splashing blood or body fluids
    c. Worn if you have an eye infection
    d. All of the above

24. Which part of the gown is "clean"?
    a. The neck strings
    b. The waist strings
    c. The sleeves
    d. The back

25. Work practice controls reduce the risk of exposure to bloodborne pathogens. Which is *wrong*?
    a. Hands are washed when gloves are removed
    b. Sharp objects are discarded into containers with the "biohazard" symbol
    c. Food and blood can be stored in the same places
    d. You cannot eat or drink in areas of occupational exposure

26. Proper use of personal protective equipment involves all of the following *except*
    a. Washing disposable gloves for reuse
    b. Removing protective equipment before leaving the work area
    c. Discarding cracked or torn utility gloves
    d. Wearing gloves when touching contaminated items or surfaces

27. When are contaminated work surfaces cleaned?
    a. After completing a procedure
    b. Immediately when there is obvious contamination
    c. After blood or other potentially infectious material is spilled
    d. All of the above

28. You have been exposed to bloodborne pathogen. Which is *true*?
    a. You do not have to report the incident.
    b. You pay for any required laboratory tests.
    c. You can refuse HBV and HIV testing.
    d. Only you are informed of your medical evaluation.

Answers

1. True	8. True	15. d	22. c
2. True	9. True	16. d	23. b
3. True	10. False	17. d	24. a
4. True	11. True	18. c	25. c
5. False	12. False	19. c	26. a
6. False	13. d	20. a	27. d
7. False	14. a	21. d	28. c

9

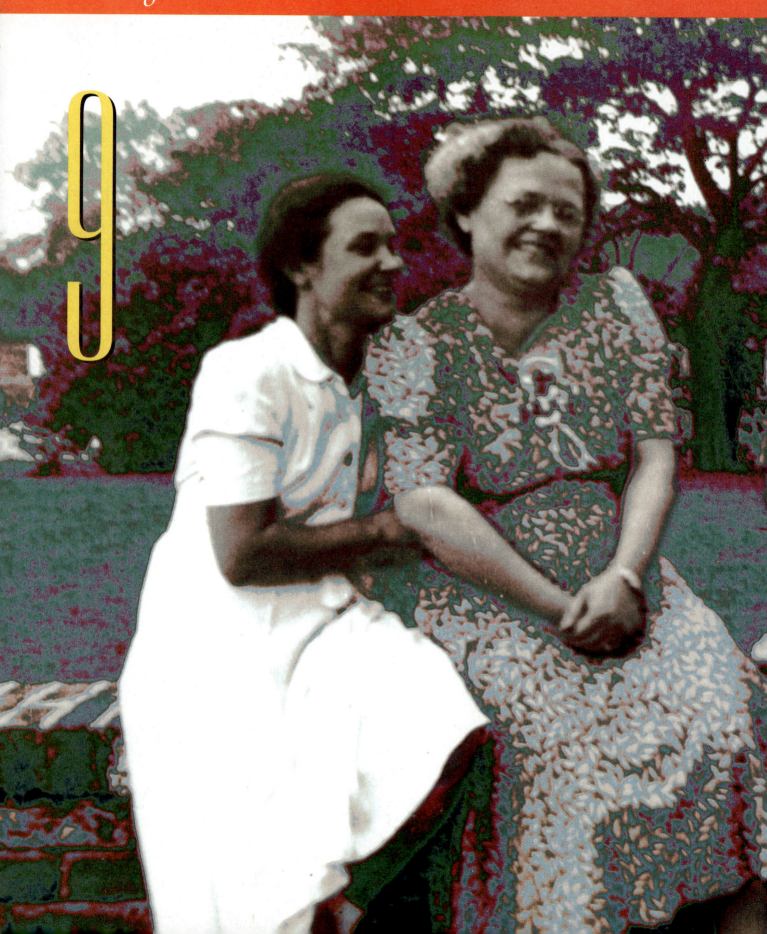

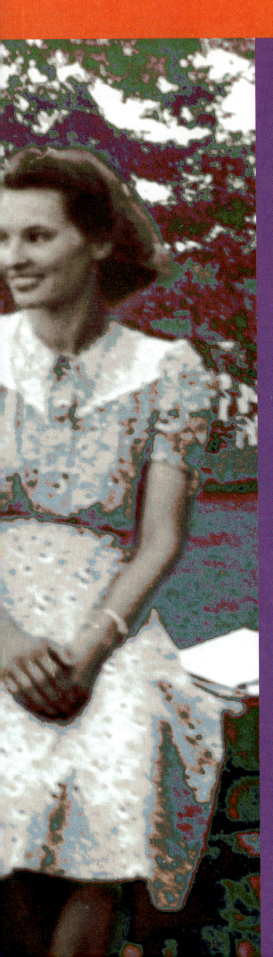

What You Will LEARN

- The key terms listed in this chapter

- The purpose for and rules of using good body mechanics

- Comfort and safety measures for lifting, turning, and moving residents in bed

- The purpose of a transfer belt (gait belt)

- Comfort and safety measures for using a stretcher to transport a resident

- Why good body alignment and position changes are important for residents

- Comfort and safety measures for positioning residents

- How to position residents in good body alignment

- How to perform the procedures described in this chapter

base of support
The area upon which an object rests

body alignment
The way in which body parts are aligned with one another; posture

body mechanics
Using the body in an efficient and careful way

dorsal recumbent position
The back-lying or supine position

Fowler's position
A semisitting position in which the head of the bed is elevated 45 to 60 degrees

friction
The rubbing of one surface against another

gait belt
A transfer belt

lateral position
The side-lying position

logrolling
Turning the resident as a unit in alignment with one motion

posture
The way in which the body parts are aligned with one another; body alignment

prone position
Lying on the abdomen with the head turned to one side

shear
That which occurs when skin sticks to a surface and the bones move forward or backward within the skin; blood supply to the skin is affected

side-lying position
The lateral position

Sims' position
A side-lying position in which the upper leg is sharply flexed so that it does not rest on the lower leg and the lower arm is behind the resident

supine position
The back-lying or dorsal recumbent position

transfer belt
A belt used to hold onto a resident during a transfer or when a worker is walking with the resident; a gait belt

Jim is so nice. He's gentle when he moves me, and he gives me time to catch my breath when he helps me to the chair.

You will move residents often. A resident may be moved or turned in bed or transferred from the bed to a chair, wheelchair, or stretcher. During these and other activities, you must use your body correctly to protect yourself from injury. Using your body correctly also protects residents from the dangers of not being held or supported properly.

BODY MECHANICS

Body mechanics is using the body in an efficient and careful way. It involves the use of good posture, balance, and the strongest and largest muscles of the body to perform work. Fatigue, muscle strain, and injury can result from improper use and positioning of the body during activity or rest. You must be concerned with both your own body mechanics and those of your residents.

The body's major movable parts are the head, trunk, arms, and legs. **Posture,** or **body alignment,** is the way the body parts are aligned with one another. Good body alignment (posture) allows the body to move and function with strength and efficiency. Good alignment is necessary when standing, sitting, or lying down.

Base of support is the area upon which an object rests. The feet provide the base of support for human beings. A good base of support is needed for balance. If you stand on one foot, it will be hard to balance yourself. If you stand with your feet apart, you will have a wider base of support. You will feel more balanced and stable. Therefore a wider base of support gives more balance and stability (Fig. 9-1).

The strongest and largest muscle groups are located in the shoulders, upper arms, hips, and thighs. These muscles are used to lift and move heavy objects. If smaller and weaker muscle groups are used, strain and exertion are placed on them, causing fatigue and injury (Fig. 9-2, A). Use the strong muscles of your thighs and hips by bending your knees or squatting to lift a heavy object (Fig. 9-2, B). Avoid bending over from the waist when lifting. Bending from the waist involves the small muscles of the back. Holding objects close to the body and base of support involves using upper arm and shoulder muscles (Fig. 9-3). If the object is held away from the body, strain is placed on the smaller muscles of the lower arms.

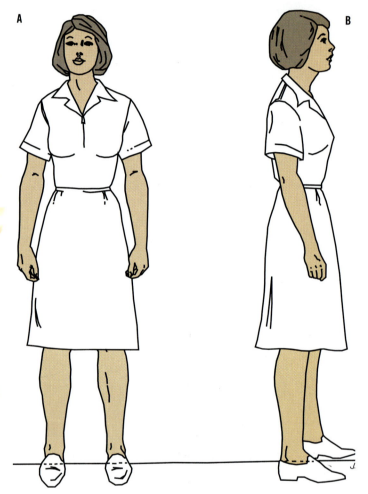

FIGURE 9-1 *A,* Anterior view of adult in good body alignment, with feet apart for a wide base of support. *B,* Lateral view of adult with good posture and alignment.

General Rules

You should use good body mechanics in all activities. Cleaning, laundry, getting in and out of a car, picking up a baby, mowing, and shoveling snow all require good body mechanics. The following rules will help you use good body mechanics to lift and move residents and heavy objects safely and efficiently.

158

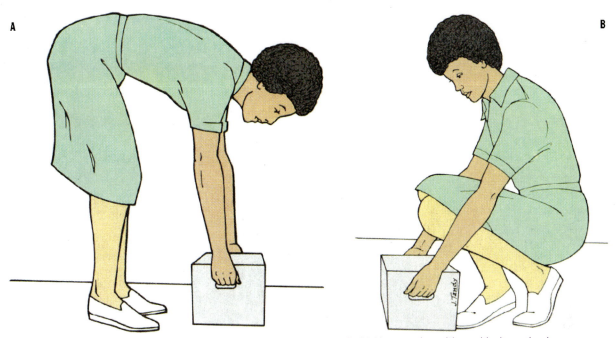

FIGURE 9-2 *A, Picking up a box with poor body mechanics. B, Picking up a box with good body mechanics.*

1. Stand in good alignment and with a wide base of support.
2. Use the stronger and larger muscles of your body. They are in the shoulders, upper arms, thighs, and hips.
3. Keep objects close to your body when you lift, move, or carry them.
4. Avoid unnecessary bending and reaching. If possible, have the height of the bed and overbed table level with your waist when you give care. Adjust the bed and table to the proper height (see Chapter 10).
5. To prevent unnecessary twisting, face the area in which you are working.
6. Push, slide, or pull heavy objects whenever possible rather than lift them.
7. Use both hands and arms when you lift, move, or carry heavy objects.
8. Turn your whole body when you change the direction of your movement.
9. Work with smooth and even movements. Avoid sudden or jerky motions.
10. Get help from a co-worker to move heavy objects or residents.
11. Squat to lift heavy objects from the floor (see Fig. 9-2, *B*). Push against the strong hip and thigh muscles to raise yourself to a standing position.

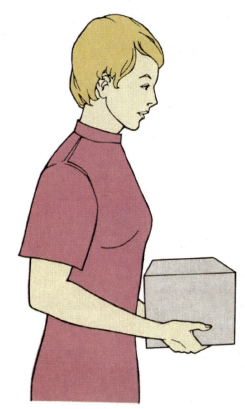

FIGURE 9-3 *The box is being carried close to the body and base of support.*

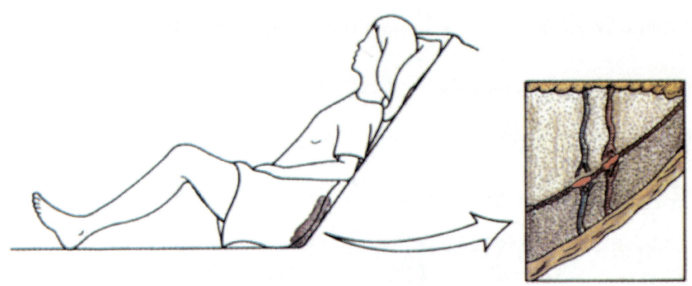

FIGURE 9-4 *When the head of the bed is raised to a sitting position, skin on the buttocks stays in place. However, the hip bones move forward as the resident slides down in bed. The skin is pinched between the mattress and the hip bones. (Courtesy Potter/Perry: Fundamentals of Nursing, 1993 Mosby.)*

LIFTING AND MOVING RESIDENTS IN BED

Some residents can move and turn in bed. Others need help from at least one person for position changes. Residents who are unconscious, paralyzed, on complete bed rest, in casts, or weak from illness or surgery need assistance. Sometimes 2 or 3 persons or a mechanical lift is needed.

You must follow the rules of body mechanics when you move and lift residents in bed. The resident must be protected from injury during the move by being kept in good body alignment. Then the resident is positioned in good body alignment after being moved. Proper positioning of the resident in bed is described on pp. 186-188.

You must protect the resident's skin from friction and shear. **Friction** is the rubbing of one surface against another. When the resident is moved in bed, his or her skin rubs against the sheet. This can cause scratching and skin tears, especially in elderly persons. **Shear** occurs when skin sticks to a surface and the bones move forward or backward within the skin. The skin is pinched between the bones and the surface. Blood supply to the skin is affected. For example, when the head of the bed is raised to a sitting position, skin on the buttocks stays in place. The hip bones, however, move forward as the resident slides

down in bed. The skin is pinched between the mattress and the hip bones (Fig. 9-4). An infection or pressure sore can develop from friction and shear (see Chapter 12). You can reduce friction and shear by rolling or lifting residents instead of sliding them. A cotton drawsheet (see Chapter 11) can be used as a *lifting sheet* (turn or pull sheet) to move the resident in bed and thereby reduce friction and shear.

Other comfort and safety measures need to be considered before residents are moved in bed.

1. Consult the nurse for any limitations or restrictions in positioning or moving the resident. These may be doctor's orders or part of the resident's care plan.
2. Decide how to move the resident and how many helpers you will need.
3. Get enough co-workers to help you before beginning the procedure.
4. Keep the person covered and screened to protect the right to privacy.
5. Protect any tubes or drainage containers connected to the resident.
6. Use caution when moving residents with severe arthritis or osteoporosis (see Chapter 23). Always ask for help when moving them to avoid causing pain or injury.

Raising the Resident's Head and Shoulders

You may have to raise a resident's head and shoulders to tie the back of a gown, to turn or remove a pillow, or to give care. You can raise the resident's shoulders easily and safely by locking arms with the resident. It is best to have help with elderly residents to prevent pain or injury to fragile joints and bones. You may need help if the resident is heavy or difficult to move.

PROCEDURE

Raising the Resident's Head and Shoulders by Locking Arms with the Resident

1. Ask a co-worker to help if assistance is needed.

2. Wash your hands.

3. Identify the resident. Check the ID bracelet and call the resident by name.

4. Explain what you are going to do.

5. Provide for privacy.

6. Lock the bed wheels.

7. Raise the bed to the best level for good body mechanics.

8. Ask your helper to stand on the other side of the bed. Lower the side rails if they are up.

9. Ask the resident to put the near arm under your near arm and behind your shoulder. His or her hand should rest on top of your shoulder. If you are standing on the right side, the resident's right hand will rest on your right shoulder (Fig. 9-5, *A*). If you have assistance, have the resident do the same with your co-worker. The resident's left hand will rest on your co-workers left shoulder (Fig. 9-6, *A*). (Figs. 9-5 and 9-6 on pp. 162-163.)

10. Put your arm near the resident under his or her arm.

Your hand should be on the resident's shoulder. Have your helper do the same.

11. Put your free arm under the resident's neck and shoulders (Fig. 9-5, *B*). If you have assistance, ask your helper to do the same (Fig. 9-6, *B*).

12. Help the resident pull up to a sitting or semisitting position on the count of "3" (Figs. 9-5, *C,* and 9-6, *C*).

13. Use the arm and hand that supported the resident's neck and shoulders to straighten or remove the pillow, tie the gown, etc. (Fig. 9-5, *D*). If you have assistance, ask your co-worker to support the resident (Fig. 9-6, *D*).

14. Help the resident lie down. Provide support with your locked arms. Support his or her neck and shoulders with your other arms.

15. Make sure the resident is comfortable and in good body alignment.

16. Place the signal light within reach.

17. Raise or lower side rails as instructed by the nurse.

18. Lower the bed to its lowest position.

19. Unscreen the resident.

20. Wash your hands.

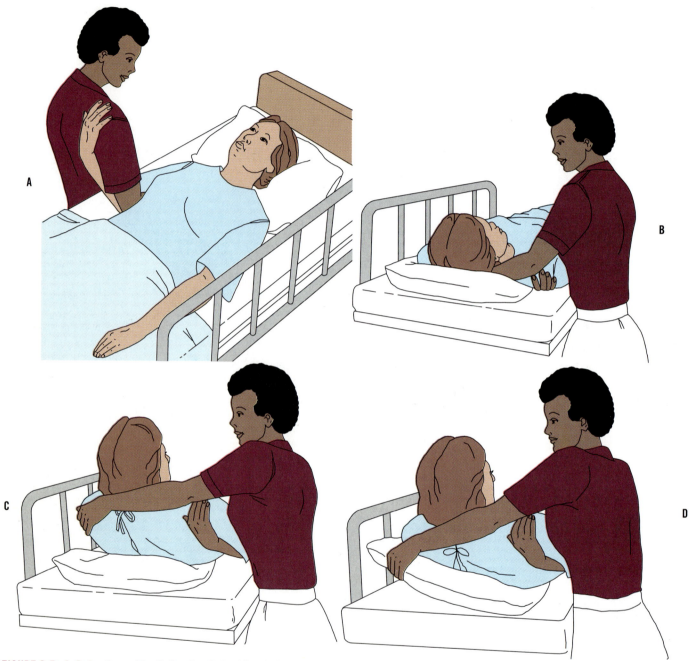

FIGURE 9-5 *A, Raise the resident's head and shoulders by locking arms with the resident. The resident's near arm is under the nursing assistant's near arm and behind the shoulder. B, The far arm of the nursing assistant is under resident's neck and shoulders, with near arm under resident's nearest arm. C, The resident is raised to semisitting position by locking arms. D, The nursing assistant lifts the pillow while the resident is raised to a semisitting position.*

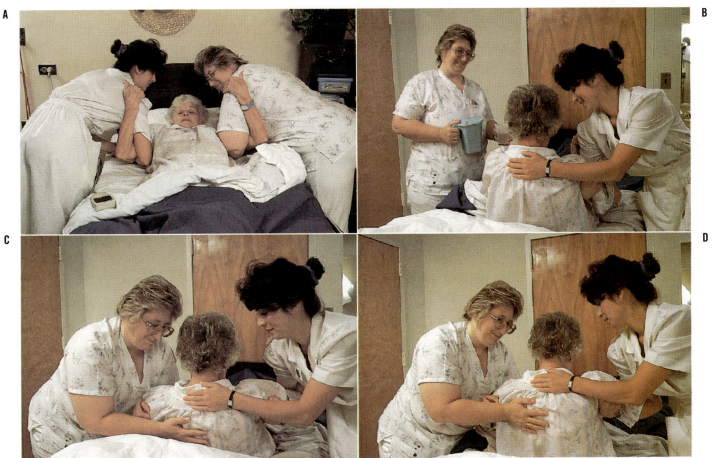

FIGURE 9-6 *A,* *The two nursing assistants lock arms with the resident.* ***B,*** *The nursing assistants have their arms under the resident's head and neck.* ***C,*** *The nursing assistants raise the resident to a semisitting position.* ***D,*** *One nursing assistant supports the resident in the semisitting position while the other gives care.*

Moving the Resident Up in Bed

When the head of the bed is raised, residents often slide down toward the middle and foot of the bed. They need to be moved up in bed to maintain good body alignment and comfort (Fig. 9-7). You can sometimes move light-weight adults up in bed without help. However, it is best to have help to protect you and the resident from pain and injury.

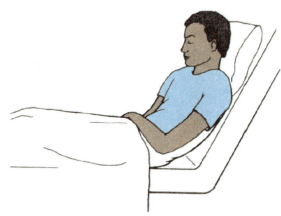

FIGURE 9-7 *A resident in poor body alignment after sliding down in bed.*

PROCEDURE

Moving the Resident Up in Bed

1. Wash your hands.

2. Identify the resident. Check the ID bracelet and call the resident by name.

3. Explain what you are going to do.

4. Provide for privacy.

5. Lock the bed wheels.

6. Raise the bed to the best level for good body mechanics.

7. Lower the head of the bed to a level appropriate for the resident. The bed should be as flat as possible.

8. Place the pillow against the headboard if the resident can be without it. This prevents his or her head from hitting the headboard when being moved up.

9. Make sure the far side rail is raised. Lower the one near you if it is up.

10. Stand with your feet about 12 inches apart. Point the foot nearest the head of the bed toward the head of the bed. Face the head of the bed.

11. Bend your hips and knees, and keep your back straight.

12. Place one arm under the resident's shoulders and the other under the resident's thighs.

13. Ask the resident to grasp the headboard and to flex both knees as in Fig. 9-8.

14. Explain that you will both move on the count of "3." Ask the resident to pull up with the hands and push against the bed with the feet. Explain what you will be doing.

15. Move the resident to the head of the bed on the count of "3." Shift your weight from your rear leg to your front leg (Fig. 9-9).

16. Put the pillow under the resident's head and shoulders. Lock arms with him or her to complete this step.

17. Straighten linens. Make sure the resident is comfortable and in good alignment.

18. Place the signal light within reach.

19. Raise or lower side rails as instructed by the nurse.

20. Raise the head of the bed to a level appropriate for the resident.

21. Lower the bed to its lowest position.

22. Unscreen the resident.

23. Wash your hands.

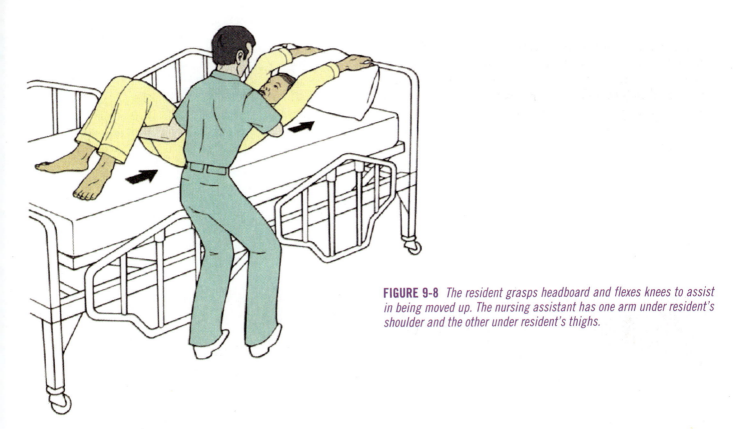

FIGURE 9-8 *The resident grasps headboard and flexes knees to assist in being moved up. The nursing assistant has one arm under resident's shoulder and the other under resident's thighs.*

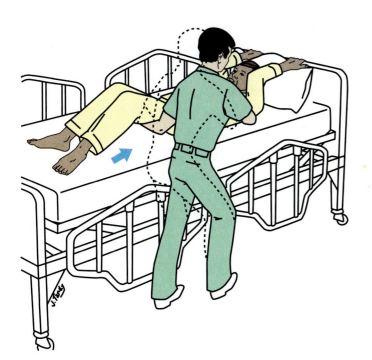

FIGURE 9-9 *The resident is moved up in bed as the nursing assistant's body weight is shifted from rear leg to front leg.*

Moving the Resident Up in Bed with Assistance

You will need assistance when a resident cannot help in being moved up in bed. At least two people are needed to move heavy, weak, or very elderly residents. Be sure to ask for help before starting the procedure. Also remember to help if a co-worker needs you.

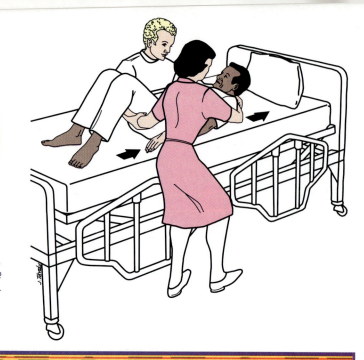

FIGURE 9-10 *A resident is moved up in bed by two nursing assistants. Each has one arm under resident's shoulder and the other under the resident's buttocks. The nursing assistants have locked arms under resident. Resident's knees are flexed.*

PROCEDURE

Moving the Resident Up in Bed with Assistance

1. Ask a co-worker to help.
2. Wash your hands.
3. Identify the resident. Check the ID bracelet and call the person by name.
4. Explain what you are going to do.
5. Provide for privacy.
6. Lock the bed wheels.
7. Raise the bed to the best level for good body mechanics.
8. Lower the head of the bed to a level appropriate for the resident. The bed should be as flat as possible.
9. Place the pillow against the headboard if the resident can be without it. This prevents his or her head from hitting the headboard when being moved up.
10. Stand on one side of the bed. Have your helper stand on the other.
11. Lower the side rails if they are up.
12. Stand with your feet about 12 inches apart. Point the foot near the head of the bed toward the head of the bed. Face that direction.
13. Bend your hips and knees, and keep your back straight.

14. Place one arm under the resident's shoulder and one arm under the buttocks. Your helper does the same. Grasp each other's forearms.
15. Ask the resident to flex both knees (Fig. 9-10).
16. Explain that you and your helper will move on the count of "3." The resident, if able, should push against the bed with the feet.
17. Move the resident to the head of the bed on the count of "3." Shift your body weight from your rear leg to your front leg.
18. Repeat steps 12 through 17 if necessary.
19. Put the pillow under the resident's head and shoulders. Straighten the linens. Make sure the resident is comfortable and in good body alignment.
20. Place the signal light within reach.
21. Raise or lower side rails as instructed by the nurse.
22. Raise the head of the bed to a level appropriate for the resident.
23. Lower the bed to its lowest position.
24. Unscreen the resident.
25. Wash your hands.

Moving the Resident Up in Bed Using a Lifting Sheet

With the help of a co-worker, you can easily and safely move a resident up in bed using a lifting sheet. Friction and shear are reduced, and the resident is lifted more evenly. You can use a flat sheet folded in half or a draw-sheet for the lifting sheet. The lifting sheet is placed under the resident. It extends from the shoulders to above the knees. Most residents should be moved up in bed with a lifting sheet, particularly those who cannot move themselves.

PROCEDURE

Moving the Resident Up in Bed Using a Lifting Sheet

1. Ask a co-worker to help.

2. Wash your hands.

3. Identify the resident. Check the ID bracelet and call the person by name.

4. Explain what you are going to do.

5. Provide for privacy.

6. Lock the bed wheels.

7. Raise the bed to the best level for good body mechanics.

8. Lower the head of the bed to a level appropriate for the resident. The bed should be as flat as possible.

9. Place the pillow against the headboard if the resident can be without it.

10. Stand on one side of the bed. Have your helper stand on the other side.

11. Lower the side rails if they are up.

12. Stand with your feet about 12 inches apart. Point the foot near the head of the bed toward the head of the bed. Face that direction.

13. Roll the sides of the lifting sheet up close to the resident (Fig. 9-11, p. 168).

14. Grasp the rolled-up lifting sheet firmly near the shoulders and buttocks.

15. Bend your hips and knees, and keep your back straight.

16. Slide the resident up in bed on the count of "3" (Fig. 9-12, p. 168). Shift your weight from your rear leg to your front leg.

17. Unroll the lifting sheet.

18. Put the pillow under the resident's head and shoulders. Straighten linens. Make sure the resident is comfortable and in good alignment.

19. Place the signal light within reach.

20. Raise or lower side rails as instructed by the nurse.

21. Raise the head of the bed to a level appropriate for the resident.

22. Lower the bed to its lowest position.

23. Unscreen the resident.

24. Wash your hands.

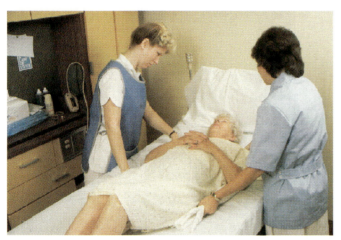

FIGURE 9-11 *The lifting sheet is rolled up close to the resident.*

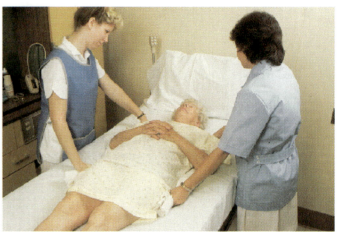

FIGURE 9-12 *Two nursing assistants move a resident up in bed with a lifting sheet. A lifting sheet is rolled close to the resident and held near the shoulders and buttocks.*

Moving a Resident to the Side of the Bed

Residents are moved to the side of the bed for repositioning and for certain procedures such as a bed bath. A resident in the middle of the bed is moved to the side of the bed before being turned. Otherwise, after turning, the resident will be lying on the side of the bed rather than in the middle. A resident should be in the middle of the bed to allow for good body alignment.

Sometimes you have to reach over to the resident. Good body mechanics can be used if reaching is minimized and if the resident is close to you.

The resident should be in the back-lying position when being moved to the side of the bed. One procedure involves moving the resident in segments. This can be done by one person. Do not use this procedure for very elderly or arthritic residents or those with spinal cord injuries or recovering from spinal surgery. For such cases, get help and use a lifting sheet. This helps prevent pain and possible skin damage.

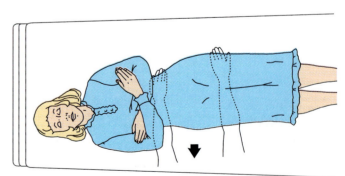

FIGURE 9-13 **A,** *The resident is moved to side of bed in segments. The upper part is moved first as the nursing assistant has one arm under resident's neck and shoulders and the other under the midportion of the resident's back.* **B,** *The nursing assistant has one arm under resident's waist and the other under the thighs to move the lower portion of the resident's body to side of the bed.* **C,** *The resident's legs and feet are moved to side of the bed. The nursing assistant has one arm under resident's thighs and the other under calves.*

PROCEDURE

Moving the Resident to the Side of the Bed in Segments

1. Wash your hands.

2. Identify the resident. Check the ID bracelet and call the person by name.

3. Explain what you are going to do.

4. Provide for privacy.

5. Lock the bed wheels.

6. Raise the bed to the best level for good body mechanics.

7. Lower the head of the bed to a level appropriate for the resident. Keep the bed as flat as possible.

8. Stand on the side of the bed to which you will be moving the resident.

9. Make sure the far side rail is raised. Lower the one near you if it is up.

10. Stand with your feet about 12 inches apart and one foot in front of the other. Flex your knees.

11. Cross the resident's arms over the chest.

12. Place your arm under the resident's neck and shoulders. Grasp the far shoulder.

13. Place your other arm under the resident's midback.

14. Move the upper part of the resident's body toward you. Rock backward and shift your weight to your rear leg (Fig. 9-13, *A*).

15. Place one arm under the resident's waist and the other under the thighs.

16. Rock backward to move the lower part of the resident's body toward you (Fig. 9-13, *B*).

17. Repeat the procedure for the legs and feet (Fig. 9-13, *C*). Your arms should be under the thighs and calves.

18. Make sure the resident is comfortable, in good body alignment, and positioned as directed by the nurse. Reposition the pillow under his or her head and shoulders.

19. Place the signal light within reach.

20. Raise or lower side rails as instructed by the nurse.

21. Lower the bed to its lowest position.

22. Unscreen the resident.

23. Wash your hands.

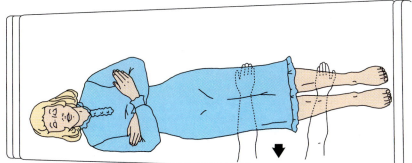

FIGURE 9-13 *C,* *The resident's legs and feet are moved to side of the bed. The nursing assistant has one arm under resident's thighs and the other under calves.*

PROCEDURE

Moving the Resident to the Side of the Bed Using a Lifting Sheet

1. Ask 1 or 2 co-workers to help you.

2. Wash your hands.

3. Identify the resident. Check the ID bracelet and call the person by name.

4. Explain what you are going to do.

5. Provide for privacy.

6. Lock the bed wheels.

7. Raise the bed to the best level for good body mechanics.

8. Lower the head of the bed to a level appropriate for the resident. Keep the bed as flat as possible.

9. Stand on one side of the bed with one helper on the other. Have the other helper stand at the foot of the bed to hold and guide the feet if the resident is very heavy or tall.

10. Lower both side rails if they are up.

11. Stand with your feet about 12 inches apart and with one foot in front of the other. Flex your knees.

12. Roll the sides of the lifting sheet up close to the resident.

13. Grasp the rolled-up lifting sheet firmly near the resident's shoulders and buttocks.

14. Rock backward on the count of "3," moving the resident toward you. Your partner rocks backward slightly and then forward toward you while keeping the arms straight (Fig. 9-14).

15. Unroll the lifting sheet.

16. Make sure the resident is comfortable, in good alignment, and positioned as directed by the nurse.

17. Place the signal light within reach.

18. Raise or lower side rails as instructed by the nurse.

19. Lower the bed to its lowest position.

20. Unscreen the resident.

21. Wash your hands.

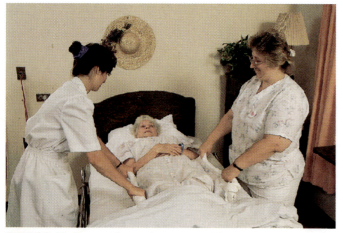

FIGURE 9-14 *Two nursing assistants use a lifting sheet to move a resident to the side of the bed. The lifting sheet lifts some of the resident's weight off the bed. Friction is reduced as the resident is moved.*

Turning Residents

Residents are turned onto their sides to prevent complications from bed rest and to receive care. Certain medical and nursing procedures require the side-lying position. Residents are turned toward or away from you. The direction depends on the person's condition and the situation. Methods for turning residents toward or away from you are described in this chapter. However, logrolling with the lifting sheet should be used for turning most residents in long-term care. It helps prevent pain in arthritic spines and hips.

PROCEDURE

Turning the Resident Toward You

1. Wash your hands.

2. Identify the resident. Check the ID bracelet and call the person by name.

3. Explain what you are going to do.

4. Provide for privacy.

5. Lock the bed wheels.

6. Raise the bed to the best level for good body mechanics.

7. Lower the head of the bed to a level appropriate for the resident. Keep the bed as flat as possible.

8. Stand on the side of the bed opposite that to which you will turn the resident. Make sure the far side rail is up. Lower the side rail near you if it is up.

9. Move the resident to the side of the bed near you.

10. Cross the resident's arms over the chest. Cross the leg near you over the far leg.

11. Raise the side rail.

12. Go to the other side. Lower the side rail.

13. Stand with your feet 12 inches apart. Flex your knees and keep your back straight.

14. Place one hand on the resident's far shoulder and the other on the far hip.

15. Roll the resident toward you gently (Fig. 9-15).

16. Make sure the resident is comfortable and in good alignment. Use pillows for support as in Fig. 9-16.

17. Place the signal light within reach.

18. Raise or lower side rails as instructed by the nurse.

19. Lower the bed to its lowest position.

20. Unscreen the resident.

21. Wash your hands.

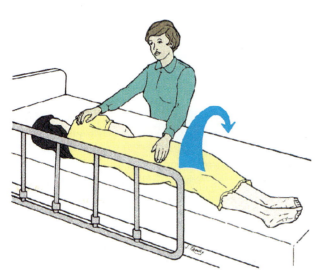

FIGURE 9-15 *The resident is turned toward the nursing assistant. Resident's arms and legs are crossed. The nursing assistant has one hand on resident's far shoulder and the other on the far hip.*

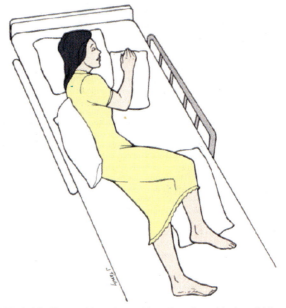

FIGURE 9-16 *The resident is positioned on her side in middle of the bed. A pillow is placed in front of bottom leg, with top leg on pillow in flexed position; note pillow against the back. A small pillow supports arm and hand; note pillow under head and shoulder.*

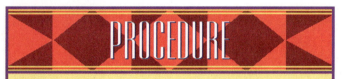

PROCEDURE

Turning the Resident Away From You

1. Follow steps 1 to 10 as in *Turning the Resident Toward You* (p. 171).

2. Stand with your feet about 12 inches apart. Flex your knees, and keep your back straight.

3. Place one hand on the resident's shoulder and the other on the buttocks near you.

4. Push the resident gently toward the other side of the bed (Fig. 9-17). Shift your weight from your rear leg to your front leg.

5. Make sure the resident is comfortable and in good body alignment. Use pillows for support (see Fig. 9-16, p. 171).

6. Raise or lower side rails as instructed by the nurse.

7. Place the signal light within reach.

8. Lower the bed to its lowest position.

9. Unscreen the resident.

10. Wash your hands.

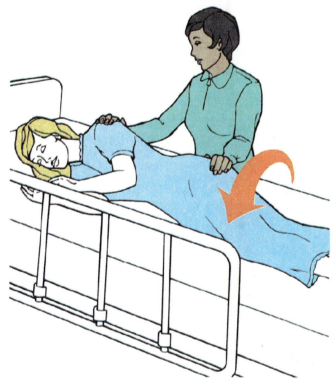

FIGURE 9-17 *The resident is turned away from the nursing assistant. Resident's arms and legs are crossed, and the nursing assistant has one hand on the resident's shoulder and the other on resident's buttocks.*

Logrolling

Logrolling is turning the resident as a unit in alignment with one motion. Elderly residents with arthritic spines and hips or those recovering from hip fractures are turned in one motion. Residents with spinal cord injuries or those recovering from spinal surgery must keep their spines straight at all times. These residents also must be rolled over in one motion. The back is kept in straight alignment when the resident is turned. Two workers are needed to logroll a resident. Three are needed if a resident is tall or heavy. A lifting sheet is used for the procedure.

PROCEDURE

Logrolling a Resident

1. Ask a nurse or a co-worker to help you.

2. Wash your hands.

3. Identify the resident. Check the ID bracelet and call the person by name.

4. Explain what you are going to do.

5. Provide for privacy.

6. Lock the bed wheels.

7. Raise the bed to the best level for good body mechanics.

8. Make sure the bed is flat.

9. Make sure the side rail is up on the side to which the resident will be turned.

10. Stand on the other side. Lower the side rail if it is up.

11. Move the resident as a unit to the side of the bed near you. (See *Moving the Resident to the Side of the Bed Using a Lifting Sheet*, p. 170.)

12. Place the resident's arms across the chest. Place a pillow between the knees (Fig. 9-18, *A*).

13. Raise the side rail. Go to the other side.

14. Lower the side rail.

15. Position yourself near the shoulders and chest. Your helper should stand by the resident's buttocks and thighs.

16. Stand with your feet about 12 inches apart. One foot should be in front of the other.

17. Ask the resident to hold his or her body rigid.

18. Roll the resident toward you using a lifting sheet (Fig. 9-18, *B*). Make sure the person is turned as a unit.

19. Make sure the resident is comfortable and in good alignment. Use pillows for support. Place:
    a. One against the back for support
    b. One under the head and neck if allowed
    c. One (or a folded bath blanket) between the legs
    d. One small pillow under the arm and hand

20. Place the signal light within reach.

21. Raise or lower side rails as instructed by the nurse.

22. Lower the bed to its lowest position.

23. Unscreen the resident.

24. Wash your hands.

A
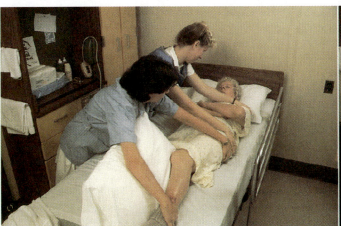
B
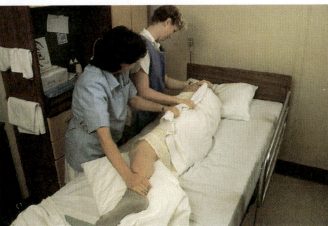

FIGURE 9-18 *Logrolling. **A,** There is a pillow between resident's legs. Arms are crossed on the chest. Resident is on far side of bed. **B,** A turning sheet is used to logroll a resident.*

SITTING ON THE SIDE OF THE BED (DANGLING)

Residents are helped to sit on the side of the bed *(dangle)* for many reasons. Many elderly persons become dizzy or faint if they get out of bed too fast. They may need to sit on the side of the bed for 1 to 5 minutes before walking or transferring. Some residents gradually increase activity in stages. They progress from bed rest, to sitting on the side of the bed, and then to sitting in a chair. Walking about in the room and then in the hallway are the next steps. While dangling, they cough, deep breathe, and move their legs back and forth and in circles to stimulate circulation.

Two workers may be needed to help a resident dangle. If there is a problem with balance or coordination, the resident must be supported. This is especially true if the person has had a stroke. Stroke victims often have problems with sitting balance. If fainting occurs, the resident is laid down. You must make certain observations while the resident is dangling. Take the resident's pulse and respirations. Observe for difficulty in breathing, pallor, or cyanosis. Also note complaints of dizziness or light-headedness.

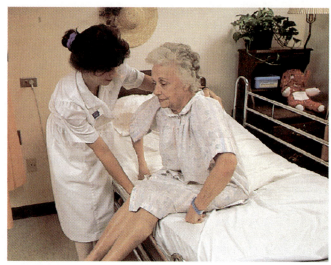

FIGURE 9-20 *The resident is upright, with legs over edge of mattress.*

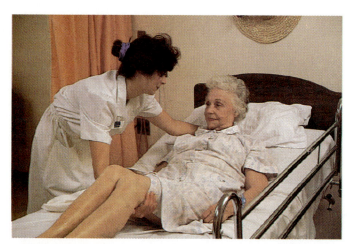

FIGURE 9-19 *The resident prepares to sit on side of bed. Resident is in Fowler's position, and nursing assistant grasps resident's far shoulder and far knee with arms.*

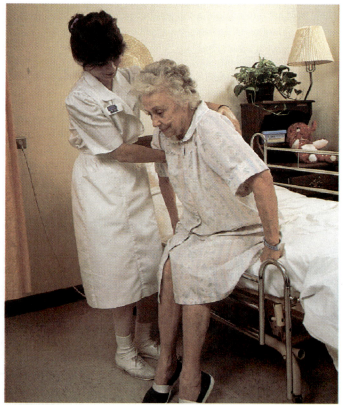

FIGURE 9-21 *The resident is supporting self with fists pushed into mattress.*

Helping the Resident to Sit on the Side of the Bed (Dangle)

1. Explain what you are going to do and how the resident can help.

2. Collect the following:
   a. Clothing or a robe and shoes
   b. Paper or sheet
   c. A footstool if the resident is very short

3. Wash your hands.

4. Identify the resident. Check the ID bracelet and call the person by name.

5. Decide which side of the bed to use.

6. Move furniture to provide moving space for you and the resident.

7. Provide for privacy.

8. Position the resident supine. Lock the bed wheels.

9. Raise the bed to the best level for good body mechanics.

10. Help the resident to move up in bed.

11. Prepare the resident to get out of bed:
    a. Fan-fold top linens to the foot of the bed.
    b. Help with clothing if the resident is to dress (see pp. 272-273).
    c. Place the paper or sheet under the resident's feet. This protects bottom linen from shoes.
    d. Put shoes on the resident.

12. Ask the resident to move to the side of the bed. Assist if necessary.

13. Raise the side rail if the bed is manually operated. Stand near the resident's waist if the bed is an electric one. This protects the resident from falling out of bed.

14. Raise the head of the bed so that the resident is sitting.

15. Lower the side rail.

16. Slide one arm under the resident's neck and shoulders. Grasp the far shoulder. Place your other hand under the far knee (Fig. 9-19).

17. Turn the resident a quarter of a turn. As the resident's legs go over the edge of the mattress, the trunk will be upright (Fig. 9-20).

18. Ask the resident to push both fists into the mattress (Fig. 9-21). This supports the person in the sitting position.

19. Do not leave the resident alone. Provide support if necessary.

20. Ask how the resident feels. Check pulse and respirations. Help the resident lie down if necessary.

21. Help the resident put on a robe or clothing.

22. Lower the bed to its lowest possible position if the resident will get out of bed.

23. Reverse the procedure to return the resident to bed.

24. Lower the head of the bed after the resident has returned to bed. Help him or her move to the center of the bed.

25. Remove the shoes and the paper or sheet protecting the bottom linen.

26. Make sure the resident is comfortable and in good alignment. Cover the resident.

27. Place the signal light within reach.

28. Lower the bed to its lowest position.

29. Raise or lower side rails as instructed by the nurse.

30. Put the robe or clothing away.

31. Return furniture to its proper location.

32. Unscreen the resident.

33. Wash your hands.

34. Report the following to the nurse:
    a. How well the activity was tolerated
    b. The length of time dangled
    c. Pulse and respiratory rates while dangling
    d. The amount of assistance needed
    e. Other observations or resident complaints

TRANSFERRING RESIDENTS

Residents often need to be moved from their beds to chairs, wheelchairs, or stretchers. Some need only a little assistance. Others need help from at least one person. Some residents are transferred by at least 2 or 3 people. Ask the nurse how much assistance a resident needs. The rules of body mechanics and the safety and comfort considerations described for lifting and moving residents apply when transferring. The room should be arranged so that there is enough space for a safe transfer. The chair, wheelchair, or stretcher must be placed correctly for a safe and efficient transfer.

A **transfer belt** is used for transferring most residents in nursing facilities. The belt is used to hold onto the resident during the transfer. Remember, *if the resident requires assistance to transfer, a transfer belt is required.* The belt is applied around the resident's waist. The belt also is called a **gait belt** and is used when walking with a resident.

PROCEDURE

Applying a Transfer (Gait) Belt

1. Wash your hands.
2. Identify the resident. Check the ID bracelet and call the person by name.
3. Explain what you are going to do.
4. Provide for privacy.
5. Assist the resident to a sitting position.
6. Apply the belt around the waist over clothing. Do not apply it over bare skin.
7. Tighten the belt so that it is snug. It should not cause discomfort or impair breathing.
8. Make sure that a woman's breasts are not caught under the belt.
9. Place the buckle off-center in the front or in the back for the resident's comfort (Fig. 9-22).
10. Prepare to transfer the resident.

A
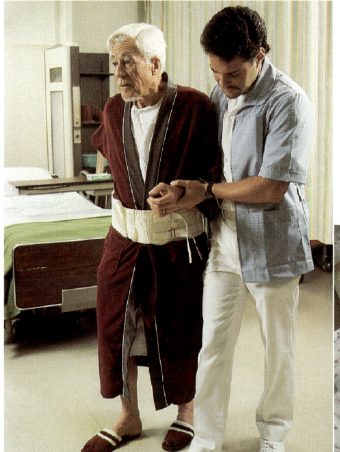

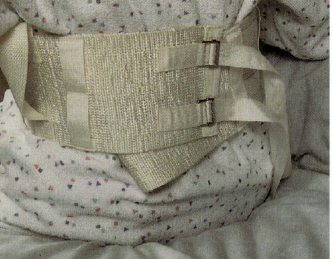
B

FIGURE 9-22 *Transfer (safety) belt.* **A,** *The belt is positioned off-center in the front.* **B,** *The belt buckle is positioned at the back.*

Transferring a resident to a chair or wheelchair
Safety is a major concern in transferring a resident to a chair or wheelchair. The resident must be protected from falling. The resident wears street shoes to prevent sliding or slipping on the floor. The chair or wheelchair must be sturdy enough to support the resident's weight. The number of helpers needed for a transfer depends on the resident's physical capabilities, condition, and size. Encourage the resident to assist in the transfer whenever possible to help increase muscle strength.

Most wheelchairs or bedside chairs have vinyl seats and backs. Vinyl holds body heat, causing the resident to become warmer and to perspire more. You can cover the back and seat with a folded bath blanket. This increases the resident's comfort in the chair. Residents who use wheelchairs often have special cushions. Check with the nurse about the proper use and placement of these cushions.

The resident is helped out of bed on his or her strong side. If the left side is weak and the right side strong, get the resident out of bed on the right side. In transferring, the strong side moves first and pulls the weaker side along. Transferring from the weak side is awkward and may be unsafe.

The nurse may ask you to take the resident's pulse before and after the transfer. The person may have a severe chronic illness and may tire with even a little exertion. The pulse rate gives some information about how the activity was tolerated. Also observe and report if the resident tires easily, complains of weakness or lightheadedness, has pain or discomfort, or has difficulty breathing (dyspnea). Also report the amount of help needed and how the resident helped in the transfer.

PROCEDURE

Transferring the Resident to a Chair or Wheelchair

1. Explain what you are going to do.
2. Collect the following:
   a. Wheelchair or armchair
   b. One or two bath blankets and a lap robe
   c. Clothing or robe and shoes
   d. Paper or sheet for the bottom linen
   e. Transfer (gait) belt if needed
   f. Special cushion if used
3. Wash your hands.
4. Identify the resident. Check the ID bracelet and call the person by name.
5. Provide for privacy.
6. Decide which side of the bed to use. Move furniture to provide moving space.
7. Place the chair or wheelchair at the head of the bed. The back must be even with the headboard (Fig. 9-23, p. 178).
8. Place the folded bath blanket or cushion on the seat. Lock the wheelchair wheels, and raise the footrests.
9. Make sure the bed is in the lowest position and the bed wheels are locked.
10. Fan-fold top linens to the foot of the bed.
11. Help the resident put on clothing or a robe.
12. Place the paper or sheet under the resident's feet to protect the bottom sheet. Put shoes on the resident.
13. Help the resident dangle. Make sure his or her feet touch the floor.
14. Apply the transfer belt.
15. Help the resident to stand. Do the following if a transfer belt is used.
    a. Stand in front of the resident.
    b. Have the resident place his or her fists on the bed by the thighs.
    c. Make sure the resident's feet are flat on the floor.
    d. Have the resident lean forward.
    e. Grasp the transfer belt at each side.
    f. Brace your knees against the resident's knees and block his or her feet with your feet (Fig. 9-24, p. 178).
    g. Ask the resident to push the fists down on the bed and to stand on the count of "3." Pull the resident into a standing position as you straighten your knees (Fig. 9-25, p. 179).

Continued.

16. Use this method if a transfer belt is not available.
    a. Stand in front of the resident.
    b. Have the resident place the fists on the bed by the thighs.
    c. Make sure the resident's feet are flat on the floor.
    d. Place your hands under his or her arms. Your hands should be around the shoulder blades (Fig. 9-26).
    e. Have the resident lean forward.
    f. Brace your knees against the resident's knees, and block his or her feet with your feet.
    g. Ask the resident to push the fists into the bed and to stand on the count of "3." Pull the resident up into a standing position as you straighten your knees.

17. Support the resident in the standing position. Hold the transfer belt or the resident's shoulder blades. Continue to block the resident's feet and knees with your feet and knees. This helps prevent falling.

18. Turn the resident so he or she can grasp the far arm of the chair. The legs will touch the edge of the chair (Fig. 9-27). Turn the resident until the other armrest is grasped.

19. Lower him or her into the chair as you bend your hips and knees (Fig. 9-28). The resident assists by leaning forward and bending the elbows and knees.

20. Make sure the buttocks are to the back of the seat. Position the resident in good alignment.

21. Position the feet on the footrests.

22. Cover the resident's lap and legs with a lap robe or bath blanket if the resident is not dressed. The blanket must be off the floor and wheels.

23. Remove the transfer belt.

24. Position the chair as the resident prefers.

25. Place the signal light and other necessary items within reach if the resident will be at the bedside. Straighten the unit.

26. Unscreen the resident.

27. Wash your hands.

28. Report the following to the nurse:
    a. Pulse rate if taken
    b. How well the activity was tolerated
    c. Complaints of lightheadedness, pain, discomfort, difficulty breathing, weakness, or fatigue
    d. The amount of assistance needed to transfer the resident

29. Reverse the procedure to return the resident to bed.

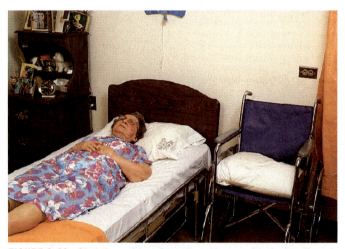

FIGURE 9-23 *Chair is positioned next to and even with the headboard.*

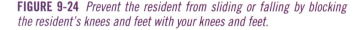

FIGURE 9-24 *Prevent the resident from sliding or falling by blocking the resident's knees and feet with your knees and feet.*

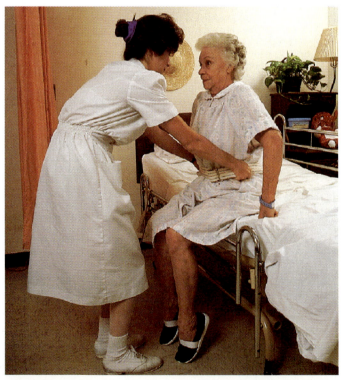

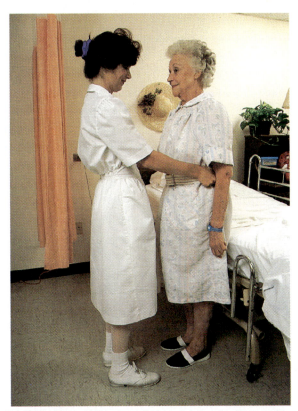

FIGURE 9-25 *The resident is pulled up into a standing position and supported by holding transfer belt and by the nurse assistant's blocking the resident's knees and feet.*

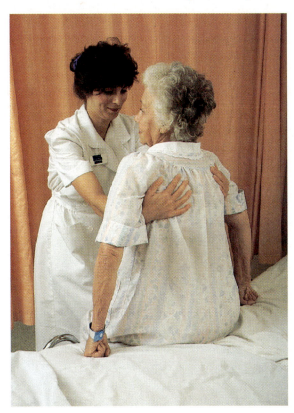

FIGURE 9-26 *The resident is being prepared to stand. The nurse assistant places hands under the resident's arms and around the shoulder blades.*

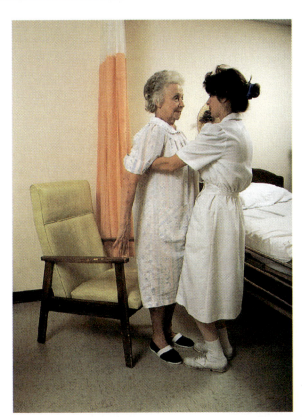

FIGURE 9-27 *The resident is supported as she grasps the far arm of the chair. Legs are against the chair.*

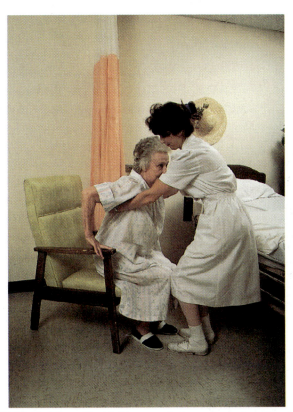

FIGURE 9-28 *The resident holds armrests, leans forward, and bends elbows and knees while being lowered into chair.*

PROCEDURE

Transferring the Resident to a Wheelchair (Two Assistants)

1. Ask a co-worker to help you.

2. Explain what you are going to do.

3. Collect the following:
   a. Wheelchair with removable armrests
   b. Bath blanket or lap robe
   c. Shoes
   d. Cushion if used

4. Wash your hands.

5. Identify the resident. Check the ID bracelet and call the person by name.

6. Provide for privacy.

7. Decide which side of the bed to use. Move furniture to provide moving space.

8. Fan-fold top linens to the foot of the bed.

9. Assist the resident to the side of the bed near you. Help him or her to a sitting position by raising the head of the bed.

10. Place the wheelchair at the side of the bed. Have the seat even with the resident's hips.

11. Remove the armrest near the bed. Place the cushion or folded bath blanket on the seat.

12. Lock wheels on the wheelchair and bed.

13. Stand behind the wheelchair. Put your arms under the resident's arms and grasp the forearms.

14. Have your helper grasp the resident's thighs and calves. This supports the lower extremities.

15. Bring the resident toward the chair on the count of "3." Lower him or her into the chair (Fig. 9-29, *A* and *B*).

16. Make sure the buttocks are to the back of the seat. Position the resident in good alignment.

17. Put the armrest back on the wheelchair.

18. Put the resident's shoes on. Position the feet on the footrests.

19. Cover the resident's lap and legs with a lap robe or a bath blanket if the resident is not dressed. The blanket must be off the floor and wheels.

20. Position the chair as the resident prefers.

21. Place the signal light and other necessary items within reach if the resident will stay at the bedside. Straighten the unit.

22. Unscreen the resident.

23. Wash your hands.

24. Report the following to the nurse:
   a. Pulse rate if taken
   b. Complaints of lightheadedness, pain, discomfort, difficulty breathing, weakness, or fatigue
   c. How well the activity was tolerated

25. Reverse the procedure to return the resident to bed.

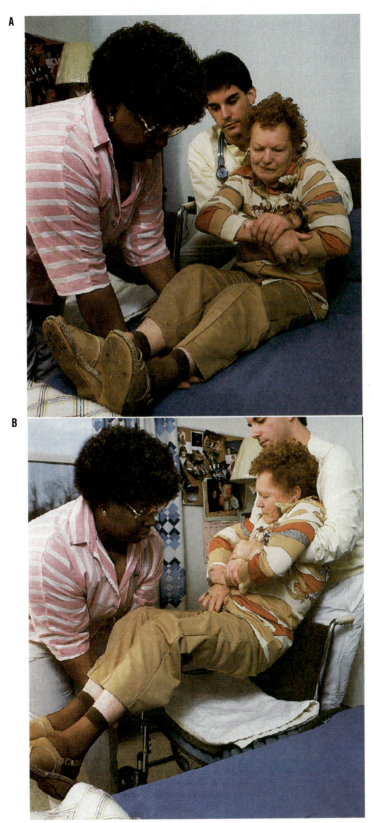

FIGURE 9-29 *Transfer to a chair by two nursing assistants. **A,** The resident is brought toward the chair. **B,** The resident is supported while being lowered into the chair.*

Using Mechanical Lifts

A mechanical lift is used to transfer helpless residents. The person may be transferred from bed to a chair, wheelchair, stretcher, bathtub, toilet, whirlpool, or car. There are many types of mechanical lifts. Be sure you know how to use the lift. Before using the lift, you need to make sure it is working. You also need to compare the resident's weight and the weight limit of the lift. Do not use the lift if the resident's weight exceeds the limit. At least two workers usually are needed when a mechanical lift is used. Be sure you know your facility's policy and procedure.

PROCEDURE

Using a Mechanical Lift

1. Ask a co-worker to help you.

2. Explain what you are going to do.

3. Collect the following:
   a. Mechanical lift
   b. Armchair or wheelchair
   c. Slippers
   d. Bath blanket

4. Wash your hands.

5. Identify the resident. Check the ID bracelet and call the person by name.

6. Provide for privacy.

7. Center the sling under the resident. Turn him or her from side to side to position the sling as if making an occupied bed (see Chapter 11). Position the sling according to the manufacturer's instruction.

8. Place the chair at the head of the bed. It should be even with the headboard and about a foot away from the bed. Place a folded bath blanket in the chair.

9. Make sure the bed wheels are locked and the bed is in its lowest position.

10. Raise the lift so it can be positioned over the resident.

11. Position the lift over the resident (Fig. 9-30, *A*).

12. Lock the lift wheels in position.

13. Attach the sling to the swivel bar (Fig. 9-30, *B*).

14. Raise the head of the bed to a sitting position.

15. Cross the resident's arms over the chest. Allow him or her to hold onto the straps, if desired, but not the swivel bar.

16. Raise the lift until the resident and sling are free of the bed (Fig. 9-30, *C*).

17. Ask your helper to support the resident's legs as you move the lift and resident away from the bed (Fig. 9-30, *D*).

18. Position the lift so the resident's back is toward the chair.

19. Gently lower the resident into the chair. (Follow the manufacturer's instructions for lowering the lift.) Guide the resident into the chair (Fig. 9-30, *E*).

20. Lower the swivel bar so the sling can be unhooked. Remove the sling if it is removable. If not, leave it under the resident.

21. Put the slippers on the resident. Position the feet on the footrests if a wheelchair is used.

22. Cover the resident's lap and legs with a lap robe or a bath blanket if the resident is not dressed. The blanket must be off the floor and wheels.

23. Position the chair as the resident prefers.

24. Place the signal light and other necessary items within reach. Straighten the unit.

25. Wash your hands.

26. Report the following to the nurse:
    a. Pulse rate if taken
    b. Complaints of lightheadedness, pain, discomfort, difficulty breathing, weakness, or fatigue
    c. How well the activity was tolerated

27. Reverse the procedure to return the resident to bed.

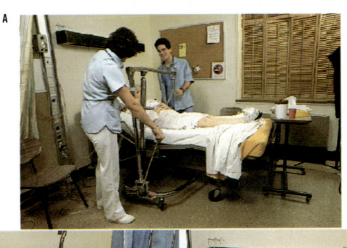

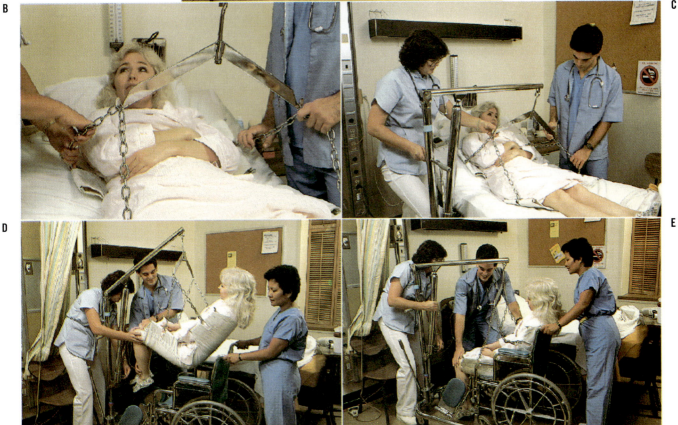

FIGURE 9-30 *A,* The lift is positioned over resident, and the legs of the lift are spread to widen base of support. *B,* The sling is attached to hooks that are turned away from the resident's body. The sling is then attached to a swivel bar. *C,* The lift is raised until the sling and the resident are off of the bed. *D,* The resident's legs are supported as resident and lift are moved away from the bed. *E,* Resident is guided into a chair.

Moving the Resident to a Stretcher

Stretchers are used to transport residents within the facility or to another facility. They are used for residents who are helpless and cannot sit up, for those who must remain in a lying position, or for those who are seriously ill. The stretcher is covered with a folded flat sheet or bath blanket. A pillow and an extra blanket should be available. To increase the resident's comfort, the head of the stretcher can be raised to a sitting or semisitting position.

Safety straps are applied once the resident is on the stretcher. The stretcher's side rails are kept up during transport. The resident is moved feet first so the helper at the head of the stretcher can watch the resident's breathing and color during the transport. A resident on a stretcher must never be left unattended.

A drawsheet can be used to transfer a resident from the bed to a stretcher. At least 3 workers are needed for a safe transfer. Remember to keep the resident in good body alignment and to use good body mechanics.

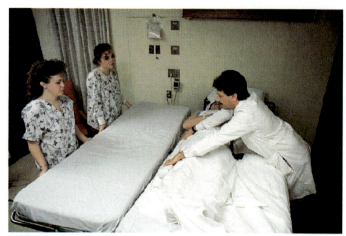

FIGURE 9-31 *The stretcher is placed against the bed and held in place by two nursing assistants.*

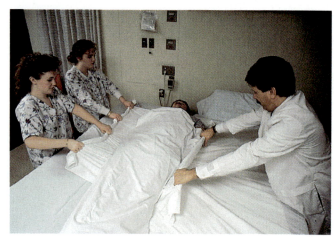

FIGURE 9-32 *The resident is lifted from the bed to a stretcher.*

PROCEDURE

Moving the Resident onto a Stretcher with a Drawsheet (Three Assistants)

1. Ask two other workers to help you.

2. Explain to the resident what you are going to do.

3. Collect the following equipment:
   a. Stretcher covered with a sheet or bath blanket
   b. Bath blanket
   c. Sheet or drawsheet
   d. Pillow(s) if needed

4. Wash your hands.

5. Identify the resident. Check the ID bracelet and call the person by name.

6. Provide for privacy.

7. Raise the bed to its highest level.

8. Cover the resident with a bath blanket. Fan-fold top linens to the foot of the bed.

9. Loosen the cotton drawsheet on each side.

10. Lower the head of the bed. It should be as flat as possible.

11. Lower the side rail on the side to which the resident will be moved.

12. Ask your helpers to help move the resident to the side of the bed by using the drawsheet.

13. Go to the other side of the bed. Lower the side rail. Protect the resident from falling by holding the far arm and leg.

14. Have your helpers position the stretcher next to the bed and stand behind the stretcher (Fig. 9-31).

15. Lock the wheels of the bed and stretcher.

16. Lay the clean sheet (or drawsheet) over the bottom sheet on the empty side of the bed.

17. Kneel on the bed at the resident's waist.

18. Roll up and grasp the drawsheet at the resident's hip and mid-chest levels.

19. Ask your helpers to roll up and grasp the drawsheet. This supports the entire length of the resident's body.

20. Transfer the resident to the stretcher on a count of "3" by lifting and pulling him or her (Fig. 9-32). Make sure the resident is centered on the stretcher.

21. Place a pillow or pillows under the resident's head and shoulders if allowed.

22. Make sure the resident is covered and comfortable.

23. Fasten the safety straps. Raise the side rails.

24. Unlock the stretcher wheels, and transport the resident as directed.

25. Wash your hands.

26. Report the following to the nurse:
   a. The time of the transport
   b. Where the resident was transported to
   c. Who accompanied the resident

27. Reverse the procedure to return the resident to bed.

POSITIONING

The resident must always be properly positioned. Comfort and well-being are promoted with regular position changes and good body alignment. Breathing is easier and circulation is promoted. Proper positioning also helps prevent many complications. These include pressure sores on bony parts (see Chapter 12) and body deformities (see Chapter 17). Residents who are in bed or in wheelchairs must be repositioned at least every 2 hours.

The doctor may order a certain position for a resident or may restrict certain positions. You need to consult with the nurse and check the resident's care plan about position changes. You need to know how often to turn a resident and to what position. Other safety measures include using good body mechanics and getting help if it is needed. If you cannot find a helper, do not try to move a resident alone. You can injure the resident or yourself. Never rush when you move a resident. Be gentle. Explain to the resident what you are going to do and protect the resident's privacy. Place the signal light within the resident's reach after repositioning.

Basic Positions for the Resident in Bed

Good body alignment and position changes are essential for the resident confined to bed. Some residents can change positions without help. Others need some assistance. Some depend entirely on nursing personnel for position changes.

Fowler's position. **Fowler's position** involves raising the head of the bed to a semisitting position. The head of the bed is raised between 45 and 60 degrees. Good body alignment for the Fowler's position involves keeping the spine straight, supporting the head with a small pillow, and supporting the arms with pillows (Fig. 9-33). Residents with heart and respiratory disorders usually can breathe more easily in the Fowler's position.

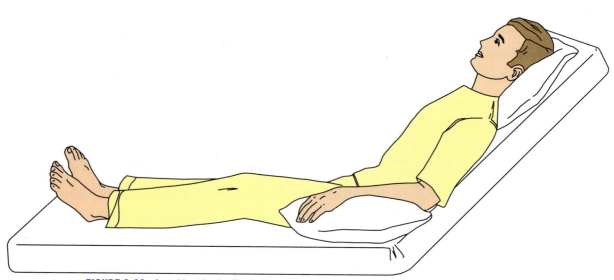

FIGURE 9-33 *A resident in the Fowler's position, with pillows used to maintain body alignment.*

Supine position. The **supine** or **dorsal recumbent position** is the back-lying position. Good body alignment involves having the bed flat, supporting the head and shoulders on a pillow, and placing the arms and hands at the resident's side. The arms may be supported with regular size pillows. The hands may be supported on small pillows with the palms down (Fig. 9-34).

The nurse may ask you to place a folded or rolled towel under the small of the resident's back. A small pillow may be placed under the resident's thighs if requested by the nurse.

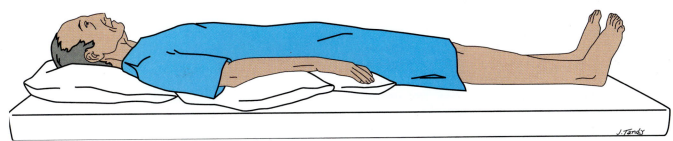

FIGURE 9-34 *A resident in the supine position.*

Prone position. Residents in the **prone position** lie on their abdomens with their heads turned to one side. Good body alignment involves placing a small pillow under the resident's head, one under the abdomen, and one under the lower legs (Fig. 9-35). The arms are flexed at the elbows with the hands near the head. You also can position residents with their feet hanging over the end of the mattress (Fig. 9-36). If that is done, a pillow is not needed under the lower legs. Most elderly residents do not tolerate the prone position well because of limited range of motion in their necks. Check with the nurse before placing any resident in the prone position.

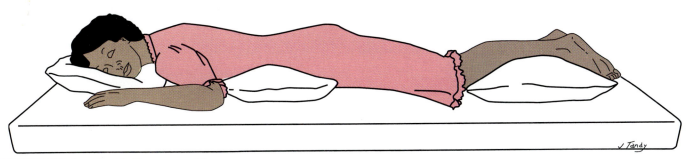

FIGURE 9-35 *A resident in the prone position.*

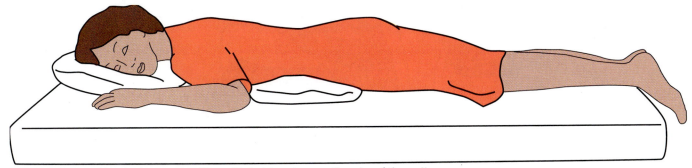

FIGURE 9-36 *A resident in the prone position, with feet hanging over the edge of the mattress.*

Lateral position. A resident in the **lateral** or **side-lying position** lies on one side (Fig. 9-37). Pillows are used to maintain good alignment. Place a pillow under the resident's head and shoulders. Place the upper leg in front of the lower leg. (The nurse may ask you to position the resident so the upper leg is behind the lower leg, not on top of it.) Support the upper leg and thigh with pillows. Place a pillow against the resident's back. Help the resident to roll back against the pillow so that his or her back is at a 45-degree angle with the mattress. Place a small pillow under the upper hand and arm.

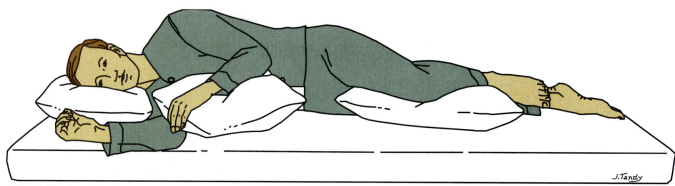

FIGURE 9-37 *A resident in the lateral position, with pillows used for support.*

Sims' position. The **Sims' position** is a side-lying position. The upper leg is sharply flexed so that it is not on the lower leg, and the lower arm is behind the resident (Fig. 9-38). Good body alignment involves placing a pillow under the resident's head and shoulder, supporting the upper leg with a pillow, and placing a pillow under the upper arm and hand. This position usually is not comfortable for elderly persons. Check with the nurse before placing a resident in this position.

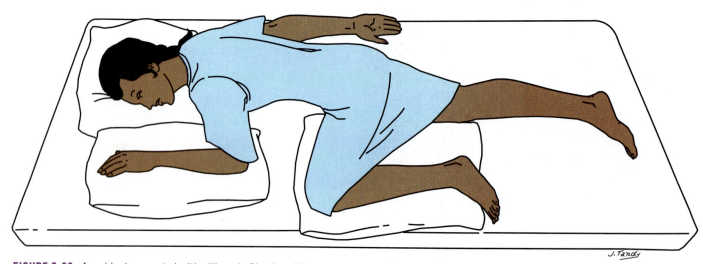

FIGURE 9-38 *A resident supported with pillows in Sims' position.*

Positioning in a Chair

Residents who sit in chairs must be able to hold the upper part of their bodies and their heads erect. Poor alignment results if the resident cannot stay in an erect position. The resident's back and buttocks should be against the back of the chair. Feet are flat on the floor or wheelchair footrests. Never leave the feet unsupported. Backs of knees and calves should be slightly away from the edge of the seat (Fig. 9-39). With the nurse's permission, you can put a small pillow between the lower part of the resident's back and the chair. This supports the lower back. Paralyzed arms are positioned on pillows. Some residents may have special foam positioners (Fig. 9-40). Ask the nurse about their proper use. Wrists are positioned at a slight upward angle.

Residents may require postural supports if they cannot keep the upper part of their bodies erect. Postural supports help keep residents in good body alignment. The jacket restraint described in Chapter 7 can be used to support posture. The jacket restraint is used for this purpose only with the nurse's approval and the resident's consent. The resident and family must clearly understand the purpose of the device. The safety rules described in Chapter 7 apply when the jacket restraint is used as a postural support.

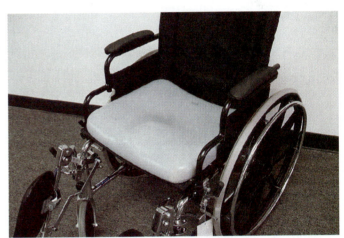

FIGURE 9-40 *Foam positioner used to keep the resident in alignment when sitting in chair.*

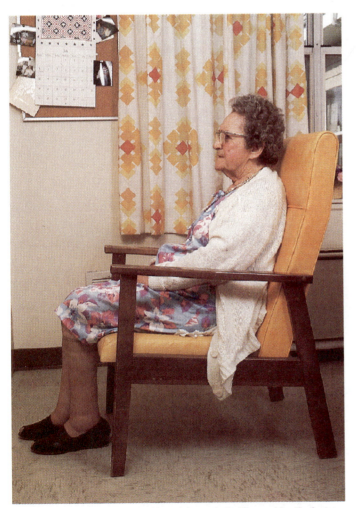

FIGURE 9-39 *A resident positioned in a chair. The resident's feet are flat on the floor, calves do not touch the chair, and the back is straight and against back of chair.*

Quality OF LIFE

OBRA requires nursing facilities to provide care in a manner that maintains and improves the quality of life, health, and safety of each resident. Proper use of body mechanics protects residents from injuries that could affect their ability to function and their health.

Remember to protect residents' rights when you lift, move, transfer, and position residents. You must protect the resident's privacy at all times. Be sure to screen the resident properly and expose only the body part involved in the procedure. Doors should be closed, curtains drawn, and shades or drapes pulled as needed to protect the resident's right to privacy.

The resident's rights also can be protected by allowing personal choice whenever possible. As long as the resident's safety is not affected, let the resident choose such things as bed positions, where the chair or wheelchair will be positioned after transfers, and when to get up or go back to bed. Be sure to check with the nurse and the resident's care plan to make sure the resident has made safe choices. Also let the resident participate in the lifting, moving, and transferring procedures to the extent possible.

The resident also has the right to be free from restraint. Side rails are considered restraints under OBRA and are used only with the resident's consent. However, side rails always must be used when the bed is raised to protect the resident from falling. Many procedures in this chapter involve raising the bed so that the nursing assistant can use good body mechanics. Therefore the procedures in this chapter include the use of side rails. Be sure to check with the nurse and the resident's care plan about the use of side rails. When you use side rails, be sure to explain to the resident why they are being used.

SUMMARY

To protect yourself and residents from injury, you must use good body mechanics whenever lifting, moving, and transferring residents. You need to keep yourself and the resident in good body alignment to promote comfort and well-being.

You have learned several ways to move, lift, transfer, and position residents. Their comfort, safety, and rights always must be considered. Be sure you know of any position restrictions ordered for a resident. Also, protect the resident's right to privacy, personal choice, and free- dom from restraint. When you work with elderly persons, work slowly and gently so you do not cause pain or injury. Encourage residents to help in repositioning or transfers to the extent possible. Finally, always protect the resident from falling.

You may need to change some lifelong habits in relation to your posture and how you move your body. As you use good body mechanics, you will feel better and work with greater efficiency. Remember to follow the general rules of body mechanics in all activities.

Review QUESTIONS

Circle *T* if the answer is true and *F* if the answer is false.

1. Body mechanics is the way body segments are aligned with one another. **T (F)**

2. Base of support is the area upon which an object rests. **(T) F**

3. Objects are held away from the body when they are lifted, moved, or carried. **T (F)**

4. Push, slide, or pull heavy objects rather than lift them. **T F**

5. Consult with the nurse for any limitations or restrictions in positioning or moving a resident. **(T) F**

6. If help is needed to move a resident, ask a co-worker to help before beginning the procedure. **T F**

7. A lifting sheet should extend from the shoulders to above the knees. **(T) F**

8. A resident is moved to the side of the bed before being turned to the side-lying position. **(T) F**

9. Logrolling involves rolling the resident in segments. **T (F)**

10. Residents with spinal cord injuries are logrolled. **(T) F**

11. A transfer belt is part of a mechanical lift. **T (F)**

12. A resident is moved from the direction of the weak side. **T (F)**

13. Safety straps are applied when a resident is on a stretcher only if left unattended. **T (F)**

14. Repositioning is essential to prevent deformities and pressure on bony parts. **(T) F**

15. The head of the bed is elevated 45 to 60 degrees for the supine position. **T (F)**

16. The Sims' position is a side-lying position. **(T) F**

Circle the *best* answer.

17. The small muscles of the body are in the
    a. Back
    b. Shoulders
    c. Upper arms
    d. Hips and thighs

18. Which will *not* reduce friction?
    a. Sliding the resident
    b. Lifting the resident
    c. Rolling the resident
    d. Using a lifting sheet

19. A resident is to be transferred from the bed to a chair. The resident should
    a. Be barefoot
    b. Wear socks
    c. Wear slippers
    d. Wear street shoes

20. A resident is to be positioned in a chair. Which is *false*?
    a. The back and buttocks should be against the back of the chair.
    b. The feet should be flat on the floor or wheelchair footrests.
    c. A paralyzed arm should rest on the resident's lap.
    d. The backs of the knees and calves should be away from the chair.

Answers

1. False	6. True	11. False	16. True
2. True	7. True	12. False	17. a
3. False	8. True	13. False	18. a
4. True	9. False	14. True	19. d
5. True	10. True	15. False	20. c

10

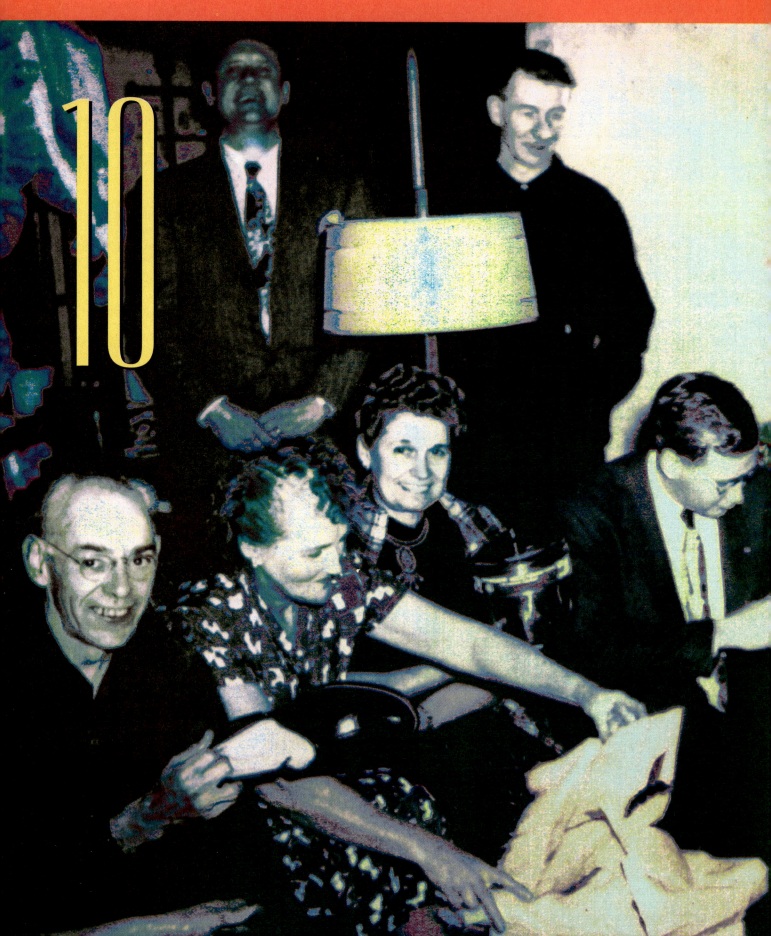

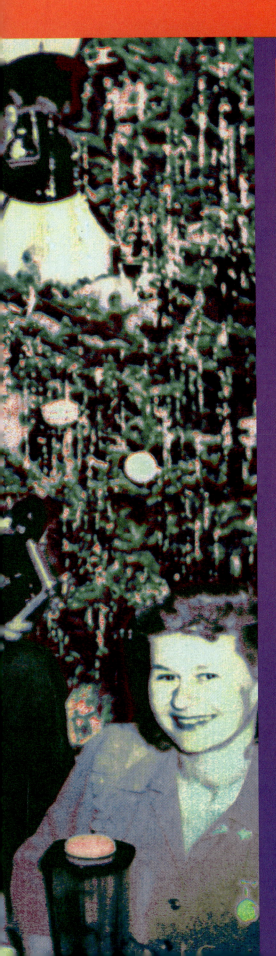

What You Will LEARN

- The key terms listed in this chapter

- The temperature ranges comfortable for most people

- How to protect residents from drafts

- Measures to prevent or reduce odors in resident rooms

- How to control the common causes of noise in health facilities

- How lighting can affect the resident's comfort

- Basic bed positions

- How equipment found in a resident unit is used

- How a bathroom is equipped for the resident's use

- Measures to help maintain the resident's unit

caster
A small wheel made of rubber or plastic

resident unit
The furniture and equipment provided for the individual by the facility

reverse Trendelenburg's position
The head of the bed is raised and the foot of the bed is lowered

semi-Fowler's position
The head of the bed is raised 45 degrees and the knee portion is raised 15 degrees; or the head of the bed is raised 30 degrees and the knee portion is not raised

Trendelenburg's position
The head of the bed is lowered and the foot of the bed is raised

I used to live in a four bedroom house. Now I share a room with another man. But I was able to bring my favorite chair from home. I used to sit in that chair with my grandchildren. They still sit on my lap when they visit me here. ✍

Residents may spend a lot of time in their rooms. Few residents have private rooms. Most share a room with another person. Each person's assigned areas within the room are considered private. The facility is their "home." They should be allowed to have and to arrange personal possessions as they choose. However, the health and safety standards of the facility must be followed. Residents must not violate the rights of other residents. The room must be comfortable and safe for all residents. There should be enough space to perform activities of daily living.

This chapter describes the conditions that influence a person's comfort and the furnishings in a resident unit. A **resident unit** is the furniture and equipment provided for the individual by the facility (Fig. 10-1).

COMFORT

Age, illness, and activity affect a resident's comfort. So do temperature, ventilation, odors, noise, and lighting. These conditions usually can be controlled to meet a person's needs.

Temperature and Ventilation

Nursing facilities have heating, air conditioning, and ventilation systems. These systems are designed to maintain a comfortable temperature and to provide fresh air in the rooms. A temperature range of 68° to 74° F usually is comfortable for most healthy people. What is comfortable for one person may be too hot or too cold for another. Elderly and chronically ill persons generally need higher room temperatures. Therefore higher temperatures usually are needed in nursing facilities. Physically active people often are more comfortable where it is cooler than are persons who cannot move without help.

Stale room air and lingering odors can affect comfort and rest. A good ventilation system provides fresh air and moves air in the room. Drafts can be created as the air moves. Those who are elderly and chronically ill are sensitive to drafts. You can help to protect these persons from drafts. Make sure they have on enough clothing. Many elderly persons choose to wear sweaters even in the summer time. Lap robes can be offered to residents in chairs and wheelchairs to cover their legs. Also make sure that residents in bed are covered with enough blankets. Residents should be moved from drafty areas whenever possible.

Odors

Many smells occur in nursing facilities. Some are pleasant, such as the aroma of food and the scent of fresh flowers. Others are unpleasant. Draining wounds, vomitus, bowel movements, and urine can cause unpleasant odors that embarrass residents. Body, breath, and smoking odors may be offensive to residents, visitors, and staff members. Visitors and some residents may be quite sensitive to odors. They may become nauseated. Other residents, especially the elderly, may not notice odors. Good nursing care and good ventilation help eliminate odors. To control odors and provide good nursing care you should:

1. Check incontinent residents often.
2. Change and promptly wash residents who are wet or soiled.
3. Dispose of soiled linen or clothing as soon as you have finished the change.
4. Empty and wash bedpans and emesis basins promptly.
5. Use a room deodorizer when necessary. Do not use spray deodorizers around residents with breathing problems. Ask the nurse if you are unsure.
6. Provide good personal hygiene for your residents to help prevent body and breath odors.

Smoking presents special problems. Make sure residents smoke only in designated areas. If you smoke, you must observe your facility's smoking policy. Wash your hands after handling smoking materials and before giving resident care. Careful attention must be given to your uniforms, hair, and breath because of clinging smoke odors.

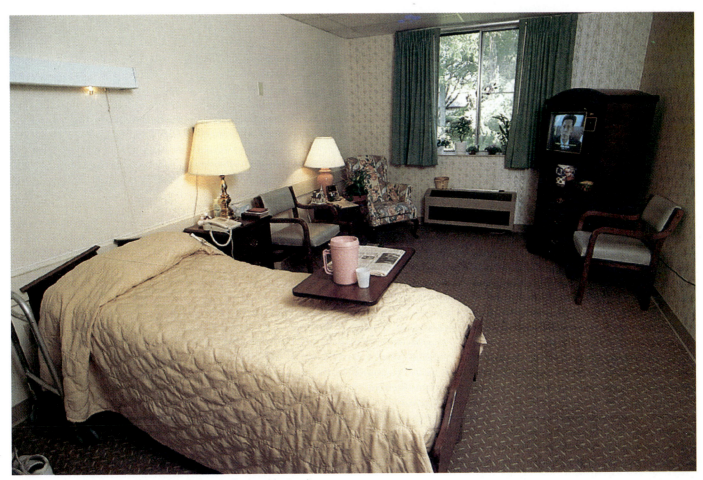

FIGURE 10-1 *Furniture and equipment in a typical resident unit.*

Remember, the facility is the residents' home. Keep it as free of unpleasant odors as possible.

Noise

Chronically ill people, especially the elderly, may be sensitive to the noises and sounds around them. Residents may be easily disturbed by common health care sounds. The clanging of metal equipment (bedpans, urinals, and wash basins) and the clatter of dishes and meal trays can be annoying. Residents may hear loud talking and laughter in hallways and at the nurse's station. They may think that staff members are talking and laughing about them. Televisions and radios, ringing telephones, and buzzing intercoms can be irritating. So is noise from equipment that needs repair or oil. Wheels on stretchers, wheelchairs, utility carts, and other similar equipment must be oiled properly.

When in an strange environment—such as a nursing facility—people try to figure out the cause and meaning of new sounds. This relates to the basic need to feel safe and secure. Residents, especially if confused, may find sounds to be dangerous, frightening, or irritating. As a result, they may become upset, anxious, and uncomfortable. Remember that what is noise to one person may not be noise to another. For example, a teenager's loud stereo music may be quite irritating to parents.

Nursing facilities are designed to reduce noise. Drapes, carpeting, and acoustical tiles all help absorb noise. Plastic equipment has replaced some metal equipment (bedpans, urinals, and wash basins). Health care workers can reduce noise and increase resident comfort by controlling the loudness of their voices and by handling equipment carefully. Keeping equipment in good working order and promptly answering telephones and intercoms also decrease noise.

Lighting

Good lighting is necessary for the safety and comfort of residents and health care workers. Glares, shadows, and dull lighting can cause falls, headaches, and eyestrain. People usually relax and rest better in dim light. A bright room is more cheerful and stimulating.

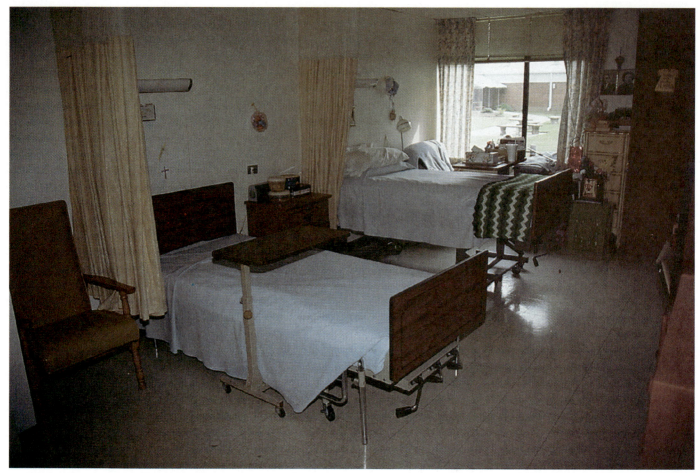

FIGURE 10-2 *One bed in the highest horizontal position and the other bed in the lowest horizontal position.*

Lighting in most rooms can be adjusted to meet the changing needs of the resident. Shades can be pulled or drapes drawn to control natural light. The light above the bed usually can be adjusted to provide soft, medium, and bright lighting. Some facilities also have ceiling lights over the beds. These provide very soft and low to extremely bright lighting. Residents with poor vision need very bright light to see. This is especially important at mealtime and when they are moving about the facility. Bright lighting also helps when health care workers are performing procedures. Light controls should be within the resident's reach to allow for the right of personal choice.

ROOM FURNITURE AND EQUIPMENT

Rooms are furnished and equipped for the resident's basic needs. There are furniture and equipment for comfort, sleep, elimination, nutrition, personal hygiene, and activity. There also is equipment for communicating with the nursing team, relatives, and friends. The right to privacy is considered when the room is equipped.

The Bed

Hospital beds are adjusted electrically or manually. They can be raised horizontally so that care can be given without unnecessary bending or reaching. The lowest horizontal position allows the resident to get out of bed with ease (Fig. 10-2). The head of the bed can be kept flat or raised in varying degrees.

Electric beds are used in many nursing facilities. Others use manually operated beds. Electric beds have hand controls. Staff members and residents can easily change the bed's position with the hand controls. The controls may be on a side panel, attached to the bed by a cable, or on a panel at the foot of the bed (Fig. 10-3). Residents are taught how to use the controls. They must be warned not to raise the bed to the high position or to adjust the bed to harmful positions. They should be told if they are limited or restricted to certain positions.

Most electric beds can be "locked" by the staff into any position. Confused residents may need to have their beds locked. This prevents them from adjusting their beds to unsafe positions.

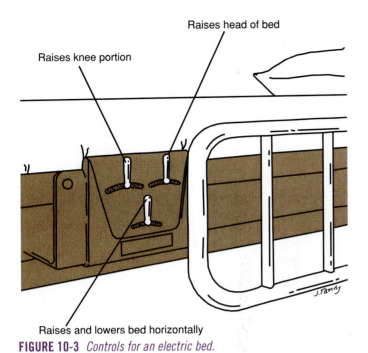

FIGURE 10-3 *Controls for an electric bed.*

Manually operated beds have hand cranks at the foot of the bed (Fig. 10-4). The left crank raises or lowers the head of the bed. The right crank adjusts the knee portion. The center crank raises or lowers the entire bed horizontally. The cranks are pulled up during use and kept down at all other times. Cranks left in the up position are a safety hazard. They can be bumped into by anyone walking past them.

Bed positions. There are four basic bed positions—Fowler's, semi-Fowler's, Trendelenburg's, and reverse Trendelenburg's.

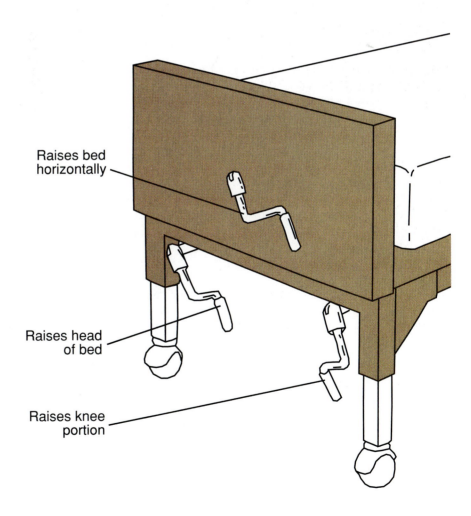

FIGURE 10-4 *Manually operated hospital bed.*

Fowler's position is a semisitting position. The head of the bed is raised 45 to 60 degrees (Fig. 10-5). Reasons for positioning a resident in Fowler's position were described in Chapter 9.

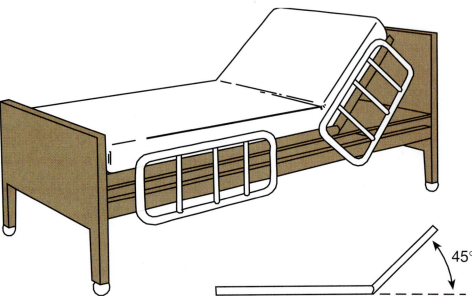

FIGURE 10-5 *Fowler's position.*

In **semi-Fowler's position,** the head of the bed is raised 45 degrees and the knee portion is raised 15 degrees (Fig. 10-6). This position is comfortable and prevents residents from sliding down in bed. Raising the knee portion, however, can interfere with circulation. Consult with the nurse before positioning a resident in the semi-Fowler's position. Many facilities define semi-Fowler's position as the position in which the head of the bed is raised 30 degrees and the knee portion is *not* raised. You must know the definition used by your employer so you can give safe care.

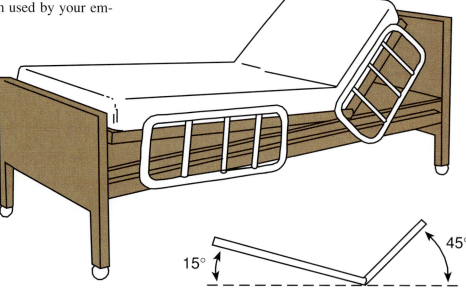

FIGURE 10-6 *Semi-Fowler's position.*

Trendelenburg's position involves lowering the head of the bed and raising the foot of the bed (Fig. 10-7). This position is not used unless ordered by the doctor or nurse. Blocks are placed under the lower legs of the bed. Some beds are made so that the entire bed frame can be tilted into Trendelenburg's position.

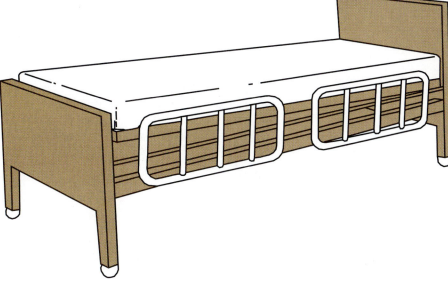

FIGURE 10-7 *Trendelenburg's position.*

Reverse Trendelenburg's position is the opposite of Trendelenburg's position. The head of the bed is raised, and the foot of the bed is lowered (Fig. 10-8). Blocks are put under the legs at the head of the bed or the bed frame is tilted. This position requires a doctor's order.

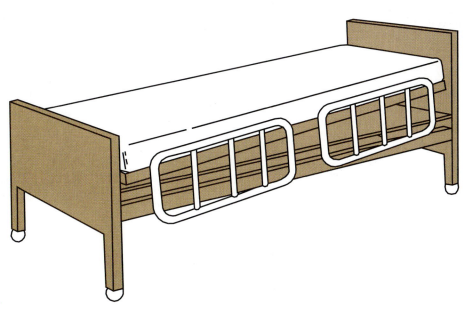

FIGURE 10-8 *Reverse Trendelenburg's position.*

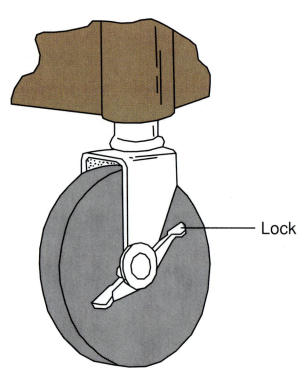

FIGURE 10-9 *Lock on a bed wheel.*

Safety considerations. Bed legs usually have wheels or casters. A **caster** is a small wheel made of rubber or plastic that allows the bed to move easily. Each wheel or caster has a lock that prevents the bed from moving (Fig. 10-9). The bed wheels must be locked before bedside care is performed. The wheels are locked at all times except when the bed is moved. Many residents get into and out of bed without help. They can be hurt if the bed moves.

The importance of side rails on hospital beds was discussed in Chapter 7.

The Overbed Table

The overbed table (see Fig. 10-1, p. 195) can be positioned over the bed by sliding the base under the bed. It can be raised or lowered to a comfortable height for the resident in bed or in a chair. The overbed table is used for meals, writing, reading, and other activities.

Some overbed tables have movable tops with a storage area underneath. The storage area often is used for beauty, hair care, or shaving items. Many also have a flip-up mirror useful for personal grooming.

The nursing team uses the overbed table as a work area. Only clean and sterile items are placed on the table. Never place bedpans, urinals, or soiled linen on the overbed table. The table is cleaned after being used as a working surface.

The Bedside Stand

The bedside stand is next to the resident's bed. The stand is a storage area for the resident's personal belongings and personal care equipment. It has a drawer at the top and a lower cabinet with a shelf (Fig. 10-10). The drawer can be used for money, eyeglasses, books, and other personal items. The first shelf is used for the wash basin, which can hold personal care items. These include soap and soap dish, powder, lotion, deodorant, towels, washcloth, bath blanket, and a clean gown or pajamas. An emesis or kidney basin (shaped like a kidney) often is used to hold oral hygiene equipment. The kidney basin can be stored in the top shelf or in the drawer. The bedpan and its cover, the urinal, and toilet paper are on the lower shelf.

The top of the stand often is used for tissues and other personal items. The resident may want to put a radio, clock, pictures, and other important items there. Some stands have a side or back rod for towels and washcloths.

Chairs

The resident unit always has at least one chair for resident and visitor use. The chair usually is an upholstered chair with armrests (Fig. 10-11). It must be comfortable for the resident. The chair also must be sturdy so that it does not move easily or tip over during transfers. The resident should be able to get in and out of the chair easily. Therefore it should not be too low or too soft.

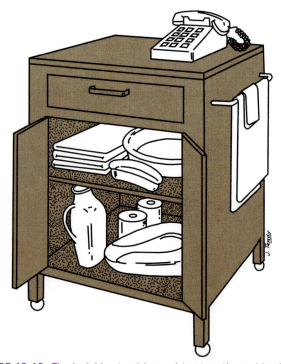

FIGURE 10-10 *The bedside stand is used to store the resident's personal care equipment.*

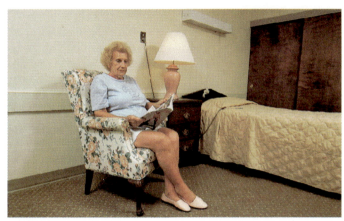

FIGURE 10-11 *The resident's chair provides comfort and support.*

Curtains or Screens

Rooms with more than one bed have a curtain between the resident units. The curtain can be pulled around either bed to provide privacy (Fig. 10-12). It is *always* pulled completely around the bed when care is given. If a portable screen is used (Fig. 10-13, p. 202), it is placed between the beds. Curtains and screens protect the resident from being seen by others. However, they do not block sound or prevent conversations from being heard.

Personal Care Equipment

Personal care equipment refers to the items needed for hygiene and elimination. Most facilities provide a wash basin, emesis or kidney basin, bedpan, urinal, water pitcher and glass, and soap and soap dish. Powder, lotion, toothbrush, toothpaste, mouthwash, tissues, a comb, and deodorant also may be provided. Usually residents bring their own oral hygiene equipment, hair care supplies, and deodorant. Some also prefer their own soap, lotion, and powder. Be sure to respect the resident's personal choice in personal care products.

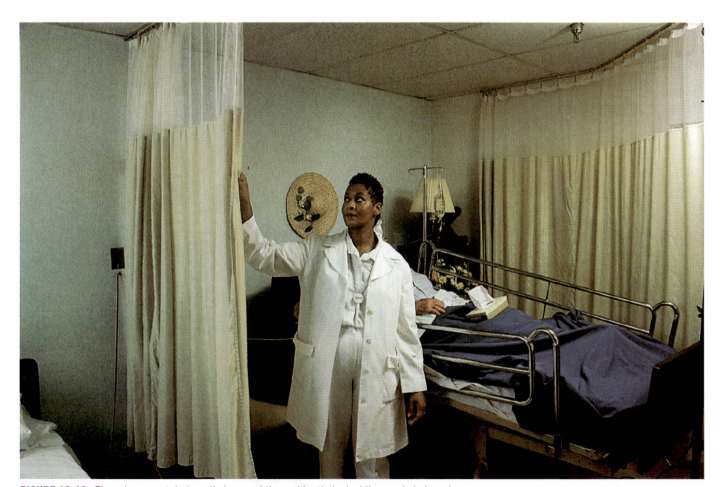

FIGURE 10-12 *The privacy curtain is pulled around the resident's bed while care is being given.*

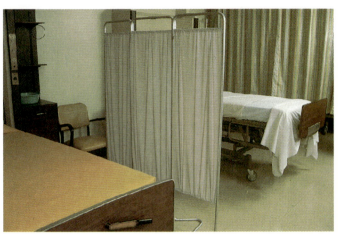

FIGURE 10-13 *A portable screen between two resident units.*

Call System

The call system lets the resident signal for assistance. The signal light is at the end of a long cord that can be attached to the bed or chair (Fig. 10-14). It must always be within the resident's reach. The resident presses a button at the end of the signal light to get assistance. The signal light at the bedside is connected to a light above the room door (Fig. 10-15, *A*) and to a light panel or intercom system at the nurse's station (Fig. 10-15, *B*). These tell the nursing staff that the resident needs help. The nurse or nursing assistant shuts off the light at the bedside when the help has been given.

An intercom system lets the resident and nursing staff member talk from the room to the nurse's station. The resident can tell the staff member what is needed. Hearing-impaired residents may have difficulty using an intercom.

Sometimes a tap bell is used instead of a signal light (Fig. 10-16). The signal light or tap bell always should be on the resident's strong side. Be sure to show residents how to use the call system when they are admitted. Be

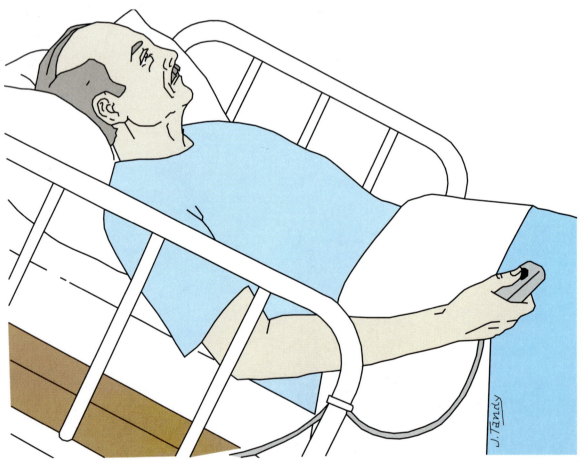

FIGURE 10-14 *The resident presses the signal light button when assistance is needed.*

A

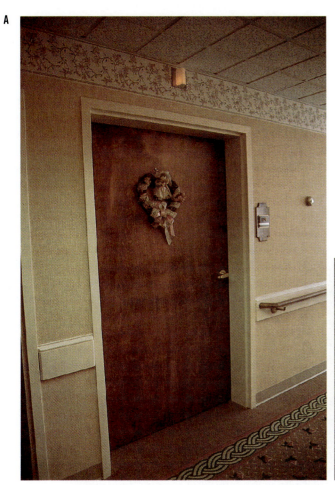

B

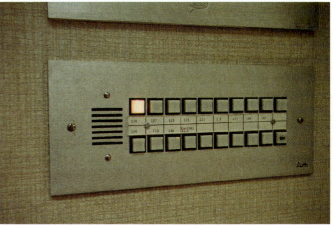

FIGURE 10-15 *A,* *The light above the door of resident's room.* *B,* *Light panel or intercom system at the nurse's station.*

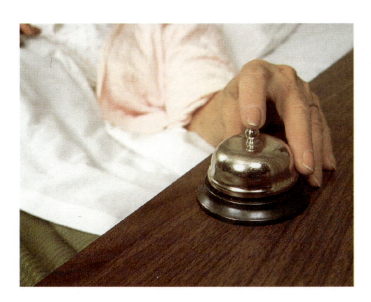

FIGURE 10-16 *Tap bell.*

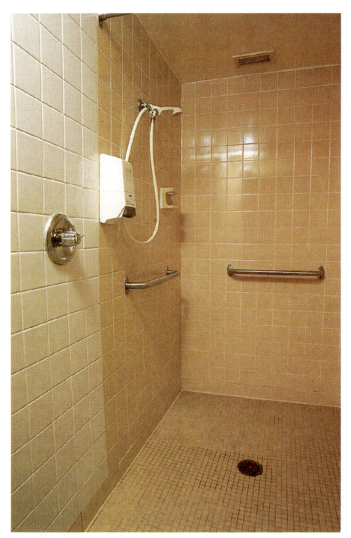

FIGURE 10-17 *A resident bathroom in a nursing facility.*

Towel racks, toilet paper, soap, paper towel dispenser, and wastebasket also are in the bathroom. They are placed within easy reach of the resident.

Closet and Drawer Space

Closet and drawer space are provided for the resident's clothing. Some residents bring in additional small chests of drawers for personal belongings. OBRA requires nursing facilities to provide each resident with closet space. The closet space must have shelves and a clothes rack (Fig. 10-18). The resident must have free access to the closet and its contents.

Items in the closet or drawers are the resident's private property. You must not search the closet or drawers without the person's permission.

Sometimes people hoard items in drawers. Elderly persons often save such things as napkins, straws, food and packets of sugar, salt, and pepper. Such hoarding can cause safety or health risks. Facility representatives can inspect a person's closet or drawers if hoarding is suspected. The person must be informed of the inspection and be present when it takes place.

Other Equipment

Facilities may allow residents to bring furniture or other items from home. Some residents like to bring favorite chairs and footstools. Televisions, radios, clocks, pictures, and other small items may be brought from home to help the residents feel "at home" in their own units. Telephones are available in some facilities.

sure to remind residents to signal when help is needed. Some residents cannot use the call light or tap bell. Be sure to check the resident's care plan for any special communication measures. You must check these residents often to make sure their needs are met.

The Bathroom

Many facilities have a bathroom in each room. Some have a bathroom that adjoins two resident rooms. A toilet, sink, call system, and mirror are standard equipment. There also may be a shower (Fig. 10-17). Handrails are installed by the toilet for the resident's safety. The resident uses them for support to sit on or get up from the toilet. Toilets in some facilities are higher than the standard toilet. The higher toilets make transfers from wheelchairs easier. They also are helpful for residents who have restricted joint movement.

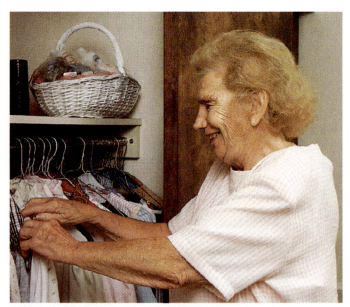

FIGURE 10-18 *The resident has access to items in her closet.*

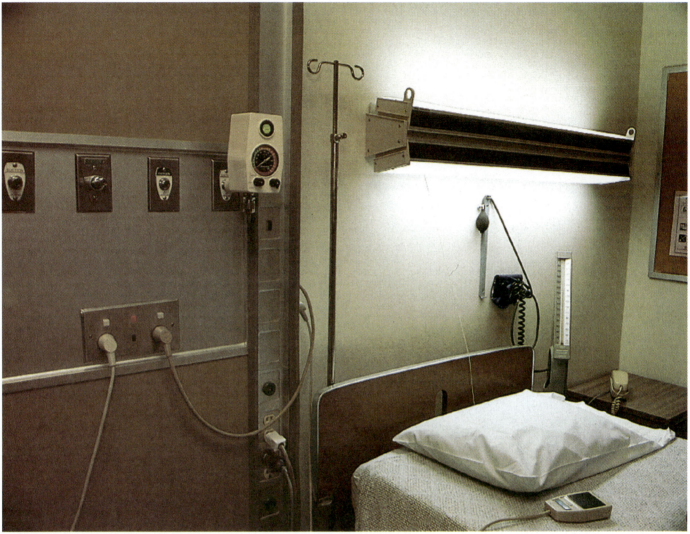

FIGURE 10-19 *This room has blood pressure equipment, an IV pole, and an oxygen outlet.*

Some rooms have equipment for measuring blood pressure mounted on the wall. Some beds are equipped with poles that are used to hang intravenous (IV) infusion bottles or bags. The poles are stored in a special part of the bed frame. The IV pole may be a separate piece of equipment that is brought in only when needed. There also may be wall outlets for oxygen and suction. Fig. 10-19 shows blood pressure equipment, an IV pole, and an oxygen outlet.

General Rules

All health care workers are responsible for keeping the resident unit clean, neat, safe, and comfortable. The following rules will help guide you in maintaining resident units.

1. Make sure the resident can reach the overbed table and the bedside stand.
2. Arrange personal belongings as the resident prefers. Make sure they are easily reached.
3. Keep the signal light within the resident's reach at all times.
4. Meet the needs of residents who cannot use the call system.
5. Provide the resident with enough tissues and toilet paper.
6. Adjust lighting, temperature, and ventilation for the resident's comfort.
7. Handle equipment carefully to prevent unnecessary noise.
8. Reassure the resident by explaining the causes of strange noises.
9. Use room deodorizers if necessary.
10. Empty the resident's wastebasket as often as needed or at least once a day.

Quality OF LIFE

Remember that the resident once had a home or apartment with furniture, appliances, a private bathroom, and many personal belongings and treasures. Now the person must live in a strange place and probably share a room with another resident. Leaving one's home is a difficult part of growing old with poor health. Therefore it is important to make the resident's unit as homelike as possible.

The resident may be allowed to bring some furniture and personal belongings. A chair, footstool, lamp, or small table are among the items that may be allowed. Residents always can bring such things as family photos, religious items, and books. Some may have plants to care for.

The resident must be allowed personal choice in arranging personal possessions. The health care team must make sure that such choices are safe and will not cause falls or other accidents. In addition, the resident's choices must not interfere with the rights of others. You may have to help the resident in choosing the best location for personal items.

Remember, the facility is now the resident's home. You and other members of the health team must help the resident feel safe, secure, and comfortable. A homelike environment will help the resident's quality of life.

SUMMARY

The resident unit is designed and equipped to meet the resident's basic needs. A homelike environment is provided to the extent possible. There is equipment for the person's comfort, hygiene, elimination, and activity. The overbed table is helpful for meals and other table activities such as writing, puzzles, sewing, or crafts. Side rails, handrails, and the call system are provided for resident safety. The resident's safety also can be promoted by controlling temperature, ventilation, lighting, noise, and odors. Curtains or screens provide privacy and help the resident feel safe and secure. Television and radio provide entertainment, relaxation, and contact with the world.

Review QUESTIONS

Circle the *best* answer.

1. Which is a comfortable temperature range for most people?
   a. 60° to 66° F
   b. 68° to 74° F
   c. 74° to 80° F
   d. 80° to 86° F

2. A resident can be protected from drafts by
   a. Wearing enough clothing
   b. Being covered with adequate blankets
   c. Being moved out of a drafty area
   d. All of the above

3. Which does not prevent or reduce odors in the resident's room?
   a. Placing fresh flowers in the room
   b. Emptying bedpans promptly
   c. Using room deodorizers
   d. Practicing good personal hygiene

4. Which will *not* control noise?
   a. Using equipment made of plastic
   b. Handling dishes and metal items with care
   c. Speaking softly
   d. Talking with others in the hallway

5. The overbed table is not used
   a. For eating
   b. As a working surface
   c. To store the urinal
   d. To store shaving items

Circle *T* if the answer is true and *F* if the answer is false.

T F 6. In Fowler's position, the head of the bed is raised 45 to 60 degrees.

T F 7. The curtain is pulled around the resident's bed to provide privacy when talking.

T F 8. Soft and dim lighting usually is more relaxing and comfortable.

T F 9. The signal light always must be within the resident's reach except when he or she is in the bathroom.

T F 10. The resident must be able to reach items in the closet.

Answers

1. b	4. d	7. False	10. True
2. d	5. c	8. True	
3. a	6. True	9. False	

11

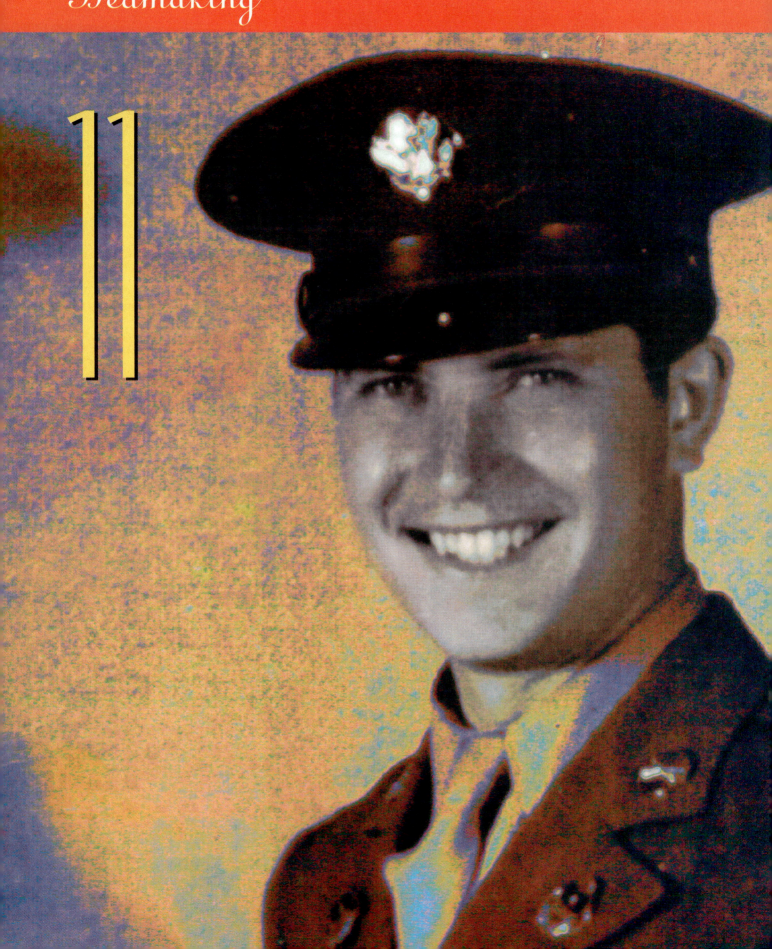

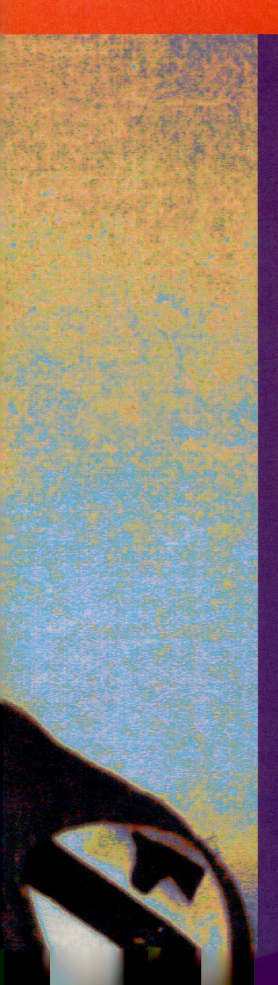

What You Will

LEARN

- The key terms listed in this chapter

- The differences among closed, open, occupied, and surgical beds

- When to change bed linens

- The purposes of plastic drawsheets and cotton drawsheets

- When to make the different types of beds

- How to handle linens following the rules of medical asepsis

- How to make a closed bed, an open bed, an occupied bed, and a surgical bed

drawsheet
A small sheet placed over the middle of the bottom sheet; it helps keep the mattress and bottom linens clean and dry; can be used to turn and move residents in bed; the "cotton drawsheet"

plastic drawsheet
A drawsheet made of plastic; it is placed between the bottom sheet and the cotton drawsheet to keep the mattress and bottom linens clean and dry

Some days I spend most of the time in bed. The staff makes sure the bed is neat and straightened. Wrinkles are uncomfortable.

Most residents are out of bed most of the day. Some are in bed all the time, and they are fed and bathed in bed. Some residents cannot get up to use the bathroom, and many are incontinent. Incontinent residents cannot control the passage of urine from their bladders or control bowel movements. They must have their bed linens changed often. Many treatments also must be done in bed.

Bedmaking is a very important part of your job. Clean, neat beds help make your residents more comfortable. Residents depend on you for their comfort and well-being. By keeping beds clean, dry, and wrinkle-free, you help prevent skin breakdown and pressure sores (see Chapter 12). These can be fatal to elderly persons.

Bed linens usually are changed every day in hospitals. In nursing facilities a complete linen change is made on the resident's bath day. Elderly persons are less active than younger people and have drier skin. Therefore they do not need a full bath every day. The resident will be scheduled for a bath or shower on certain days. The complete linen change will be made after the bath or shower when the resident is up for the day. Residents like to have beds made and rooms cleaned before visitors arrive.

Your bedmaking responsibilities include straightening linens, making beds, or making beds with complete linen changes on bath days. For incontinent residents, linens are changed throughout the day whenever they become wet, soiled, or damp. Be sure to wear gloves and use universal precautions when handling the linens of incontinent residents.

Beds are made in the following ways.

1. A *closed bed* is not being used by the resident until bedtime. A closed bed also is one that is ready for a new resident. The top linens are not folded back (Fig. 11-1).
2. An *open bed* is being used by a resident. Top linens are folded back so that the resident can get into bed. A closed bed becomes an open bed by folding back the top linens (Fig. 11-2).
3. An *occupied bed* is made with the resident in it (Fig. 11-3).
4. A *surgical bed* is made so that a resident can be moved from a stretcher to the bed. This bed is made for residents who are admitted by ambulance (Fig. 11-4).

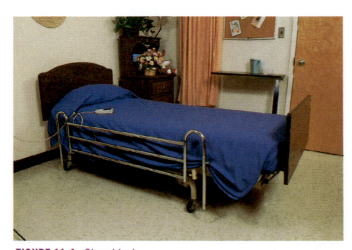

FIGURE 11-1 *Closed bed.*

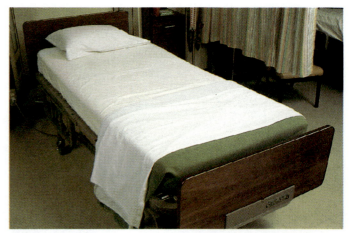

FIGURE 11-2 *Open bed. Top linens are folded to the foot of the bed.*

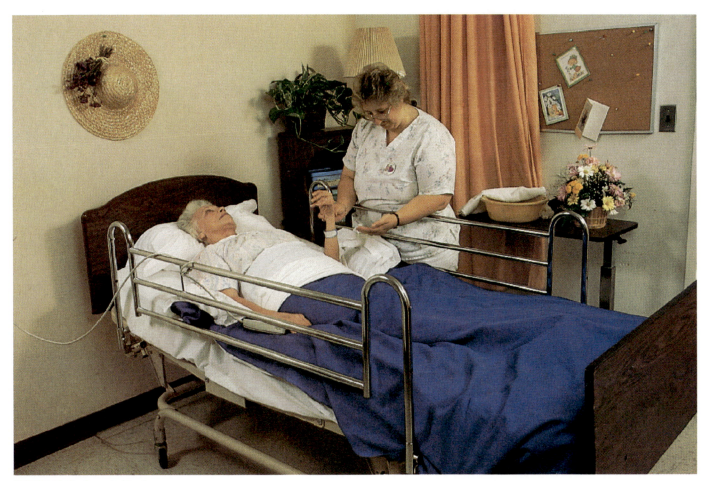

FIGURE 11-3 *Occupied bed.*

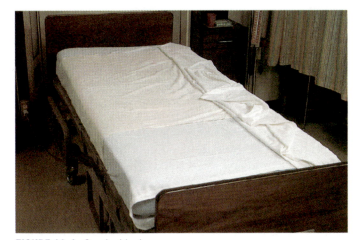

FIGURE 11-4 *Surgical bed.*

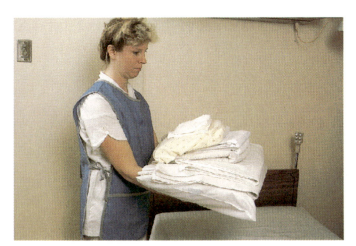

FIGURE 11-5 *Linens are held away from the body and uniform.*

LINENS

Special attention is given to the care and use of linens. The rules of medical asepsis are followed in handling linens and making beds. Because your uniform is considered dirty, always hold linens away from your body and uniform (Fig. 11-5). Never shake linens in the air. Shaking them causes the spread of microcrobes. Clean linens are placed on a clean surface. Never put dirty linen on the floor.

Clean linens are collected in the order they will be used. Linens for the resident's personal care also are collected. Be sure to collect enough linens. If your resident has 2 pillows, take 2 pillowcases. Extra blankets may be needed for warmth. You must make sure that you have necessary linens. However, you must not bring unneeded linens to a resident's room. Extra linens in a resident's room are considered contaminated and cannot be used for another resident.

You should collect linens in the following order:
1. Mattress pad
2. Bottom sheet (flat sheet or contour sheet)
3. Plastic drawsheet or disposable bed protectors
4. Cotton drawsheet
5. Top sheet (flat sheet)
6. Blanket
7. Bedspread
8. Pillowcase(s)
9. Bath towel(s)
10. Hand towel
11. Washcloth
12. Hospital gown if the resident uses one
13. Bath blanket

Use one arm to hold the linens and the other hand to pick them up. The item to be used first is at the bottom of your stack. (You picked up the mattress pad first; therefore it is at the bottom. The bath blanket is on top.) You need the mattress pad first. To get it on top, simply place your arm over the bath blanket. Then turn the stack over to the arm on the bath blanket (Fig. 11-6). The arm that had been holding the linens will be free. Place the clean linens on a clean surface.

Linens are pressed and folded to prevent the spread of microbes and to make bedmaking easy. They are pressed with a center crease, which is placed in the center of the bed from the head to the foot. The linens unfold easily.

When removing dirty linens from the bed, roll them away from you. The side of the linen that touched the resident is inside the roll. The side that has not touched the resident is on the outside (Fig. 11-7).

Not all linens are changed every time the bed is made. The mattress pad, plastic drawsheet, blanket, and bedspread may be reused for the same resident. They can be reused if not soiled, wet, damp, or excessively wrinkled. Some facilities use only flat sheets. The flat top sheet can

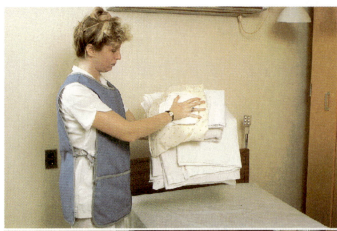
A

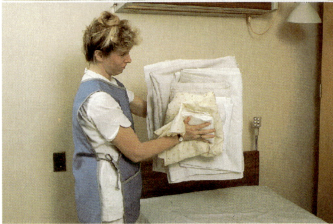
B

FIGURE 11-6 *A, Arm placed over the top of the stack of linens. B, Stack of linens turned over onto the arm.*

be reused as the bottom sheet. If a resident has been discharged, all linens are removed and a closed bed is made. Make sure the bed has been washed before it is made. Check your facility's policy about linen changes. *Remember, wet, damp, or soiled linens must be changed right away. You must wear gloves and use universal precautions.*

A bed may have a plastic drawsheet and a cotton drawsheet. A **drawsheet** (cotton drawsheet) is a small sheet placed over the middle of the bottom sheet. It helps keep the mattress and bottom linens clean and dry. A **plastic drawsheet** protects the mattress and bottom linens from becoming damp or soiled. It is placed between the bottom sheet and cotton drawsheet. Although the bottom linen and mattress are protected, resident discomfort and skin breakdown may occur. This is because of heat retention and the difficulty in keeping the drawsheets tight and wrinkle-free.

Most mattresses made for clinical use are covered with plastic. Plastic mattress covers may be used. Disposable waterproof bed protectors can be used. Plastic and cotton drawsheets may be used only for certain resi-

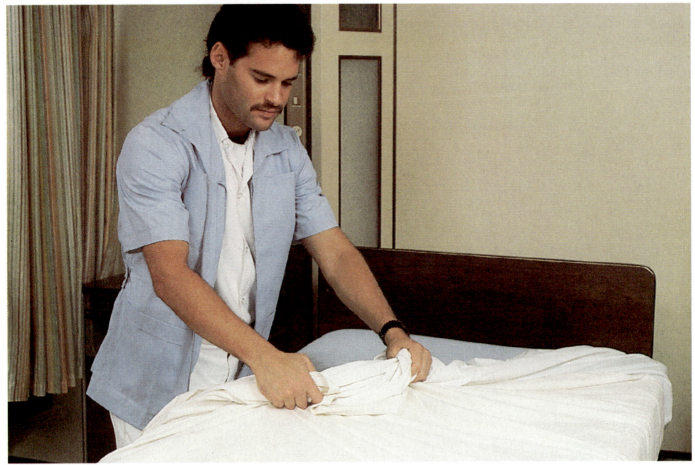

FIGURE 11-7 *Roll linens away from you when removing them from the bed.*

dents. They include those with bowel or bladder control problems or those who have excessive wound drainage.

A cotton drawsheet may be used without a plastic drawsheet. Plasticized mattresses cause some residents to perspire heavily and can cause discomfort. A cotton drawsheet helps to reduce heat retention and absorbs moisture. Cotton drawsheets often are used to move and position residents in bed (see Chapter 9). When used for this purpose, the drawsheet is not tucked in at the sides. The bedmaking procedures in this chapter include both plastic and cotton drawsheets. Consult with the nurse about their use. Also, you need to know your employer's policies about the use of plastic and cotton drawsheets.

GENERAL RULES

Remember these rules when making beds.

1. Use good body mechanics at all times.
2. Follow the rules of medical asepsis, universal precautions, and the bloodborne pathogens standard.
3. Always wash your hands before handling clean linen and after handling dirty linen.
4. Bring enough linen to the resident's room.
5. Never shake linens. This causes the spread of microorganisms.
6. Extra linen in the resident's room is considered contaminated. Do not use it for other residents. Put it in the dirty laundry so staff members do not use it for other residents.
7. Hold linens away from your uniform. Neither dirty nor clean linen should ever touch your uniform.
8. Never put dirty linen on the floor or on top of clean linen.
9. Linens the resident lies on (bottom linens) should be tight and free of wrinkles.
10. A cotton drawsheet must completely cover the plastic drawsheet. A plastic drawsheet should never touch the resident's body.
11. Change the linen of incontinent residents promptly. Be sure to wear gloves, use universal precautions, and follow the bloodborne pathogens standard.
12. Make as much of one side of the bed as possible before going to the other side. This saves time and energy.

213

THE CLOSED BED

A closed bed is made if the resident will be out of bed for most of the day or after a resident has been discharged. After a resident has been discharged, the bed frame and mattress must be cleaned before you make the bed. They should be cleaned according to facility policy.

PROCEDURE

Making A Closed Bed

1. Wash your hands.

2. Collect gloves and clean linen:
   a. Mattress pad
   b. Bottom sheet (flat or contour sheet)
   c. Plastic drawsheet
   d. Cotton drawsheet
   e. Top sheet (flat sheet)
   f. Blanket
   g. Bedspread
   h. Pillowcase(s)
   i. Bath towel(s)
   j. Hand towel
   k. Washcloth
   l. Hospital gown
   m. Bath blanket

3. Place linen on a clean surface.

4. Raise the bed to the best level for using good body mechanics.

5. Make sure the bed and bed frame have been cleaned if the resident has been discharged. If making the bed for a current resident, remove dirty linen one piece at a time. Roll linen away from you so that the surface that touched the resident is inside the roll. Wear gloves if linens are soiled with urine, feces, or other body fluids or substances. Remove and discard the gloves after removing soiled linen.

6. Move the mattress to the head of the bed.

7. Put the mattress pad on the mattress. It should be even with the top of the mattress.

8. Place the bottom sheet on the mattress pad (Fig. 11-8, p. 216).
   a. Unfold it lengthwise.
   b. Place the center crease in the middle of the bed.
   c. Position the lower edge even with the bottom of the mattress.
   d. Place the larger hem at the top and the small hem at the bottom.
   e. Face the hem stitching downward.

9. Pick the sheet up from the side to open it. Fan-fold it toward the other side of the bed as in Fig. 11-9 on p. 216.

10. Go to the head of the bed. Tuck the top of the sheet under the mattress. You will have to lift the mattress slightly. Make sure the sheet is tight and smooth.

11. Make a mitered corner as in Fig. 11-10 on p. 216.

12. Place the plastic drawsheet, on the bed about 14 inches from the top of the mattress.

13. Open the plastic drawsheet, and fan-fold it toward the other side of the bed.

14. Place a cotton drawsheet over the plastic drawsheet. It must cover the entire plastic drawsheet (Fig. 11-11, p. 217).

15. Open the cotton drawsheet, and fan-fold it toward the other side of the bed.

16. Tuck both drawsheets under the mattress. You may tuck each in separately.

17. Go to the other side of the bed.

18. Miter the top corner of the bottom sheet.

19. Pull the bottom sheet tight so there are no wrinkles. Tuck in the sheet.

20. Pull the plastic and cotton drawsheets tight so there are no wrinkles. Tuck them in together, or pull each tight and tuck in separately (Fig. 11-12, p. 217).

21. Go to the other side of the bed.

22. Put the top sheet on the bed.
    a. Unfold it lengthwise.
    b. Place the center crease in the middle of the bed.
    c. Place the large hem at the top, even with the top of the mattress.
    d. Open the sheet, and fan-fold the extra part toward the other side of the bed.
    e. Face the hem stitching outward.
    f. Do not tuck the bottom sheet in yet.
    g. Never tuck top linens in on the sides.

23. Place the blanket on the bed.
    a. Unfold it so the center crease is in the middle.
    b. Put the upper hem about 6 to 8 inches from the top of the mattress.
    c. Open the blanket, and fan-fold the extra part toward the other side.
    d. Do not tuck the blanket in yet.

24. Turn the top sheet down over the blanket. Hem stitching should be down.

25. Place the bedspread on the bed.
    a. Unfold it so the center crease is in the middle.
    b. Place the spread so that about 18 inches extends beyond the top of the mattress. This will be used to cover the pillow.
    c. Open the spread, and fan-fold the extra part toward the other side.
    d. Make sure the side of the spread facing the door is even and covers all top linens.
    e. Turn about 24 inches of the bedspread back from the head of the bed (Fig. 11-13, p. 217).

26. Tuck in top linens together at the foot of the bed. They should be smooth and tight. Make a mitered corner.

27. Go to the other side.

28. Straighten all top linen, working from the head of the bed to the foot.

29. Tuck in top linens together. Make a mitered corner.

30. Place the pillow on the bed.

31. Open the pillowcase so it lies flat on the bed.

32. Put the pillowcase on the pillow as in Fig. 11-14 on p. 218. Fold any extra material under the pillow at the seam end of the pillowcase.

33. Place the pillow on the bed so the open end is away from the door. The seam of the pillowcase is toward the head of the bed.

34. Cover the pillow with the bedspread. Tuck the spread under the front edge of the pillow.

35. Attach the signal light to the bed.

36. Lower the bed to its lowest position.

37. Put towels, washcloth, gown, and bath blanket in the bedside stand.

38. Wash your hands.

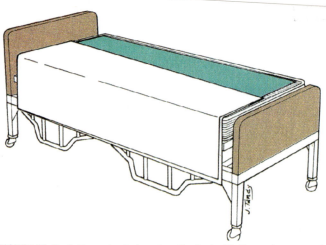

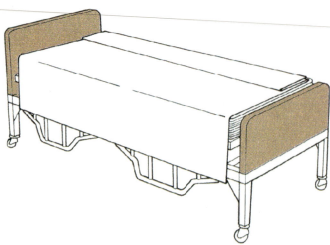

FIGURE 11-8 *Bottom sheet placed on the bed with the center crease in the middle of the bed. The lower edge of the sheet is even with the bottom of the mattress, and the hem stitching is toward the mattress pad.*

FIGURE 11-9 *Bottom sheet fan-folded to the other side of the bed.*

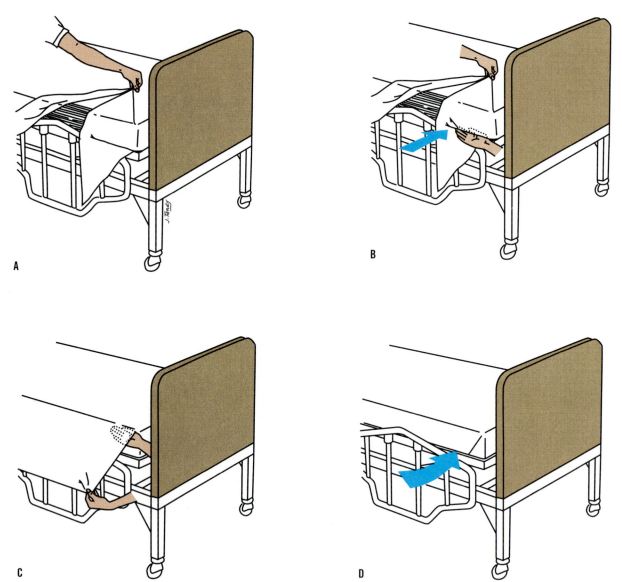

A

B

C

D

FIGURE 11-10 *Making a mitered corner.* **A,** *Bottom sheet is tucked under mattress, and side of sheet is raised onto mattress.* **B,** *Remaining portion of sheet is tucked under mattress.* **C,** *Raised portion of sheet is brought off the mattress.* **D,** *Entire side of sheet is tucked under mattress.*

216

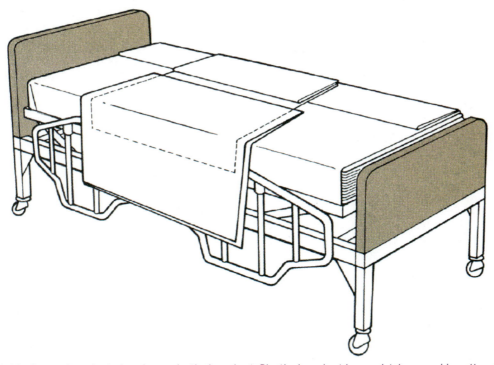

FIGURE 11-11 *Cotton drawsheet placed over plastic drawsheet. Plastic drawsheet is completely covered by cotton drawsheet.*

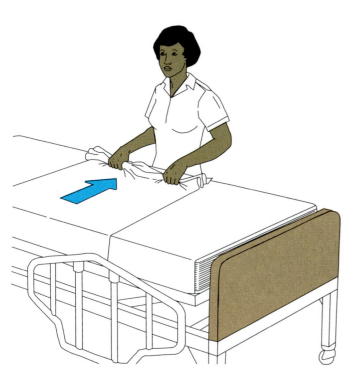

FIGURE 11-12 *Drawsheet pulled tight to remove wrinkles*

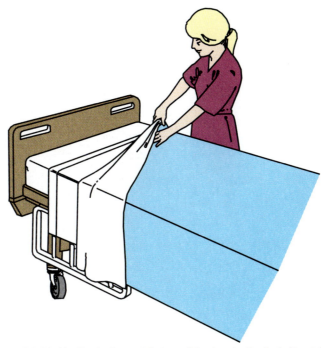

FIGURE 11-13 *The bedspread is turned back onto the bed. About 24 inches of the spread will be used to cover the pillow.*

THE OPEN BED

The open bed is an unoccupied bed. The linens are folded back so the resident can get into bed with ease. An open bed is made when your resident will be out of bed for a short time only. A closed bed easily becomes an open bed by folding back the top linens.

A

B

C

D

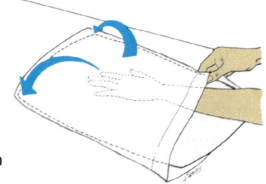

PROCEDURE

Making an Open Bed

1. Wash your hands.
2. Collect gloves and linen as for a closed bed.
3. Make a closed bed.
4. Fan-fold the bedspread to the foot of the bed.
5. Fan-fold the rest of the top linens to the foot of the bed (see Fig. 11-2, p. 210).
6. Attach the signal light to the bed.
7. Lower the bed to its lowest position.
8. Put towels, washcloth, gown, and bath blanket in the bedside stand.
9. Place the dirty linen in the linen hamper.
10. Wash your hands.

FIGURE 11-14 *Putting a pillowcase on the pillow.* **A,** *Grasp the corners of the pillow at the seam end and form a "V" with the pillow.* **B,** *Pillowcase flat on the bed, the nursing assistant opening the pillowcase with the free hand.* **C,** *"V" end of the pillow is guided into the pillowcase.* **D,** *"V" end of the pillow falls into the corners of the pillowcase.*

THE OCCUPIED BED

An occupied bed is made when a resident cannot be out of bed because of illness or injury. When making an occupied bed, you must keep the resident in good body alignment. You also must know of restrictions or limitations in the resident's movement or positioning. Check with the nurse before you make the bed. Be sure to explain each step of the procedure to the resident before it is done. This is important even if the resident is comatose or cannot respond to you.

PROCEDURE

Making an Occupied Bed

1. Explain the procedure to the resident.

2. Wash your hands.

3. Collect gloves and linen as for a closed bed (see p. 214).

4. Place linen on a clean surface.

5. Provide for privacy.

6. Remove the call signal.

7. Raise the bed to the best level for good body mechanics.

8. Lower the head of the bed to a level appropriate for the resident. It should be as flat as possible.

9. Lower the side rail near you if it is up. Make sure the far one is up and secure.

10. Wear gloves, and follow universal precautions if linens are soiled with urine, feces, or other body fluids or body substances. Also follow the bloodborne pathogens standard.

11. Loosen top linens at the foot of the bed.

12. Remove the bedspread and blanket separately. Fold them as in Fig. 11-15 (p. 221) if they are to be reused.

13. Cover the resident with a bath blanket to provide warmth and privacy.
    a. Unfold a bath blanket over the top sheet.
    b. Ask the resident to hold onto the bath blanket. If he or she cannot help, tuck the top of the bath blanket under the shoulders.

   c. Grasp the top sheet under the bath blanket at the resident's shoulders. Bring the sheet down to the foot of the bed. Remove the sheet from under the blanket (Fig. 11-16, p. 221).

14. Move the mattress to the head of the bed.

15. Position the resident on the side of the bed away from you. Adjust the pillow for the resident's comfort. It should be on the far side of the bed.

16. Loosen bottom linens from the head to the foot of the bed.

17. Fan-fold bottom linens one at a time toward the resident: cotton drawsheet, plastic drawsheet, bottom sheet, and mattress pad (Fig. 11-17, p. 222). Do not fan-fold the mattress pad if it is to be reused.

18. Place a clean mattress pad on the bed. Unfold it lengthwise so the center crease is in the middle. Fan-fold the top part toward the resident. If reusing the mattress pad, straighten and smooth any wrinkles.

19. Place the bottom sheet on the mattress pad so the hem stitching is away from the resident. Unfold the sheet so the center crease is in the middle. The small hem should be even with the bottom of the mattress. Fan-fold the top part toward the resident.

20. Make a mitered corner at the head of the bed. Tuck the sheet under the mattress from the head to the foot.

Continued.

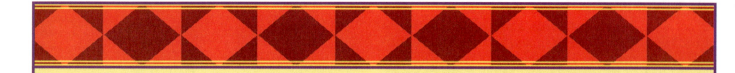

21. Pull the fan-folded plastic drawsheet toward you over the bottom sheet. Tuck the excess drawsheet under the mattress. Do the following if using a clean plastic drawsheet (Fig. 11-18, p. 223).
    a. Place the plastic drawsheet on the bed about 14 inches from the top of the mattress.
    b. Fan-fold the top part toward the resident.
    c. Tuck in the excess material.

22. Place the cotton drawsheet over the plastic drawsheet. It must cover the entire plastic drawsheet. Fan-fold the top part toward the resident. Tuck in excess material.

23. Raise the side rail. Go to the other side and lower the side rail.

24. Position the resident on the side of the bed away from you. Explain to the resident that he or she will roll over a "big bump." As you roll the resident, assure the resident that he or she will not fall. (Some residents become frightened as they roll over the stack of linen. They feel that they are rolling off the bed.) Adjust the pillow for the resident's comfort.

25. Loosen bottom linens. Remove soiled linen one piece at a time. Remove and discard the gloves if worn.

26. Straighten and smooth the mattress pad.

27. Pull the clean bottom sheet toward you. Make a mitered corner at the top. Tuck the sheet under the mattress from the head to the foot of the bed.

28. Pull the drawsheets tightly toward you. Tuck both under together or separately.

29. Position the resident in the supine position in the center of the bed. Adjust the pillow for comfort.

30. Put the top sheet on the bed. Unfold it lengthwise. Make sure the center crease is in the middle, the large hem is even with the top of the mattress, and the hem stitching is on the outside.

31. Ask the resident to hold onto the top sheet so you can remove the bath blanket. You may have to tuck the top sheet under the shoulders. Remove the bath blanket.

32. Place the blanket on the bed. Unfold it so the crease is in the middle. Unfold the blanket so it covers the resident. The upper hem should be 6 to 8 inches from the top of the mattress.

33. Place the bedspread on the bed, unfolding it so the center crease is in the middle. Unfold it so it covers the resident. The top hem should be even with the mattress top.

34. Turn the top hem of the bedspread under the blanket to make a cuff.

35. Bring the top sheet down over the bedspread to form a cuff.

36. Go to the foot of the bed.

37. Lift the mattress corner with one arm. Tuck all top linens under the mattress together. Be sure linens are loose enough to allow movement of the resident's feet. Make a mitered corner.

38. Raise the side rail. Go to the other side and lower the side rail.

39. Straighten and smooth top linens.

40. Tuck top linens under the mattress as in step 37. Make a mitered corner.

41. Change the pillowcase(s).

42. Place the signal light within reach.

43. Raise the head of the bed to a level appropriate for the resident. Make sure the resident is comfortable.

44. Lower the bed to its lowest position.

45. Raise or lower side rails as instructed by the nurse.

46. Put towels, washcloth, gown, and bath blanket in the bedside stand.

47. Unscreen the resident. Thank him or her for cooperating.

48. Place the dirty linen in the linen bag.

49. Wash your hands.

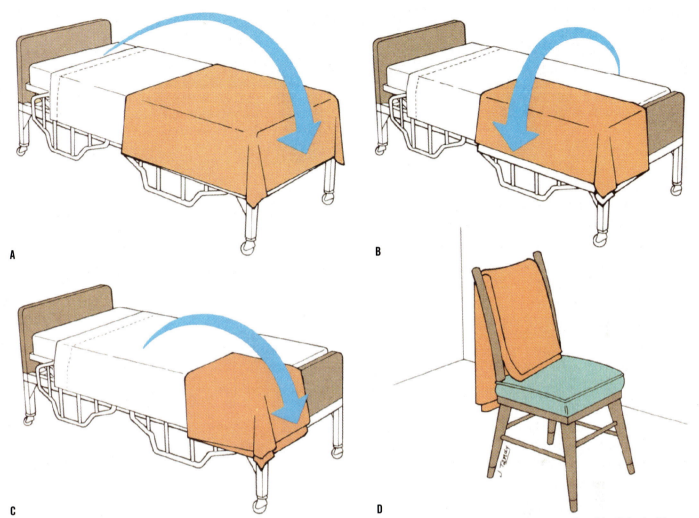

A

B

C

D

FIGURE 11-15 *Folding linen for reuse.* **A,** *Top edge of blanket folded down to the bottom edge.* **B,** *Blanket folded on the far side of the bed to near side.* **C,** *Top edge of blanket folded down to bottom edge again.* **D,** *Folded blanket placed over back of straight chair.*

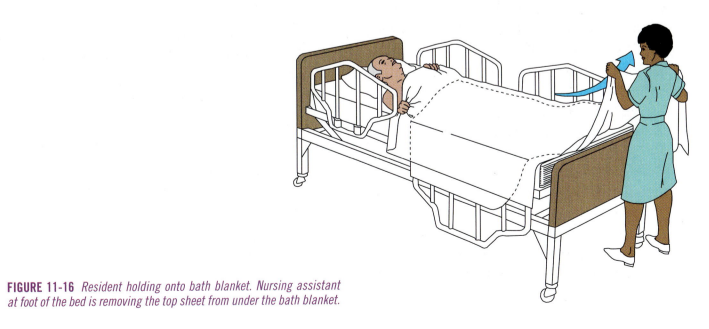

FIGURE 11-16 *Resident holding onto bath blanket. Nursing assistant at foot of the bed is removing the top sheet from under the bath blanket.*

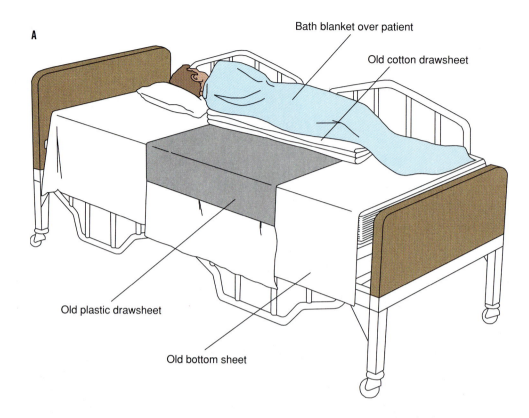

A

Bath blanket over patient

Old cotton drawsheet

Old plastic drawsheet

Old bottom sheet

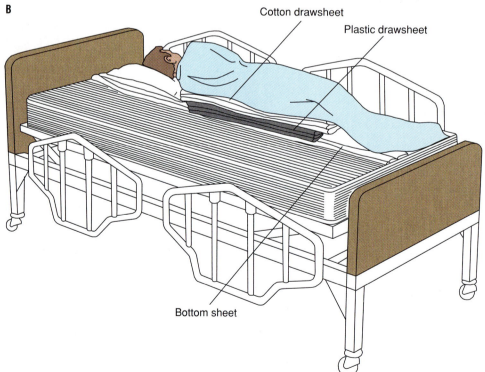

B

Cotton drawsheet

Plastic drawsheet

Bottom sheet

FIGURE 11-17 *Occupied bed.* **A,** *Cotton drawsheet fan-folded and tucked under resident.* **B,** *All bottom linens tucked under resident.*

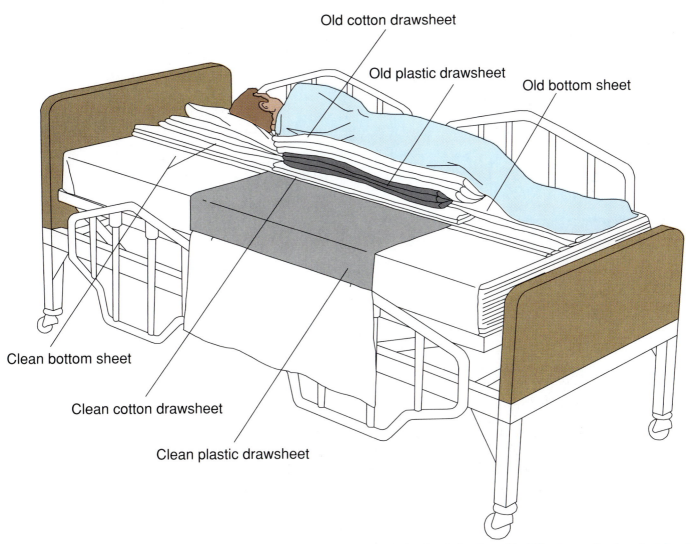

Old cotton drawsheet

Old plastic drawsheet

Old bottom sheet

Clean bottom sheet

Clean cotton drawsheet

Clean plastic drawsheet

FIGURE 11-18 *Clean bottom sheet and plastic drawsheet on bed, with both fan-folded and tucked under resident. The clean cotton drawsheet is put in step 22 (see text).*

THE SURGICAL BED

The surgical bed (recovery bed, postoperative bed, or anesthetic bed) is a form of the open bed. Top linens are folded so that the resident can be transferred from a stretcher to the bed. The surgical bed and its other names imply that the resident has had surgery. Surgery is not performed in long-term care facilities. In nursing facilities, surgical beds are used for residents who are arriving at the facility by ambulance. They also are used when residents are taken to treatment rooms or physical therapy by stretcher or when portable tubs are used.

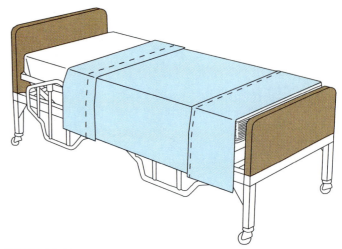

FIGURE 11-19 *Surgical bed. Bottom of the top linens folded back onto the bed. The fold is even with the edge of the mattress.*

PROCEDURE

Making a Surgical Bed

1. Wash your hands.

2. Collect gloves and linen as for a closed bed (see p. 214).

3. Place linen on a clean surface.

4. Remove the signal light.

5. Raise the bed to the best level for good body mechanics.

6. Remove all linen from the bed. Wear gloves, and use universal precautions if necessary and follow the bloodborne pathogens standard.

7. Make a closed bed (see *Making A Closed Bed*, p. 214). Do not tuck top linens under the mattress.

8. Fold all linen at the foot of the bed back onto the bed. The fold should be even with the edge of the mattress (Fig. 11-19).

9. Use one of these methods to fold the top linen.
   a. Fan-fold linen lengthwise to the side of the bed farthest from the door (Fig. 11-20).
   b. Fan-fold top linens from the head of the bed to the foot (Fig. 11-21).

10. Put the pillowcase(s) on the pillow(s).

11. Place the pillow(s) on a clean surface.

12. Leave the bed in its highest position.

13. Make sure both side rails are down.

14. Put towels, washcloth, gown, and bath blanket in the bedside stand.

15. Move the furniture away from the bed. Make sure there is room for the stretcher and for staff members to move about.

16. Do not attach the signal light to the bed.

17. Place dirty linen in the linen bag.

18. Wash your hands.

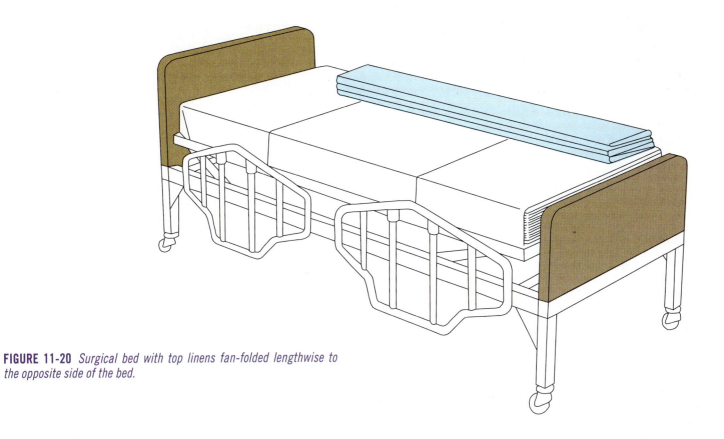

FIGURE 11-20 *Surgical bed with top linens fan-folded lengthwise to the opposite side of the bed.*

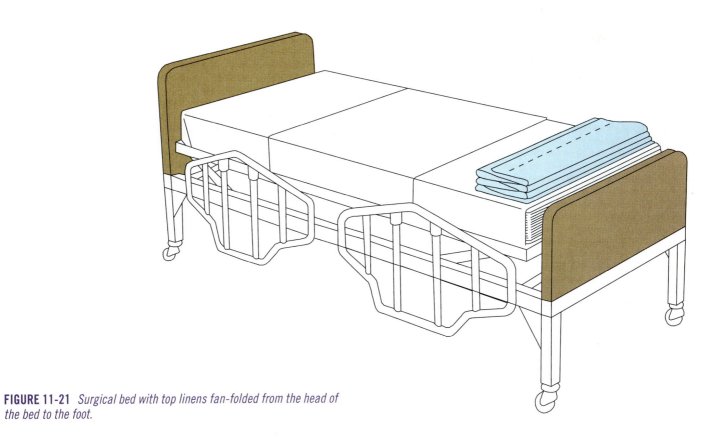

FIGURE 11-21 *Surgical bed with top linens fan-folded from the head of the bed to the foot.*

Quality OF LIFE

The bed is the largest piece of equipment in the resident's unit. It is the focus of the resident's unit. The resident, family, and visitors will question the quality of care, and thus the resident's quality of life, if the bed is unmade or messy. The bed must be neat and well-made so the resident's environment is orderly and pleasant. If the resident stays in bed, you need to straighten and tighten loose sheets and other linen whenever necessary.

Some residents choose to bring their own bedspreads, pillows, blankets, or afghans from home. Remember to use these when making the bed. Because such items are the resident's property, be sure to handle them with care and respect. Make sure the items are properly marked with the resident's name to prevent them from becoming lost or confused with the property of other residents.

Be sure to allow the resident personal choice whenever possible. The facility may use white, blue, yellow, pink, or other colored or printed linens. If so, let the resident choose which linen to use. Also, let the resident decide how many pillows or blankets to use. If possible, the resident also should be able to choose when the bed will be made. The more choices you allow the resident, the greater the person's sense of usefulness and quality of life.

SUMMARY

You have learned different ways to make beds. You also have learned the principles of bedmaking and of handling linens. Facility policies and procedures or a resident's condition may require changes in these procedures. However, the principles must be followed. Resident comfort and safety must be the focus of bedmaking. Therefore the bed must be neat, clean, and free of wrinkles. A well-made bed helps make your resident more comfortable.

Be sure to handle linens properly so that you do not spread microorganisms. Also follow the rules of medical asepsis, universal precautions, the bloodborne pathogens standard, bedmaking, and good body mechanics so you can make a bed safely and easily. Be sure to protect the resident's rights and to allow personal choice as much as possible.

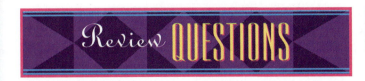

Review **QUESTIONS**

1. False	5. False	9. False	13. True
2. False	6. True	10. True	14. True
3. True	7. False	11. True	15. False
4. False	8. True	12. False	16. True

Circle *T* if the statement is true and *F* if the statement is false.

T F **1.** An open bed is made after a resident has been discharged.

T F **2.** A surgical bed is only for residents who have had surgery.

T F **3.** Linens are held away from your body and uniform.

T F **4.** Dirty linens can be put on the floor to avoid contact with clean linen.

T F **5.** Extra linen in a resident's room can be used for another resident.

T F **6.** A cotton drawsheet always is used when a plastic drawsheet is used.

T F **7.** Shake linens in the air to remove crumbs from the bed.

T F **8.** Hem stitching of the bottom sheet should be downward, away from the resident.

T F **9.** The plastic drawsheet is placed 6 to 8 inches from the top of the mattress.

T F **10.** A cotton drawsheet must completely cover the plastic drawsheet.

T F **11.** The large hem of the sheet should be even with the top of the mattress.

T F **12.** An occupied bed is made for resident who will be up.

T F **13.** A resident is screened when an occupied bed is made.

T F **14.** During the making of an occupied bed, the far side rail must be up at all times.

T F **15.** After a surgical bed is made, it is left in the lowest horizontal position.

T F **16.** Facilities usually allow residents to bring such things as comforters and afghans from home.

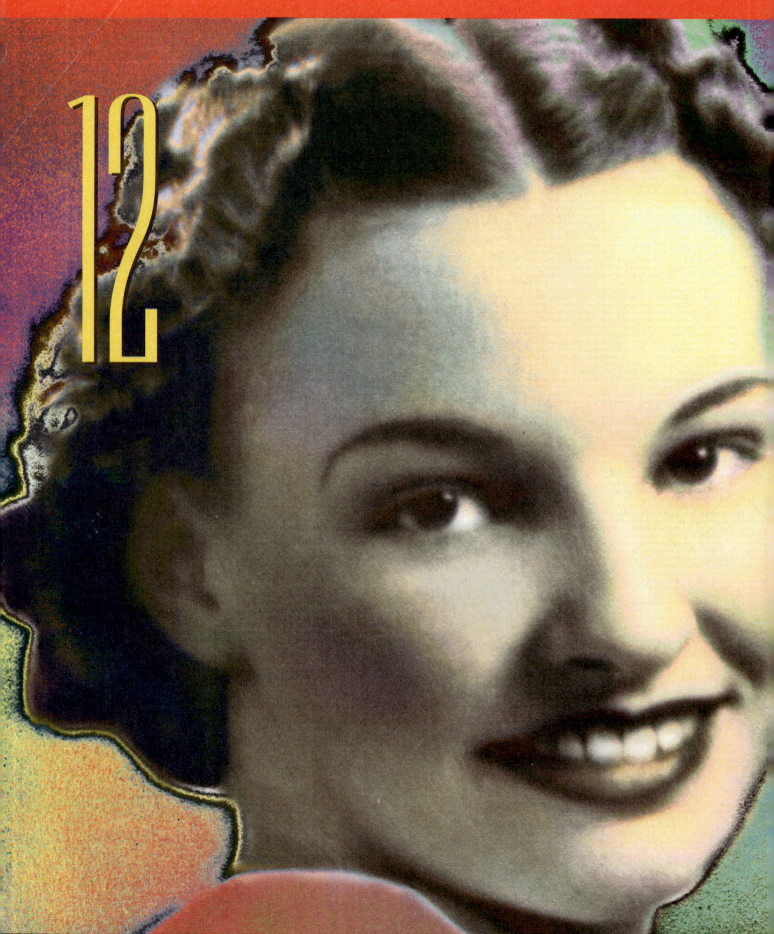

12

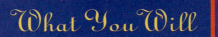

What You Will LEARN

- The key terms listed in this chapter

- The importance of cleanliness and skin care

- Routine care performed for residents before and after breakfast, after lunch, and in the evening

- The importance of oral hygiene and the observations to report to the nurse about oral hygiene

- The rules related to bathing and the observations you should make when bathing a resident

- Safety precautions for residents taking tub baths or showers

- The purposes of a back massage

- The purposes of perineal care

- The importance of hair care, shaving, and nail and foot care

- How to dress and undress residents

- The signs, symptoms, and causes of pressure sores

- The pressure points of the body in the prone, supine, lateral, Fowler's, and sitting positions

- How to prevent pressure sores

- How to perform the procedures described in this chapter

AM care
Care performed before breakfast; early morning care

aspiration
Breathing fluid or an object into the lungs

bedsore
A decubitus ulcer; a pressure sore

decubitus ulcer
A bedsore; a pressure sore

early morning care
AM care

HS care
Care given in the evening at bedtime

morning care
Care given after breakfast; cleanliness and skin care measures are more thorough at this time

oral hygiene
Measures performed to keep the mouth and teeth clean; mouth care

perineal care
Cleansing the genital and anal areas of the body; pericare

pressure sore
An area where the skin and underlying tissues are eroded as a result of a lack of blood flow; a bedsore or decubitus ulcer

My appearance has always been important to me. I need to feel clean and to smell nice. I put make-up and perfume on after my bath. I like nail polish, too.

Cleanliness and skin care are necessary for comfort, safety, and health. The skin is the body's first line of defense against disease. Intact skin prevents microorganisms from entering the body and causing infection. Likewise, the mucous membranes of the mouth, genital areas, and anus need to be kept clean and intact. In addition to cleansing, hygiene practices prevent body and breath odors, promote relaxation, and increase circulation.

Culture and personal choice influence hygiene practices. Some people like to shower. Others like tub baths. One person may bathe at bedtime. Another may bathe in the morning. The frequency of bathing also varies. Some people do not have water for bathing. Others cannot afford such items as soap, deodorant, shampoo, a toothbrush, or toothpaste.

Residents often need some help with personal hygiene. Weakness from illness and body changes from aging affect the ability to practice hygiene. The need for cleanliness and skin care is affected by perspiration, urinary and bowel elimination, vomiting, drainage from wounds or body openings, bed rest, and activity. The nurse decides the amount and type of personal hygiene you need to provide for an individual.

DAILY CARE OF THE RESIDENT

Personal hygiene is performed as often as necessary to stay clean and comfortable. People who can care for themselves practice hygiene routinely and out of habit. They brush their teeth and wash their face and hands after rising in the morning. These and other hygiene measures may be done routinely before and after meals and at bedtime. Weak or disabled residents need help with hygiene. Routine care is given throughout the day. Remember to assist a resident with personal hygiene whenever necessary. Also remember to protect the resident's rights, especially the right to privacy and the right to personal choice.

Before Breakfast

Routine care performed before breakfast often is called early morning or **AM care**. The night- or day-shift staff members are responsible for this care. They get residents ready for breakfast or for special tests scheduled for early in the day. Hygiene measures performed at this time include:

1. Assisting residents to the bathroom or offering the bedpan or urinal
2. Cleaning incontinent residents and changing any soiled linen
3. Helping residents wash their faces and hands
4. Assisting residents with oral hygiene
5. Assisting residents to dress for breakfast in the dining room. Some are assisted into Fowler's position or to bedside chairs for breakfast.
6. Assisting residents to the dining room for breakfast
7. Straightening linens or making beds
8. Straightening resident units

After Breakfast

Morning care is given after breakfast. Cleanliness and skin-care measures are more thorough at this time. Routine morning care usually involves:

1. Assisting residents to the bathroom or offering the bedpan or urinal
2. Cleaning incontinent residents and changing any soiled linen
3. Helping residents wash their faces and hands
4. Assisting with oral hygiene
5. Shaving residents
6. Providing showers, tub baths, or complete or partial bed baths
7. Performing range-of-motion exercises (see Chapter 17)
8. Assisting residents to dress in street clothes or to change into clean gowns or pajamas
9. Brushing and combing hair
10. Assisting with ambulation
11. Changing bed linens or making beds
12. Straightening resident units

Afternoon Care

Routine personal hygiene measures are performed after lunch and supper. Many residents like to have afternoon care completed before having visitors or attending activity programs. Afternoon care consists of:

1. Assisting residents to the bathroom or offering the bedpan or urinal before and after naps
2. Cleaning incontinent residents and changing any soiled linen before and after naps
3. Helping residents wash their faces and hands
4. Assisting residents to lie down for a nap
5. Assisting residents up after the nap
6. Assisting with ambulation
7. Providing range-of-motion exercises
8. Straightening resident units

Evening Care

Care given to residents in the evening at bedtime is called **HS care.** Hygiene measures are performed just before the resident is ready for sleep. They help increase comfort and the ability to relax. HS care involves:

1. Assisting residents to the bathroom or offering bedpans or urinals
2. Cleaning incontinent residents and changing any soiled linen
3. Helping residents wash their faces and hands
4. Assisting with oral hygiene
5. Helping residents in street clothes to undress and put on gowns or pajamas
6. Giving back massages
7. Straightening resident units

ORAL HYGIENE

Oral hygiene (mouth care) involves keeping the mouth and teeth clean. This prevents mouth odors and infections, increases comfort, and makes food taste better. Illness and disease may cause the resident to have bad tastes in the mouth. Some drugs and diseases cause a whitish coating on the mouth and tongue. Others may cause redness and swelling of the mouth and tongue.

The nurse decides the type of mouth care and amount of assistance a resident needs. Oral hygiene is provided upon awakening, after each meal, and at bedtime. Many persons also practice oral hygiene before meals.

Equipment

A toothbrush, toothpaste, dental floss, and mouthwash are needed for oral hygiene. The toothbrush should have soft or medium bristles. Residents with dentures need denture cleaner, a denture cup, and a denture brush or regular toothbrush. Toothettes or other applicators are used for residents with sore and tender mouths and for unconscious residents. A *toothette* is a piece of spongy foam attached to a stick. You need to be careful when using toothettes. Check the foam pad to make sure it is tight on the stick. The resident could choke on the foam pad if it comes off the stick. Other needed items include a kidney basin, water glass, straw, tissues, towels, and gloves. Nursing unit supply rooms usually have such items. Many residents choose to bring their own oral hygiene equipment from home.

Universal precautions are necessary when you give oral care. You will have contact with the resident's mucous membranes. Gums may bleed during oral hygiene. Also, many pathogens are present in the mouth. Pathogens spread through sexual contact may remain in the mouths of some persons.

Brushing Teeth

Many residents perform oral hygiene themselves. Others need help in gathering and setting up the equipment. You may have to brush the teeth of residents who are very weak or cannot use or move their arms. Some residents are too confused to brush their own teeth. You need to provide oral hygiene for them. The following are reported to the nurse if observed when teeth are brushed:

1. Dry, cracked, swollen, or blistered lips
2. Redness, swelling, irritation, sores, or white patches in the mouth or on the tongue
3. Bleeding, swelling, or excessive redness of the gums

Assisting the Bed Resident to Brush the Teeth

1. Explain the procedure to the resident.

2. Wash your hands.

3. Collect the following:
   a. Toothbrush
   b. Toothpaste or dentifrice
   c. Mouthwash
   d. Dental floss
   e. Water glass with cool water
   f. Straw
   g. Kidney basin
   h. Face towel
   i. Paper towels
   j. Gloves

4. Place the paper towels on the overbed table. Arrange other items on top of them.

5. Identify the resident. Check the ID bracelet and call the resident by name.

6. Provide for privacy.

7. Raise the head of the bed to a comfortable level for the resident.

8. Place the towel over the resident's chest to protect the gown and linens from spills.

9. Lower the side rail if up.

10. Move the overbed table in front of the resident. Adjust the height so the resident can work with ease.

11. Allow the resident to brush the teeth.

12. Move overbed table next to the bed when the resident is done. Lower it to an appropriate level for the resident.

13. Make sure the resident is comfortable.

14. Place the signal light within reach.

15. Raise or lower side rails as instructed by the nurse.

16. Clean and return equipment to its proper place.

17. Wipe the overbed table with paper towels. Discard paper towels.

18. Unscreen the resident.

19. Place soiled linen in the linen hamper.

20. Wash your hands.

21. Report your observations to the nurse.

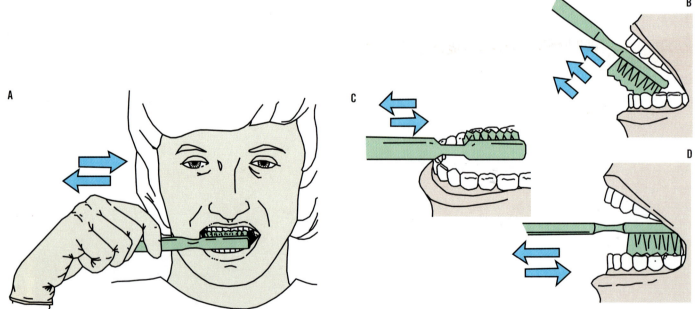

FIGURE 12-1 *A, Position the brush horizontally as shown, and brush back and forth with short strokes. B, Position the brush at a 45-degree angle against the inside of the front teeth. Brush from the gum to the crown of the tooth with short strokes. Reposition the brush until all of the front teeth have been brushed. C, Hold the brush horizontally against the inner surfaces of the teeth, and brush back and forth. D, Position the brush on the biting surfaces of the teeth as shown, and brush back and forth.*

Brushing the Resident's Teeth

1. Explain the procedure to the resident.

2. Wash your hands

3. Collect equipment (see *Assisting the Bed Resident to Brush the Teeth*, p. 232).

4. Place the paper towels on the overbed table. Arrange items on top of them.

5. Identify the resident. Check the ID bracelet and call the resident by name.

6. Provide for privacy.

7. Raise the bed to the best level for good body mechanics. Make sure side rails are up.

8. Raise the head of the bed so the resident can sit comfortably. Position the resident in the side-lying position near you if he or she cannot sit up.

9. Lower the side rail near you.

10. Place the towel over the resident's chest.

11. Position the overbed table so you can reach it with ease. Adjust the height as needed.

12. Put on the gloves.

13. Apply toothpaste to the toothbrush.

14. Hold the toothbrush over the kidney basin. Pour some water over the brush.

15. Brush the resident's teeth gently as described in Fig. 12-1.

16. Let the resident rinse the mouth with water. Hold the kidney basin under the resident's chin (Fig. 12-2).

17. Floss the resident's teeth (see *Flossing the Resident's Teeth*, p. 234).

18. Let the resident use mouthwash. Hold the kidney basin under the chin.

19. Remove and discard the gloves.

20. Make sure the resident is comfortable.

21. Place the signal light within reach.

22. Lower the bed to its lowest position.

23. Raise or lower side rails as instructed by the nurse.

24. Clean and return equipment to its proper place.

25. Wipe off the overbed table with the paper towels and discard them.

26. Lower the overbed table to a level appropriate for the resident.

27. Unscreen the resident.

28. Place soiled linen in the linen hamper.

29. Wash your hands.

30. Report your observations to the nurse.

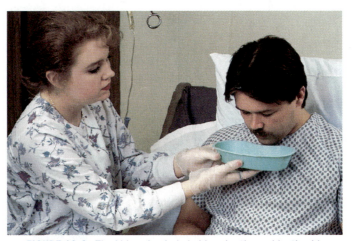

FIGURE 12-2 *The kidney basin is held under the resident's chin.*

Flossing

Flossing teeth is part of good oral hygiene. It removes plaque and tartar from the teeth. These substances can cause serious gum disease that leads to the loosening and loss of teeth. Therefore, flossing is a preventive measure. Flossing also is done to remove food between the teeth. Flossing usually is performed after brushing but can be done at other times. Some people floss after meals. If done only once a day, bedtime is the best time to floss.

There is waxed and unwaxed floss. Waxed floss does not fray as easily as the unwaxed type. Waxed floss is easier to use because it slides between the teeth. However, particles on tooth surfaces are more likely to attach to unwaxed floss. Many dentists recommend the unwaxed type, which is thinner than waxed floss.

You will need to floss for any resident who cannot tend to oral hygiene. Some elders have never flossed their teeth. Respect their wishes if they refuse to have it done. Be sure to report this to the nurse so the information can be noted on the resident's care plan.

PROCEDURE

Flossing the Resident's Teeth

1. Explain the procedure to the resident.

2. Wash your hands.

3. Collect the following:
   a. Kidney basin
   b. Water glass with cool water
   c. Dental floss
   d. Face towel
   e. Paper towels
   f. Disposable gloves

4. Place the paper towels on the overbed table. Arrange other items on top of them.

5. Identify the resident. Check the ID bracelet and call the resident by name.

6. Provide for privacy.

7. Raise the bed to the best level for good body mechanics. Make sure the side rails are up.

8. Raise the head of the bed so the resident can sit comfortably. Position the resident in a side-lying position near you if he or she cannot sit up.

9. Place the towel over the resident's chest.

10. Position the overbed table for easy access. Adjust the height as needed.

11. Lower the side rail near you.

12. Put on gloves.

13. Break off an 18-inch piece of floss from the dispenser.

14. Hold the floss between the middle fingers of each hand (Fig. 12-3).

15. Stretch the floss with your thumbs.

16. Start at the upper back tooth on the right side and work around to the left side.

17. Move the floss gently up and down between the teeth (Fig. 12-4).

18. Move to another section of floss after every second tooth.

19. Hold the floss with your index fingers (Fig. 12-5).

20. Floss the lower teeth. Use back-and-forth motions, and go under the gum as for the upper teeth. Start at the right side and work around to the left side.

21. Let the resident rinse the mouth. Hold the kidney basin under the chin. Repeat rinsing as necessary.

22. Follow steps 19 through 30 for *Brushing the Resident's Teeth* on p. 233.

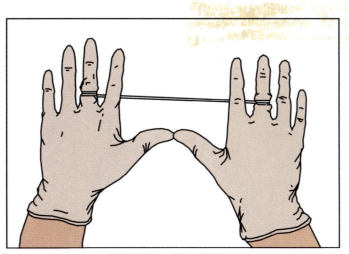

FIGURE 12-3 *Dental floss is held between the middle fingers to floss the upper teeth.*

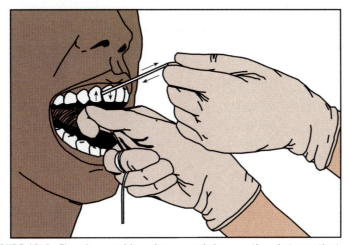

FIGURE 12-4 *Floss is moved by using up-and-down motions between the teeth.*

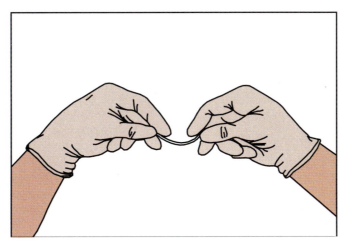

FIGURE 12-5 *Floss is held with the index fingers to floss the lower teeth.*

Mouth Care for the Unconscious Resident

Unconscious residents need special mouth care. They cannot eat and drink, and they breathe with their mouths open. Many receive supplemental oxygen. These factors cause the mouth to become dry and crusts to form on the tongue and mucous membranes. Good mouth care helps keep the mouth clean and moist and helps prevent infection.

Lemon glycerine swabs sometimes are used to give mouth care to these special residents. They have a drying effect, however, and may cause mouth ulcers. Use them only if ordered by the nurse. Toothettes dipped in a small amount of mouthwash, hydrogen peroxide, or a salt solution can be used to clean the mouth. To prevent cracking, petrolatum or other lubricant is applied to the lips after cleaning.

Unconscious residents usually cannot swallow. They must be protected from choking and aspiration. **Aspiration** is the breathing of fluid or an object into the lungs. To prevent aspiration, position the resident on one side with the head turned well to the side (Fig. 12-6). This position allows excess fluid to run out of the mouth, reducing the danger of aspiration. Using only a small amount of fluid also reduces the possibility of aspiration.

The resident's mouth needs to be kept open for mouth care. A padded tongue blade can be used for this purpose. (Fig. 12-7 shows how to make a padded tongue blade.) Do not use your fingers to hold the mouth open. The resident may bite down on them. Microorganisms can enter your body through the broken skin and cause an infection.

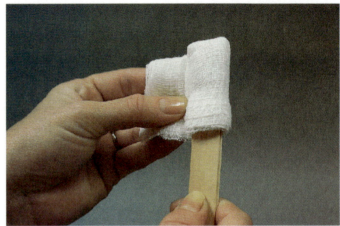

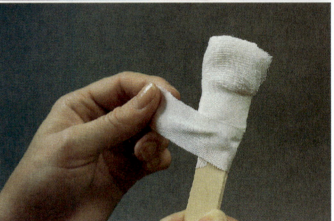

FIGURE 12-7 *Padded tongue blade.* **A,** *Place two wooden tongue blades together and wrap gauze around the top half.* **B,** *Tape the gauze in place.*

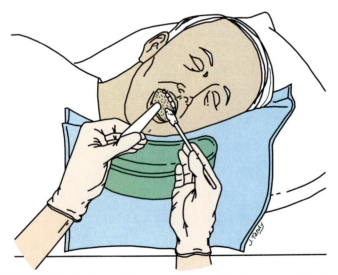

FIGURE 12-6 *The head of the unconscious resident is turned well to the side to prevent aspiration. A padded tongue blade is used to keep the mouth open while the mouth is cleaned with applicators.*

Unconscious residents cannot speak or respond to what is happening. However, they may be able to hear. Always assume that unconscious residents can hear. Explain what you are doing step by step. Also tell the resident when you have finished and when you are leaving the room.

Mouth care usually is given every 2 hours. Check with the nurse and the resident's care plan to see how often it is done and the solution to use. Unconscious residents also should be repositioned every 2 hours. Combining mouth care, skin care, and other comfort measures at this time increases comfort and safety. The possibility of forgetting mouth care is reduced if it is part of a routine care given every 2 hours.

PROCEDURE

Providing Mouth Care for an Unconscious Resident

1. Wash your hands.
2. Collect the following:
   a. Lemon glycerine swabs (if ordered by the nurse)
   b. Antiseptic mouthwash or other solution
   c. Toothettes or other applicators
   d. Padded tongue blade
   e. Water glass with cool water
   f. Face towel
   g. Kidney basin
   h. Petrolatum jelly
   i. Paper towels
   j. Disposable gloves
3. Place the paper towels on the overbed table. Arrange items on top of them.
4. Identify the resident. Check the ID bracelet and call the resident by name.
5. Explain the procedure to the resident.
6. Provide for privacy.
7. Raise the bed to the best level for good body mechanics.
8. Lower the side rail near you.
9. Put on the gloves.
10. Position the resident in the side-lying position. Turn his or her head well to the side.
11. Place the towel under the resident's face.
12. Place the kidney basin under the chin.
13. Position the overbed table for easy access. Adjust the height as needed.
14. Separate the upper and lower teeth with the padded tongue blade.

15. Clean the mouth using the toothettes or applicators moistened with mouthwash or other solution (see Fig. 12-6).
    a. Clean the chewing and inner surfaces of the teeth.
    b. Swab the roof of the mouth, inside of the cheeks, and the lips.
    c. Swab the tongue.
    d. Moisten a clean applicator with water, and swab the mouth to rinse.
    e. Place used applicators in the kidney basin.
16. Repeat step 15 using the glycerine swabs (if ordered by the nurse).
17. Apply petrolatum jelly to the resident's lips.
18. Remove and discard the gloves.
19. Explain that the procedure is done and that you will reposition the resident.
20. Reposition the resident.
21. Raise the side rails.
22. Make sure the signal light is within reach.
23. Lower the bed to its lowest position.
24. Clean and return equipment to its proper place. Discard disposable items.
25. Unscreen the resident.
26. Tell the resident that you are leaving the room.
27. Place soiled linen in the linen hamper.
28. Wash your hands.
29. Report your observations to the nurse.

237

Denture Care

Dentures are cleaned for residents who cannot do this for themselves. Mouth care is provided and dentures are cleaned as often as natural teeth. Remember that dentures are the resident's property and are expensive. Losing or damaging them is negligent conduct.

Dentures are slippery when wet. They can easily break or chip if dropped. You must hold them firmly. Clean them over a basin of water lined with a towel.

Hot water causes them to warp. Never use hot water to clean or store dentures. Some residents do not regularly wear their dentures. Most residents remove them at bedtime. When not being worn, dentures are stored in a container filled with cool water. Dentures can dry out and warp if they are not stored in water. Residents who can clean their own dentures may need your help. They may need help getting to the bathroom and in gathering supplies.

PROCEDURE

Denture Care

1. Explain the procedure to the resident.
2. Wash your hands.
3. Collect the following:
   a. Denture brush or toothbrush
   b. Denture cup labeled with the resident's name and room number
   c. Denture cleaner or toothpaste
   d. Water glass with cool water
   e. Straw
   f. Mouthwash
   g. Kidney basis
   h. Two face towels
   i. Gauze squares
   j. Disposable gloves
4. Identify the resident. Check the ID bracelet and call the resident by name.
5. Provide for privacy.
6. Lower the side rail if up.
7. Place a towel over the resident's chest.
8. Put on gloves.
9. Ask the resident to remove the dentures. Carefully place them in the kidney basin.
10. Remove the dentures using gauze if the resident cannot do so. (The gauze lets you get a good grip on the slippery dentures.)
    a. Grasp the upper denture with the thumb and index finger of one hand (Fig. 12-8). Move the denture up and down slightly to break the seal. Gently remove the denture once the seal is broken. Place it in the kidney basin.
    b. Remove the lower denture by grasping it with your thumb and index finger. Turn it slightly, and lift it out of the mouth. Place it in the kidney basin.
11. Raise or lower side rails as instructed the nurse.
12. Take the kidney basin, denture cup, brush, and denture cleaner or toothpaste to the sink.
13. Rinse each denture under warm running water. Return them to the denture cup.
14. Line the sink with a towel and fill it with water.
15. Apply denture cleaner or toothpaste to the brush.
16. Brush the dentures as in Fig. 12-9.
17. Rinse the dentures under warm running water. Handle them carefully; do not drop them.
18. Place them in the denture cup. Fill it with cool water until the dentures are covered.
19. Clean the kidney basin.
20. Bring the denture cup and kidney basin to the bedside.
21. Raise or lower side rails as instructed by the nurse.
22. Position the resident for oral hygiene.
23. Ask the resident to rinse his or her mouth with mouthwash. Hold the kidney basin under the chin.

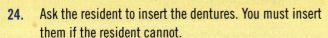

24. Ask the resident to insert the dentures. You must insert them if the resident cannot.
    a. Grasp the upper denture firmly with your thumb and index finger. Raise the upper lip with the other hand and insert the denture. Use your index fingers to press gently on the upper denture to make sure that it is securely in place.
    b. Grasp the lower denture securely with your thumb and index finger. Pull down slightly on the lower lip and insert the denture. Gently press down on the denture to make sure it is in place.
25. Put the denture cup in the top drawer of the bedside stand if the dentures are not reinserted.

26. Remove and discard the gloves.
27. Make sure the resident is comfortable.
28. Place the signal light within reach.
29. Raise or lower side rails as instructed by the nurse.
30. Unscreen the resident.
31. Clean and return equipment to its proper place. Wear gloves if necessary. Discard disposable items.
32. Place soiled linen in the linen hamper.
33. Wash your hands.
34. Report your observations to the nurse.

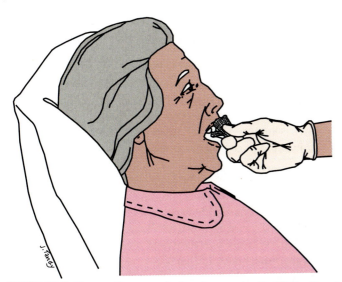

FIGURE 12-8 *Remove the upper denture by grasping it with the thumb and index finger of one hand. Use a piece of gauze to grasp the slippery denture.*

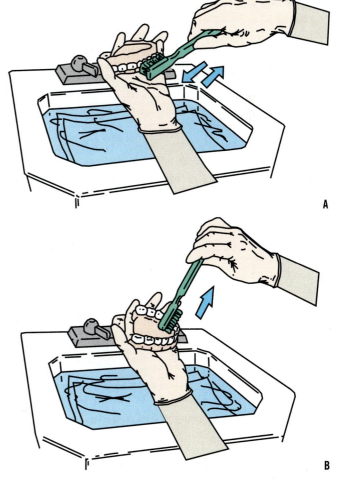

FIGURE 12-9 ***A,*** *Outer surfaces of the upper denture are brushed with back and forth motions. Note that the denture is held over the sink, which is filled halfway with water and lined with a towel.* ***B,*** *Position the brush vertically to clean the inner surfaces of the denture. Use upward strokes.*

BATHING

Bathing has other purposes besides cleansing. A bath is refreshing and relaxing. Circulation is stimulated and body parts exercised. The bath also gives you time to talk with and get to know the resident. In addition, you can make important observations during the bath.

A resident may have a complete or partial bath in bed, a tub bath, or a shower. The method depends on the resident's condition, ability to provide self-care, and personal choice. In nursing facilities, bathing usually occurs after breakfast or the evening meal. Bath time also should be a matter of personal choice.

Certain factors influence how often a person bathes. Personal choice is one factor. Some people bathe at least daily. Others take a complete bath only once or twice a week. Illness is another factor. Many illnesses increase the need for bathing because of fever and perspiration. Others prevent frequent bathing. Age is also a factor. Elderly people tend to have dry, fragile skin that is easily injured. Frequent bathing can increase the dryness. For elderly persons, a complete bath twice a week usually is enough. However, a partial bath should be given daily.

Skin Care Products

There are many kinds of skin care products. Some clean the skin. Others protect the skin from drying or friction. The products used depend on personal choice and cost.

Soaps cleanse the skin. They remove dirt, dead skin, skin oil, some microorganisms, and perspiration. However, they tend to dry and irritate skin. Dry skin can be itchy, uncomfortable, and easily injured. Skin must be rinsed well to remove all soap.

Soap is not needed for every bath. Plain water can clean the skin. Plain water often is used for elderly persons because of their dry skin. Those with dry skin may prefer soaps that contain bath oils. Soaps should not be used if a person has very dry skin.

Bath oils keep the skin soft and prevent drying. Some soaps contain bath oils, or liquid bath oil can be added to bath water. Showers and tubs become slippery from bath oils. Safety precautions must be taken to prevent falls.

Creams and lotions protect the skin from the drying effect of air and evaporation. They do not feel greasy but leave an oily film on the skin. Most are scented. Lotion is used for the back massage. Applying lotion to bony points helps prevent skin breakdown. You can apply lotion to the elbows, knees, and heels after the bath or shower.

Powders absorb moisture and prevent friction when two skin surfaces rub together. They usually are applied under the breasts, under the arms, and in the groin area. Sometimes powders are applied between the toes. Pow-der is applied to dry skin in a thin, even layer. Excessive powder causes caking and crusts that can irritate the skin.

Deodorants and antiperspirants are applied to the axillae (underarms) after bathing. *Deodorants* mask and control body odors. *Antiperspirants* reduce perspiration. Deodorants and antiperspirants should not be applied to irritated skin. They do not take the place of bathing.

Observations

When bathing a resident or assisting a resident to bathe, you must observe the skin. The following observations are reported to the nurse:

1. Color of the skin, lips, nail beds, and sclera (whites of the eyes)
2. Location and description of rashes
3. Dry skin
4. Bruises or open areas of skin
5. Pale or reddened areas, especially over bony parts
6. Drainage or bleeding from wounds or body openings
7. Skin temperature
8. Resident complaints of pain or discomfort

General Rules

Certain rules must be followed for bed baths, showers, or tub baths.

1. Ask the nurse what type of bath a resident is to have. Find out which skin care products to use. Allow personal choice whenever possible.
2. Collect necessary equipment before beginning the procedure.
3. Protect the resident's privacy. Properly screen the resident and close doors, shades, or drapes.
4. Make sure the resident is adequately covered for warmth and privacy.
5. Reduce drafts by closing doors and windows.
6. Protect the resident from falling.
7. Use good body mechanics at all times.
8. Make sure water temperature is not too hot, particularly for elderly persons.
9. Keep soap in the soap dish between latherings. This prevents the water from becoming too soapy. If a tub bath is taken, it reduces the chance of slipping and falls.
10. Wash from the cleanest to the dirtiest areas.
11. Encourage the resident to help as much as is safely possible.
12. Rinse the skin thoroughly to remove the soap.
13. Pat the skin dry to avoid irritating or breaking the skin.
14. Bathe the skin whenever fecal material or urine is on the skin. Be sure to wear gloves, follow universal precautions, and follow the bloodborne pathogen standard.

The Complete Bed Bath

The *complete bed bath* involves washing the resident's entire body in bed. Residents who are unconscious, paralyzed, in casts or traction, or weak from illness or surgery usually need bed baths. Complete bed baths are given to residents who cannot bathe themselves.

Ask the nurse about a resident's ability to assist in the bath. Also ask about any limitations in activity or position and the need for universal precautions. You also should check the resident's care plan and ask the resident for any personal choices about bathing.

Many residents have never had a bed bath. They may be embarrassed to have another person see their body and may fear being exposed. Each resident must get an explanation about how a bed bath is given and how the body is covered to protect privacy.

PROCEDURE

Giving a Complete Bed Bath

1. Identify the resident. Check the ID bracelet and call the resident by name.

2. Explain the procedure to the resident.

3. Offer the bedpan or urinal (see Chapter 13). Screen the resident if the bedpan or urinal is used.

4. Wash your hands.

5. Collect clean linen as for the closed bed. Place linen on a clean surface.

6. Collect the following:
   a. Wash basin
   b. Soap dish with soap
   c. Bath thermometer
   d. Orange stick or nail file
   e. Washcloth
   f. Two bath towels and two face towels
   g. Bath blanket
   h. Gown, pajamas, or clothing
   i. Equipment for oral hygiene
   j. Deodorant or antiperspirant
   k. Body lotion
   l. Brush and comb
   m. Other toilet articles as requested
   n. Paper towels
   o. Disposable gloves

7. Arrange the equipment on the overbed table (use the bedside stand if necessary). Adjust the height if necessary.

8. Close doors and windows to prevent drafts.

9. Provide for privacy.

10. Raise the bed to the best level for good body mechanics. Make sure the side rails are up.

11. Remove the signal light.

12. Lower the side rail near you.

13. Provide oral hygiene.

14. Remove top linens and cover the resident with a bath blanket (see *Making an Occupied Bed*, p. 219).

15. Lower the head of the bed to a level appropriate for the resident. Keep it as flat as possible. Allow the resident at least one pillow.

16. Place the paper towels on the overbed table.

17. Raise the side rail.

18. Fill the wash basin 2/3 full with water. Water temperature should be 110° to 115° F (43° to 46° C).

19. Place the wash basin on the overbed table on top of the paper towels.

20. Lower the side rail.

21. Place a face towel over the resident's chest.

22. Make a mitt with the washcloth (Fig. 12-10, p. 243). Use a mitt throughout the procedure.

23. Wash the eyes with water only. Do not use soap. Gently wipe from the inner aspect with a corner of the mitted washcloth (Fig. 12-11, p. 244). Clean the eye farthest from you first. Repeat this step for the other eye.

Continued.

24. Ask the resident if you should use soap for the face.

25. Wash the face, ears, and neck. Rinse and dry well with the towel on the chest.

26. Help the resident move to the side of the bed near you.

27. Remove the gown. Do not expose the resident.

28. Place a bath towel lengthwise under the far arm.

29. Support the arm with the palm of your hand under the resident's elbow. His or her forearm should rest on your forearm.

30. Wash the arm, shoulder, and underarm with long, firm strokes (Fig. 12-12, p. 244). Rinse and pat dry.

31. Place the basin on the towel. Put the resident's hand into the water and wash it well (Fig. 12-13, p. 244). Clean under the fingernails with an orange stick or nail file.

32. Encourage the resident to exercise the hand and fingers.

33. Remove the basin and dry the hand well. Cover the arm with the bath blanket.

34. Repeat steps 28 through 33 for the near arm.

35. Place a bath towel over the resident's chest crosswise. Hold the towel in place, and pull the bath blanket from under the towel to the waist.

36. Lift the towel slightly and wash the chest (Fig. 12-14, p. 245). Do not expose the resident. Rinse and pat dry. Dry well under the breasts of a woman.

37. Place the towel lengthwise over the chest and abdomen. Do not expose the resident. Pull the bath blanket down to the pubic area.

38. Lift the towel slightly and wash the abdomen (Fig. 12-15, p. 245). Rinse and pat dry.

39. Pull the bath blanket up to the shoulders, covering both arms. Remove the towel.

40. Change the water if it is soapy or cool. Raise the side rail before you leave the bedside. Lower it when you return.

41. Uncover the far leg. Do not expose the genital area. Place a towel lengthwise under the foot and leg.

42. Bend the knee and support the leg with your arm. Wash it with long, firm strokes. Rinse and pat dry.

43. Place the basin on the towel by the foot.

44. Lift the leg slightly. Slide the basin under the foot.

45. Place the foot in the basin (Fig. 12-16, p. 246). Use an orange stick or nail file to clean under toenails if necessary.

46. Remove the basin. Dry the leg, foot, and between the toes. Cover the leg with the bath blanket. Remove the towel.

47. Repeat steps 41 through 46 for the other leg.

48. Change the water. Raise the side rail before leaving the bedside. Lower it when you return.

49. Turn the resident onto the side away from you. Keep him or her covered with the bath blanket.

50. Uncover the back and buttocks. Do not expose the resident. Place a towel lengthwise on the bed along the back.

51. Wash the back, working from the back of the neck to the buttocks. Use long, firm continuous strokes (Fig. 12-17, p. 246). Rinse and dry well.

52. Give a back massage. (The resident may prefer the back massage after the bath.)

53. Turn the resident onto his or her back.

54. Change the water for perineal care. Raise the side rail before leaving the bedside. Lower it when you return.

55. Have the resident wash the genital area. Adjust the overbed table so that the wash basin, soap, and towels can be reached. Place the signal light within reach. Ask the resident to signal when through. Make sure he or she understands what to do. Answer the signal light promptly. Provide perineal care if the resident cannot do so (see pp. 256-259).

56. Give a back massage if you have not already done so. Apply lotion to the elbows, knees, and heels.

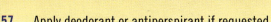

57. Apply deodorant or antiperspirant if requested.

58. Put a clean gown or pajamas on the resident.

59. Comb and brush the hair.

60. Make the bed. Attach the signal light.

61. Make sure the resident is comfortable.

62. Lower the bed to its lowest position.

63. Raise or lower side rails as instructed by the nurse.

64. Empty and clean the basin. Return it and other supplies to their proper place.

65. Wipe off the overbed table with the paper towels and discard them.

66. Unscreen the resident.

67. Place soiled linen in the linen hamper.

68. Wash your hands.

69. Report your observations to the nurse (see p. 240).

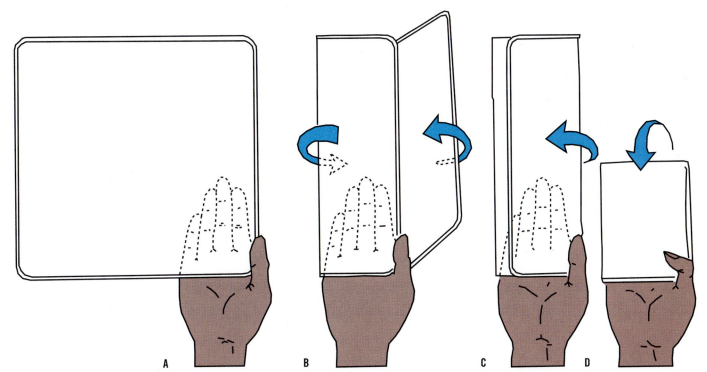

FIGURE 12-10 *A, Make a mitt with a washcloth by grasping the near side of the washcloth with your thumb. B, Bring the washcloth around and behind your hand. C, Fold the side of the washcloth over your palm as you grasp it with your thumb. D, Fold the top of the washcloth down and tuck it under next to your palm.*

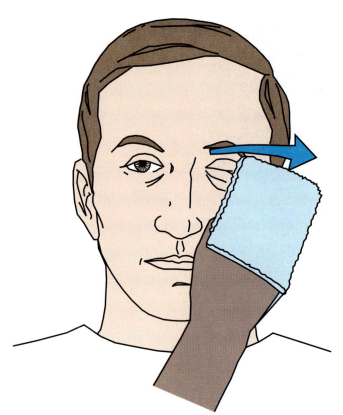

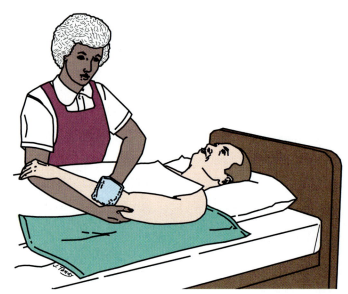

FIGURE 12-11 *Wash the resident's eye with a mitted washcloth. Wipe from the inner to the outer aspect of the eye.*

FIGURE 12-12 *Using a mitted washcloth, wash the resident's arm with firm, long strokes.*

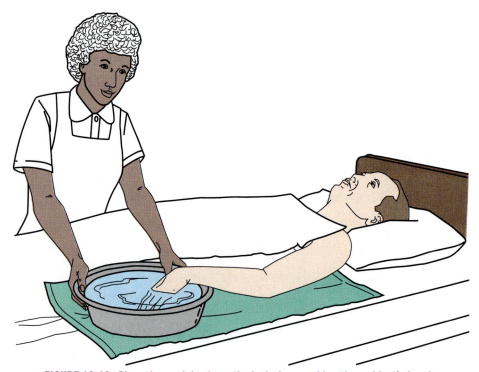

FIGURE 12-13 *Place the wash basin on the bed when washing the resident's hands.*

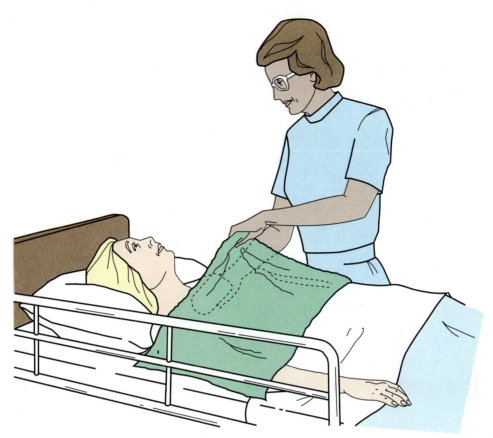

FIGURE 12-14 *The resident's breasts are not exposed during the bath. A bath towel is placed horizontally over the chest area. The nursing assistant lifts the towel slightly and reaches under it to wash the breasts and chest.*

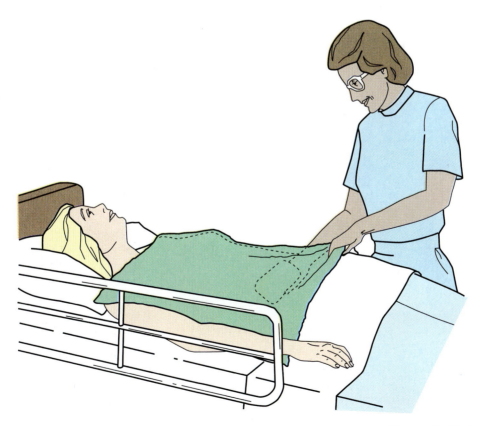

FIGURE 12-15 *The bath towel is turned to the vertical position so that it covers the breasts and abdomen. The towel is lifted slightly to bathe the abdomen. The bath blanket covers the pubic area.*

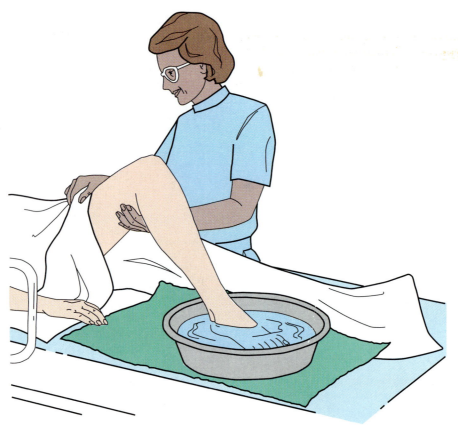

FIGURE 12-16 *The foot is washed by placing it in the wash basin on the bed.*

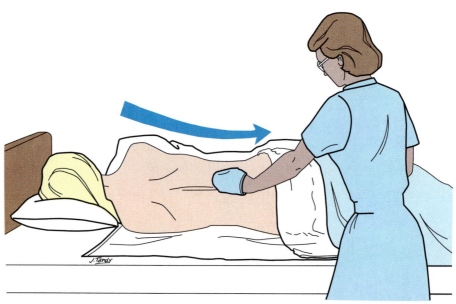

FIGURE 12-17 *The back is washed with long, firm, continuous strokes. Note that the resident is in a side-lying position. A towel is placed lengthwise on the bed to protect the linens from water.*

The Partial Bath

The *partial bath* involves bathing the resident's face, hands, axillae (underarms), genital area, back, and buttocks. These areas may develop odors or cause discomfort if not clean. Partial bed baths are given to residents unable to help themselves. Some residents can bathe themselves in bed or at the sink. Nursing staff members assist as needed, particularly in washing the back.

The same rules for bathing apply when giving a partial bed bath. So do the considerations involved in giving a complete bath.

PROCEDURE

Giving a Partial Bath

1. Follow steps 1 through 9 in *Giving a Complete Bed Bath,* p. 241.

2. Make sure the bed is in the lowest position.

3. Place the paper towels on the overbed table.

4. Fill the basin with water 110° to 115° F (43° to 46° C).

5. Place the basin on the overbed table on top of the paper towels.

6. Raise the head of the bed to a level where the resident can bathe comfortably. Assist the resident to sit at bedside if he or she is safe in this position.

7. Position the overbed table so the resident can easily reach the basin and supplies. The side rail should be down.

8. Assist the resident in removing gown or pajamas.

9. Ask the resident to wash the parts of the body that can be easily reached (Fig. 12-18, p. 248). Explain that you will wash the back and other areas that cannot be reached.

10. Place the signal light within reach. Ask the person to signal when help is needed or when bathing is complete.

11. Leave the room after washing your hands.

12. Return when the signal light is on. Knock before entering.

13. Change the bath water.

14. Ask what was washed. Wash areas not done. The face, hands, axillae, genital area, back, and buttocks are washed for a partial bath.

15. Give a back massage. Apply lotion to the elbows, knees, and heels.

16. Apply deodorant or antiperspirant if requested.

17. Help the resident put on a clean gown, pajamas, or clothing.

18. Assist with hair care, makeup, and shaving.

19. Assist the resident to a chair or wheelchair if the activity is allowed. Otherwise, turn the resident onto the side away from you.

20. Make the bed. Then lower it to its lowest position.

21. Help the resident return to bed if indicated.

22. Make sure the resident is comfortable.

23. Place the signal light within reach.

24. Raise or lower side rails as instructed by the nurse.

25. Empty and clean the basin. Return it and other supplies to their proper place.

26. Wipe off the overbed table with the paper towels. Then discard them.

27. Unscreen the resident.

28. Place soiled linen in the linen hamper.

29. Wash your hands.

30. Report your observations to the nurse (see p. 240).

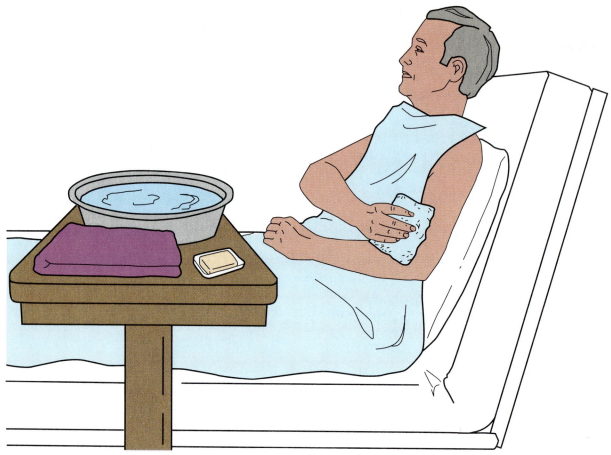

FIGURE 12-18 *The resident is bathing himself in bed. Necessary equipment is within his reach.*

The Tub Bath

Many people prefer tub baths to showers, especially elderly persons. Most residents find them relaxing. However, they need to be protected from falling when getting in and out of the tub. Burns caused by hot water also must be prevented. A tub bath can cause a person to feel faint, weak, or tired. A bath should not last longer than 20 minutes. Do not let a resident take a tub bath without the nurse's approval.

You need to reserve the tub room. The tub must be clean before it is used. The resident's safety is important. You must prevent slipping and falls. Check to see if the tub has a nonskid surface. If not, place a bath mat on the bottom of the tub to prevent falls. After the bath, it is safer to drain the tub before the person gets out. Be sure to keep the resident covered and protected from exposure and chilling while the tub is draining. Changes in this procedure may be necessary for some residents. If the resident is very weak or large, two workers may be needed to safely perform the procedure. Consult with the nurse for any special instructions before assisting a resident with a tub bath.

Some facilities have portable tubs. The sides are lowered to transfer the resident from the bed to the tub (Fig. 12-19). After the transfer, the sides are raised into position. The resident is then transported to the tub room. The tub is filled and the resident bathed in the usual manner.

Whirlpool tubs also may be available (Fig. 12-20). They have special hydraulic lifts. A resident is placed in a special wheeled chair at the bedside and taken to the tub room. The chair is attached to the lift and unlocked from the wheeled base. The chair and resident are lifted into the tub. The tub has a whirlpool action that cleans the resident. The nursing assistant washes the upper portion of the resident's body.

Some tubs have special gurneys (stretchers) for residents who cannot sit up. The resident is transferred from the bed to the gurney and wheeled into the tub room. The resident is lowered into a tub on the gurney (Fig. 12-21). The tub has a whirlpool action that cleans the resident.

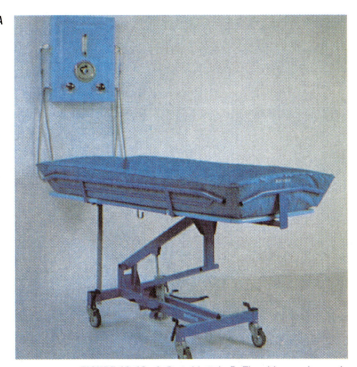

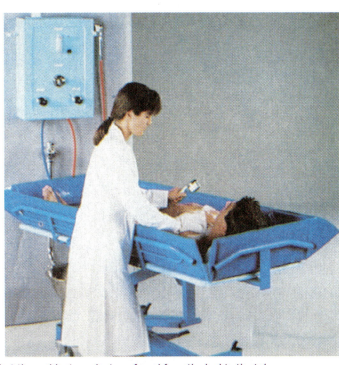

FIGURE 12-19 *A,* *Portable tub.* **B,** *The sides are lowered so that the resident can be transferred from the bed to the tub.*

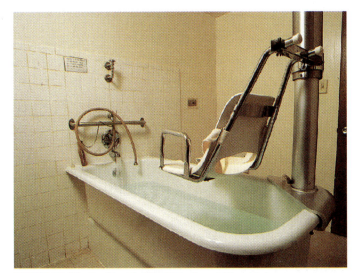

FIGURE 12-20 *Resident is lifted into the whirlpool tub.*

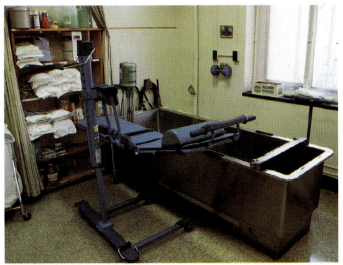

FIGURE 12-21 *A resident can be placed on a special gurney that is lowered into a tub. This tub has whirlpool action.*

Mosby's Textbook for Long-Term Care Assistants

PROCEDURE

Assisting the Resident With a Tub Bath

1. Reserve use of the bathtub if necessary.

2. Identify the resident. Check the ID bracelet and call the resident by name.

3. Explain the procedure to the resident.

4. Wash your hands.

5. Collect the following:
   a. Washcloth
   b. Two bath towels
   c. Soap
   d. Bath thermometer
   e. Gown, pajamas, or clothing
   f. Deodorant or antiperspirant
   g. Lotion
   h. Other toilet items as requested

6. Place supplies in the bathroom in the space provided or on a chair.

7. Clean the tub if indicated.

8. Place a rubber bath mat in the tub.

9. Place a disposable bath mat or towel in front of the tub.

10. Place the "occupied" sign on the bathroom door.

11. Return to the resident's room. Provide for privacy.

12. Help the resident sit on the side of the bed.

13. Help the resident put on a robe and shoes.

14. Assist the resident to the bathroom. Use a wheelchair if necessary.

15. Have the resident sit on the chair next to the tub.

16. Fill the tub halfway with water. Water temperature should be 105° F (41° C).

17. Help the resident remove shoes, robe, and gown.

18. Ask the resident to step into the tub (Fig. 12-22). Give needed support. Have the resident use the handbar for support. If the resident cannot step into the tub, have him or her sit on the edge of the tub. Then have the resident transfer into the tub.

19. Let the resident bathe. Assist as needed. Remember, the bath should not last longer than 20 minutes.

20. Do not leave the resident alone in the tub or in the tub room.

21. Place a towel across the chair.

22. Help the resident out of the tub and onto the chair.

23. Help the resident dry off; pat gently.

24. Apply lotion to the resident's back and to the elbows, knees, and heels.

25. Help the resident dress. Or help the resident put on a clean gown or pajamas, bathrobe, and shoes.

26. Help the resident return to the room. Assist with hair care and other grooming needs as requested by the resident.

27. Assist the resident back to bed if indicated.

28. Make sure the resident is comfortable and the signal light is within reach.

29. Raise or lower side rails as instructed by the nurse.

30. Clean the tub. Remove soiled linen and discard disposable items. Put the "unoccupied" sign on the door. Return supplies to their proper place.

31. Place soiled linen in the linen hamper.

32. Wash your hands.

33. Report your observations to the nurse (see p. 240).

250

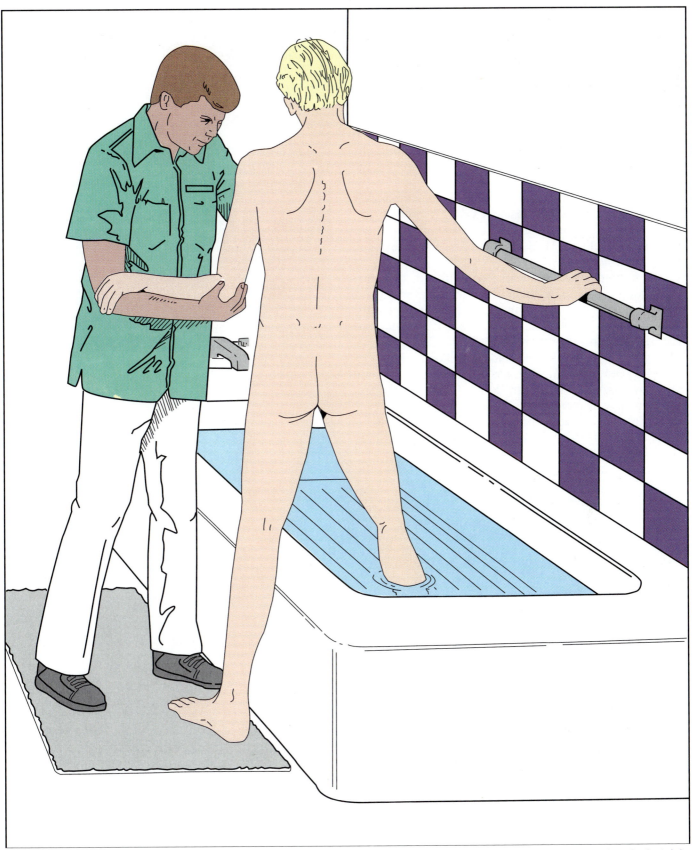

FIGURE 12-22 *The nursing assistant helps the resident into the tub to protect the resident from falling. A bath mat is placed in the tub; the tub is filled halfway with water, and a floor mat is in front of the tub.*

The Shower

Most nursing facilities have shower rooms with shower stalls (Fig. 12-23). Shower stalls have advantages over bathtub-shower units. The resident does not have to step into the tub. The resident simply walks into the stall or is wheeled in on a shower chair. Shower chairs have wheels on the legs. A round open area on the plastic seat lets water drain off the chair (Fig. 12-24). The chair can be used to transport the person to and from the shower room. The wheels must be locked during the shower to prevent the chair from moving.

The shower room may have more than one shower stall. You must protect the resident's right to privacy. Remember, the resident has the right not to have his or her body seen by others. Make sure you properly screen and cover the resident.

You need to protect residents from falls and chills during showers. Encourage the use of handrails for support while the resident is showering. Like tubs, shower stalls may have nonskid surfaces. If not, a bathmat needs to be used in the stall. Never let weak or unsteady residents stand in the shower. They need to use a shower chair. Privacy also must be protected. Be sure to close doors and the shower curtain. However, do not leave any resident alone in shower room. Stay in the shower room in case the resident needs help or becomes weak or faint. Residents are not allowed to shower unless the nurse gives approval.

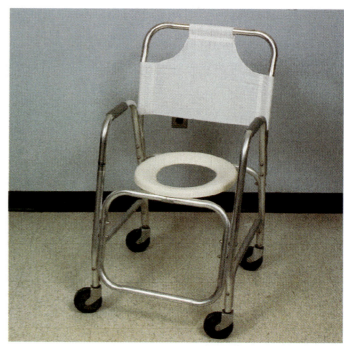

FIGURE 12-24 *A shower chair has a round opening in the center of the seat. The legs have wheels with locks to allow the chair to be used for transfers.*

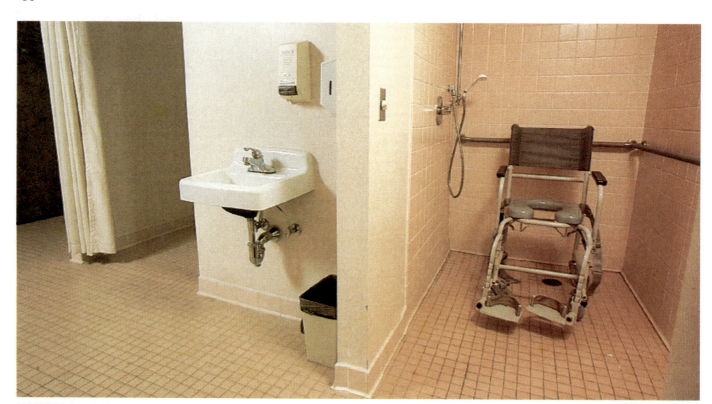

FIGURE 12-23 *A shower room has several shower stalls.*

PROCEDURE

Assisting the Resident to Shower

1. Reserve use of the shower.

2. Identify the resident. Check the ID bracelet and call the resident by name.

3. Explain the procedure to the resident.

4. Wash your hands.

5. Collect items as for a tub bath (p. 250).

6. Place items on a chair or space provided in the shower.

7. Clean the shower if needed.

8. Place a rubber bath mat if needed. Do not block the drain.

9. Place a disposable bath mat or towel in front of the shower.

10. Place the "occupied" sign on the door.

11. Return to the resident's room. Provide for privacy.

12. Help the resident sit on the side of the bed.

13. Help the resident put on a robe and shoes. Or transfer the resident to a shower chair. Cover the resident well with a bath blanket.

14. Assist the resident to the shower room. Use a wheelchair or shower chair if necessary.

15. Turn the shower on. Adjust the water temperature and pressure.

16. Provide help in removing shoes, gown, and robe. Or remove the bath blanket.

17. Help the resident into the shower. If a shower chair is used, place it in position and lock the wheels.

18. Assist the resident in washing if necessary.

19. Place a towel across the chair outside the shower.

20. Turn the shower off.

21. Assist the resident out of the shower and onto the chair if a shower chair is not used.

22. Help the resident dry off. Pat gently.

23. Apply lotion to the resident's back, elbows, knees, and heels.

24. Help him or her dress. Or help the resident put on a clean gown, pajamas, robe, and shoes.

25. Help the resident back to the room. Use the wheelchair or shower chair if necessary.

26. Assist with hair care and other grooming needs as requested by the resident.

27. Assist the resident back to bed if indicated.

28. Make sure the resident is comfortable and the signal light is within reach.

29. Raise or lower side rails as instructed by the nurse.

30. Clean the shower. Remove soiled linen and discard disposable items. Put the "unoccupied" sign on the door. Return supplies to their proper place.

31. Place soiled linen in the linen hamper.

32. Wash your hands.

33. Report your observations to the nurse (see p. 240).

THE BACK MASSAGE

The back massage (back rub) relieves tension, is relaxing, and stimulates circulation. It is given after a bath and as a part of HS care. It should last 4 to 6 minutes. You need to observe the skin for abnormalities before beginning.

Lotion is used to reduce friction during a massage. It should be warmed before being applied. Place the lotion bottle in the bath water or hold it under warm running water to warm. You also can rub some lotion between your hands.

The prone position is best for a massage. However, many elderly persons find this uncomfortable or impossible. The side-lying position is acceptable. Firm strokes are used, and always keep your hands in contact with the resident's skin.

Some residents should not have back massages as described in this procedure. They may be dangerous for those with certain heart diseases, back injuries, back surgeries, skin diseases, and some lung disorders. Check with the nurse before giving a back massage to residents with these conditions.

PROCEDURE

Giving a Back Massage

1. Identify the resident. Check the ID bracelet and call the resident by name.

2. Explain the procedure to the resident.

3. Wash your hands.

4. Collect the following:
   a. Bath blanket   c. Lotion
   b. Bath towel

5. Provide for privacy.

6. Raise the bed to the best level for good body mechanics. Make sure the side rails are up.

7. Lower the side rail near you.

8. Position the resident prone or in the side-lying position with the back toward you.

9. Expose the back, shoulders, upper arms, and buttocks. Cover the rest of the body with the bath blanket.

10. Lay the towel on the bed along the back.

11. Warm the lotion bottle under running water, or rub some lotion between your hands.

12. Explain that the lotion may feel cool and wet.

13. Apply lotion to the lower back areas.

14. Stroke upward from the buttocks to the shoulders. Then stroke down over the upper arms. Stroke up the upper arms, across the shoulders, and down the back to the buttocks (Fig. 12-25). Use firm strokes. Keep your hands in contact with the resident's skin.

15. Repeat step 14 for at least 3 minutes.

16. Knead by grasping tissue between the thumb and fingers as in Fig. 12-26. Knead very gently on elderly residents to avoid skin damage or bruising. Knead half of the back starting at the buttocks and moving upward to the shoulder. Then knead downward from the shoulder to the buttocks. Repeat on the other half of back.

17. Massage bony areas. Use circular motions with the tips of your index and middle fingers.

18. Use fast movements to stimulate and slow movements to relax the resident.

19. Stroke with long, firm movements to end the massage. Tell the resident you are finishing.

20. Apply lotion to the elbows, knees, and heels.

21. Cover the resident. Remove the towel and bath blanket.

22. Make sure the resident is comfortable.

23. Lower the bed to its lowest position.

24. Raise or lower side rails as instructed by the nurse.

25. Place the signal light within reach.

26. Return the lotion to its proper place.

27. Unscreen the resident.

28. Place soiled linen in the linen hamper.

29. Wash your hands.

30. Report your observations to the nurse.

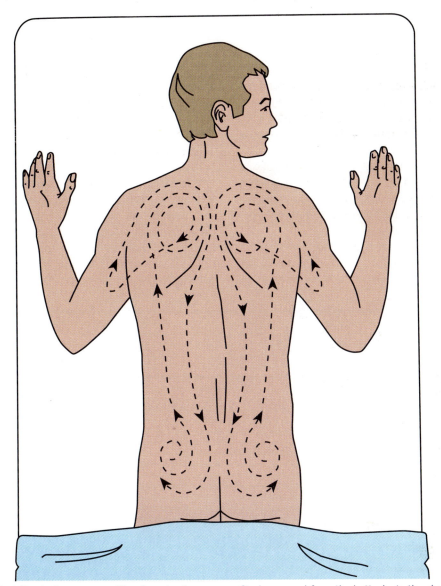

FIGURE 12-25 *The resident lies in the prone position for a back massage. Stroke upward from the buttocks to the shoulders, down over the upper arms, back up the upper arms, across the shoulders, and down the back to the buttocks.*

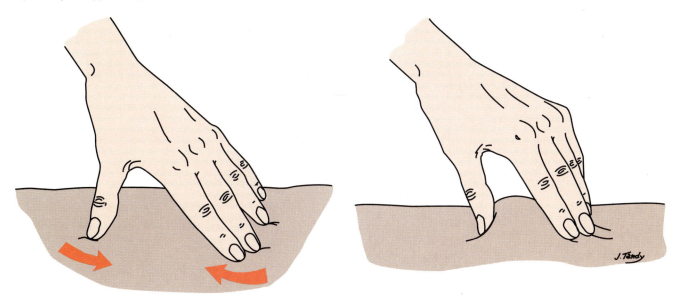

FIGURE 12-26 *Kneading is done by picking up tissue between the thumb and fingers.*

PERINEAL CARE

Perineal care (pericare) involves cleaning the genital and anal areas. These areas are warm, moist, and dark. They provide a place for microorganisms to grow. Perineal care prevents infection and odors and promotes comfort.

Perineal care is done at least daily as part of the bath. The procedure also is done whenever the area is contaminated with urine or feces. The nurse may ask you to give perineal care at other times. Residents with certain disorders need more frequent perineal care.

Residents should do their own perineal care if able. Otherwise it is given by the nursing staff. Many residents and nursing personnel find the procedure embarrassing, especially when given to someone of the opposite sex. Most residents do not know the terms perineum and perineal. They probably understand "privates," "private parts," "crotch," "genitals," or "the area between your legs." Be sure to use terms that the resident understands. The term should be in good taste professionally.

Universal precautions, the rules of medical asepsis, and the bloodborne pathogen standard are followed. You will work from the cleanest area to the dirtiest. The urethral area is the cleanest, the anal area dirtiest. Therefore clean from the urethra to the anal area. The perineal area is very delicate and easily injured. Use warm water, not hot. The area must be rinsed thoroughly. Pat dry after rinsing to reduce moisture and promote comfort.

PROCEDURE

Giving Female Perineal Care

1. Explain the procedure to the resident.

2. Wash your hands.

3. Collect the following:
   a. Soap dish with soap
   b. Three to ten disposable washcloths or a small package of cotton balls
   c. Bath towel
   d. Bath blanket
   e. Bath thermometer
   f. Waterproof pad
   g. Disposable gloves
   h. Paper towels
   i. Disposable bag (for used washcloths or cotton balls)

4. Arrange items on the overbed table.

5. Identify the resident. Check the ID bracelet and call her by name.

6. Provide for privacy.

7. Raise the bed to the best level for good body mechanics. Make sure the side rails are up.

8. Lower the side rail near you.

9. Cover the resident with a bath blanket. Move top linens to the foot of the bed.

10. Position the resident on her back.

11. Place a waterproof pad under her buttocks.

12. Drape the resident as in Fig. 12-27.

13. Raise the side rail.

14. Fill the basin with water. Water temperature should be about 105° to 109° F (41° to 43° C).

15. Place the basin on the overbed table on top of the paper towels.

16. Put the washcloths in the wash basin.

17. Lower the side rail.

18. Help the resident flex her knees and spread her legs, if she is able. Otherwise, help her spread her legs as much as possible with her knees straight.

19. Put on the gloves.

20. Fold the corner of the bath blanket between the resident's legs onto her abdomen.

21. Apply soap to a washcloth.

22. Separate the labia. Clean downward from front to back with one stroke (Fig. 12-28, p. 258). Discard the washcloth.

23. Repeat steps 21 and 22 until the area is clean.

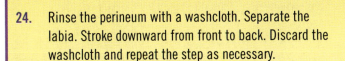

24. Rinse the perineum with a washcloth. Separate the labia. Stroke downward from front to back. Discard the washcloth and repeat the step as necessary.

25. Pat the area dry with the towel.

26. Fold the blanket back between the resident's legs.

27. Help the resident lower her legs and turn onto her side away from you.

28. Apply soap to a washcloth.

29. Clean the anal area. Clean from the vagina to the anus with one stroke (Fig. 12-29, p. 258). Discard the washcloth.

30. Repeat steps 28 and 29 until the area is clean.

31. Rinse the anal area with a washcloth. Stroke from the vagina to the anus. Discard the washcloth. Repeat the step as necessary.

32. Pat the area dry with the towel.

33. Remove the gloves and discard.

34. Position the resident so she is comfortable.

35. Return the bed linens to their proper position and remove the bath blanket.

36. Lower the bed to its lowest position.

37. Raise or lower side rails as instructed by the nurse. Place the signal light within reach.

38. Empty and clean the basin. Return it and other supplies to their proper place.

39. Wipe off the overbed table with the paper towels and then discard them.

40. Unscreen the resident.

41. Take soiled linen and the disposable bag to the "dirty" utility room.

42. Wash your hands.

43. Report your observations to the nurse:
    a. Odors
    b. Redness, swelling, discharge, or irritation
    c. Resident complaints of pain, burning, or other discomfort

A   B

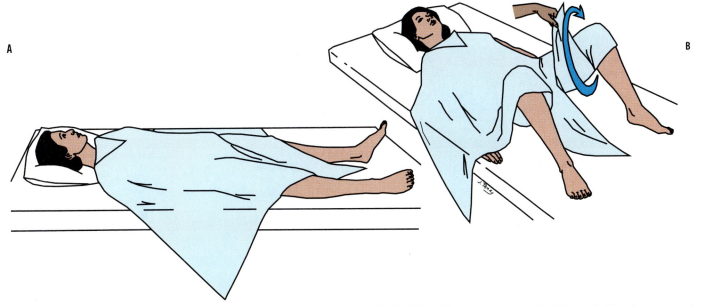

FIGURE 12-27 *A,* Drape the resident for perineal care by positioning the bath blanket like a diamond: one corner is at the neck; there is a corner at each side, and one corner is between the resident's legs. *B,* Wrap the blanket around the leg by bringing the corner around under the leg and over the top. Tuck the corner under the hip.

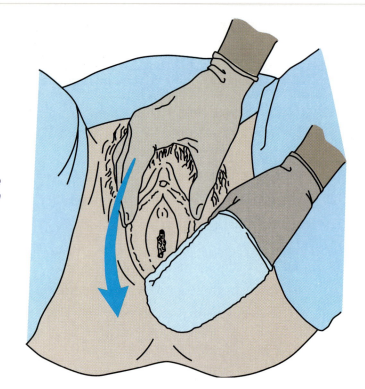

FIGURE 12-28 *Perineal care is given to the female by separating the labia with one hand. The nursing assistant uses a mitted washcloth to cleanse between the labia with downward strokes.*

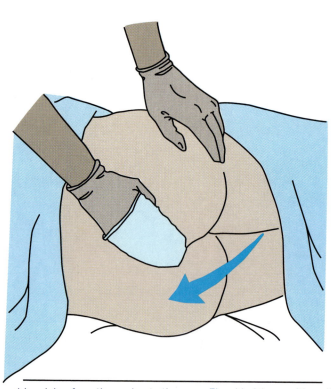

FIGURE 12-29 *The anal area is cleansed by wiping from the vagina to the anus. The side-lying position allows the anal area to be cleaned more thoroughly.*

PROCEDURE

Giving Male Perineal Care

1. Follow steps 1 through 21 as for *Giving Female Perineal Care*, pp. 256.

2. Retract the foreskin if the resident is uncircumcised (Fig. 12-30).

3. Grasp the penis.

4. Clean the tip using a circular motion. Start at the urethral opening and work outward (Fig. 12-31). Discard the washcloth. Repeat this step as necessary.

5. Rinse the area with another washcloth.

6. Return the foreskin to its natural position if the resident is uncircumcised.

7. Clean the shaft of the penis with firm downward strokes. Rinse the area.

8. Help the resident flex his knees and spread his legs if he is able. Otherwise, help him spread his legs as much as possible with his knees straight.

9. Cleanse the scrotum and rinse well.

10. Pat dry the penis and scrotum.

11. Fold the corner of the bath blanket back between his legs.

12. Help the resident lower his legs and turn onto his side away from you.

13. Clean the anal area (see *Giving Female Perineal Care*, p. 257). Rinse and dry well.

14. Follow steps 33 through 43 in *Female Perineal Care*.

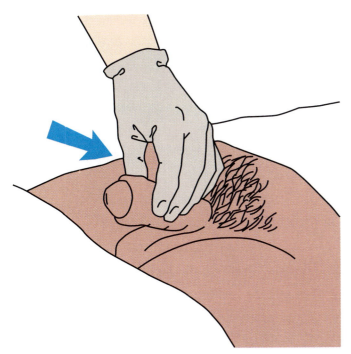

FIGURE 12-30 *The foreskin of the uncircumcised male is pulled back for perineal care. It is returned to the normal position immediately after cleaning.*

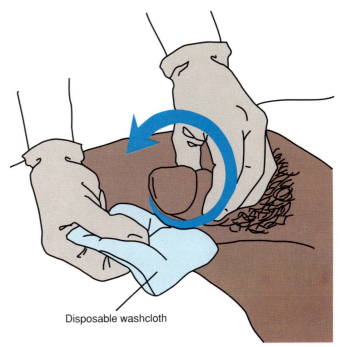

Disposable washcloth

FIGURE 12-31 *The penis is cleaned with circular motions starting at the urethra.*

HAIR CARE

Appearance and mental well-being are affected by how the hair looks and feels. Residents may be unable to care for their own hair. You need to assist them with hair care whenever necessary. Some facilities have a barber and a beautician to cut and shampoo hair. Daily hair care, however, is your responsibility.

Brushing and Combing Hair

Brushing and combing hair are part of morning care. They are also done whenever needed. Encourage residents to do their own hair care. However, provide assistance as necessary. You must provide hair care for residents who cannot do it themselves. Let the resident choose how hair is to be brushed, combed, and styled.

Long hair is easily matted and tangled during bed rest. Daily brushing and combing helps prevent this problem. Braiding does too. Do not braid hair without the resident's permission. Never cut hair to remove mats or tangles.

When giving hair care, protect the resident's gown or clothing by placing a towel across the shoulders. If given when the resident is in bed, do it before changing the pillowcase. If done after a linen change, place a towel across the pillow for falling hair.

PROCEDURE

Brushing and Combing the Resident's Hair

1. Identify the resident. Check the ID bracelet and call the resident by name.

2. Explain the procedure to the resident.

3. Collect the following:
   a. Comb and brush
   b. Bath towel
   c. Other toilet items as requested

4. Arrange items on the bedside stand.

5. Wash your hands.

6. Provide for privacy.

7. Lower the side rail if up.

8. Help the resident to the chair or to a semi-Fowler's position if allowed. The resident is dressed or has on a robe and slippers if he or she is to be up.

9. Place the towel across the resident's shoulders. Place the towel across the pillow if he or she is in bed.

10. Ask the resident to remove eyeglasses. Put them in the glass case. Put the glass case in the bedside stand.

11. Part the hair into 2 main sections (Fig. 12-32, *A*). Then divide one side into 2 sections (Fig. 12-32, *B*).

12. Brush the hair. Start at the scalp and brush toward the hair ends (Fig. 12-33).

13. Style the hair as the resident prefers.

14. Remove the towel.

15. Let the resident put eyeglasses on again.

16. Assist him or her to a comfortable position.

17. Raise or lower side rails as instructed by the nurse.

18. Place the signal light within reach.

19. Unscreen the resident.

20. Clean and return equipment to its proper place. Place soiled linen in the linen hamper.

21. Wash your hands.

A

B

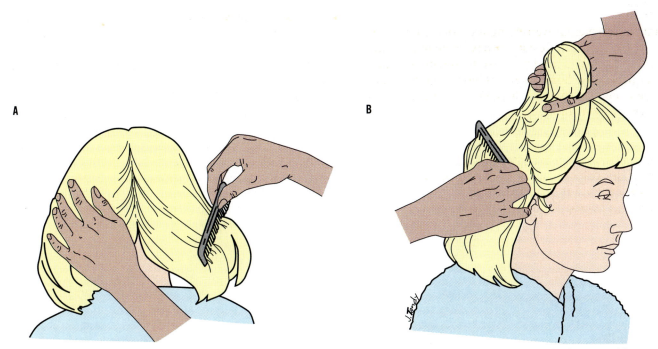

FIGURE 12-32 *A, The hair is parted down the middle and divided into two main sections. B, The main section is then parted into two smaller sections.*

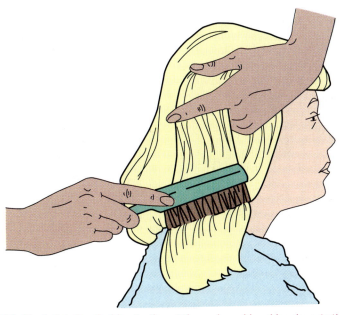

FIGURE 12-33 *The hair is brushed by starting at the scalp and brushing down to the hair ends.*

Shampooing

Residents usually need help shampooing. Shampooing usually is done weekly on the resident's tub or shower day. Some residents use special shampoos or conditioners. Others may have a doctor's order for a medicated shampoo. Ask the nurse about the type of shampoo or conditioner to use. If a woman has her hair done by the beautician, do not shampoo her hair. Protect her hair with a shower cap during her tub bath or shower.

There are several shampooing methods. The method used depends on the person's condition, safety factors, and personal choice. The nurse decides which method to use. Hair is dried and styled as quickly as possible after shampooing. Women may want their hair curled or rolled up before drying. Consult with the nurse before curling or rolling up a resident's hair.

Shampooing during the shower or tub bath. The resident's hair usually is shampooed during the shower or tub bath. A hand-held shower nozzle is used. The resident tips his or her head back to keep shampoo and water out of the eyes. This is especially important if a medicated shampoo is used. Support the back of the resident's head with one hand as you shampoo with the other. Some residents cannot tip their heads back. Have them lean forward and hold a folded washcloth over the eyes. Support the resident's forehead with one hand as you shampoo with the other. Be sure that the resident can breathe easily. If a medicated shampoo or conditioner is used, return it to the nurse. Never leave it at the bedside unless instructed to do so.

Shampooing at the sink. Some people prefer to sit in front of a sink for a shampoo. This is done at the resident's request and with the nurse's permission. Many elderly or disabled residents have limited range-of-motion in their necks and upper backs. They cannot tolerate this procedure.

The resident is positioned in a chair or wheelchair facing away from the sink. A folded towel placed over the edge of the sink protects the resident's neck. The person's head is tilted back over the edge of the sink. A water pitcher or hand-held nozzle is used to wet and rinse the hair.

Shampooing a resident on a stretcher. Hair can be washed with the person on a stretcher (Fig. 12-34). The stretcher is positioned in front of the sink. A pillow is placed under the resident's head and neck. The head is tilted over the edge of the sink. The water pitcher or hand-held nozzle is used to wet and rinse the hair. Be sure to lock the stretcher wheels and use the safety straps. Make sure the far side rail is up. Do not use this method for residents with limited range-of-motion in the neck or upper back. Check with the nurse before using this method.

Shampooing a resident in bed. A shampoo can be given to a resident in bed. This method is used for those who cannot sit in a chair or be shampooed on a stretcher. The resident's head and shoulders are moved to the edge of the bed if this position is allowed. A rubber or plastic trough is placed under the resident's head to protect the linens and mattress from water. The trough also drains water into a basin placed on a chair next to the bed (Fig. 12-35). Use a water pitcher to wet and rinse the hair.

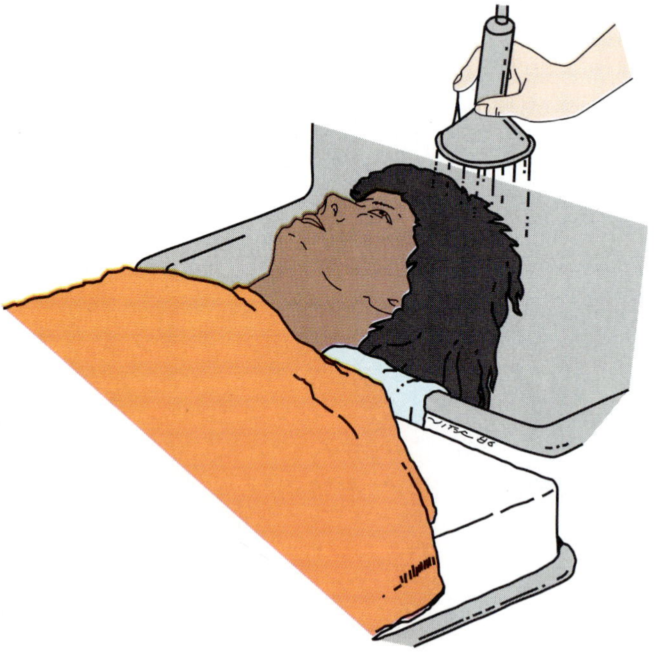

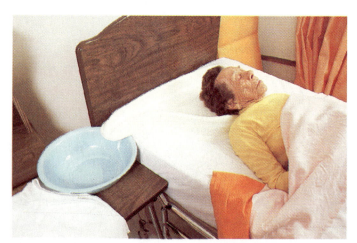

FIGURE 12-34 *Shampooing while the resident is on a stretcher. The stretcher is in front of the sink.*

FIGURE 12-35 *A trough is placed under the head of the resident when shampooing the resident in bed. The trough is directed to the side of the bed to allow water to drain into a collecting basin.*

PROCEDURE

Shampooing the Resident's Hair

1. Explain the procedure to the resident.

2. Wash your hands.

3. Collect the following:
   a. Two bath towels
   b. Face towel or washcloth folded lengthwise
   c. Shampoo
   d. Hair conditioner if requested
   e. Bath thermometer
   f. Pitcher or hand-held nozzle
   g. Equipment for the shampoo in bed (if needed)
      (1) Trough
      (2) Basin or pail
      (3) Waterproof bed protector
   h. Comb and brush
   i. Hair dryer

4. Arrange equipment in a convenient place.

5. Identify the resident. Check the ID bracelet and call the resident by name.

6. Provide for privacy.

7. Position the resident for the method you are going to use.

8. Place a bath towel across the shoulders or across the pillow under the resident's head.

9. Brush and comb hair thoroughly to remove snarls and tangles.

10. Raise side rails of the bed or stretcher if you need to leave to get water.

11. Obtain water. Water temperature should be about 110° F (43° to 44° C).

12. Lower the side rail.

13. Ask the resident to hold the face towel or washcloth over the eyes. Make sure it does not slip down over the nose or mouth.

14. Use the pitcher or nozzle to wet the hair completely.

15. Use a small amount of shampoo.

16. Work up a lather with both hands. Start at the hairline and work toward the back of the head.

17. Massage the scalp with your fingertips. Do not scratch the scalp with your fingernails.

18. Rinse the hair.

19. Repeat steps 15 through 18.

20. Apply conditioner and rinse as directed on the container.

21. Wrap the resident's head with a bath towel.

22. Dry his or her face with the towel or washcloth used to protect the eyes.

23. Help the resident raise his or her head if appropriate.

24. Rub the hair and scalp with the towel. Use the second towel if the first becomes too wet.

25. Comb hair to remove snarls and tangles. A woman may want her hair curled or rolled up.

26. Dry the hair as quickly as possible.

27. Make sure the resident is comfortable.

28. Raise or lower side rails as instructed by the nurse.

29. Place the signal light within reach.

30. Clean and return equipment to its proper place. Discard disposable items. Place soiled linen in the linen hamper.

31. Wash your hands.

SHAVING

A clean-shaven face is important for the comfort and mental well-being of many men. Many elderly women have a growth of coarse hair on their faces. They may prefer to have such hair shaved off. Younger women usually shave their legs and underarms.

Some residents use electric shavers. They usually are required to have their own electric shavers. If the facility's shaver is used for residents, the shaver must be cleaned between each use. Follow facility policy for cleaning electric shavers. Also be sure to practice the safety precautions for using electrical equipment.

Some residents like blade shavers (razor blades). Razor blades can cause nicks or cuts. Be sure to wear gloves and practice universal precautions to prevent contact with the resident's blood. Residents should have their own blade shavers. If not, disposable shavers are used. Remember, razor blades are extremely sharp. You must protect the resident and yourself from nicks or cuts. Be sure to follow the bloodborne pathogen standard.

Some residents take medication that affects blood clotting. They bleed easily from even a small nick or cut. Avoid using razor blades to shave these residents. Electric shavers are safer for these individuals. Check the resident's care plan and ask the nurse what type of shaver to use.

The beard and skin are softened before shaving with a blade. Soften the beard by applying a warm washcloth or face towel to the face for a few minutes. Then lather the face with soap and water or shaving cream. Take care not to cut or irritate the skin while shaving. Women's legs and underarms can be shaved after the bath when the skin is soft. Soap and water, shaving cream, or lotion also can provide a lather for shaving legs and underarms.

Many men have beards and mustaches that need daily grooming. Ask the resident how he wants his beard or mustache cared for.

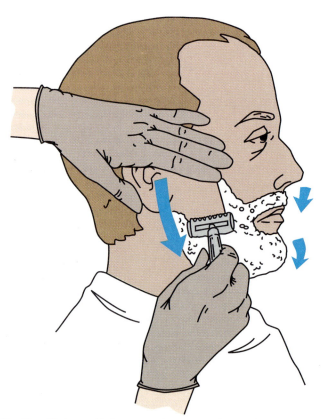

FIGURE 12-36 *Shaving is done in the direction of hair growth. Longer strokes are used on the larger areas of the face. Short strokes are used around the chin and lips.*

PROCEDURE

Shaving the Resident with a Blade Shaver

1. Explain the procedure to the resident.

2. Wash your hands.

3. Collect the following:
    a. Wash basin
    b. Bath towel
    c. Face towel
    d. Washcloth
    e. Bath thermometer
    f. Disposable razor
    g. Mirror
    h. Shaving cream, soap, or lotion
    i. Shaving brush
    j. After-shave lotion (male residents only)
    k. Tissues
    l. Paper towels
    m. Disposable gloves

4. Arrange the equipment on the overbed table.

5. Identify the resident. Check the ID bracelet and call the resident by name.

6. Provide for privacy.

7. Raise the bed to the best level for good body mechanics. Make sure the side rails are up.

8. Fill the basin with water. Water temperature should be about 115° F (46° C).

9. Place the basin on the overbed table on top of the paper towels.

10. Lower the side rail near you.

11. Position the resident in a semi-Fowler's position, if allowed, or on his or her back.

12. Adjust lighting so you can clearly see the resident's face.

13. Place the bath towel over the chest.

14. Position the overbed table within easy reach and at a comfortable working height.

15. Wash the resident's face. Do not dry.

16. Place a washcloth or face towel in the basin and wet thoroughly. Wring it out.

17. Apply the washcloth or towel to the resident's face for 3 to 5 minutes.

18. Put on the gloves.

19. Apply shaving cream with your hands. Or use a shaving brush to apply lather.

20. Hold the skin taut with one hand.

21. Shave in the direction of hair growth. Use shorter strokes around the chin and lips (Fig. 12-36).

22. Rinse the razor frequently and wipe with tissues.

23. Apply direct pressure to any bleeding area.

24. Wash off any remaining shaving cream or soap. Dry with a towel.

25. Apply after-shave lotion if requested.

26. Move the overbed table to the side of the bed.

27. Make sure the resident is comfortable.

28. Place the signal light within reach.

29. Lower the bed to its lowest position.

30. Raise or lower side rails as instructed by the nurse.

31. Clean and return equipment and supplies to their proper place. Discard disposable items. Remove and discard the gloves.

32. Wipe off the overbed table with the paper towels. Position the table as appropriate for the resident. Discard paper towels.

33. Unscreen the resident.

34. Place soiled linen in the linen hamper.

35. Wash your hands.

36. Report any nicks or bleeding to the nurse.

CARE OF NAILS AND FEET

Nails and feet need special attention to prevent infection, injury, and odors. Hangnails, ingrown nails (nails that grow in at the side), and nails torn away from the skin cause breaks in the skin. Those breaks let microorganisms enter the body. Long or broken nails can scratch the skin or snag clothing. Dirty feet, socks, or stockings can harbor microorganisms and cause foot odors.

Cleaning and trimming nails are easier right after they have been soaked. After a tub bath or shower also is a good time because the nails already are soft. Nail clippers are used to cut fingernails. Do not use scissors. Extreme caution must be taken to prevent damage to surrounding tissue when fingernails are clipped and trimmed. Nursing assistants do not cut or trim toenails.

PROCEDURE

Giving Nail and Foot Care

1. Explain the procedure to the resident.

2. Wash your hands.

3. Collect the following:
    - a. Wash basin
    - b. Bath thermometer
    - c. Bath towel
    - d. Face towel
    - e. Washcloth
    - f. Kidney basin
    - g. Nail clippers
    - h. Orange stick
    - i. Emery board or nail file
    - j. Lotion or petrolatum
    - k. Paper towels
    - l. Disposable bath mat

4. Arrange the equipment on the overbed table.

5. Identify the resident. Check the ID bracelet and call the resident by name.

6. Provide for privacy.

7. Assist the resident to the bedside chair. Place the signal light within reach.

8. Place the bath mat under the resident's feet.

9. Fill the basin. Water temperature should be 109° F (42° C).

10. Place the wash basin on the floor on the towel. Help the resident put the feet into the basin.

11. Position the overbed table in front of the resident. It should be low and close to the resident.

12. Fill the kidney basin. See step 9 for water temperature.

13. Place the kidney basin on the overbed table on top of the paper towels.

14. Put the resident's fingers into the basin. Position the arms so that he or she is comfortable (Fig. 12-37).

15. Let the feet and fingernails soak for 15 to 20 minutes. Rewarm the water in 10 to 15 minutes.

16. Clean under fingernails with the orange stick.

17. Remove the kidney basin. Dry fingers thoroughly.

18. Clip fingernails straight across with nail clippers (Fig. 12-38).

19. Shape nails with an emery board or nail file.

20. Push cuticles back with a washcloth or orange stick (Fig. 12-39).

21. Move the overbed table from in front of the resident.

22. Scrub callused areas of the feet with the washcloth.

23. Remove the feet from the basin. Dry thoroughly, especially between the toes.

24. Apply lotion or petrolatum to the tops and soles of the feet. Do not apply between the toes.

25. Help the resident back to bed (if indicated) and to a comfortable position. Place the signal light within reach.

26. Raise or lower side rails as instructed by the nurse.

27. Put socks and shoes or slippers on residents who will stay up.

28. Clean and return equipment and supplies to their proper places. Discard disposable supplies.

29. Unscreen the resident.

30. Take soiled linen to the linen hamper.

31. Wash your hands.

32. Report your observations to the nurse:
    - a. Reddened, irritated, or callused areas
    - b. Breaks in the skin

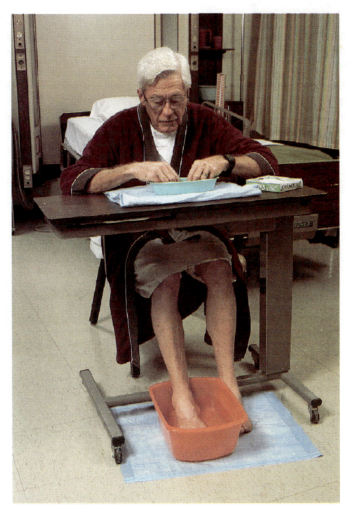

FIGURE 12-37 *Nail and foot care. The feet soak in a foot basin, and the fingers soak in the emesis basin.*

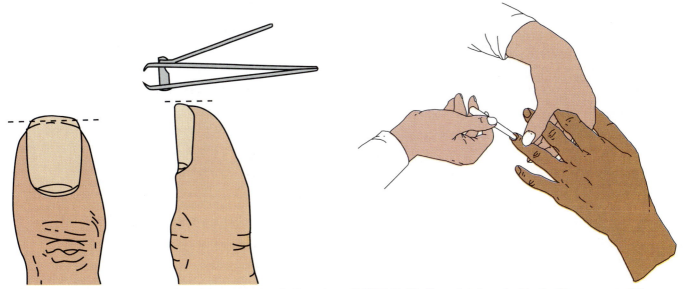

FIGURE 12-38 *Fingernails are clipped straight across. A nail clipper is used.*

FIGURE 12-39 *The cuticle is pushed back with an orange stick.*

CHANGING CLOTHING AND HOSPITAL GOWNS

Dressing and undressing occur at least daily. Residents change from gowns or pajamas into clothing after morning care. They undress and put on gowns or pajamas at bedtime. Clothing changes may be more frequent for incontinent residents. Some residents cannot dress and undress themselves. Others need some help. The change is easy for residents who can move their arms and legs. Arm or leg injuries or paralysis also requires special measures.

Some residents wear hospital gowns. Gowns usually are worn by those receiving IV therapy. If so, gowns are put on and removed in a certain way.

Certain rules are followed when changing gowns or clothing.

1. Provide for privacy. Do not expose the resident.
2. Encourage the resident to do as much as possible.
3. Allow the resident personal choice in clothing selections.
4. Remove clothing from the strong or "good" side first.
5. Put clothing on the weak side first.
6. Support the arm or leg when removing or putting on a garment.

PROCEDURE

Undressing the Resident

1. Explain the procedure to the resident.

2. Wash your hands.

3. Get a bath blanket.

4. Identify the resident. Check the ID bracelet and call the resident by name.

5. Provide for privacy.

6. Raise the bed to a level for good body mechanics.

7. Lower the side rail on the resident's weak side.

8. Position the resident supine.

9. Cover the resident with the bath blanket. Fan-fold linens to the foot of the bed. Do not expose the resident.

10. Remove garments that open in the back.
    a. Raise the head and shoulders (see *Raising the Resident's Head and Shoulders by Locking Arms with the Resident*, p. 161). Or turn him or her onto the side away from you.
    b. Undo buttons, zippers, ties, or snaps.
    c. Bring the sides of the garment to the resident's sides (Fig. 12-40). Do the following if he or she is in a side-lying position.
       (1) Tuck the far side under the resident.
       (2) Fold the near side onto the chest (Fig. 12-41).
    d. Position the resident supine.

    e. Slide the garment off the shoulder on the strong side. Remove the garment from the arm (Fig. 12-42, p. 270).
    f. Repeat step 10e for the weak side.

11. Remove garments that open in the front.
    a. Undo buttons, zippers, snaps, or ties.
    b. Slide the garment off the shoulder and arm on the strong side.
    c. Raise the resident's head and shoulders. Bring the garment over to the weak side (Fig. 12-43, p. 270). Lower the resident's head and shoulders.
    d. Remove the garment from the weak side.
    e. Do the following if you cannot raise the resident's head and shoulders:
       (1) Turn the resident toward you. Tuck the removed part under the resident.
       (2) Turn him or her onto the side away from you.
       (3) Pull the side of the garment out from under the resident. Make sure he or she will not lie on it when supine.
       (4) Return the resident to the supine position.
       (5) Remove the garment from the weak side.

12. Remove pullover garments.
    a. Undo any buttons, zippers, ties, or snaps.
    b. Remove the garment from the strong side.

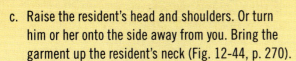

    c. Raise the resident's head and shoulders. Or turn him or her onto the side away from you. Bring the garment up the resident's neck (Fig. 12-44, p. 270).

    d. Remove the garment from the weak side.

    e. Bring the garment over the resident's head.

    f. Position the resident in the supine position.

13. Remove pants or slacks.

    a. Remove shoes or slippers.

    b. Position the resident supine.

    c. Undo buttons, zippers, ties, snaps, or buckles.

    d. Remove the belt if one is worn.

    e. Ask the resident to lift the buttocks off the bed. Slide the pants down over the hips and buttocks (Fig. 12-45, p. 271). Have the resident lower the hips and buttocks.

    f. Do the following if the resident cannot raise the hips off the bed.

      (1) Turn the resident toward you.

      (2) Slide the pants off the hip and buttock on the strong side (Fig. 12-46, p. 271).

      (3) Turn the resident away from you.

      (4) Slide the pants off the hip and buttock on the weak side (Fig. 12-47, p. 271).

    g. Slide the pants down the legs and over the feet.

14. Dress or put a clean gown on the resident (see *Dressing the Resident,* p. 272).

15. Help the resident get out of bed if he or she is to be up.

16. Do the following for the resident who will stay in bed:

    a. Cover the resident and remove the bath blanket.

    b. Make sure the resident is comfortable.

    c. Lower the bed to its lowest position.

    d. Raise or lower the side rails as instructed by the nurse.

    e. Place the signal light within reach.

17. Unscreen the resident.

18. Place soiled clothing in the appropriate place.

19. Report your observations to the nurse.

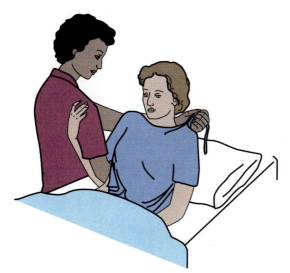

FIGURE 12-40 *The sides of the garment are brought from the back to the sides of the resident.*

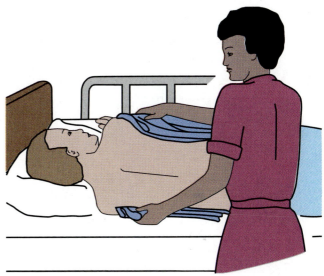

FIGURE 12-41 *A garment that opens in the back is removed from the resident in the side-lying position. The far side of the garment is tucked under the resident. The near side is folded onto the resident's chest.*

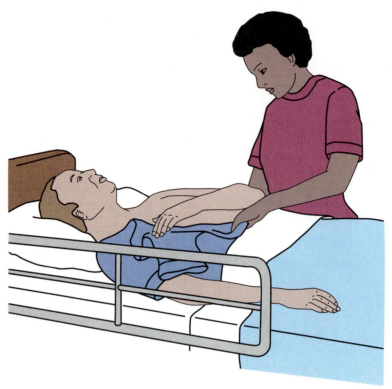

FIGURE 12-42 *The garment is removed from the strong side first.*

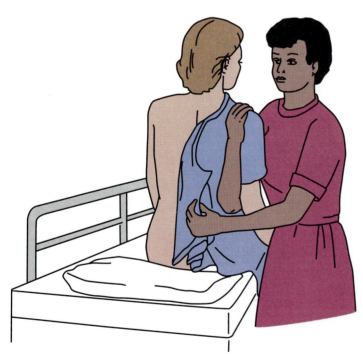

FIGURE 12-43 *A front-opening garment is removed with the resident's head and shoulders raised. The garment is removed from the strong side first. Then it is brought around the back to the weak side.*

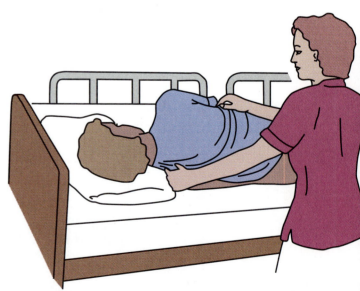

FIGURE 12-44 *A pullover garment is removed from the strong side first. Then the garment is brought up to the resident's neck so that it can be removed from the weak side.*

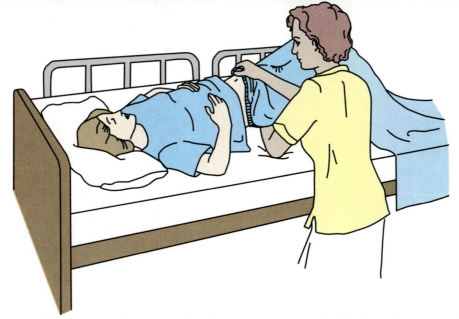

FIGURE 12-45 *The resident lifts the hips and buttocks so that the pants can be removed. Slide the pants down over the hips and buttocks.*

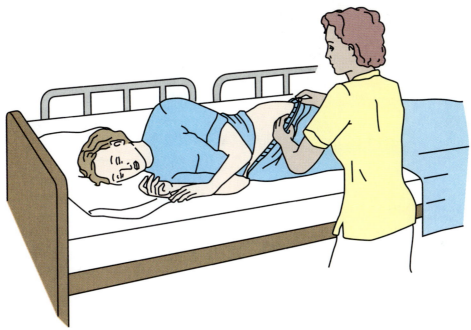

FIGURE 12-46 *Pants are removed in the side-lying position. They are removed from the strong side first. Slide the pants over the hips and buttocks.*

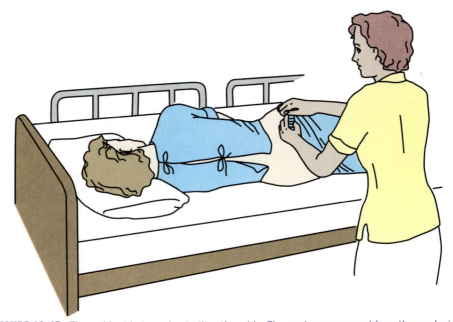

FIGURE 12-47 *The resident is turned onto the other side. The pants are removed from the weak side.*

PROCEDURE

Dressing the Resident

1. Explain the procedure to the resident.

2. Wash your hands.

3. Get a bath blanket and necessary clothing.

4. Identify the resident. Check the ID bracelet and call the resident by name.

5. Provide for privacy.

6. Raise the bed to the best level for good body mechanics.

7. Undress the resident (see *Undressing the Resident*, pp. 268-269).

8. Lower the side rail on the resident's strong side.

9. Position the resident supine.

10. Cover the resident with the bath blanket. Fan-fold linens to the foot of the bed. Do not expose the resident.

11. Put on garments that open in the back.
    a. Slide the garment onto the arm and shoulder of the weak side.
    b. Slide the garment onto the arm and shoulder of the strong side.
    c. Raise the resident's head and shoulders.
    d. Bring the sides of the garment to the back.
    e. Do the following if the resident is in a side-lying position:
       (1) Turn the resident toward you.
       (2) Bring the side of the garment to the resident's back (Fig. 12-48, *A*).
       (3) Turn the resident away from you.
       (4) Bring the other side of the garment to the resident's back (Fig. 12-48, *B*).
    f. Fasten buttons, snaps, ties, or zippers.
    g. Position the resident supine.

12. Put on garments that open in the front.
    a. Slide the garment onto the arm and shoulder on the weak side.
    b. Raise the head and shoulders by locking arms with the resident. Bring the side of the garment around to the back. Lower the resident to the supine position. Slide the garment onto the arm and shoulder of the strong arm.
    c. Do the following if the resident is unable to raise the head and shoulders:
       (1) Turn the resident toward you.
       (2) Tuck the garment under him or her.
       (3) Turn the resident away from you.
       (4) Pull the garment out from under the resident.
       (5) Turn the resident back to the supine position.
       (6) Slide the garment over the arm and shoulder of the strong arm.
    d. Fasten buttons, snaps, ties, or zippers.

13. Put on pullover garments.
    a. Position the resident supine.
    b. Bring the neck of the garment over the head.
    c. Slide the arm and shoulder of the garment onto the weak side.
    d. Raise the resident's head and shoulders.
    e. Bring the garment down.
    f. Slide the arm and shoulder of the garment onto the strong side.
    g. Do the following if the resident cannot assume a semisitting position:
       (1) Turn the resident toward you.
       (2) Tuck the garment under the resident.
       (3) Turn the resident away from you.
       (4) Pull the garment out from under him or her.
       (5) Return the resident to the supine position.
       (6) Slide the arm and shoulder of the garment onto the strong side.
    h. Fasten buttons, snaps, ties, or zippers.

14. Put on pants or slacks.
    a. Slide the pants over the feet and up the legs.

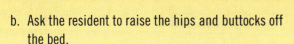

b. Ask the resident to raise the hips and buttocks off the bed.

c. Bring the pants up over the buttocks and hips.

d. Ask the resident to lower the hips and buttocks.

e. Do the following if the resident cannot raise the hips and buttocks.

   (1) Turn the resident onto the strong side.

   (2) Pull the pants over the buttock and hip on the weak side.

   (3) Turn the resident onto the weak side.

   (4) Pull the pants over the buttock and hip on the strong side.

   (5) Position the resident supine.

f. Fasten buttons, ties, snaps, the zipper, and belt buckle.

15. Put socks and shoes or slippers on the resident.

16. Help the resident get out of bed if he or she is to be up.

17. Do the following for the resident who will stay in bed.

   a. Cover the resident and remove the bath blanket.

   b. Make sure the resident is comfortable.

   c. Lower the bed to its lowest position.

   d. Raise or lower the side rails as instructed by the nurse.

   e. Place the signal light within reach.

18. Unscreen the resident.

19. Place soiled clothing in the appropriate place.

20. Report your observations to the nurse.

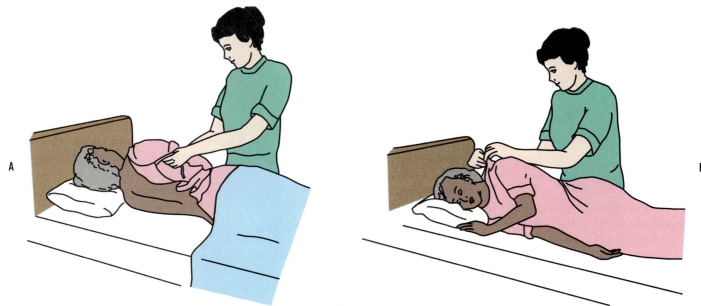

FIGURE 12-48 *A, The side-lying position can be used to put on garments that open in the back. The resident is turned toward the nursing assistant after the garment is put on the arms. The side of the garment is brought to the resident's back. B, The resident is then turned away from the nursing assistant. The other side of the garment is brought to the back and fastened.*

PROCEDURE

Changing the Gown of a Resident With an IV

1. Explain the procedure to the resident.

2. Wash your hands.

3. Get a clean gown.

4. Identify the resident. Check the ID bracelet and call the resident by name.

5. Provide for privacy.

6. Raise the bed to the best level for good body mechanics. Make sure the side rails are up.

7. Lower the side rail if up.

8. Untie the back of the gown. Free parts that the resident is lying on.

9. Remove the gown from the arm with no IV.

10. Gather up the sleeve of the arm with the IV. Slide it over the IV site and tubing. Remove the arm and hand from the sleeve (Fig. 12-49, *A*).

11. Keep the sleeve gathered. Slide your arm along the tubing to the bottle (Fig. 12-49, *B*).

12. Remove the IV bottle from the pole. Slide the bottle and tubing through the sleeve (Fig. 12-49, *C*). Do not pull on the tubing. Keep the bottle above the resident's arm.

13. Hang the IV bottle on the pole.

14. Gather the sleeve of the clean gown that will go on the arm with the IV infusion.

15. Remove the bottle from the pole. Quickly slip the gathered sleeve over the bottle at the shoulder part of the gown (Fig. 12-49, *D*). Hang the bottle on the pole.

16. Slide the gathered sleeve over the tubing, hand, arm, and IV site. Then slide the sleeve onto the resident's shoulder.

17. Put the other side of the gown on and fasten the back.

18. Make sure the resident is comfortable. Place the signal light within reach.

19. Lower the bed to its lowest position.

20. Raise or lower side rails as instructed by the nurse.

21. Unscreen the resident.

22. Take the soiled linen to the linen hamper.

23. Wash your hands.

24. Ask the nurse to check the IV flow rate.

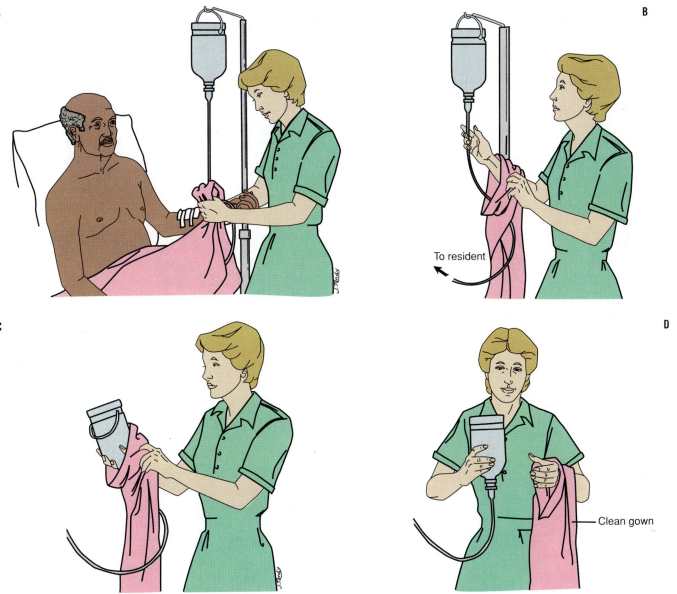

FIGURE 12-49 *A,* The gown is removed from the uninvolved arm. The sleeve on the arm with the IV is gathered up, slipped over the IV site and tubing, and removed from the arm and hand. *B,* The gathered sleeve is slipped along the IV tubing to the bottle. *C,* The IV bottle is removed from the pole and passed through the sleeve. *D,* The gathered sleeve of the clean gown is slipped over the IV bottle at the shoulder part of the gown.

Mosby's Textbook for Long-Term Care Assistants

PRESSURE SORES

Pressure sores (**decubitus ulcers,** [decubiti] **bedsores**) are areas where the skin and underlying tissues are eroded from lack of blood flow (Fig. 12-50). Pressure sores are seen most often in elderly, paralyzed, obese, or very thin and malnourished residents. The first sign is pale or white skin or a reddened area. The resident may complain of pain, burning, or tingling in the area. Some may not feel any abnormal sensations.

Sites

Pressure sores usually occur over bony areas. The bony areas also are called pressure points because they bear the weight of the body in a particular position. Fig. 12-51 shows the pressure points for the bed positions and the sitting position. Pressure from body weight can reduce blood flow to the area. In obese persons, pressure sores

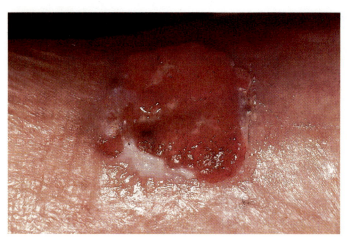
FIGURE 12-50 *A pressure sore.*

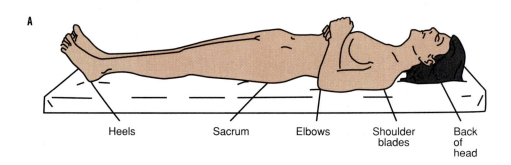

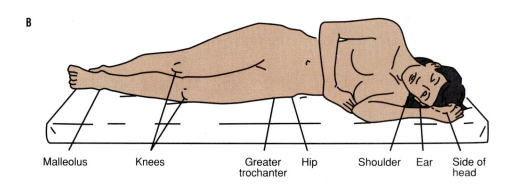

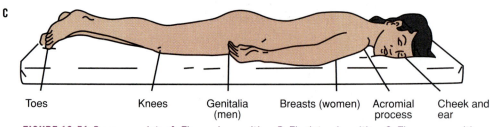

FIGURE 12-51 *Pressure points.* **A,** *The supine position.* **B,** *The lateral position.* **C,** *The prone position.*

276

can develop in areas where skin touches skin. Friction results when this occurs. Pressure sores can develop between abdominal folds, the legs, and the buttocks, and under the breasts.

Causes

Pressure, shear, and friction are common causes of skin breakdown. Shear occurs when skin sticks to a surface and bones move forward or backward inside the skin (see p. 160). This pinches the skin between the surface and the bones. Blood supply is affected.

Friction occurs when a person is pulled across a surface. For example, a resident is pulled up in bed without a lift sheet. The skin rubs across the bottom sheet, causing small open areas. These open areas can develop into pressure sores. Pressure sores can become quite severe.

Other causes include skin breakdown, poor circulation to an area, moisture, dry skin, and irritation by urine and feces. These can cause pressure sores and make existing pressure sores worse. Persons who are inactive or cannot move or change position are at greater risk for pressure sores.

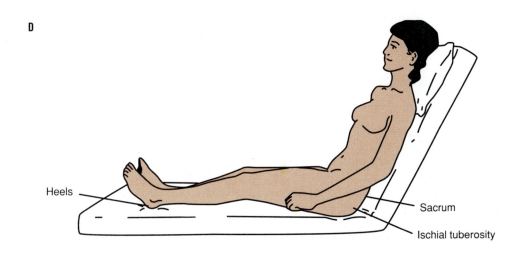

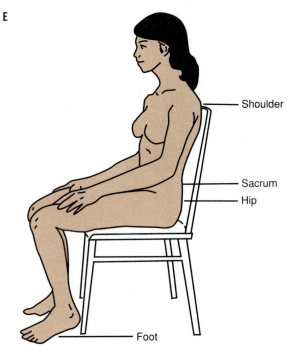

FIGURE 12-51 *D, Fowler's position.* *E, The sitting position.*

277

Prevention

Preventing pressure sores is much easier than trying to heal them. Good nursing care, cleanliness, and skin care are essential. The following measures help prevent skin breakdown and pressure sores.

1. Reposition residents in good alignment at least every 2 hours. This includes those in wheelchairs. Use pillows for support.
2. Provide good skin care. The skin must be clean and dry after bathing. Make sure skin is free of urine, feces, and perspiration.
3. Apply lotion to dry areas such as the hands, elbows, legs, ankles, and heels.
4. Give a back massage when the resident is repositioned.
5. Do not massage pale or reddened pressure points. Massaging these areas increases tissue damage. Be careful when applying lotion or giving a back massage.
6. Keep linens clean, dry, and free of wrinkles and crumbs.
7. Apply powder to areas where skin touches skin.
8. Do not irritate the skin. Avoid scrubbing or vigorous rubbing when bathing or drying the resident.
9. Use pillows and blankets to prevent skin being in contact with skin and to reduce moisture and friction.
10. Use lift sheets when positioning residents in bed.
11. Report any signs of skin breakdown or pressure sores immediately to the nurse.

Treatment

Treatment of pressure sores is directed by the doctor. Drugs, treatments, and special equipment may be ordered to promote healing. The nurse and the resident's care plan will tell you about the person's treatment. The following equipment may be used to treat and prevent pressure sores. (See also the discussion of trochanter rolls in Chapter 17).

Sheepskin. Sheepskin (lamb's wool) is placed on the bottom sheet (Fig. 12-52). It protects the skin from the irritating bed linens and reduces friction between the skin and the bottom sheet. Air circulates between the tufts to help keep the skin dry. Sheepskin comes in various sizes for use under the shoulders, buttocks, or heels.

Bed cradle. A bed cradle (Anderson frame) is a metal frame placed on the bed and over the resident. Top linens are brought over the cradle to prevent pressure on the legs and feet (Fig. 12-53). Top linens are tucked in at the bottom of the mattress and mitered. They also are tucked under both sides of the mattress to protect the resident from air drafts and chilling.

Heel and elbow protectors. Heel and elbow protectors are made of foam rubber or sheepskin. They fit the shape of the heel or elbow (Fig. 12-54) and are secured in place with straps. Friction is prevented between the bed and the heel or elbow.

Flotation pads. Flotation pads or cushions are like water beds (Fig. 12-55). They are filled with a gel-like substance. The outer case is heavy plastic. They are used for chairs and wheelchairs. The pad is placed in a pillowcase to prevent contact between the plastic and the skin.

Egg crate mattresses and wheelchair pads. The egg crate mattress is a foam pad that looks like an egg carton (Fig. 12-56). Peaks in the mattress distribute the resident's weight more evenly. The egg crate mattress is placed inside a lightweight plastic sleeve or tube. The sleeve and tube help keep out moisture and prevent soiling. The egg crate mattress is placed on top of the regular mattress. Only a bottom sheet covers both the egg crate mattress and the regular mattress.

Text continued on p. 280.

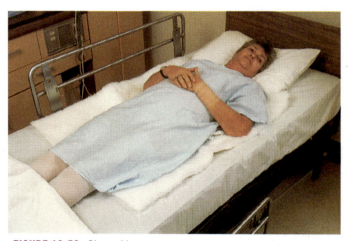

FIGURE 12-52 *Sheepskin.*

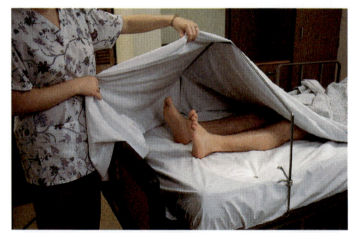

FIGURE 12-53 *A bed cradle is placed on top of the bed. Linens are brought over the top of the bed and then over the top of the cradle.*

A

B

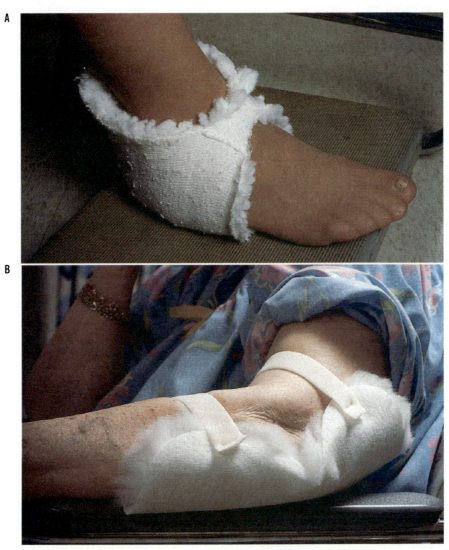

FIGURE 12-54 *A,* *Heel protector.* ***B,*** *Elbow protectors.*

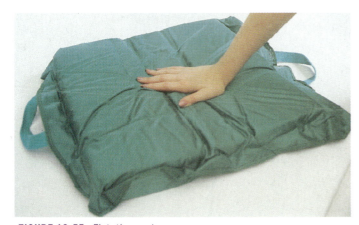

FIGURE 12-55 *Flotation pad.*

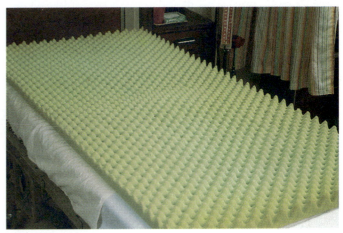

FIGURE 12-56 *Egg crate mattress on the bed.*

279

There also are wheelchair pads like the egg crate mattress. They are covered with a lightweight plastic. The pad is put into a pillowcase and placed in the wheelchair.

Egg crate mattresses and pads are never washed. If soiled, they are thrown away. Washing removes the fire retardant and creates a fire hazard.

Water beds. Water beds are used in many facilities. The resident "floats" on top of the mattress. Body weight is distributed along the entire length of the body. Therefore pressure on bony points is reduced.

Alternating pressure mattresses. An alternating pressure mattress is electrically operated. It has vertical tubelike sections (Fig. 12-57). Every other section is inflated with air. The others are deflated. Every 3 to 5 minutes the sections deflate or inflate automatically. With this mattress, constant pressure on any area is avoided.

Only a bottom sheet is used with an alternating pressure mattress. Drawsheets and waterproof bed protectors are avoided. They add layers of material between the resident and air tubes. The air tubes should not be kinked. Pins should not be used.

Clinitron beds. The Clinitron bed has a specially designed mattress. Air flows through the mattress. The air is kept at a controlled temperature. The mattress is solid when the air is off and like a water bed when the air is on. The resident "floats" on the mattress. Body weight is distributed evenly. Pressure on bony parts in minimal.

Air flotation beds. The mattress of the air flotation bed actually consists of many individual air bags. Each bag is the same width as the bed frame. The bags are placed side-by-side the length of the bed. Air flows through the bags continuously. Each bag is connected separately to an air flow unit. Like the Clinitron bed, body weight is distributed evenly. The pressure on the body parts is minimal.

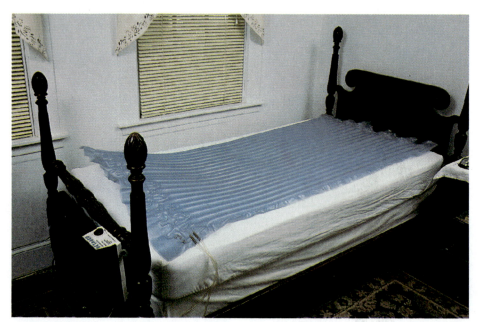

FIGURE 12-57 *Alternating pressure mattress.*

Quality OF LIFE

Remember, resident rights are protected by OBRA. Such rights are intended to improve the resident's quality of life, health, and safety. You must provide personal hygiene in a manner that maintains or improves the resident's quality of life, health, and safety. You must protect the resident's rights when performing personal hygiene activities.

The right to privacy and confidentiality is very important. The resident must not be exposed during personal hygiene. Ask visitors to leave the room when care is to be given. A family member or friend may want to help give care. The resident must give permission for this. Remember to close doors, privacy curtains, shades, and drapes before beginning procedures. Only the body part involved in the procedure can be exposed. Remember to properly cover residents who are taken to and from tub or shower rooms. If the shower room has more than one shower stall, you must protect the resident from being exposed to others who may be present.

Residents also have the right to personal choice. This means that they have the right to be involved in planning their care and treatment. Hygiene is a very personal matter. Whenever possible, the resident should be allowed to make choices. Allow the person to be involved in deciding when and how personal hygiene is done. The resident should be allowed personal choice in such matters as bath time, the products to use, what to wear, and hair styling.

Residents have the right to keep and use personal possessions. You will be handling the resident's property in personal hygiene procedures. Dentures and eyeglasses must be protected from loss or breakage. If jewelry or religious medals are removed for care, make sure you protect them from loss, damage, or theft. You must carefully handle the resident's personal hygiene products, shaver, hair dryer, brush and comb, perfumes, and other items used for personal care. The resident's clothing also needs your attention. Be careful not to break zippers, tear clothing, or lose buttons. Remember to treat all of the resident's property with care and respect.

Freedom from restraint is another resident right. Side rails are considered physical restraints under OBRA. Hygiene procedures include steps on raising and lowering side rails. Side rails must always be up when the bed is raised. They prevent the resident from *falling* out of bed when giving care. They are considered to be restraints when used to prevent a resident from *getting* out of bed. Side rails are lowered after the bed has been lowered to its lowest position. Keep the side rails up if instructed to do so by the nurse.

SUMMARY

Promoting cleanliness and providing skin care are important responsibilities. The resident's physical and mental well-being are affected by good personal hygiene. Cultural and personal choice influence hygiene practices. Whenever possible you should respect the resident's choices. Personal choice is a resident right. You must protect the right to personal choice and the other resident rights.

The skin must be kept clean and intact. This promotes comfort and prevents infection. Oral hygiene, bathing, back massages, perineal care, hair care, and nail and foot care also are important. Shaving and wearing a clean gown, pajamas, or clothing are appreciated. Residents should be allowed and encouraged to perform as much self-care as possible. You need to assist as necessary. Giving personal care provides a good time to get to know the person and to observe the skin.

Pressure sores and skin breakdown can result from poor nursing and skin care. They are very difficult to heal. The resident faces increased discomfort and prolonged nursing and medical care. Pressure sores are very serious and can even cause death. Follow the measures needed to prevent them. If they occur, follow the directions outlined by the nurse. Remember, it is easier to prevent pressure sores than to treat and heal them.

Review QUESTIONS

Circle *T* if the answer is true and *F* if the answer is false.

T F   1. A back massage is part of morning care and HS care.

T **F**   2. The unconscious resident should be supine for mouth care.

T **F**   3. You can use your fingers to keep the mouth of an unconscious resident open during mouth care.

T **F**   4. Dentures are washed in warm water over a hard surface.

T F   5. Powders absorb moisture and prevent friction.

T **F**   6. A tub bath should last 20 minutes or more.

T **F**   7. You can give permission for tub baths or showers.

T **F**   8. Residents can be left alone in the shower if they are sitting.

T F   9. A back massage relaxes muscles and stimulates circulation.

T F   10. Perineal care helps prevent infection.

T **F**   11. You can use scissors to cut fingernails and toenails.

T F   12. Clothing is removed from the strong side first.

T F   13. White or reddened skin is the first sign of a pressure sore.

T F   14. Pressure sores usually occur over bony areas.

T **F**   15. Pressure is the only cause of pressure sores.

T F   16. Poor nursing care can lead to the development of pressure sores.

T F   17. Side rails are raised to prevent the resident from falling out of bed when giving care.

Circle the *best* answer.

18. Oral hygiene is part of
    a. AM care and HS care
    b. Morning care
    c. Care given after lunch
    d. All of the above

19. Which is *not* a purpose of bathing?
    a. Increasing circulation
    b. Promoting drying of the skin
    c. Exercising body parts
    d. Refreshing and relaxing the resident

20. Soaps do the following *except*
    a. Remove dirt and dead skin
    b. Remove pathogens
    c. Remove skin oil and perspiration
    d. Dry the skin

21. Which action is *incorrect* when bathing a person?
    a. Cover the resident to provide warmth and privacy.
    b. Rinse the skin thoroughly to remove all soap.
    c. Wash from the dirtiest to the cleanest areas.
    d. Pat the skin dry.

22. Bath water for a complete bed bath should be
    a. 100° F
    b. 105° F
    c. 110° F
    d. 120° F

23. You are to give a back massage. Which is *false*?
    a. It should last about 4 to 6 minutes.
    b. Lotion is warmed before being applied.
    c. The hands should always be in contact with the skin.
    d. The prone position is always used.

24. Before shaving a resident's face you should
    a. Dry the face thoroughly
    b. Apply a cold washcloth to the face
    c. Soften the skin
    d. Apply after-shave lotion

25. Which does *not* prevent pressure sores?
    a. Repositioning the resident every 2 hours
    b. Applying lotion to dry areas
    c. Scrubbing and rubbing the skin
    d. Keeping bed linens clean, dry, and free of wrinkles

26. Which are *not* used to treat pressure sores?
    a. Clinitron bed
    b. Water bed and flotation pad
    c. Plastic drawsheet and waterproof pad
    d. Heel and elbow protectors

Answers

1. True	8. False	15. False	22. c
2. False	9. True	16. True	23. d
3. False	10. True	17. True	24. c
4. False	11. False	18. d	25. c
5. True	12. True	19. b	26. c
6. False	13. True	20. b	
7. False	14. True	21. c	

283

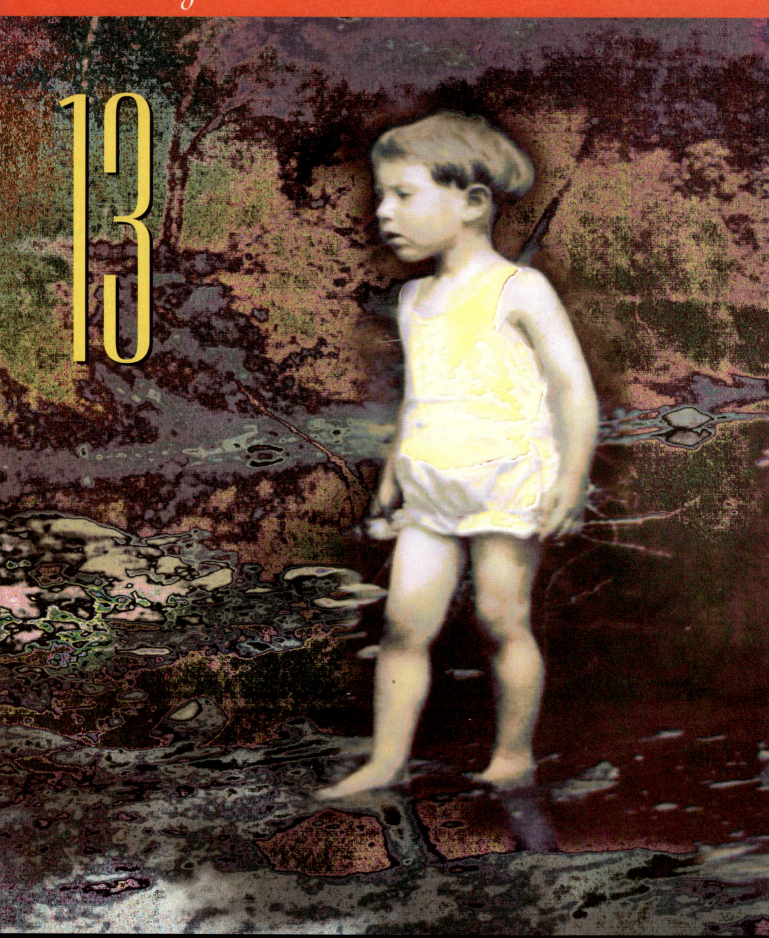

13

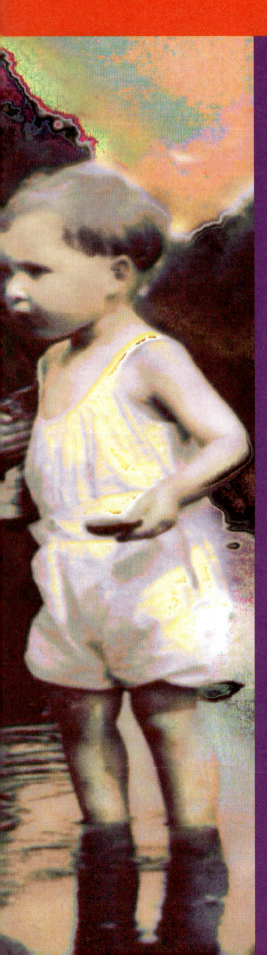

catheter
A tube used to drain or inject fluid through a body opening

catheterization
The process of inserting a catheter

condom catheter
A rubber sheath that slides over the penis; an external catheter

continent
Having control of bladder or bowel function

dysuria
Painful or difficult (dys) urination (uria)

Foley catheter
A catheter that is left in the urinary bladder so that urine drains continuously into a collection bag; an indwelling or retention catheter

fracture pan
A bedpan with a thin rim and that is shallow at one end

glucosuria
Sugar (glucos) in the urine (uria)

indwelling catheter
A retention or Foley catheter

micturition
The process of emptying the bladder; urination or voiding

retention catheter
A Foley or indwelling catheter

urinary incontinence
The inability to control the passage of urine from the bladder

urination
The process of emptying the bladder; micturition or voiding

voiding
Urination or micturition

The urinary system removes much of the waste from the body and regulates the amount of water in the body. The kidneys, ureters, urinary bladder, and urethra are the major structures of the urinary tract (see Chapter 5). Blood passes through the two kidneys, where urine is formed. Urine consists of wastes and excess fluids filtered out of the blood. Urine is carried through two ureters to the urinary bladder where it is stored until urination. The urethra is the tube that connects the urinary bladder to the outside of the body. Urine is eliminated from the body through the urethra. **Urination, micturition,** and **voiding** all mean the process of emptying the bladder.

NORMAL URINATION

The healthy adult excretes about 1000 to 1500 ml (milliliters) (2 to 3 pints) of urine a day. Many factors affect the amount of urine produced. These include the amount and kinds of fluid ingested, age, the amount of salt in the diet, illnesses, and drugs being taken. Certain substances increase urine production. Examples are coffee, tea, alcohol, and some drugs. A diet high in salt causes the body to retain water. When water is retained, less urine is produced. Urine production also is influenced by body temperature, the amount of perspiration, and the external temperature.

Urinary frequency depends on many factors. The amount of fluid ingested, personal habits, and available toilet facilities affect frequency. So do activity, work, and illness. People usually urinate before going to bed and after getting up. Some people urinate every 2 to 3 hours. Others void every 8 to 12 hours. Sleep may be disturbed if large amounts of urine are being produced. Elderly persons may have to urinate at night. Many cannot retain urine as long as younger persons do.

MAINTAINING NORMAL URINATION

Residents often need help to maintain normal elimination. Some need help getting to the bathroom. Others use bedpans, urinals, or commodes.

General Rules

You need to follow certain rules to help residents maintain normal urinary elimination. The rules of medical asepsis, universal precautions, and the bloodborne pathogen standard also are practiced.

1. Help the resident to the bathroom, or provide the bedpan, urinal, or commode as soon as requested. The need to void may be urgent.
2. Help the person assume a normal position for voiding if possible. Women use the sitting or squatting position. Men stand to urinate.
3. Make sure the bedpan or urinal is warm.
4. Cover the person for warmth and privacy.
5. Provide for privacy. Pull the curtain around the bed, close doors to the room and bathroom, and pull drapes or window shades. Leave the room if the person is strong enough to be alone.
6. Remain nearby if the person is weak, unsteady, or confused.
7. Place the signal light and toilet paper within reach.
8. Allow the person enough time to void.
9. Run water in a nearby sink if the person has difficulty starting the stream. You also can place the person's fingers in warm water.
10. Provide perineal care as needed. Be sure to wear gloves and follow universal precautions.
11. Let the resident wash at the sink. Provide a wash basin, soap, washcloth, and towel if the bedpan or urinal was used. Assist as necessary.
12. Assist the resident to the bathroom, or offer the bedpan or urinal at regular intervals. Some persons are embarrassed or too weak or too confused to ask.

What to Report to the Nurse

Before disposing of urine, the nursing assistant observes it carefully. Urine is observed for color, clarity, odor, amount, and particles. Urine is normally yellow, straw- or amber-colored, and clear. It usually has a faint odor and has no particles. Urine that looks abnormal is saved for the nurse to observe. Complaints of urgency, burning on urination, or dysuria are reported. **Dysuria** means painful or difficult (dys) urination (uria). Also report if the resident has trouble starting the urine stream or voids frequently in small amounts.

Bedpans

Bedpans are used by persons confined to bed. Women use bedpans for urination and bowel movements. Men

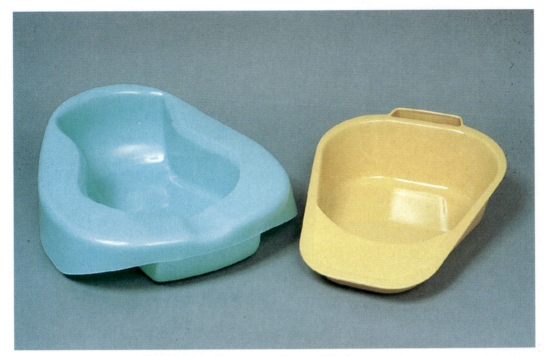

FIGURE 13-1 *The regular bedpan and the fracture pan.*

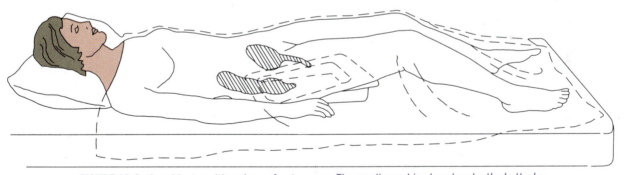

FIGURE 13-2 *A resident positioned on a fracture pan. The smaller end is placed under the buttocks.*

use them for bowel movements only. Bedpans usually are made of plastic or stainless steel. Stainless steel bedpans tend to be cold and are warmed before being given to residents.

Fracture pans also are available. They have thinner rims and are only about 1/2 inch deep at one end (Fig. 13-1). The smaller end goes under the buttocks (Fig. 13-2). Fracture pans are used for elderly residents with lim-

ited range-of-motion in their backs and for those with casts or in traction.

The bedpan is covered after being used and taken to the toilet or "dirty" utility room. There it is emptied, rinsed, and cleaned with a disinfectant. Then it is returned to the bedside stand with a clean cover. Universal precautions are important in handling bedpans.

PROCEDURE

Giving the Bedpan

1. Provide for privacy.

2. Collect the following:
   a. Bedpan
   b. Bedpan cover
   c. Toilet tissue
   d. Disposable gloves

3. Arrange equipment on the chair or bed.

4. Explain the procedure to the resident.

5. Raise the bed to the best level for good body mechanics. Make sure the side rails are up.

6. Warm and dry the bedpan.

7. Lower the side rail near you.

8. Position the resident supine. Elevate the head of the bed slightly.

9. Fold the top linens and gown out of the way. Keep the lower portion of the body covered.

10. Ask the resident to flex the knees and raise the buttocks by pushing against the mattress with his or her feet.

11. Slide your hand under the lower back, and help the resident raise the buttocks.

12. Slide the bedpan under the resident (Fig. 13-3).

13. Do the following if the resident cannot assist in getting on the bedpan.
    a. Turn the resident onto his or her side away from you.
    b. Place the bedpan firmly against the buttocks (Fig. 13-4, *A*, p. 290).
    c. Push the bedpan down and toward the resident (Fig. 13-4, *B*, p. 290).
    d. Hold the bedpan securely. Turn the resident onto the back. Center the bedpan under the resident.

14. Return top linens to their proper position.

15. Raise the head of the bed so the resident is in a sitting position.

16. Make sure the resident is correctly positioned on the bedpan (Fig. 13-5, p. 290).

17. Raise the side rail.

18. Place the toilet tissue and signal light within reach.

19. Ask the resident to signal when through or when assistance is needed.

20. Leave the room and close the door. Wash your hands.

21. Return when the resident signals. Knock before entering.

22. Lower the side rail and the head of the bed.

23. Put on gloves.

24. Ask the resident to raise the buttocks. Remove the bedpan. You also may need to hold the bedpan securely and turn him or her onto the side away from you.

25. Clean the genital area if the resident cannot do so. Clean from front to back with toilet tissue. Provide perineal care if necessary.

26. Cover the bedpan. Take it to the bathroom or "dirty" utility room. Raise the side rail before you leave the bedside.

27. Measure urine if the resident is on intake and output (I&O) (see Chapter 15). Collect a urine specimen if needed. Note the color, amount, and character of the urine or feces.

28. Empty and rinse the bedpan. Clean it with a disinfectant.

29. Return the bedpan and clean cover to the bedside stand.

30. Remove the gloves.

31. Help the resident wash the hands.

32. Make sure the resident is comfortable.

33. Raise or lower the bed to its lowest position.

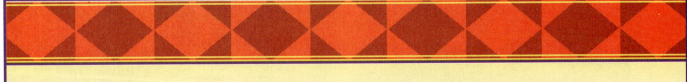

34.	Place the signal light within reach.	**37.**	Place soiled linen in the linen hamper.
35.	Lower the side rails as instructed by the nurse.	**38.**	Wash your hands.
36.	Unscreen the resident.	**39.**	Report your observations to the nurse.

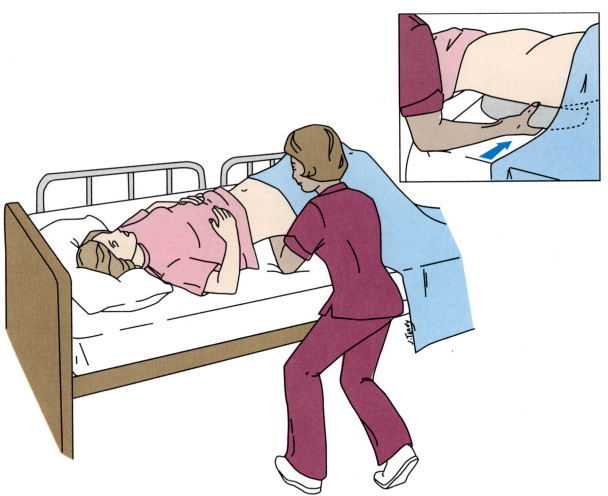

FIGURE 13-3 *The resident raises the buttocks off the bed with the help of the nursing assistant. The bedpan is slid under the resident.*

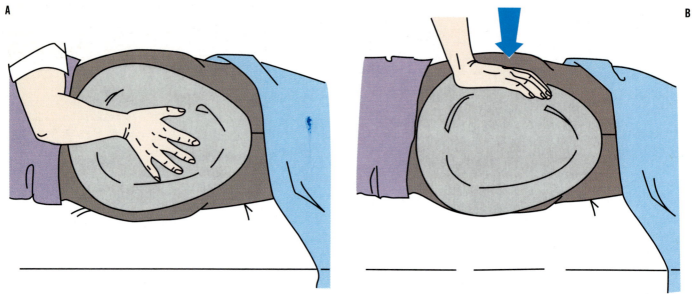

FIGURE 13-4 *A, Position the resident on one side, and place the bedpan firmly against the buttocks. B, Push downward on the bedpan and toward the resident.*

Urinals

Urinals (Fig. 13-6, *A*) are used by men for urination. They are made of the same materials as bedpans. Plastic urinals have caps at the top and hook type of handles. The hook is used to hang the urinal from the side rail within the resident's reach (Fig. 13-6, *B*). Men can use the urinal while lying in bed, sitting on the edge of the bed, or standing at the bedside. If possible, the man should stand. Provide support if he is weak. If necessary, ask someone to help you support the resident. You may have to place and hold the urinal for some men.

Urinals are emptied promptly to prevent odors and the spread of microbes. A filled urinal can easily spill and cause safety hazards. Urinals are cleaned like bedpans.

After using urinals, many men place them on nearby tables until someone empties them. This practice is to be discouraged. They should hang the urinal from the side rail after use. They should be reminded to signal when urinals need to be emptied.

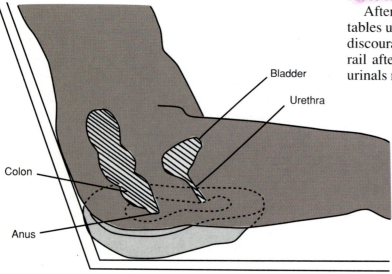

Bladder

Urethra

Colon

Anus

FIGURE 13-5 *The resident is positioned on the bedpan so that the urethra and anus are directly over the opening.*

PROCEDURE

Giving the Urinal

1. Provide for privacy.
2. Determine if the man will stand or use the urinal in bed.
3. Give him the urinal if he will stay in bed. Remind him to tilt the bottom down to prevent spills.
4. Do the following if he will stand:
    a. Help him sit on the side of the bed.
    b. Put slippers on him.
    c. Assist him to a standing position.
    d. Provide support if he is unsteady.
    e. Give him the urinal.
5. Position the urinal between his legs if necessary. Position his penis in the urinal if he cannot hold the urinal. (Wear gloves for this step.)
6. Cover him to provide for privacy.
7. Place the signal light within reach. Ask him to signal when through or when he needs assistance.
8. Wash your hands. Leave the room and close the door if it is safe to leave him alone.
9. Return when he signals for you. Knock before entering.
10. Put on gloves.
11. Cover the urinal. Take it to the bathroom or "dirty" utility room.
12. Measure urine if he is on I&O. Collect a urine specimen if needed. Note the color, amount, and character of the urine.
13. Empty the urinal and rinse it with cold water. Clean it with a disinfectant. Return it to the bedside stand.
14. Remove the gloves.
15. Help him wash his hands.
16. Make sure he is comfortable.
17. Raise or lower side rails as instructed by the nurse.
18. Place the signal light within reach.
19. Unscreen the resident.
20. Wash your hands.
21. Report your observations to the nurse.

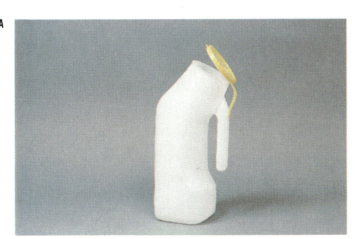 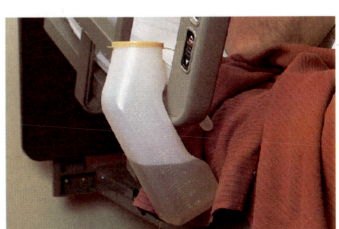

FIGURE 13-6 *A, Urinal for a male. B, The urinal hangs from the side rail within the resident's reach.*

Commodes

A bedside commode is a portable chair or wheelchair with a center opening for a bedpan or similar receptacle (Fig. 13-7). Residents unable to walk to the bathroom may be allowed to use the commode. The commode lets the resident assume the normal position for elimination. The arms and back of the commode support the resident and prevent falls. The bedpan or receptacle is cleaned after use like a regular bedpan.

Some commodes can be wheeled into the bathroom and placed over the toilet. This provides privacy and safety for residents who cannot walk to the bathroom or who cannot sit unsupported on the toilet. The receptacle is removed if the commode is used with the toilet. Make sure the wheels are locked after the commode has been positioned over the toilet.

PROCEDURE

Helping the Resident to the Commode

1. Explain the procedure to the resident.

2. Provide for privacy.

3. Collect the following:
   a. Commode
   b. Toilet tissue
   c. Bath blanket
   d. Disposable gloves

4. Bring the commode next to the bed. Remove the seat and lid from the container.

5. Help the resident sit on the side of the bed.

6. Help the resident put on a robe and slippers.

7. Assist the resident to the commode.

8. Place a bath blanket over his or her lap for warmth.

9. Place the toilet tissue and signal light within reach.

10. Ask him or her to signal when through or when assistance is needed.

11. Wash your hands. Leave the room and close the door if the resident can be alone.

12. Return when the resident signals. Knock before entering.

13. Put on gloves.

14. Help the resident clean the genital area if indicated. Remove the gloves.

15. Help the resident back to bed. Remove the robe and slippers.

16. Raise the side rail if instructed by the nurse.

17. Put on another pair of gloves. Cover and remove the container. Clean the commode if necessary.

18. Take the container to the bathroom or "dirty" utility room.

19. Check urine and any feces for color, amount, and character. Measure urine if the resident is on I&O. Collect a specimen if one is needed.

20. Clean and disinfect the container. Return it to the commode. Remove the gloves.

21. Return other supplies to their proper place.

22. Help the resident wash the hands.

23. Make sure he or she is comfortable and the signal light is within reach.

24. Raise or lower the side rails as instructed by the nurse.

25. Unscreen the resident.

26. Place soiled linen in the linen hamper.

27. Wash your hands.

28. Report your observations to the nurse.

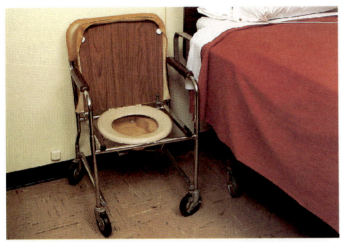

FIGURE 13-7 *The bedside commode has a toilet seat with a container. The container slides out from under the toilet seat for emptying.*

URINARY INCONTINENCE

Urinary incontinence is the inability to control the passage of urine from the bladder. There are several causes. Injuries, diseases, urinary tract infections, reproductive or urinary tract surgeries, medications, aging, and fecal impaction or constipation (see Chapter 14) are some causes. Inability to get to the bathroom is another cause. This can result from immobility, restraint, or not knowing where to find the bathroom in a new or strange environment. Difficulty removing clothes in time may be another cause. Incontinence may be temporary or permanent.

There are different types of incontinence. Persons with spinal cord injuries, central nervous system disorders, or severe dementia (see Chapters 23 and 24) may not know when their bladders are full. Their bladders empty automatically. Catheters may be ordered.

Women may have *stress incontinence*. They dribble or leak urine while laughing, sneezing, coughing, lifting, or straining in any way. Stress incontinence usually is caused by multiple childbirths, weak pelvic muscles, or aging. These women may be wet constantly during illnesses that cause coughing. They may be very embarrassed. Be sensitive to their needs. Offer them garment protectors or incontinent pads or briefs (Fig. 13-8). Make sure they know how to use them. Stress incontinence also may occur in men.

With *urge incontinence* the person has little warning of the need to urinate. The need is very strong when it occurs. The person starts to urinate and cannot stop. The person cannot hold the urine long enough to get to the toilet. Urinary frequency and urinating at night often occur with urge incontinence. It can be caused by urinary tract infection, tumors, fecal impaction or constipation,

and reproductive disorders. A bladder training program usually is planned (see p. 299).

Functional incontinence occurs when a resident cannot get to the bathroom in time. Immobility, restraints, darkness, and a strange environment are among the causes. The person who needs assistance may not get needed help or may be unable to alert a staff member that help is needed. Unanswered signal lights or not having signal lights within reach can cause functional incontinence. This type of incontinence is easy to treat.

1. Answer signal lights promptly.
2. Make sure the signal light is always within the resident's reach.
3. Respond promptly to requests from residents in dining rooms or activity areas. Do not ignore a resident's need to urinate.
4. Meet the basic needs of restrained residents (see Chapter 7).
5. Keep a night light on in the resident's room.
6. Show new residents their surroundings. You may have to do this several times.
7. Follow the rules for maintaining normal elimination.
8. Follow the resident's care plan for preventing incontinence.

Incontinence can occur in residents who usually are continent. You must report the event to the nurse. It may indicate a urinary tract infection, fecal impaction, or dehydration. Medications and certain diseases are other causes.

Incontinence is embarrassing. Clothing becomes wet, odors develop, and the person is uncomfortable. Irrita-

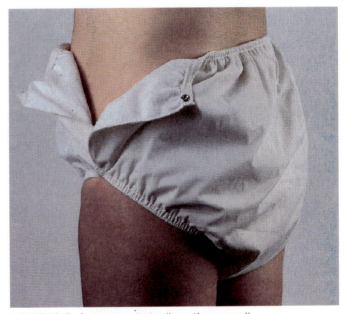

FIGURE 13-8 *Garment protector (incontinence pad).*

tion, infection, and pressure sores also can occur. Good skin care is essential.

Incontinent care is given every 2 hours or as often as noted on the resident's care plan. Incontinent residents are checked to see if they are wet. Wet or soiled garments are changed and perineal care is given. If residents are dry, they are taken to the bathroom or commode or given the urinal or bedpan.

Following the rules for maintaining normal urinary elimination will prevent incontinence in some people. Others need bladder training programs. Some wear garment protectors or incontinent pads or briefs. Never call these items "diapers." The resident's sense of esteem is affected by incontinence. The term *diapering* will only add to the loss of esteem.

CATHETERS

A **catheter** is a rubber or plastic tube used to drain or inject fluid through a body opening. A urinary catheter is inserted through the urethra into the bladder to drain urine. An **indwelling catheter (retention** or **Foley catheter)** is left in the bladder so that urine drains continuously into a drainage bag. A balloon near the tip is inflated after the catheter is inserted. The balloon prevents the catheter from slipping out of the bladder (Fig. 13-9). Tubing connects the catheter to the drainage (collection) bag. Catheter insertion (**catheterization**) is done by a nurse or doctor.

Catheters may be used postoperatively to keep the bladder empty. After surgery a full bladder can cause pressure on nearby organs. Residents who have had surgery may be admitted to the facility with a catheter in place. A catheter also may be used for urinary incontinence.

General Rules

You may care for residents with indwelling catheters. The following rules help promote comfort and safety.

1. Make sure urine flows freely through the catheter or tubing. Tubing should not be kinked.
2. Keep the drainage bag below the level of the bladder. This prevents urine from flowing backward into the bladder. Attach the drainage bag to the bed frame (never the side rail) or wheelchair.
3. Coil connecting tubing on the bed, and pin it to the bottom linen (Fig. 13-10). Tubing also can be attached to the chair or wheelchair (Fig. 13-11). This lets urine flow freely.
4. Tape the catheter to the inner thigh as in Fig. 13-10, or tape the catheter to the man's abdomen. This prevents excessive movement of the catheter and reduces friction at the insertion site. Some facilities use abdominal or leg straps for securing catheters. Know your facility's policy.
5. Provide catheter care in addition to perineal care. Catheter care is performed daily and may be done twice a day in some facilities (see *Catheter Care*, p. 296).
6. Empty the drainage bag at the end of the shift or at time intervals directed by the nurse. Measure and record the amount of urine (see *Emptying a Urinary Drainage Bag*, p. 297).
7. Report complaints to the nurse immediately. These include complaints of pain, burning, the need to urinate, or irritation. Also report the color, clarity, and odor of urine.
8. Follow the rules of universal precautions, medical asepsis, and the bloodborne pathogen standard at all times.

A
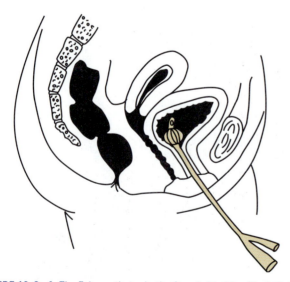
B
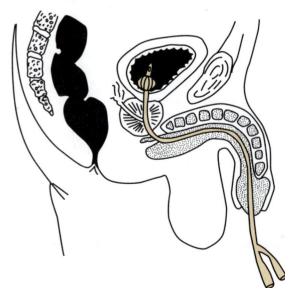

FIGURE 13-9 *A, The Foley catheter in the female bladder. The inflated balloon at the top prevents the catheter from slipping out through the urethra. B, A Foley catheter with the balloon inflated in the male bladder.*

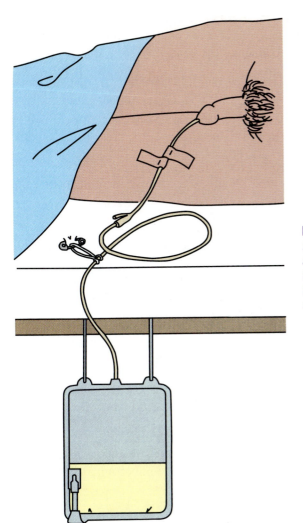

FIGURE 13-10 *The drainage tubing is coiled on the bed and pinned to the bottom linens so that urine flows freely. A rubber band is placed around the tubing with a clove hitch. The safety pin is passed through the loops and pinned to the linens. The catheter is taped to the inner thigh. Enough slack is left on the catheter to prevent friction at the urethra.*

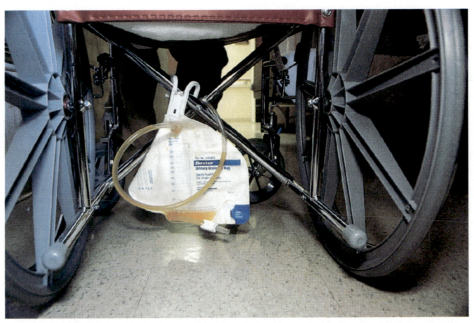

FIGURE 13-11 *Drainage tubing is coiled and attached to the wheelchair.*

Catheter Care

1. Explain the procedure to the resident.

2. Wash your hands.

3. Collect the following:
   a. Equipment for perineal care
   b. Disposable gloves
   c. Disposable bed protector

4. Identify the resident. Check the resident's ID bracelet and call the resident by name.

5. Provide for privacy.

6. Raise the bed to the best level for good body mechanics. Make sure side rails are up.

7. Lower the side rail near you.

8. Cover the resident with a bath blanket. Fan-fold top linens to the foot of the bed.

9. Drape the resident as for perineal care (see Fig. 12-27, p. 257).

10. Put on the gloves.

11. Perform perineal care (see *Giving Female Perineal Care*, p. 256 or *Giving Male Perineal Care*, p. 259).

12. Place the bed protector under the buttocks.

13. Separate the labia (female) see Fig 12-28, or retract the foreskin (uncircumcised male) see Fig 12-30. Check for any crusts, abnormal drainage, or secretions.

14. Clean the catheter from the meatus down the catheter about 4 inches (Fig. 13-13). Use soap, water, and a clean washcloth. Repeat if necessary using a clean washcloth each time.

15. Tape the catheter properly. The tubing should be properly coiled and secured to the bed as in Fig. 13-10 on p. 295.

16. Remove the bed protector.

17. Remove and discard gloves.

18. Cover the resident and remove the bath blanket.

19. Make sure the resident is comfortable.

20. Lower the bed to its lowest position.

21. Raise or lower side rails as instructed by the nurse.

22. Place the signal light within reach.

23. Clean and return equipment to its proper place. Discard disposable items.

24. Unscreen the resident.

25. Take soiled linen to the "dirty" utility room.

26. Wash your hands.

27. Report your observations to the nurse.

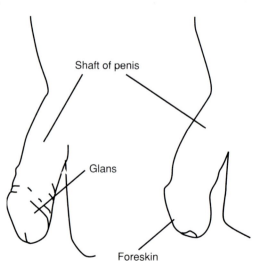

FIGURE 13-12 *A, Circumcised male. B, Uncircumcised male.*

Shaft of penis

Glans

Foreskin

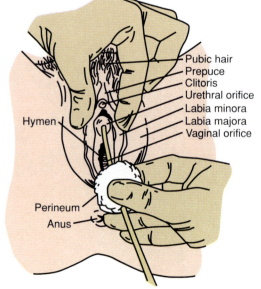

FIGURE 13-13 *The catheter is cleaned beginning at the meatus. About 4 inches of the catheter is cleaned.*

Pubic hair
Prepuce
Clitoris
Urethral orifice
Labia minora
Labia majora
Vaginal orifice

Hymen

Perineum
Anus

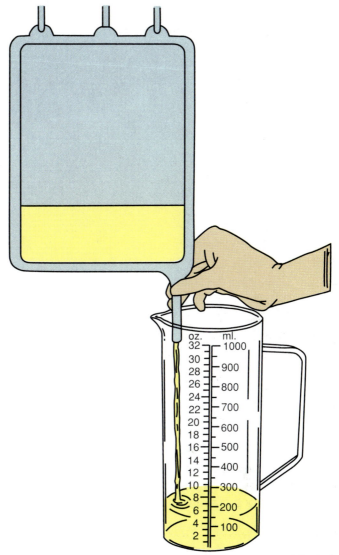

PROCEDURE

Emptying a Urinary Drainage Bag

1. Collect equipment:
   a. Disposable gloves
   b. Graduate

2. Wash your hands.

3. Explain the procedure to the resident.

4. Identify the resident. Check the ID bracelet and call the resident by name.

5. Provide for privacy.

6. Put on the gloves.

7. Place the graduate so that urine can be collected when the drain is opened.

8. Open the clamp on the bottom of the drainage bag.

9. Let all urine drain into the graduate. Do not let the drain touch the graduate (Fig. 13-14).

10. Close the clamp. Replace the clamped drain in the holder on the bag (see Fig. 13-11, p. 295).

11. Measure the urinary output.

12. Rinse the graduate and return it to its proper place.

13. Remove the gloves and wash your hands.

14. Record the time and amount on the I&O record.

15. Unscreen the resident.

16. Report the amount and other observations to the nurse.

FIGURE 13-14 *The clamp on the drainage bag is opened, and the drain is directed into the graduate. The drain must not touch the inside of the graduate.*

297

The Condom Catheter

Condom catheters (external, Texas catheter) often are used for incontinent men. A condom catheter is a soft, rubber sheath that slides over the penis. Tubing connects the condom catheter and the drainage bag. Residents may prefer leg bags during the day (Fig. 13-15).

A new condom catheter is applied daily. The penis is thoroughly washed with soap and water and dried before a new catheter is applied. The penis is observed for reddened or open areas. These are reported to the nurse before a new catheter is applied. Universal precautions are followed in removing or applying condom catheters.

PROCEDURE

Applying a Condom Catheter

1. Explain the procedure to the male resident.

2. Wash your hands.

3. Collect the following:
   - a. Condom catheter
   - b. Drainage bag or leg bag
   - c. Skin barrier as ordered by the nurse
   - d. Basin of warm water
   - e. Soap
   - f. Towel
   - g. Washcloths
   - h. Bath blanket
   - i. Disposable gloves
   - j. Disposable bed protector
   - k. Bag for disposable supplies
   - l. Paper towels

4. Arrange paper towels and equipment on the overbed table.

5. Provide for privacy.

6. Raise the bed to the best level for good body mechanics. Make sure side rails are up.

7. Lower the side rail near you.

8. Cover the resident with a bath blanket. Bring top linens to the foot of the bed.

9. Ask the resident to raise his buttocks off the bed. You may need to turn the resident onto his side away from you.

10. Slide the bed protector under his buttocks.

11. Have him lower his buttocks, or turn him onto his back.

12. Bring top linens up to cover his knees and lower legs.

13. Secure the drainage bag to the bed frame.

14. Raise the bath blanket to expose the genital area.

15. Put on the gloves.

16. Remove the condom catheter:
    - a. Roll the sheath off the penis.
    - b. Disconnect drainage tubing from the condom.
    - c. Place the condom in the bag.

17. Provide perineal care (see *Giving Male Perineal Care*, p. 259).

18. Apply skin barrier to the shaft of the penis. Follow the nurse's instruction for application. Allow 15 seconds to dry.

19. Hold the penis firmly. Roll the condom onto the penis. Leave a 1-inch space between the penis and the end of the catheter (Fig. 13-16).

20. Secure the condom according to the manufacturer's instructions.

21. Connect the condom to the drainage tubing. Coil tubing as in Fig. 13-10, or attach the leg bag.

22. Remove the bed protector.

23. Remove the gloves.

24. Return top linens, and remove the bath blanket.

25. Make sure the resident is comfortable. Place the signal light within reach. Lower the bed.

26. Raise or lower side rails as instructed by the nurse.

27. Clean and return the basin and other equipment to their proper place.

28. Unscreen the resident.

29. Take the bag, used drainage bag, and disposable items to the "dirty" utility room. Measure and record the amount of urine in the bag. Make sure you use universal precautions.

30. Wash your hands.

31. Report your observations.

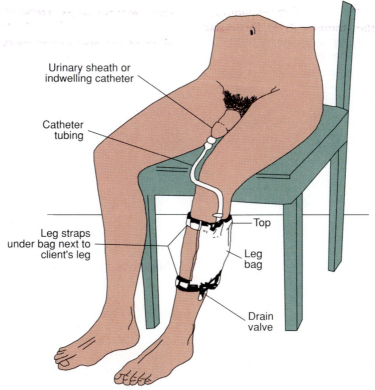

FIGURE 13-15 *A condom catheter attached to a leg bag. (From Hoeman SP: Rehabilitation/restorative care in the community, St Louis, 1990, Mosby–Year Book.)*

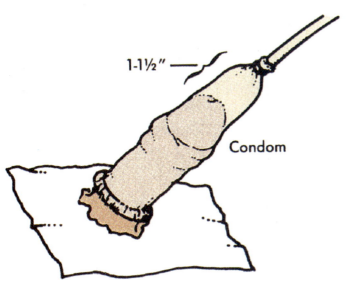

FIGURE 13-16 *A condom catheter applied to the penis. There is a 1-inch space between the penis and the end of the catheter. (From Hoeman SP: Rehabilitation/restorative care in the community, St Louis, 1990, Mosby–Year Book.)*

BLADDER TRAINING

Bladder training programs may be developed for residents with urinary incontinence. Voluntary control of urination is the goal. With the doctor's approval, the nurse develops a plan for bladder training. The plan becomes part of the resident's care plan. You will assist in the bladder training program as directed by the nurse.

The resident uses the toilet, commode, bedpan, or urinal at scheduled intervals. At first the resident may be asked to void every 60 to 90 minutes. Time is slowly increased. The person may be asked to void every 1½ to 2 hours. The goal is for the person to be **continent** (have control of bladder function) for 3- to 4-hour intervals. The person is given 15 or 20 minutes to start voiding. The rules for helping to maintain normal urination are followed. The normal position for urination should be assumed if possible. Privacy is important.

COLLECTING AND TESTING URINE SPECIMENS

Urine specimens (samples) are collected for laboratory study. Urine is examined to help the doctor diagnose a problem or evaluate treatments. There are many types of specimens. A laboratory requisition slip is completed for each specimen sent to the laboratory. The nurse is responsible for completing the requisition. It contains the resident's identifying information and the test to be done. Nursing assistants often collect specimens.

General Rules

Practice the following rules when collecting urine specimens.

1. Wash your hands before and after collecting the specimen.
2. Use universal precautions and follow the blood-borne pathogen standard.
3. Use a clean container for each specimen.
4. Use a container appropriate for the specimen.
5. Label the container accurately with requested information. Most request the resident's full name, room and bed number, date, and time the specimen was collected.
6. Do not touch the inside of the container or lid.
7. Collect the specimen at the specified time.
8. Ask the resident not to have a bowel movement while the specimen is being collected. The specimen must be free of fecal material.
9. Ask the resident to put toilet tissue in the toilet or wastebasket. The specimen should not contain tissue.
10. Take the specimen to the designated storage place.

The Routine Urine Specimen

The routine urine specimen also is called the *random urine sample* or *routine urinalysis*. The test is done as a part of many physical examinations. Some residents can collect the specimen themselves. Weak, very ill, and confused residents need assistance.

PROCEDURE

Collecting a Routine Urine Specimen

1. Explain the procedure to the resident.
2. Wash your hands.
3. Collect the following:
   a. Bedpan and cover, urinal, or disposable specimen pan
   b. Specimen container and lid
   c. Label
   d. Disposable gloves
4. Fill out the label. Put it on the container.
5. Put the container and lid in the bathroom or "dirty" utility room.
6. Identify the resident. Check the ID bracelet and call the resident by name.
7. Provide for privacy.
8. Ask the resident to urinate in the receptacle. Remind him or her to put toilet tissue into the wastebasket or toilet, not into the bedpan or specimen pan.
9. Put on the gloves.
10. Take the bedpan, urinal, or specimen pan to the bathroom or "dirty" utility room.
11. Measure urine if the resident is on I&O.
12. Pour urine into the specimen container until it is about ¾ full. Dispose of excess urine.
13. Place the lid on the specimen container.
14. Clean the bedpan or urinal. Remove the gloves.
15. Return it to its proper place.
16. Help the resident to wash the hands.
17. Make sure he or she is comfortable.
18. Raise or lower the side rails as instructed by the nurse.
19. Place the signal light within reach.
20. Unscreen the resident.
21. Take the specimen to the designated area.
22. Wash your hands.
23. Report your observations to the nurse.

The Clean-Catch Urine Specimen

The clean-catch urine specimen also is called a *midstream specimen* or *clean-voided specimen*. The perineal area is cleaned before collecting the specimen. This reduces the number of microbes in the urethral area when the specimen is collected. The resident voids into the toilet, bedpan, urinal, or commode. Then the stream is stopped and the specimen container positioned. The resident then voids into the specimen container until enough urine is obtained.

Many residents find it hard to stop the stream of urine. You may need to position and hold the specimen container in place for the resident. Be sure to wear gloves, practice universal precautions, and follow the blood-borne pathogen standard.

PROCEDURE

Collecting a Clean-Catch Urine Specimen

1. Explain the procedure to the resident.

2. Wash your hands.

3. Collect the following:
   a. Clean-catch specimen kit
   b. Disposable gloves
   c. Bedpan, urinal, or commode if the resident cannot use the bathroom

4. Label the container with the requested information.

5. Identify the resident. Check the ID bracelet and call the resident by name.

6. Provide for privacy.

7. Let the resident complete the procedure if able. Make sure the signal light is within reach.

8. Assist the resident if necessary.

9. Offer the bedpan, or provide assistance to the bathroom or commode. Be sure the resident has on a robe and slippers if he or she will be up.

10. Open the kit. Remove the specimen container and towelettes. Put on the gloves.

11. Clean the penis or perineal area with towelettes or other specified solution (see *Giving Male Perineal Care*, p. 259 or *Giving Female Perineal Care*, p. 256).

12. Keep the female labia separated until the specimen is collected. For an uncircumcised male, keep the foreskin retracted until the specimen is collected.

13. Collect the specimen:
    a. Ask the resident to urinate into the receptacle.
    b. Ask him or her to stop the stream.
    c. Hold the specimen container under the resident. The container must not touch the resident.
    d. Ask him or her to start urinating again.
    e. Ask the resident to stop the stream when urine has been collected.
    f. Let him or her finish urinating.

14. Put the lid on the container immediately. Do not touch the inside of the lid.

15. Help the resident clean the perineal area. Return the foreskin to its natural position.

16. Clean the bedpan or commode. Remove the gloves.

17. Return equipment to its proper place. Discard disposable items.

18. Help the resident wash the hands.

19. Make sure the resident is comfortable.

20. Raise or lower side rails as instructed by the nurse.

21. Place the signal light within reach.

22. Unscreen the resident.

23. Take the specimen to the designated area.

24. Wash your hands.

25. Report your observations to the nurse.

The 24-Hour Urine Specimen

All urine voided during a 24-hour period is collected for a 24-hour urine specimen. The urine is chilled on ice or refrigerated during the collection period. This prevents the growth of microorganisms. For some tests a preservative is added to the collection container.

The resident voids to begin the test. This voiding is discarded. *All* voidings during the next 24 hours are collected. The procedure and time period for the test must be clearly understood by the resident and everyone involved in the person's care. The rules for collecting urine specimens also must be followed.

PROCEDURE

Collecting a 24-Hour Urine Specimen

1. Review the procedure with the nurse. Ask if a preservative is to be used and if urine is to be preserved on ice.

2. Explain the procedure to the resident.

3. Wash your hands.

4. Collect the following:
   a. Urine container for a 24-hour collection
   b. Preservative if ordered
   c. Bucket with ice if needed
   d. Two labels stating a 24-hour urine specimen is being collected
   e. Funnel
   f. Bedpan, urinal, commode, or specimen pan
   g. Disposable gloves

5. Write the requested information on the specimen container.

6. Identify the resident. Check the ID bracelet and call the resident by name.

7. Arrange the equipment in the resident's bathroom or "dirty" utility room.

8. Put one label in the appropriate place in the bathroom or "dirty" utility room. Place the other near the bed.

9. Offer the bedpan or urinal, or help the resident to the bathroom or commode. Be sure the resident has on a robe and slippers when up.

10. Ask the resident to void.

11. Put on the gloves.

12. Discard the specimen and note the time. This begins the 24-hour collection period.

13. Clean the bedpan, urinal, commode, or specimen pan.

14. Remove the gloves.

15. Mark the time the test began and when it will end on the labels in the room and bathroom. Also mark the specimen container.

16. Ask the resident to use the bedpan, urinal, commode, or specimen pan during the next 24 hours. Ask him or her to signal when there is urine to be emptied. Remind him or her not to have a bowel movement at the same time and not to put toilet tissue in the receptacle.

17. Measure all urine if the resident's I&O is being recorded.

18. Use the funnel (wear gloves) to pour urine into the specimen container. Do not spill any urine. The test must be restarted if urine is spilled or discarded.

19. Add ice to the bucket as necessary.

20. Ask the resident to void at the end of the 24-hour period. Pour the urine into the specimen container.

21. Take the specimen and requisition to the designated area.

22. Remove the labels from the room and bathroom. Clean and return equipment to its proper place. Discard any disposable items.

23. Thank the resident for cooperating.

24. Make sure he or she is comfortable.

25. Raise or lower side rails as instructed by the nurse.

26. Place the signal light within reach.

27. Wash your hands.

28. Report your observations to the nurse.

The Fresh-Fractional Urine Specimen

Double-voided specimen is another term for a fresh-fractional urine specimen. It is so called because the resident voids twice. The resident voids to empty the bladder that contains "stale" urine. In 30 minutes, the resident voids again. "Fresh" urine has collected in the bladder since the first voiding. This second voiding usually is a very small or "fractional" amount of urine. Fresh-fractional urine specimens are used for some urine tests.

Testing Urine

Various urine tests used to be done for residents with *diabetes mellitus*. Diabetes mellitus is a chronic disease in which the pancreas fails to secrete enough insulin. Without enough insulin the body cannot use sugar for energy.

Sugar builds up in the blood if it cannot be used. Some sugar appears in the urine. **Glucosuria** is the medical term for sugar (glucos) in the urine (uria).

Urine tests for sugar used to be done several times a day. Blood glucose monitoring, however, is now preferred over urine testing. This test is done by the nurse. A small amount of blood is obtained from the resident's finger. The blood is tested to determine the blood glucose level. You will not be responsible for blood glucose monitoring.

There may be occasions when urine testing is ordered for a resident. The nurse will ask you to collect a fresh-fractional urine specimen. If you are allowed to perform the test, the nurse will give you necessary instructions.

PROCEDURE

Collecting a Fresh-Fractional Urine Specimen

1. Explain the procedure to the resident.
2. Wash your hands.
3. Collect the following:
   a. Bedpan, urinal, commode, or disposable specimen pan
   b. Two specimen containers
   c. Urine testing equipment
   d. Disposable gloves
4. Identify the resident. Check the ID bracelet and call the resident by name.
5. Provide for privacy.
6. Offer the bedpan or urinal, or assist the resident to the bathroom or commode. Be sure he or she has on a robe and slippers when up.
7. Ask the resident to urinate.
8. Put on gloves.
9. Take the receptacle to the bathroom or "dirty" utility room.
10. Measure urine if the resident's I&O is being recorded. Pour some urine into the specimen container.
11. Tell the nurse there is urine for testing.
12. Clean the receptacle and return it to its proper place. Remove the gloves.
13. Help the resident wash the hands.
14. Make sure the resident is comfortable.
15. Raise or lower side rails as instructed by the nurse.
16. Place the signal light within reach.
17. Unscreen the resident.
18. Wash your hands.
19. Return to the room in 20 to 30 minutes.
20. Repeat steps 5 through 18.
21. Report your observations to the nurse.

Straining Urine

Stones (calculi) can develop in the urinary system. They may be present in the kidneys, ureters, or bladder. Stones may be as small as a pinhead or as large as an orange. Stones that cause severe pain and damage to the urinary system may be surgically removed. A stone may exit the body through urine. When a stone is suspected, all urine must be strained. If a stone is passed, it is sent to the laboratory to be examined.

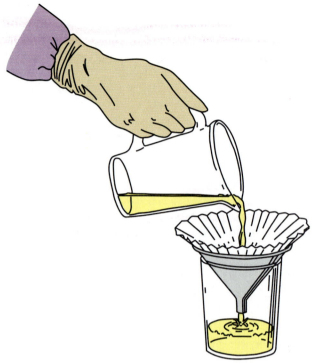

FIGURE 13-17 *A disposable strainer is placed in a specimen container. Urine is poured through the strainer into the specimen container.*

PROCEDURE

Straining Urine

1. Explain the procedure to the resident. Also explain that the urinal, bedpan, commode, or specimen pan is used for voiding.

2. Wash your hands.

3. Collect the following:
   a. Disposable strainer or 4 x 4 gauze
   b. Specimen container
   c. Urinal, bedpan, commode, or specimen pan
   d. Labels for the resident's room and bathroom (labels state that all urine is strained)
   e. Disposable gloves

4. Identify the resident. Check the ID bracelet and call the resident by name.

5. Arrange the equipment in the resident's bathroom.

6. Place one label in the bathroom. Place the other near the bed.

7. Provide for privacy.

8. Offer the bedpan or urinal, or assist the resident to the commode or bathroom. Be sure the resident has on a robe and slippers when up.

9. Ask the resident to signal after voiding.

10. Return when the resident has signaled. Knock before entering.

11. Put on the gloves.

12. Place the strainer or gauze into the specimen container.

13. Pour the urine into the specimen container. Urine will pass through the strainer or gauze (Fig. 13-17).

14. Discard the urine.

15. Place the strainer or 4 × 4 gauze in the specimen container if any crystals, stones, or particles appear.

16. Help the resident clean the perineal area if necessary.

17. Help the resident wash the hands.

18. Clean and return equipment to its proper place. Remove and dispose of gloves.

19. Make sure the resident is comfortable.

20. Place the signal light within reach.

21. Raise or lower side rails as instructed by the nurse.

22. Unscreen the resident.

23. Label the specimen container with the requested information.

24. Take the specimen and to the designated area.

25. Wash your hands.

26. Report your observations to the nurse.

Quality OF LIFE

Elimination is a very private act. People usually do not urinate in front of others. Unfortunately, illness, disease, and aging can affect this very private act. Residents often need to depend on the nursing staff to assist with elimination needs. They may be so weak and disabled that they cannot be left alone to use the bathroom, commode, bedpan, or urinal.

You must do all you can to protect the person's privacy. Pull privacy curtains and close doors, shades, and drapes. If you must stay in the room, position yourself so that the resident has as much privacy as possible. Maybe you need to stand just outside the bathroom door in case the resident needs you. Or maybe it is safe to stand on the other side of the privacy curtain. The nurse will help you with ways to protect the resident's privacy.

Privacy and confidentiality are important for incontinent residents. Remember, incontinence is embarrassing and affects the person's esteem. Only those involved in the resident's care need to know about the incontinence.

Incontinence has been linked to abuse, mistreatment, and neglect of residents. Caring for these residents can be very stressful. They need frequent care and may wet again just after you have provided incontinent care. You must not lose patience with these residents. Their needs are great and your role is to meet their needs. If you find yourself becoming short-tempered and impatient, discuss the situation with the nurse immediately. The nurse may need to reassign you to other residents for a while. Residents have the right to be free from abuse, mistreatment, or neglect. Remember, incontinence is beyond the resident's control. It is not something he or she chooses to let happen. Kindness, empathy, understanding, and patience are very important.

SUMMARY

You are responsible for helping residents maintain normal urination. You also assist with incontinent residents, bladder training, and collecting specimens. You must follow the rules of medical asepsis, universal precautions, the bloodborne pathogen standard, cleanliness, and skin care. Your observations of the person's urine are valuable to doctors and nurses. They use them to plan and evaluate the person's treatment and progress.

Urination is considered a private function. Normal position and privacy are important for urinary elimination. However, you must never leave a weak or confused resident alone in the bathroom or on the commode. Be sure to provide assistance as needed.

Review QUESTIONS

Circle the *best* answer.

1. Which statement is *false*?
   a. Urine is normally clear and yellow or amber in color.
   b. Urine normally has an ammonia odor.
   c. People normally urinate before going to bed and upon rising.
   d. A person normally urinates about 1000 to 1500 ml a day.

2. Which is *not* a rule for maintaining normal elimination?
   a. Help the person assume a normal position for urination.
   b. Provide for the person's privacy.
   c. Help the person to the bathroom or commode, or provide the bedpan or urinal as soon as requested.
   d. Always stay with the person who is on a bedpan.

3. The best position for using a bedpan is
   a. Fowler's position
   b. The supine position
   c. The prone position
   d. The side-lying position

4. After a man uses the urinal, you should ask him to
   a. Cover the urinal
   b. Put the signal light on
   c. Put the urinal on the overbed table
   d. Empty the urinal

5. A woman leaks urine when laughing or sneezing. This is
   a. Stress incontinence
   b. Urge incontinence
   c. Functional incontinence
   d. Fecal incontinence

6. You can prevent functional incontinence by doing all of the following *except*
   a. Answering signal lights promptly.
   b. Keeping the signal light within the resident's reach.
   c. Catheterizing the resident.
   d. Following the rules for normal elimination.

7. A resident has a catheter. Which is *incorrect*?
   a. Keep the drainage bag above the level of the bladder.
   b. Make sure the drainage tubing is free of kinks.
   c. Coil drainage tubing on the bed.
   d. Tape the catheter to the inner thigh.

8. A resident has a catheter. Which is *false*?
   a. Daily perineal care is sufficient.
   b. The rules of medical asepsis are followed.
   c. The drainage bag is emptied at the end of each shift.
   d. Complaints of pain, burning, the need to urinate, or irritation are reported immediately.

9. The goal of bladder training is to
   a. Remove the catheter
   b. Allow the person to walk to the bathroom
   c. Gain voluntary control of urination
   d. All of the above

10. When collecting a urine specimen, you should
    a. Label the container with the requested information
    b. Use the appropriate container
    c. Collect the specimen at the time specified
    d. All of the above

11. The perineal area is cleaned immediately before collecting a
    a. Routine urine specimen
    b. Clean-catch urine specimen
    c. 24-hour urine specimen
    d. Fresh-fractional urine specimen

12. A 24-hour urine specimen involves
    a. Collecting all urine voided by a resident during a 24-hour period
    b. Collecting a routine urine specimen every hour for 24 hours
    c. Straining urine
    d. Having the person void once in 24 hours

Answers

1. b	4. a	7. a	10. d
2. d	5. a	8. a	11. b
3. a	6. c	9. c	12. a

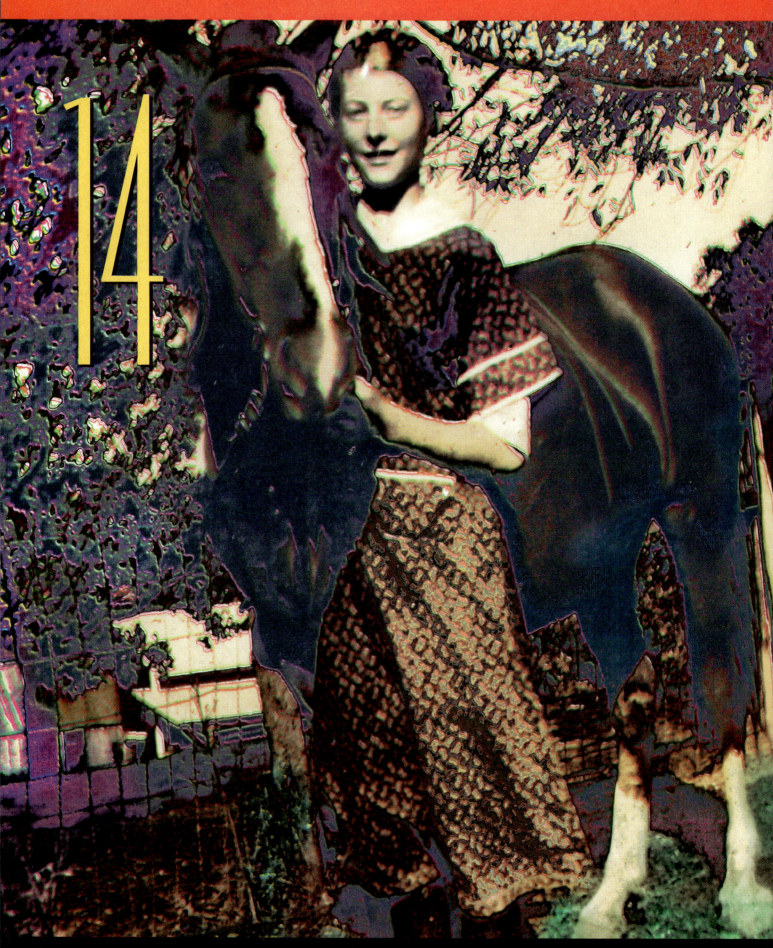

14

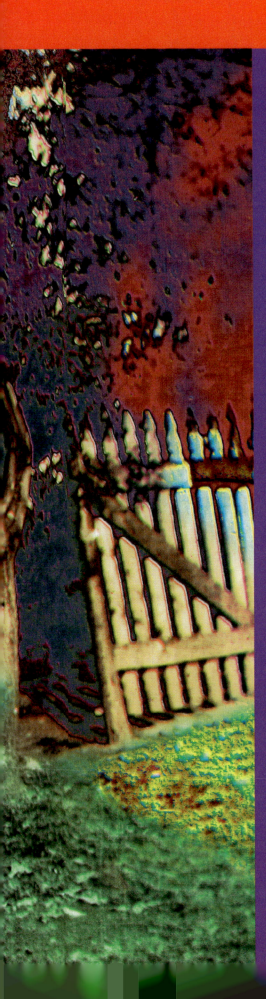

What You Will LEARN

- The key terms listed in this chapter

- Characteristics of normal stools and the normal patterns and frequency of bowel movements

- Observations about defecation that are reported to the nurse

- Factors that affect bowel elimination

- Common problems relating to defecation

- Measures that promote comfort and safety during defecation

- Why enemas are given

- The common enema solutions

- Rules for the administration of enemas

- The purpose of rectal tubes

- How to care for a resident with a colostomy or ileostomy

- How to perform the procedures described in this chapter

anal incontinence
The inability to control the passage of feces and gas through the anus; fecal incontinence

bowel movement
Defecation

chyme
Partially digested food and fluid that pass from the stomach into the small intestine

colostomy
An artificial opening between the colon and abdomen

constipation
The passage of a hard, dry stool

defecation
The process of excreting feces from the rectum through the anus; a bowel movement

diarrhea
The frequent passage of liquid stools

enema
The introduction of fluid into the rectum and lower colon

fecal impaction
The prolonged retention and accumulation of fecal material in the rectum

fecal incontinence
Anal incontinence

feces
The semisolid mass of waste products in the colon

flatulence
The excessive formation of gas in the stomach and intestines

flatus
Gas or air in the stomach or intestines

ileostomy
An artificial opening between the ileum (small intestine) and the abdomen

ostomy
The surgical creation of an artificial opening

peristalsis
The alternating contraction and relaxation of intestinal muscles

stoma
An opening; see *colostomy* and *ileostomy*

stool
Feces that have been excreted

suppository
A cone-shaped solid medication that is inserted into a body opening; it melts at body temperature

I don't like those enemas. So I try to eat a lot of vegetables and fruit. I also try to take a walk every day in the garden. It all seems to help keep me regular.

Bowel elimination is the excretion of wastes from the gastrointestinal system. Foods and fluids normally are taken in through the mouth and are partially digested in the stomach. The partially digested foods and fluids are called **chyme.** Chyme passes from the stomach and into the small intestine. Further digestion and absorption of nutrients occur as chyme passes through the small bowel. The chyme eventually enters the large intestine (large bowel or colon) where fluid is absorbed. There chyme becomes less fluid and more solid in consistency. **Feces** refers to the semisolid mass of waste products in the colon.

Feces move through the intestines by **peristalsis,** the alternating contraction and relaxation of intestinal muscles. Feces move through the large intestine to the rectum. Feces are stored in the rectum until excreted from the body (Fig. 14-1). **Defecation (bowel movement)** is the process of excreting feces from the rectum through the anus. **Stool** is the term for feces that have been excreted.

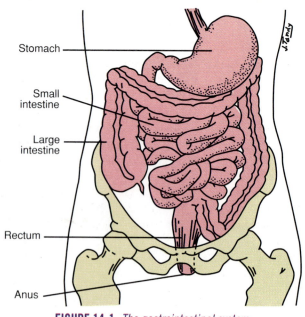

Stomach

Small intestine

Large intestine

Rectum

Anus

FIGURE 14-1 *The gastrointestinal system.*

NORMAL BOWEL MOVEMENTS

The frequency of bowel movements is highly individual. Some people have a bowel movement every day. Others have a bowel movement every 2 to 3 days. Some people have 2 or 3 bowel movements a day. The pattern of elimination also involves the time of day. Many people defecate after breakfast; others do so in the evening.

Stools normally are brown in color. Bleeding in the stomach, intestines, or colon affects the color of stools. Color also is affected by certain diseases and foods. A diet high in beets causes red feces. A diet high in green vegetables can cause green stools.

Feces normally are soft, formed, and shaped like the rectum. Feces that move rapidly through the intestine are watery and unformed. This is called **diarrhea.** Stools that move slowly through the intestines are harder than normal. **Constipation** is the excretion of a hard, dry stool.

Feces have a characteristic odor. The odor is due to the bacterial action in the intestines. Certain foods and drugs can affect the odor of stools.

What to Report to the Nurse

Stools are carefully observed before disposal. Note the color, amount, consistency, and odor. The shape and size of feces and frequency of defecation are reported. Also report any complaints of pain. Abnormal stools should be observed by the nurse.

Many people, especially the elderly, believe they must have a bowel movement daily. They may demand enemas. Report such demands to the nurse. Never give an enema without a nurse's order.

FACTORS AFFECTING BOWEL ELIMINATION

Normal defecation is affected by many factors. Regularity, frequency, consistency, color, and odor of stools can be affected by both psychological and physical factors.

Privacy

Like urination, bowel elimination is a private act. Lack of privacy may prevent a person from defecating even though there is an urge. The odors and sounds that accompany a bowel movement can be embarrassing. Imagine what it is like to use a bedpan or commode for bowel elimination in a semiprivate room. Some residents may ignore the urge to defecate to avoid having a bowel movement in the presence of others.

Disability

Many paraplegic residents lack voluntary control of bowel movements. Defecation occurs whenever feces enter the rectum. Special bowel training programs may be used for these residents. The goal is to have a bowel movement at the same time each day. This keeps the rectum empty and prevents anal incontinence (see p. 312).

Aging

Anal incontinence in elderly persons is due to changes in the body as a result of aging or chronic illness. Confused residents may have anal incontinence because they cannot find the bathroom. Demented residents may not remember how to use the toilet. These residents may have bowel training programs to prevent incontinence. Aging and illness also can slow down the passage of feces through the intestine. This results in constipation.

Diet

A well-balanced diet helps maintain normal bowel elimination. A certain amount of bulk is needed. Foods high in fiber are not completely digested and leave a residue that provides needed bulk. A diet low in fiber reduces the frequency of defecation, causing constipation. Fruits and vegetables are high in fiber.

Many elderly persons do not eat enough fruits and vegetables. They may not have teeth or their dentures may fit poorly. Therefore they cannot chew these foods. Some people believe they cannot digest fruits and vegetables and refuse to eat them. Bran often is added to cereal, prunes, or prune juice in nursing facilities. These foods are a good source of fiber and help prevent constipation.

Individual reaction to certain foods can cause diarrhea and constipation. Milk may cause constipation in some people and diarrhea in others. Chocolate and other foods can cause similar reactions.

Gas-forming foods can stimulate peristalsis. Increased peristalsis aids defecation. Gas-forming foods include onions, beans, cabbage, cauliflower, radishes, and cucumbers. Elderly persons often avoid gas-forming foods. Gas may cause "stomach aches" or "bloating."

Fluids

Fecal material contains a certain amount of water. Water is absorbed as feces move through the large intestine. Stool consistency depends on how much water is absorbed. The amount of fluid ingested and the amount of urine both affect the amount of water absorbed by the large intestine. Drinking fluids (unless fluids are limited) helps prevent constipation.

Activity

Exercise and activity maintain muscle tone and stimulate peristalsis. Irregular bowel elimination and constipation often are due to inactivity and bed rest. Inactivity may result from chronic illness, disease, injury, surgery, or aging.

Medications

Medications can control diarrhea or prevent constipation. Some medications are unrelated to bowel elimination. However, they may have the side effects of diarrhea or constipation. Drugs for pain relief often cause constipation. Antibiotics, used to fight or prevent infection, often cause diarrhea. Diarrhea results because antibiotics kill normal bacteria in the large intestine. Normal bacteria are necessary for the formation of stool.

COMMON PROBLEMS

Many factors can affect normal bowel elimination. Common problems include constipation, fecal impaction, diarrhea, anal incontinence, and flatulence.

Constipation

Constipation is the passage of a hard, dry stool. The person usually strains to have a bowel movement. The stool may be large or marble-sized. Large stools can cause pain as they pass through the anus. Constipation occurs when feces move through the intestine slowly, allowing more time for the absorption of water. Causes of constipation include ignoring the urge to defecate, diet, decreased fluid intake, inactivity, medications, aging, and certain diseases.

Fecal Impaction

A **fecal impaction** is the prolonged retention and accumulation of feces in the rectum. Feces become hard or puttylike in consistency. A fecal impaction results if constipation is not relieved. The person cannot defecate, and more water is absorbed from the already hardened feces. Liquid seeping from the anus is a sign of fecal impaction. Liquid feces pass around the hardened fecal mass in the rectum.

The person with a fecal impaction may try several times to have a bowel movement. Abdominal discomfort, nausea, and rectal pain may be reported. Poor appetite or mental confusion may be signs of fecal impaction in elderly persons. Be sure to report these symptoms to the nurse. The doctor may order medications and enemas to remove the impaction. The nurse may have to remove the fecal mass with a gloved finger.

Diarrhea

Diarrhea is the frequent passage of liquid stools. Feces move through the intestines rapidly, reducing the time for fluid absorption. There is an urgent need to defecate. Some people have difficulty controlling elimination. Abdominal cramping, nausea, and vomiting also may occur.

Causes include infections, certain medications, irritating foods, and microorganisms in food and water. Medical treatment involves reducing peristalsis by diet or medication. You must provide the bedpan or commode promptly for a person with diarrhea. Prompt disposal of stool is necessary to reduce odors and prevent the spread of microbes. Be sure to use universal precautions, and follow the bloodborne pathogen standard. Good skin care is essential. Liquid feces are very irritating to the skin. Frequent wiping of the anal area with toilet tissue also is irritating. Pressure sores may develop if cleanliness and good skin care are not practiced. Report diarrhea to the nurse.

Anal Incontinence

Anal incontinence *(fecal incontinence)* is the inability to control the passage of feces and gas through the anus. Diseases or injuries to the nervous system are causes. Sometimes it results from an unanswered signal light when the person needs the bedpan or help getting to the commode or bathroom.

The person with fecal incontinence needs good skin care. Providing the bedpan or assisting the resident to the commode or bathroom after meals and every 2 to 3 hours may be helpful. A bowel training program may be planned. Consider the psychological impact of anal incontinence on the person. Frustration, embarrassment, anger, and humiliation are a few of the emotions that may be experienced.

Flatulence

Gas or air in the stomach or intestines is called **flatus**. Swallowing air while eating and drinking and bacterial action in the intestines are the common sources of flatus. Normally flatus is expelled through the mouth and anus.

Flatulence is the excessive formation of gas in the stomach and intestines. If gas is not expelled, the intestines distend. That is, they swell or enlarge from the pressure of the gases. The person may have abdominal cramping, shortness of breath, and a swollen abdomen. Flatulence may be caused by gas-forming foods, constipation, medications, and abdominal surgery. In addition, tense or anxious people may swallow large amounts of air when drinking. People who drink through straws also may swallow large amounts of air. Doctors may order enemas, medications, or rectal tubes to relieve distention.

COMFORT AND SAFETY DURING ELIMINATION

Certain measures help promote normal bowel elimination. The health care team plans measures that involve diet, fluids, and exercise. The following actions should be practiced routinely to promote bowel elimination, comfort, and safety.

1. Assist the resident to the toilet or commode or provide the bedpan as soon as requested. Whenever possible, wheel the resident into the bathroom on the commode. Place it over the toilet. This provides privacy for the resident who cannot walk to the bathroom or sit safely on the toilet.
2. Provide for privacy. Close doors, pull curtains around the bed, and pull window curtains or shades. Remember that defecation is a private act. Leave the room if the resident can be alone.
3. Ask visitors to leave the room when a resident asks to use the bedpan, commode, or toilet.
4. Make sure the bedpan is warm.
5. Position the resident in a normal sitting or squatting position.
6. Make sure the person is covered for warmth and privacy.
7. Allow enough time for defecation.
8. Place the signal light and toilet tissue within the person's reach.
9. Stay nearby if the resident is weak or unsteady.
10. Provide perineal care.
11. Dispose of feces promptly. This reduces odors and prevents the spread of microbes.
12. Let residents wash their hands after defecating and wiping with toilet tissue.
13. Offer the bedpan or assist the resident to the commode or bathroom after meals if there is the problem of incontinence.
14. Use universal precautions and follow the bloodborne pathogen standard if contact with feces is possible.

BOWEL TRAINING

Bowel training involves two aspects. One is gaining control of bowel movements. The other is developing a regular pattern of elimination. Fecal impaction, constipation, and anal incontinence are prevented.

The urge to defecate usually is felt after a meal, particularly breakfast. Therefore the use of the toilet, commode, or bedpan is encouraged at this time. The time of day that the resident normally has a bowel movement should be noted on the Kardex. Offer the toilet, commode, or bedpan at that time. Other factors that influence elimination are included on the Kardex, resident's care plan, and bowel training program. These include diet, fluids, activity, and privacy. The nurse will give you instructions about a person's bowel training program.

...tory to stimulate defe-
...ped solid medication
... It melts at body tem-
...inserted into the rec-
...out 30 minutes before
...ovement. Enemas also

... of fluid into the rectum and
...ered by doctors. They are
...elieve constipation or fecal
...ered to clean the bowel of
...ocedures. Sometimes ene-
...tus and to relieve intestinal
...ograms often involve ene-

...by the doctor depends on the
...he solution may be *tap water*
...uds enema (SSE) is prepared by
...soap to 1000 ml of water. A *saline*
enema is a solu... f salt and water. These solutions are
used for cleansing enemas. Cleansing enemas involve
the removal of feces from the rectum and colon.

Oil is used to give oil-retention enemas. They are
given for constipation or fecal impaction. The oil is retained in the rectum for 30 to 60 minutes. This softens
the feces and lubricates the rectum. This allows feces to
pass with ease. Mineral oil, olive oil, or a commercial
oil–retention enema may be used.

Commercial enemas often are ordered for constipated
residents. They also are ordered when complete cleansing of the bowel is not indicated. The enema contains
about 120 ml (4 ounces) of a solution. It causes defecation by irritating and distending the rectum.

Other enema solutions may be ordered. Consult with
the nurse and use the facility's procedure manual to
safely prepare and give uncommon enemas.

Equipment

Disposable enema kits are available from the supply
area. The kit (Fig. 14-2) includes a plastic enema bag,
tubing, a clamp for the tubing, and a waterproof bed protector. The enema bag holds the solution. Most kits have
packets of castile soap for soap suds enemas. A lubricant
is needed if the tubing end is not prelubricated. A bath
thermometer is needed to measure the solution temperature. Some solutions are obtained from the supply area.
If a commercial enema has been ordered, you need the
enema and a waterproof bed protector. A bedpan usually
is needed for an enema. Enema procedures also require
gloves for universal precautions.

General Rules

Giving an enema generally is a safe procedure. Many
people give themselves enemas at home. However, enemas are dangerous for persons with certain heart and kidney diseases. Give an enema only after receiving clear
instructions and after reviewing the procedure with the
nurse.

Comfort and safety measures need to be practiced in
giving an enema. In addition, these rules must be followed.

1. Solution temperature should be 105° F (40.5° C).
    Measure temperature with a bath thermometer.
2. The amount of solution to be given depends on the
    purpose of the enema and the person's age. Adults
    generally receive 750 to 1000 ml. Some elderly resi-
    dents, however, cannot retain more than 500 ml.
3. The left Sims' position usually is used (see Fig. 9-38,
    p. 188). Elderly persons may be more comfortable in
    the left side–lying position.
4. The enema bag is raised no more than 18 inches
    above the level of the mattress.
5. The lubricated enema tubing is inserted only 2 to 4
    inches into the rectum. The bowel can be injured if
    the tube is inserted any deeper.
6. The solution is given slowly. Usually it takes 10 to
    15 minutes to give 750 to 1000 ml.
7. The solution should be retained in the bowel for a
    certain length of time. The length of time depends on
    the amount and type of solution. Some residents can-
    not retain the enema. Place them on the bedpan im-
    mediately.
8. The enema tube is held in place while the solution is
    being administered.
9. The bathroom must be vacant when the person has
    the urge to defecate. Make sure the bathroom will
    not be used by another resident.
10. Ask the nurse to observe the results of the enema.
11. Universal precautions are used and the boodborne
    pathogen standard is followed.

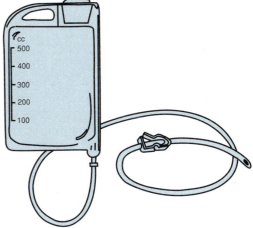

FIGURE 14-2 *An enema kit contains a plastic enema bag, tubing, and a clamp.*

The Cleansing Enema

Cleansing enemas often are given to clean the bowel of feces and flatus. The doctor may order a soap suds, tap water, or saline enema. The doctor may order "enemas until clear." Enemas are given until the return solution is clear and free of fecal material. Check with the nurse to see how many enemas can be given. The facility may only allows enemas to be repeated only 2 or 3 times. This is especially important for elderly residents.

Tap water enemas can be dangerous. The large intestine may absorb some of the water into the bloodstream. This creates a fluid imbalance in the body. Repeated enemas increase the danger of excessive fluid absorption. Soap suds enemas are very irritating to the bowel's mucous lining. Bowel damage can result with repeated enemas. Using more than 5 ml of castile soap and using stronger soaps also can damage the bowel. The saline solution is similar to body fluid. Some persons, however, may absorb some of the salt in the solution.

PROCEDURE

Giving a Cleansing Enema

1. Explain the procedure to the resident.

2. Wash your hands.

3. Collect the following:
   a. Bedpan or commode
   b. Disposable enema kit (enema bag, tubing, and clamp)
   c. Bath thermometer
   d. Waterproof bed protector
   e. Water-soluble lubricant
   f. Disposable gloves (3 pairs)
   g. Material for enema solution: 5 ml castile soap or 2 teaspoons of salt
   h. Toilet tissue
   i. Bath blanket
   j. IV pole
   k. Large measuring container
   l. Robe and slippers
   m. Specimen container (if needed)
   n. Paper towels

4. Identify the resident. Check the ID bracelet with the treatment order.

5. Provide for privacy.

6. Raise the bed to the best level for good body mechanics. Make sure the side rails are up.

7. Lower the side rail near you.

8. Cover the resident with a bath blanket. Fan-fold top linens to the foot of the bed.

9. Position the IV pole so the enema bag will be 12 inches above the anus or 18 inches above the level of the mattress.

10. Raise the side rail.

11. Prepare the enema.
    a. Close the clamp on the enema tubing.
    b. Adjust water flow until it is lukewarm.
    c. Fill the measuring container with water to the 1000 ml mark or as otherwise ordered.
    d. Measure water temperature. It should be 105° F (40.5° C).
    e. Prepare the enema solution:
       (1) Saline: add 2 teaspoons of salt
       (2) Soap suds: add 5 ml of castile soap
       (3) Tap water: add nothing to the water
    f. Stir the solution with the bath thermometer. Scoop off any suds (SSE), using the bath thermometer.
    g. Pour the solution into the enema bag.
    h. Seal the top of the bag.
    i. Hang the enema bag on the IV pole.

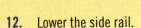

12. Lower the side rail.

13. Position the resident in the left Sims' or a comfortable left side–lying position.

14. Place the waterproof pad under the buttocks.

15. Expose the anal area.

16. Put on the gloves.

17. Place the bedpan behind the resident.

18. Position the enema tubing in the bedpan. Open the clamp. Let solution flow through the tubing to remove air. Clamp the tubing.

19. Lubricate the tubing with lubricant. Lubricate 2 to 4 inches up from the tip.

20. Separate the buttocks to see the anus.

21. Ask the resident to take a deep breath through the mouth.

22. Insert the tubing gently 2 to 4 inches into the rectum when the resident is exhaling (Fig. 14-3, p. 316). Stop if he or she complains of pain or if you feel resistance.

23. Check how much solution is in the bag.

24. Unclamp the tubing, and administer the solution slowly (Fig. 14-4, p. 316).

25. Ask the resident to take slow deep breaths. This helps the resident relax while the enema is being given.

26. Clamp the tubing if the resident expresses a desire to defecate, complains of abdominal cramping, or begins to expel the solution. Unclamp the tubing when symptoms subside.

27. Give at least 750 ml or the desired amount. Stop if the resident cannot tolerate the procedure.

28. Clamp the tubing before it is empty of solution. This prevents air from entering the bowel.

29. Hold several thicknesses of toilet tissue around the tubing and against the anus. Remove the tubing.

30. Discard soiled tissue into the bedpan.

31. Wrap the tubing tip with paper towels, and place inside the enema bag.

32. Help the resident onto the bedpan. Raise the head of the bed. Or lower the side rail and assist the resident to the bathroom or commode. The resident wears a robe and slippers when up.

33. Place the signal light and toilet tissue within reach. Remind the resident not to flush the toilet.

34. Leave the room if the resident can be alone. Discard disposable items and remove the gloves. Wash your hands.

35. Return when the resident signals. Knock before entering.

36. Observe enema results for amount, color, consistency, and odor.

37. Put on the gloves.

38. Obtain a stool specimen if ordered.

39. Help the resident clean the perineal area if indicated.

40. Empty, clean, and disinfect the bedpan or commode container. Do not flush the toilet until the nurse observes the results. Return equipment to its proper place.

41. Remove the waterproof bed protector. Remove gloves.

42. Help the resident wash the hands.

43. Return top linens and remove the bath blanket.

44. Make sure the resident is comfortable and the signal light is within reach.

45. Lower the bed to its lowest position.

46. Raise or lower side rails as instructed by the nurse.

47. Unscreen the resident.

48. Discard disposable items. Place soiled linen in the linen bag. Wear gloves for this step if necessary.

49. Wash your hands.

50. Report your observations to the nurse.

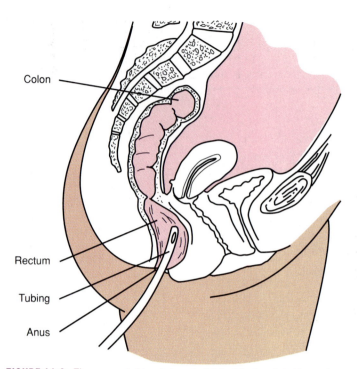

Colon

Rectum

Tubing

Anus

FIGURE 14-3 *The enema tubing is inserted 2 to 4 inches into the rectum.*

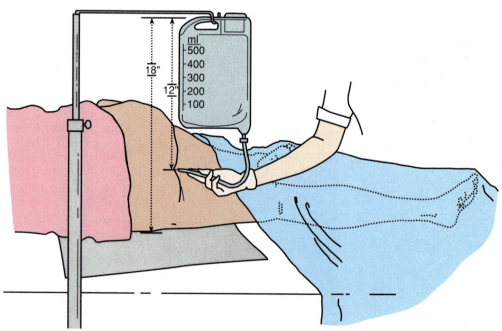

FIGURE 14-4 *An enema is given in the left Sims' position. The IV pole is positioned so that the enema bag is 12 inches above the anus and 18 inches above the mattress.*

The Commercial Enema

The commercial enema is ready to be given (Fig. 14-5). The solution usually is given at room temperature. However, the nurse may have you warm the enema in a basin of warm water. The left Sims' or left side–lying position is used. The nurse will tell you how to position the resident.

The plastic bottle is squeezed and rolled up from the bottom to give the solution. Squeezing and rolling are continued until all of the solution has been given. Do not release pressure on the bottle. If pressure is released, solution is withdrawn from the rectum back into the bottle. Encourage the resident to retain the solution until the urge to defecate is felt. Remaining in the Sims' or side-lying position will help the person retain the enema longer.

A commercial enema is considered a medication in some states. Nursing assistants are not allowed to give medications. Therefore you may not be allowed to give commercial enemas. Check facility policy and know the state law before you give such an enema.

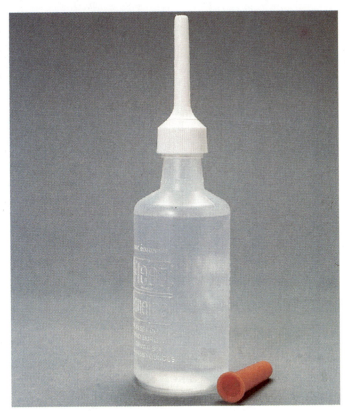

FIGURE 14-5 *A commercial enema.*

PROCEDURE

Giving a Commercial Enema

1. Explain the procedure to the resident.

2. Wash your hands.

3. Collect the following:
   a. Commercial enema
   b. Bedpan, commode, or specimen pan
   c. Waterproof bed protector
   d. Toilet tissue
   e. Disposable gloves (3 pair)
   f. Robe and slippers
   g. Specimen container (if needed)
   h. Bath blanket

4. Identify the resident. Check the ID bracelet with the treatment order.

5. Provide for privacy.

6. Raise the bed to the best level for using good body mechanics. Make sure the side rails are up.

7. Lower the side rail near you.

8. Cover the resident with a bath blanket. Fan-fold top linens to the foot of the bed.

9. Position the resident in the left Sims' or a comfortable side-lying position.

10. Place the bed protector under the buttocks.

11. Expose the anal area.

12. Position the bedpan near the resident.

13. Put on the gloves.

14. Remove the protective cap from the enema.

Continued.

Giving a Commercial Enema——cont'd

15. Separate the buttocks to see the anus.

16. Ask the resident to take a deep breath through the mouth.

17. Insert the enema tip 2 inches into the rectum when the resident is exhaling (Fig. 14-6). Insert the tip gently.

18. Squeeze and roll the bottle gently. Do not release pressure until all of the solution has been given.

19. Remove the tip from the rectum. Put the bottle back into the box tip first.

20. Remove the gloves.

21. Lower the bed to its lowest position.

22. Help the resident to the bathroom or commode or onto the bedpan. The resident has on a robe and slippers when up.

23. Place the signal light and toilet tissue within reach. Remind the resident not to flush the toilet.

24. Leave the room if the resident can be alone. Discard disposable items. Wash your hands.

25. Return when the resident signals. Knock before entering.

26. Put on gloves.

27. Observe enema results for amount, color, consistency, and odor.

28. Obtain a stool specimen if ordered.

29. Help the resident clean the perineal area if indicated.

30. Empty, clean, and disinfect the bedpan or commode container. Flush the toilet after the nurse observes the results. Return equipment to its proper place.

31. Remove the waterproof bed protector.

32. Remove the gloves.

33. Help the resident wash the hands.

34. Return top linens and remove the bath blanket.

35. Make sure the resident is comfortable and the signal light is within reach.

36. Lower the bed to its lowest position.

37. Raise or lower side rails as instructed by the nurse.

38. Unscreen the resident.

39. Place soiled linen in the linen bag. Wear gloves if necessary.

40. Wash your hands.

41. Report your observations to the nurse.

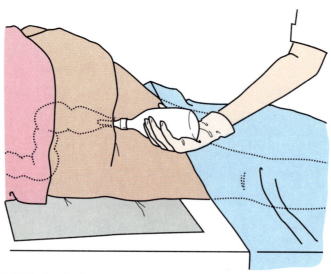

FIGURE 14-6 *The tip of the commercial enema is inserted 2 inches into the rectum.*

The Oil-Retention enema

Commercial oil-retention enemas are given like other commercial enemas. However, the solution is retained in the rectum so that feces soften. The enema is retained for a specified length of time, usually for 30 to 60 minutes. Oil-retention enemas are ordered to relieve constipation or fecal impaction.

PROCEDURE

Giving an Oil Retention Enema

1. Explain the procedure to the resident.
2. Wash your hands.
3. Collect the following:
   a. Commercial oil-retention enema
   b. Waterproof bed protector
   c. Disposable gloves
   d. Bath blanket
4. Identify the resident. Check the ID bracelet with the treatment order.
5. Provide for privacy.
6. Raise the bed to the best level for using good body mechanics. Make sure the side rails are up.
7. Lower the side rail near you.
8. Cover the resident with a bath blanket. Fan-fold top linens to the foot of the bed.
9. Position the resident in the left Sims' or a comfortable side-lying position.
10. Place the bed protector under the buttocks.
11. Expose the anal area.
12. Put on the gloves.
13. Remove the cap from the enema.
14. Separate the buttocks to see the anus.
15. Ask the resident to take a deep breath through the mouth.
16. Insert the enema tip 2 inches into the rectum when the resident is exhaling. Insert the tip gently.
17. Squeeze and roll the bottle gently. Do not release pressure until all solution has been given.
18. Remove the tip from the rectum. Put the bottle in the box, tip first.
19. Remove the gloves.
20. Cover the resident. Leave the resident lying in the Sims' or side-lying position.
21. Encourage the resident to retain the enema for the time ordered.
22. Place additional waterproof protectors on the bed if needed.
23. Lower the bed to its lowest position.
24. Raise or lower the side rail as instructed by the nurse.
25. Make sure the resident is comfortable. Place the signal light within reach.
26. Unscreen the resident.
27. Discard used disposable equipment.
28. Wash your hands.
29. Check the resident often.
30. Report your observations to the nurse.

RECTAL TUBES

A rectal tube is inserted into the rectum to relieve flatulence and intestinal distention. Flatus passes from the body without effort or straining. Disposable rectal tubes have a tube and a flatus bag (Fig. 14-7). The bag collects feces that may be expelled along with the flatus. If a flatus bag is not included with the rectal tube, place the open end of the tube in a folded waterproof pad.

The rectal tube is removed after 20 to 30 minutes. This helps prevent rectal irritation. The nurse tells you when to insert the tube and how long to leave it place.

PROCEDURE

Using a Rectal Tube

1. Explain the procedure to the resident.

2. Wash your hands.

3. Collect the following:
   a. Disposable rectal tube with flatus bag
   b. Water-soluble lubricant
   c. Adhesive tape
   d. Disposable gloves (at least two pairs)
   e. Waterproof bed protector if there is no flatus bag

4. Identify the resident. Check the ID bracelet and call the resident by name.

5. Provide for privacy.

6. Raise the bed to the best level for good body mechanics.

7. Lower the side rail.

8. Position the resident in the left Sims' or left side–lying position.

9. Expose the anal area.

10. Put on the gloves.

11. Lubricate 2 to 4 inches up from the tip of the tube.

12. Separate the buttocks to see the anus.

13. Ask the resident to take a deep breath through the mouth.

14. Insert the tube gently 2 to 4 inches into the rectum when the resident is exhaling. Stop if the resident complains of pain or you feel resistance.

15. Tape the rectal tube to the buttocks.

16. Position the flatus bag so it rests on the bed (Fig. 14-8). Remove the gloves.

17. Cover the resident.

18. Leave the tube in place for 20 minutes.

19. Lower the bed to its lowest position. Place the signal light within reach. Raise or lower side rails as instructed by the nurse.

20. Wash your hands. Leave the room. Check the resident often.

21. Return to the room after 20 minutes. Knock before entering.

22. Put on gloves.

23. Remove the rectal tube. Wipe the rectal area.

24. Ask the resident about the amount of gas expelled.

25. Make sure he or she is comfortable and the signal light is within reach.

26. Raise or lower side rails as instructed by the nurse.

27. Unscreen the resident.

28. Take used disposable items and soiled linen to the "dirty" utility room. Remove the gloves.

29. Wash your hands.

30. Report your observations to the nurse.

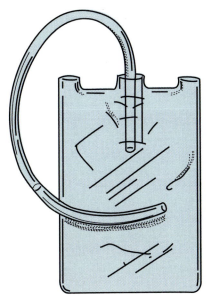

FIGURE 14-7 *A rectal tube and flatus bag.*

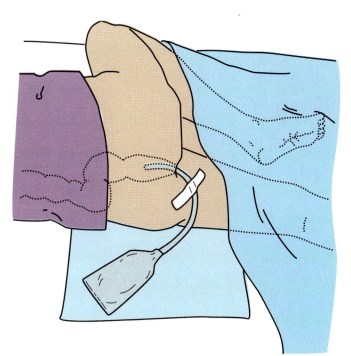

FIGURE 14-8 *After being inserted, the rectal tube is taped to the buttocks and the flatus bag rests on the bed. The tube is inserted 2 to 4 inches into the rectum.*

THE RESIDENT WITH AN OSTOMY

Sometimes it is necessary to surgically remove part of the intestines. Cancer, bowel diseases, and trauma (such as stab wounds or bullet wounds) are common reasons for intestinal surgery. An ostomy may be necessary. An **ostomy** is the surgical creation of an artificial opening. The opening is called the **stoma.** The nurse will care for the ostomy resident in the early postoperative period. However, you may care for a person who has had an ostomy for a long time.

Colostomy

A **colostomy** is the surgical creation of an artificial opening between the colon and abdomen. Part of the colon is brought out onto the abdominal wall and a stoma made. Feces and flatus pass through the stoma rather than the anus. Colostomies may be permanent or temporary. If permanent, the diseased part of the colon is removed. A temporary colostomy gives the diseased or injured portion of the bowel time to heal. After healing, surgery is performed to reconnect the bowel.

The colostomy location depends on the part of the colon that is diseased or injured. Figure 14-9 on p. 322 shows common colostomy sites. Stool consistency depends on the location of the colostomy. The stool can be liquid to formed. The more colon remaining to absorb water, the more solid and formed the stool. If the colostomy is near the beginning of the colon, stools will be liquid. A colostomy near the end of the large intestine results in formed stools.

The person wears a colostomy appliance. The appliance is a disposable plastic bag applied over the stoma. It collects feces expelled through the stoma. When the appliance becomes soiled, it is replaced with a new one. Universal precautions are essential and the bloodborne pathogen standard must be followed. Skin care is given to prevent skin breakdown around the stoma. The appliance has an adhesive backing that is applied to the skin. Many people also secure the appliance to an ostomy belt (Fig. 14-10, p. 324). Many people manage their colostomies without assistance. If able, they should be allowed to do so.

Odors should be prevented. Good hygiene is essential. A new bag is applied whenever soiling occurs. Emptying the bag of feces and avoiding gas-forming foods also help to control odors. Deodorants can be placed in the appliance. The nurse will tell you which one to use.

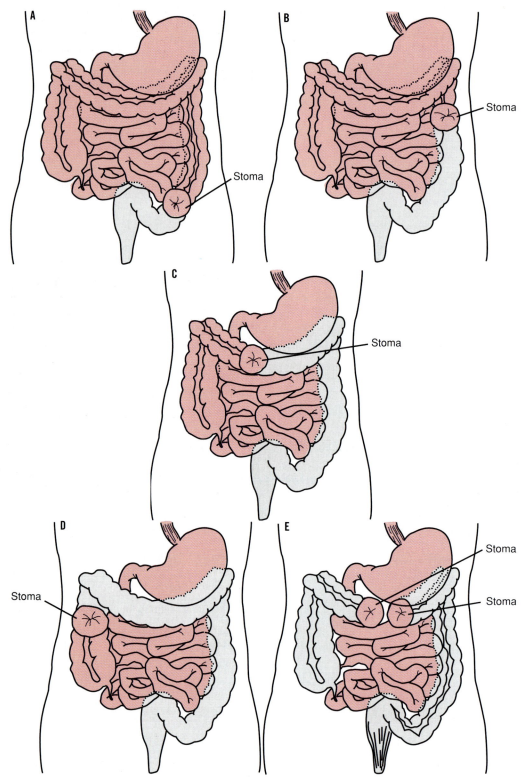

FIGURE 14-9 *Colostomy sites, with the shaded area indicating the part of the bowel that has been surgically removed.* **A,** *Sigmoid colostomy.* **B,** *Descending colostomy.* **C,** *Transverse colostomy.* **D,** *Ascending colostomy.* **E,** *Double-barrel colostomy. Two stomas are created: one allows for the excretion of fecal material. The other allows medication to be introduced to help the bowel heal. This type of colostomy usually is temporary.*

PROCEDURE

Caring for a Resident With a Colostomy

1. Explain the procedure to the resident.

2. Wash your hands.

3. Collect the following:
   a. Bedpan with cover
   b. Waterproof bed protectors
   c. Bath blanket
   d. Toilet tissue
   e. Clean colostomy appliance
   f. Clean ostomy belt
   g. Wash basin
   h. Bath thermometer
   i. Prescribed soap or cleansing agent
   j. Skin barrier as ordered
   k. Deodorant for the appliance
   l. Disposable bag
   m. Paper towels
   n. Disposable gloves

4. Identify the resident. Check the ID bracelet and call the resident by name.

5. Provide for privacy.

6. Raise the bed to the best level for using good body mechanics. Make sure the side rails are up.

7. Lower the side rail near you.

8. Cover the resident with a bath blanket. Fan-fold linens to the foot of the bed.

9. Place the waterproof pad under the buttocks.

10. Put on the gloves.

11. Disconnect the appliance from the belt.

12. Remove the colostomy belt.

13. Remove the appliance gently. Place it in the bedpan.

14. Wipe around the stoma with toilet tissue to remove any mucus or feces. Place soiled tissue in the bedpan.

15. Cover the bedpan. Take it to the bathroom.

16. Empty the appliance and bedpan into the toilet. Note color, amount, consistency, and odor of feces. Put the appliance in the disposable bag.

17. Fill the wash basin. Water temperature should be 115° F (46.1° C). Place the basin on the overbed table on top of the paper towels.

18. Clean the skin around the stoma with water. Rinse and pat dry. Use soap or other cleansing agent if ordered.

19. Apply the skin barrier.

20. Put a clean colostomy belt on the resident.

21. Add deodorant to the new appliance.

22. Remove adhesive backing on the appliance.

23. Center the appliance over the stoma. Make sure it is sealed to the skin. Apply gentle pressure to the adhesive surface from the stoma outward.

24. Connect the belt to the appliance.

25. Remove the bed protector. Remove the gloves.

26. Return top linens and remove the bath blanket.

27. Make sure the resident is comfortable.

28. Raise or lower side rails as instructed by the nurse.

29. Lower the bed to its lowest position.

30. Place the signal light within reach.

31. Unscreen the resident.

32. Put on another pair of gloves.

33. Clean the bedpan, wash basin, and other equipment. Wash the ostomy belt. Place used disposable items in the disposable bag.

34. Return the equipment to its proper place.

35. Take the disposable bag and soiled linen to the "dirty" utility room. Remove the gloves.

36. Wash your hands.

37. Report your observations to the nurse.

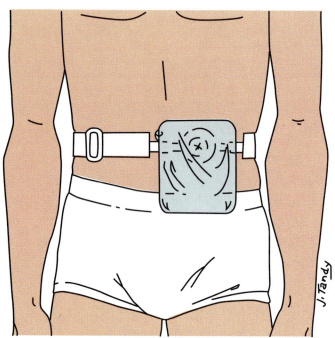

FIGURE 14-10 *A colostomy appliance is in place over the stoma and is secured with a colostomy belt.*

Ileostomy

An **ileostomy** is the surgical creation of an artificial opening between the ileum (small intestine) and the abdomen. Part of the ileum is brought out onto the abdominal wall and a stoma made. The entire large intestine is removed (Fig. 14-11). Liquid feces drain constantly from an ileostomy. Water is not absorbed because the colon has been removed. Feces in the small intestine contain digestive juices that are very irritating to the skin. The ileostomy appliance must fit well so that feces do not touch the skin. The appliance is sealed to the skin and is removed every 2 to 4 days. Good skin care is essential.

There are disposable and reusable ileostomy appliances. The appliance is clamped at the end so that feces can collect in the bag. To empty the bag, direct it into the toilet and remove the clamp (Fig. 14-12). The appliance is emptied every 4 to 6 hours or when the person urinates. Reusable bags are washed with soap and water and allowed to dry and air out. The care of a resident with an ileostomy is similar to that of one with a colostomy. Universal precautions and the bloodborne pathogen standard must be practiced.

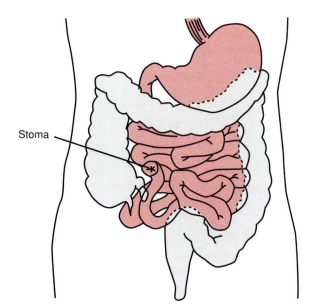

Stoma

FIGURE 14-11 *An ileostomy. The entire large intestine is removed during the surgery.*

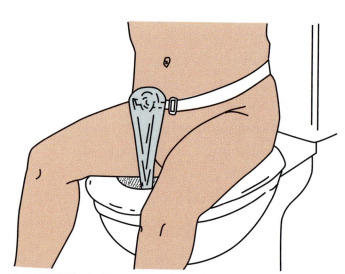

FIGURE 14-12 *An ileostomy appliance is emptied by directing it into the toilet and unclamping the end.*

PROCEDURE

Caring for a Resident with an Ileostomy

1. Explain the procedure to the resident.

2. Wash your hands.

3. Collect the following equipment:
   a. Prescribed solvent
   b. Medicine dropper
   c. Clean ileostomy appliance
   d. Clean ostomy belt
   e. Clamp for the appliance
   f. Gauze dressing
   g. Disposable washcloths
   h. Towels
   i. Cotton balls
   j. Prescribed soap or other cleansing agent
   k. Skin barrier as ordered
   l. Soft brush
   m. Deodorant
   n. Robe and slippers
   o. Disposable gloves

4. Arrange the equipment in the resident's bathroom.

5. Identify the resident. Check the ID bracelet and call the resident by name.

6. Provide for privacy.

7. Help the resident put on a robe and slippers.

8. Assist the resident to the bathroom.

9. Help him or her sit on the toilet.

10. Put on the gloves.

11. Direct the appliance into the toilet (see Fig. 14-12). Remove the clamp.

12. Let the appliance empty into the toilet. Wipe the end with toilet tissue. Discard tissue into the toilet. Observe feces for amount, color, consistency, and odor.

13. Disconnect the appliance from the belt. Remove the belt.

14. Apply a few drops of solvent to the skin around the appliance. (Use the medicine dropper.) The appliance will loosen and can be gently removed.

15. Cover the stoma with a gauze dressing to absorb the drainage.

16. Wet the skin around the stoma with a cotton ball soaked with solvent.

17. Clean the skin around the stoma with warm water. Rinse and pat dry. Use soap or other cleansing agent only if ordered.

18. Prepare the skin barrier as ordered.

19. Remove the gauze dressing from the stoma.

20. Apply the skin barrier around the stoma.

21. Add deodorant to the appliance.

22. Apply the appliance. Be sure the bottom is clamped.

23. Put a clean belt on the resident. Connect the belt to the appliance.

24. Remove the gloves.

25. Help the resident wash the hands.

26. Assist the resident back to bed or to a chair.

27. Make sure he or she is comfortable. Place the signal light within reach.

28. Raise or lower side rails as instructed by the nurse.

29. Unscreen the resident.

30. Put on another pair of gloves.

31. Clean the used appliance with soap and water using the soft brush. Wash the belt. Allow both items to dry.

32. Clean and return reusable equipment to its proper place.

33. Discard disposable items in the "dirty" utility room.

34. Remove the gloves.

35. Wash your hands, and report your observations to the nurse.

COLLECTING STOOL SPECIMENS

Stool specimens are sent to the laboratory for study. When internal bleeding is suspected, feces are checked for blood. Stools also are studied for fat, microorganisms, worms, and other abnormal contents. The rules for collecting urine specimens (see Chapter 13, p. 300)

apply when collecting stool specimens. Universal precautions also are necessary and the bloodborne pathogen standard must be followed.

The specimen must not be contaminated with urine. Some tests require a warm stool. The specimen is taken to the laboratory immediately.

PROCEDURE

Collecting a Stool Specimen

1. Explain the procedure to the resident.

2. Wash your hands.

3. Collect the following:
   a. Bedpan and cover (another bedpan may be necessary if the resident needs to urinate) or commode
   b. Urinal
   c. Specimen pan if the bathroom or commode will be used
   d. Specimen container and lid
   e. Tongue blade
   f. Disposable bag
   g. Toilet tissue
   h. Laboratory requisition slip
   i. Disposable gloves

4. Label the container with requested information.

5. Identify the resident. Check the ID bracelet and call the resident by name.

6. Provide for privacy.

7. Offer the bedpan or urinal for urination.

8. Assist the person onto the bedpan or to the commode or toilet. Place the specimen pan under the toilet seat (Fig. 14-13). The resident wears a robe and slippers when up.

9. Ask the resident not to put toilet tissue in the bedpan, commode container, or specimen pan. Provide a disposable bag for toilet tissue.

10. Place the signal light and toilet tissue within reach. Raise side rails if instructed by the nurse.

11. Leave the room if the resident can be alone. Wash your hands.

12. Return when the resident signals. Knock before entering

13. Put on the gloves. Provide perineal care if necessary.

14. Use the tongue blade to take about 2 tablespoons of feces from the bedpan to the specimen container (Fig. 14-14).

15. Put the lid on the container. Do not touch the inside of the lid or container.

16. Place the tongue blade in the bag.

17. Empty, clean, and disinfect the bedpan, commode container, or specimen pan. Return it to its proper place. Remove the gloves.

18. Help the resident wash the hands.

19. Make sure the resident is comfortable. Place the signal light within reach.

20. Raise or lower side rails as instructed by the nurse.

21. Unscreen the resident.

22. Take the specimen and laboratory requisition slip to the designated area.

23. Wash your hands.

24. Report your observations to the nurse.

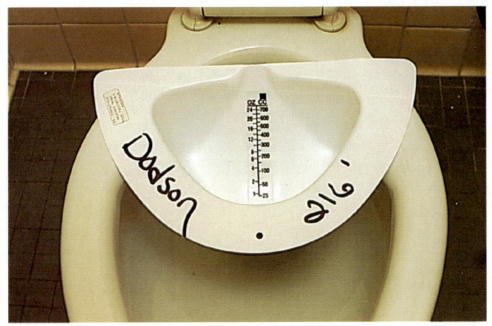

FIGURE 14-13 *A specimen pan is placed in the toilet for a stool specimen.*

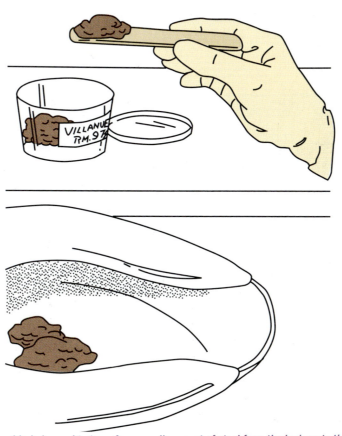

FIGURE 14-14 *A tongue blade is used to transfer a small amount of stool from the bedpan to the specimen container.*

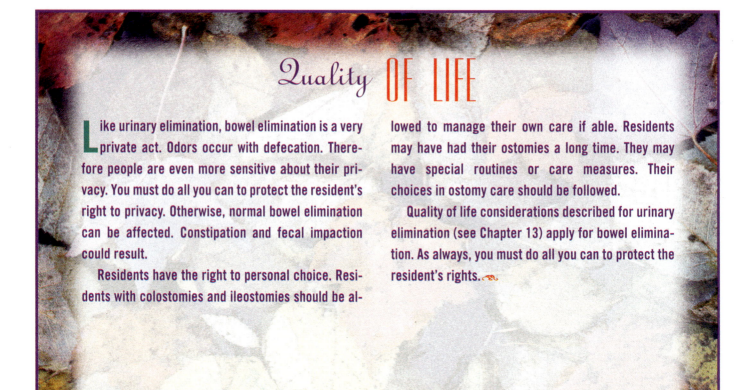

Quality OF LIFE

Like urinary elimination, bowel elimination is a very private act. Odors occur with defecation. Therefore people are even more sensitive about their privacy. You must do all you can to protect the resident's right to privacy. Otherwise, normal bowel elimination can be affected. Constipation and fecal impaction could result.

Residents have the right to personal choice. Residents with colostomies and ileostomies should be al-lowed to manage their own care if able. Residents may have had their ostomies a long time. They may have special routines or care measures. Their choices in ostomy care should be followed.

Quality of life considerations described for urinary elimination (see Chapter 13) apply for bowel elimination. As always, you must do all you can to protect the resident's rights.

SUMMARY

Your responsibilities in assisting persons with bowel elimination are like those relating to urinary elimination. The act of defecation is private. Bowel control is important to people. So are the hygiene practices that follow bowel movements. Physical and mental well-being are closely associated with maintaining normal bowel function. The personal routines related to defecation also affect well-being.

Normal bowel elimination is not always possible. Constipation, fecal impaction, diarrhea, anal incontinence, and flatulence are common problems. The doctor may order enemas, rectal tubes, medications, or dietary changes to relieve the problem. The nurse may direct you to give an enema or insert a rectal tube. The instructions and procedures need to be completely understood before they are carried out. Sometimes ileostomies or colostomies are necessary to treat bowel problems.

When assisting the person with bowel elimination, always consider the person's need for privacy and bowel control. The person's dignity and mental well-being are just as important as the physical act of defecation. In addition, the rules of medical asepsis, universal precautions, cleanliness, skin care, and safety must be followed. The boodborne pathogen standard is also important.

Review QUESTIONS

Circle the best answer.

1. Which is *false?*
   a. A person must have a bowel movement every day.
   b. Stools are normally brown, soft, and formed.
   c. Diarrhea occurs when feces move through the intestines rapidly.
   d. Constipation results when feces move through the large intestine slowly.

2. Bowel elimination is affected by
   a. Privacy and age
   b. Medications and diet
   c. Fluid intake and activity
   d. All of the above

3. The prolonged retention and accumulation of feces in the rectum is called
   a. Constipation
   b. Fecal impaction
   c. Flatulence
   d. Anal incontinence

4. Which will *not* promote comfort and safety in relation to bowel elimination?
   a. Asking visitors to leave the room
   b. Assisting the resident to assume a sitting position
   c. Offering the bedpan after meals
   d. Telling the resident you will return very soon

5. The goal of bowel training is to
   a. Gain control of bowel movements
   b. Develop a regular pattern of elimination
   c. Prevent fecal impaction, constipation, and fecal incontinence
   d. All of the above

6. Which is *not* used for a cleansing enema?
   a. Soap suds
   b. Saline
   c. Oil
   d. Tap water

7. Which is *false?*
   a. Enema solutions should be 105° F (40.5° C).
   b. The left Sims' position is used for an enema.
   c. The enema bag is held 12 inches above the anus.
   d. The enema solution is given rapidly.

8. The enema tube is inserted
   a. 1 to 2 inches
   b. 2 to 4 inches
   c. 4 to 6 inches
   d. 6 to 8 inches

9. Oil-retention enemas are retained
   a. 10 to 15 minutes
   b. 15 to 30 minutes
   c. 30 to 60 minutes
   d. 60 to 90 minutes

10. Rectal tubes are left in place no longer than
    a. 20 to 30 minutes
    b. 10 to 20 minutes
    c. 10 to 15 minutes
    d. 5 to 10 minutes

11. Which statement about colostomies and ileostomies is *false?*
    a. Good skin care around the stoma is essential.
    b. Odors can be controlled with deodorant.
    c. The individual has to wear an appliance.
    d. Feces are always liquid in consistency.

12. The ileostomy appliance usually is emptied
    a. Every 4 to 6 hours
    b. Every morning
    c. Every 2 to 3 days
    d. When the doctor gives the order to do so

Answers

1. a	4. d	7. d	10. a
2. d	5. d	8. b	11. d
3. b	6. c	9. c	12. a

15

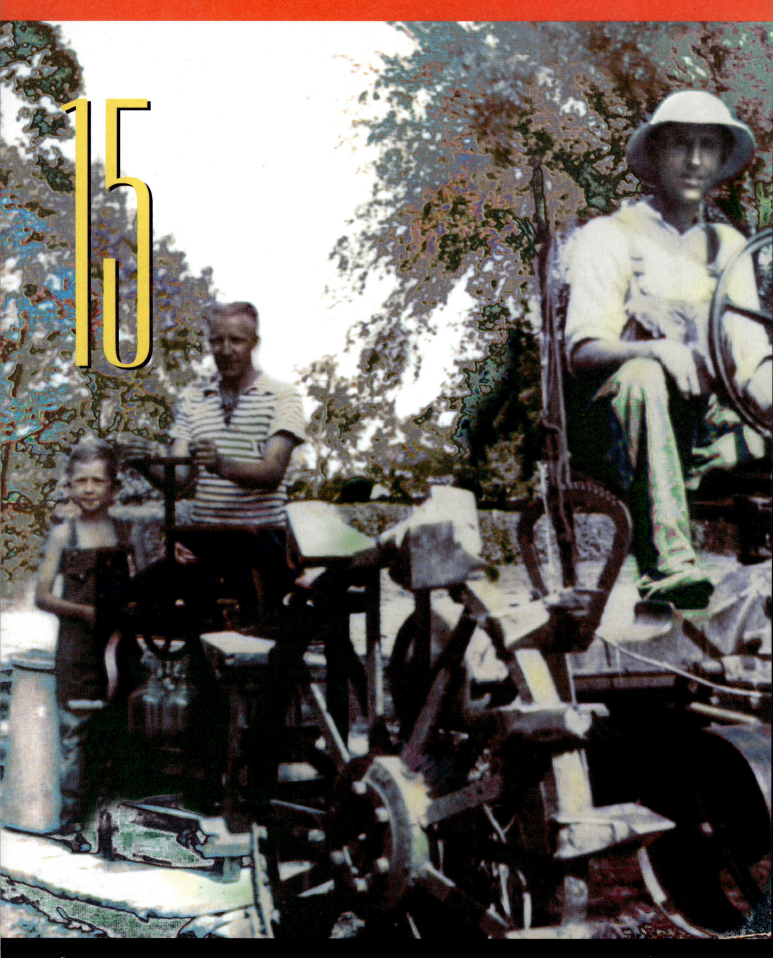

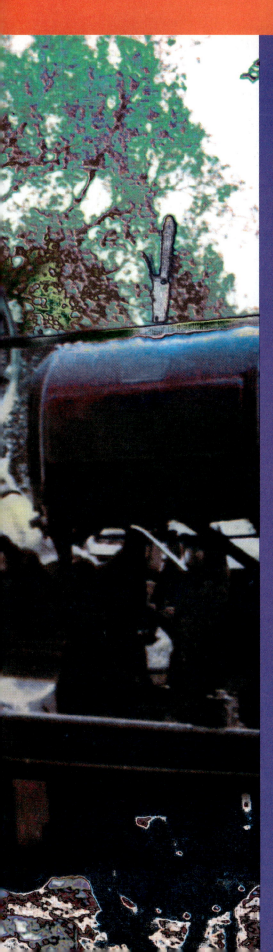

What You Will LEARN

- The key terms listed in this chapter

- How to use the Food Guide Pyramid

- The importance of protein, carbohydrates, and fats and their sources

- The functions of vitamins and minerals and their sources

- Factors that affect eating and nutrition

- Special diets

- Normal adult fluid requirements

- Common causes of dehydration

- Your responsibilities when forced fluids, restricted fluids, and nothing by mouth (NPO) are ordered

- The purpose of intake and output records

- What is counted as fluid intake

- The purpose of between-meal nourishments

- Why tube feedings, intravenous therapy, and hyperalimentation are ordered

- How to promote the resident's quality of life

- How to perform the procedures described in this chapter

anorexia
Loss of appetite

calorie
The amount of energy produced from the burning of food by the body

dehydration
A decrease in the amount of water in body tissues

dysphagia
Difficulty or discomfort in swallowing

edema
The swelling of body tissues with water

gastrostomy
Surgically created opening in the stomach

gavage
Tube feeding

graduate
A calibrated container used to measure fluid

intravenous therapy
Fluid administered through a needle inserted into a vein; IV and IV infusion

nutrient
A substance that is ingested, digested, absorbed, and used by the body

nutrition
The many processes involved in the ingestion, digestion, absorption, and use of foods and fluids by the body

My wife was such a good cook. She baked a lot, too. They try to provide a variety of ethnic meals here to please everyone. But I like when my daughter visits and we can eat together. She usually brings something my wife used to make. I like that.

The need for food and water is a basic physical need. Food and water are necessary for life. The amount and quality of foods and fluids in the diet affect physical and mental well-being. The elderly and disabled may have special dietary needs. A poor diet and poor eating habits place a person at risk for infection and chronic diseases. Chronic illnesses may become worse. Healing problems and abnormalities in physical and mental function also are related to poor diet and eating habits. Poor physical and mental functioning increases the risk for accidents and injuries.

Eating and drinking also provide pleasure. They sometimes are associated with social activity with family and friends. Elderly persons need to have a friendly, social atmosphere at meal times (Fig. 15-1). They may eat poorly if they eat alone.

Dietary practices are influenced by many factors. They include culture, religion, finances, and personal choice. These practices include food selection, preparation, and the way it is served.

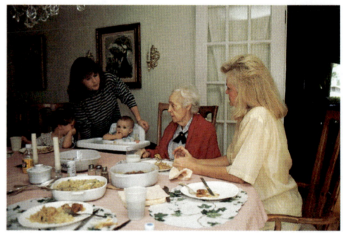

FIGURE 15-1 *Meals are more enjoyable when shared with family and friends.*

BASIC NUTRITION

Nutrition is the many processes involved in the ingestion, digestion, absorption, and use of foods and fluids by the body. Good nutrition is needed for growth, healing, and maintaining body functions. It begins with the proper selection of foods and fluids. Good selections provide a well-balanced diet and the right number of calories. A high-calorie diet will cause weight gain or obesity. Too few calories cause weight loss.

Foods and fluids contain nutrients. A **nutrient** is a substance that is ingested, digested, absorbed, and used by the body. Many nutrients are considered necessary for body functioning. They are grouped into fats, proteins, carbohydrates, vitamins, and minerals.

Fats, proteins, and carbohydrates give the body fuel for energy. The amount of energy provided by a nutrient is measured in calories. A **calorie** is the amount of energy produced when the body burns food. One gram of fat supplies the body with 9 calories. One gram of protein provides 4 calories, and one gram of carbohydrate also supplies 4 calories. Energy is needed for all body functions. Sitting in a chair requires energy. So does living in a coma. The number of calories a person needs depends on many factors. These include age, activity, climate, state of health, and the amount of sleep obtained. Men usually need more calories than women do.

Food Guide Pyramid

In the past good nutrition was based on the four basic food groups: milk and dairy products; meats and fish; fruits and vegetables; and breads and cereals. In 1992 the United States Department of Agriculture (USDA) released its "Food Guide Pyramid." The pyramid replaces the four basic food groups.

The purpose of the Food Guide Pyramid is to make wise food choices (Fig. 15-2). The pyramid has 6 food groups:

- Bread, cereal, rice, and pasta
- Vegetables
- Fruits
- Milk, yogurt, and cheese
- Meat, poultry, fish, dry beans, eggs, and nuts
- Fats, oils, and sweets

The message of the pyramid is to eat more of the foods at the bottom level and lesser amounts at each of the levels that lead to the top. The Food Guide Pyramid encourages a low fat-diet. More bread, cereal, rice, and pasta (lowest level) and more vegetables and fruits (third) level should be eaten. There should be moderate amounts from the milk, yogurt, and cheese group and also from the meat, poultry, fish, beans, eggs, and nut group (second level). Fats, oils, and sweets (top level) should be used sparingly.

Foods from each of the five groups in the lower three levels are needed in the daily diet. Essential nutrients are found in varying amounts in the lower five food groups. No one food or food group contains every nutrient needed by the body.

Note the small circles and triangles in the pyramid (see Fig. 15-2). The small circles are for fat, and the triangles are for sugar. Some sugar and fat naturally occur in all foods. They appear in all levels of the pyramid. There are fewer fats and sugars at the two lower levels of the pyramid. Therefore the bread, vegetable, and fruit groups are low in sugar and fat. More servings are allowed from these groups than from the other groups. The result is a low-fat diet.

The pyramid is for everyone older than 2 years of age. Better health is the goal. Many diseases are related to diet and the kinds of food eaten. They include heart disease, high blood pressure, stroke, adult-onset diabetes, and certain cancers. The risk for such diseases can be reduced by following the Dietary Guidelines for Americans. These seven guidelines were developed by the United States Department of Agriculture and the Department of Health and Human Services.

1. Eat a variety of foods.
2. Maintain a healthy weight.
3. Choose a diet low in fat, saturated fat, and cholesterol.
4. Choose a diet with plenty of vegetables, fruits, and grain products.
5. Use sugars only in moderation.
6. Use salt and sodium only in moderation.
7. If you drink alcoholic beverages, do so in moderation.

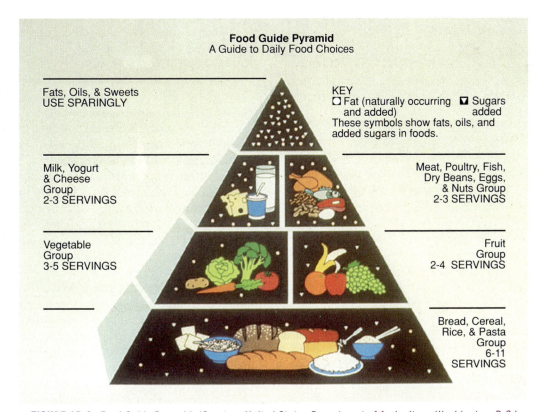

FIGURE 15-2   *Food Guide Pyramid. (Courtesy United States Department of Agriculture, Washington, D.C.)*

Food Guide Pyramid Serving Sizes

Bread Group

1 slice of bread = 1 serving
1 ounce of ready-to-eat cereal = 1 serving
½ cup of cooked cereal, rice, or pasta = 1 serving

Vegetable Group

1 cup raw leafy vegetables = 1 serving
½ cup other cooked or chopped raw vegetables = 1 serving
¾ cup vegetable juice = 1 serving

Fruit Group

1 medium apple, orange, or banana = 1 serving
½ cup chopped, cooked, or canned fruit = 1 serving
¾ cup fruit juice = 1 serving

Milk, Cheese, and Yogurt

1 cup of milk or yogurt = 1 serving
½ to 1 ounce cheese = 1 serving
2 ounces process cheese = 1 serving

Meat, Poultry, Fish, Dry Beans, Eggs, and Nuts

2 to 3 ounces cooked lean meat, poultry, or fish = 1 serving
½ cup cooked dry beans = 1 serving
1 egg = 1 serving
2 tablespoons peanut butter = 1 serving

Fats, Oils, and Sweets

Use sparingly

Breads, cereals, rice, and pasta group. The bread group forms the base of the pyramid. Most servings come from breads, cereals, rice, and pasta. The USDA recommends 6 to 11 servings a day (List 15-1). All foods in the bread group come from grain (e.g., wheat, oats, rice). Protein, carbohydrates, iron, thiamin, niacin, and riboflavin are the main nutrients in this group. Small amounts of fats and sugars also are found.

Such foods as pie, cake, cookies, pastries, doughnuts, and muffins are made from grains. However, they also are made with fats and sugars. Depending on the amount of fat and sugar added, they are high-fat food choices.

Vegetable group. The USDA recommends 3 to 5 servings a day from the vegetable group (see List 15-1). Vegetables provide fiber, vitamins A and C, carbohydrates, and minerals. They are naturally low in fat. A variety of vegetables should be eaten: dark green and yellow vegetables, tomatoes, potatoes, and vegetable juices.

Naturally low in fat, vegetables can become high in fat from food preparation. French fries are very high in fat compared with a baked or boiled potato. Butter, oil, mayonnaise, salad dressing, sour cream, and sauces often are added to vegetables. These toppings are high in fat. Small amounts of low-fat toppings will help keep vegetables low in fat.

Fruit group. Fruits naturally contain some sugar, and they are low in fat. The USDA recommends 2 to 4 servings of fruit daily (see List 15-1). Fruits provide carbohydrates, vitamins A and C, potassium, and other minerals. This group includes all fruits and fruit juices. Fresh fruits and juices are best. Frozen or canned fruits should be unsweetened. Often they are sweetened or syrupy and therefore higher in sugar and calories.

Milk, yogurt, and cheese group. Milk and milk products are high in protein, carbohydrates, fat, calcium, and riboflavin. The USDA recommends 2 to 3 daily servings from the milk group—milk, cheese, and yogurt (see List 15-1). Children and breast-feeding mothers need 3 servings a day.

Skim milk is lower in fat than whole milk. One cup of skim milk has only a trace of fat; 1 cup of whole milk has 8 grams of fat. Low-fat food choices also include cheeses made with skim milk, low or nonfat yogurts, and ice milk rather than ice cream.

Meat, poultry, fish, dry beans, eggs, and nuts group. Meat, poultry, fish, dry beans, eggs, and nuts make up the meat group. The foods in this group are higher in fat than those in the milk, fruit, vegetable, and bread groups. The USDA recommends 2 to 3 servings a day (see List 15-1). Protein, fat, iron, and thiamin are the main nutrients found in this group.

The serving size is very important in planning a well-balanced diet. This is especially important for meat and fish because they contain many calories. Serving size is influenced by many factors, including culture, appetite, personal choice, and the recipe used. A quarter-pound hamburger, a 12-ounce T-bone steak, a 10-ounce lobster tail, and a quarter of a chicken are examples of servings advertised by restaurants. *One serving* in this group is 2 to 3 ounces of boned meat, fish, or poultry. A 12-ounce steak is equal to 4 to 6 servings from this group!

Remember, foods in this group are higher in fat than foods in the other groups (except the fats, oils, and sweets group). The greater the fat, the greater the calories. Wise food choices can lower fat intake from this group. Fish and shellfish are low in fat. Chicken and turkey have less fat than veal, beef, pork, and lamb. Veal is lower in fat than beef. Lean cuts of beef and pork should be used. Egg yolks have more fat than egg whites. Low-fat egg substitutes can be used in cooking and baking.

Food preparation also is important. Fat should be trimmed from meat and poultry. Poultry should be

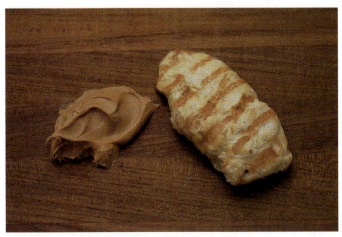

FIGURE 15-3 *Two tablespoons of peanut butter (one serving) equals this 3-ounce chicken breast (one serving).*

skinned. Roasting, broiling, and baking are better than frying. Gravies and sauces also add fat.

Nuts and peanut butter are higher in fat than the other foods in this group. They should be used wisely. As shown in Fig. 15-3, 1 serving of peanut butter (2 tablespoons) is equal to 1 serving of meat (2 to 3 ounces)! Peas and cooked dry beans are very low in fat. They should be used often.

Fats, oils, and sweets. Fats, oils, and sweets are at the very top of the pyramid. The USDA recommends that they be used sparingly. There are no recommended servings or serving sizes. They should be used as little as possible. There is little nutritional value in fats, oils, and sweets (foods with added sugar). However, they are very high in calories. Foods in this group include cooking oils, shortening, butter, margarine, salad dressing, soft drinks, all candy, sour cream, cream cheese, frosting, cookies, cake, pie, ice cream, and many desserts. Some foods are high in fat, some in added sugar, and some in both. Butter and oil are high in fat. Soft drinks, jellies, jams, and syrups are high in added sugar. So are coffee and cereal if sugar is added at the table. Chocolate and ice cream are examples of food high in both fat and added sugar.

Alcohol also is included in this group. Beer, wine, champagne, whiskey, vodka, gin, and Scotch, are examples of alcoholic drinks. If used at all, alcohol intake should be moderate.

Nutrients

No one food or food group contains every essential nutrient needed by the body. A well-balanced diet consists of servings from the five foods in the lower three levels of the Food Guide Pyramid. It ensures an adequate intake of the essential nutrients.

Protein. Protein is the most important nutrient—it is needed for tissue growth and repair. Sources of protein include meat, fish, poultry, eggs, milk and milk products, cereals, beans, peas, and nuts. Foods high in protein usually are expensive. Therefore people with low incomes often lack protein in their diets.

Each body cell is made up of protein. Excessive protein intake causes some protein to be excreted in the urine. Some protein changes into body fat and some into carbohydrates.

Carbohydrates. Carbohydrates give the body energy and provide fiber for bowel elimination. Carbohydrates are found in fruits, vegetables, breads, cereals, and sugar. These foods are rather inexpensive. Rarely are carbohydrates lacking in the diet.

Carbohydrates are broken down into sugars during digestion. The sugars are then absorbed into the blood stream. The fiber in foods that contain carbohydrates is not digested. It provides the bulky part of chyme in the elimination process. Excess carbohydrate intake results in some of the nutrient being stored in the liver. The rest changes into body fat.

Fats. Fats also provide energy. In addition to energy, fats have other functions. They add flavor to food and help the body use certain vitamins. Fats also conserve body heat and protect organs from injury. Dietary sources of fat include the fat in meats, lard, butter, shortenings, salad and vegetable oils, milk, cheese, egg yolks, and nuts. These sources are more expensive than carbohydrate sources. Dietary fat not needed by the body is stored as body fat (adipose tissue).

Vitamins. Although they do not provide calories, vitamins are essential nutrients. They are ingested through food and cannot be produced by the body. Vitamins A, D, E, and K can be stored by the body. Vitamin C and the B complex vitamins are not stored. They must be ingested daily. Each vitamin is necessary for certain body functions. The lack of a particular vitamin results in signs and symptoms of a particular disease. List 15-2 on p. 336. summarizes the sources and major functions of common vitamins.

Minerals. A well-balanced diet supplies the necessary amounts of minerals. Minerals are involved in many body processes. They are needed for bone and teeth formation, nerve and muscle function, fluid balance, and other body processes. List 15-3 on p. 336 summarizes the major functions and dietary sources of common minerals.

List 15-2

Major Functions and Sources of Common Vitamins

Vitamin	Major functions	Sources
Vitamin A	Growth; vision; healthy hair, skin, and mucous membranes; resistance to infection	Liver, spinach, green leafy and yellow vegetables, fruits, fish liver oils, egg yolk, butter, cream, milk
Vitamin B_1 (thiamin)	Muscle tone; nerve function; digestion; appetite; normal elimination; utilization of carbohydrates	Pork, liver and other organ meats, breads and cereals, potatoes, peas, beans, and soybeans
Vitamin B_2 (riboflavin)	Growth; healthy eyes; protein and carbohydrate metabolism; healthy skin and mucous membranes	Milk and milk products, organ meats, green leafy vegetables, eggs, breads and cereals
Vitamin B_3 (niacin)	Protein, fat, and carbohydrate metabolism; functioning of the nervous system; appetite; functioning of the digestive system	Meat, poultry, fish, peanut butter, breads and cereals, peas and beans, eggs, liver
Vitamin B_{12}	Formation of red blood cells; protein metabolism; functioning of the nervous system	Liver and other organ meats, meats, fish, eggs, green leafy vegetables
Folic acid	Formation of red blood cells; functioning of the intestines; protein metabolism	Liver, meats, fish, yeast, green leafy vegetables, eggs, mushrooms
Vitamin C (ascorbic acid)	Formation of substances that hold tissues together; healthy blood vessels, skin, gums, bones, and teeth; wound healing; prevention of bleeding; resistance to infection	Citrus fruits, tomatoes, potatoes, cabbage, strawberries, green vegetables, melons
Vitamin D	Absorption and metabolism of calcium and phosphorus; healthy bones	Fish liver oils, milk, butter, liver, exposure to sunlight
Vitamin E	Normal reproduction; formation of red blood cells; muscle function	Vegetable oils, milk, eggs, meats, fish, cereals, green leafy vegetables
Vitamin K	Blood clotting	Liver, green leafy vegetables, margarine, soybean and vegetable oils, eggs

List 15-3

The Major Functions and Sources of Common Minerals

Mineral	Major function	Source
Calcium	Formation of teeth and bones; blood clotting; muscle contraction; heart function; nerve function	Milk and milk products, green leafy vegetables
Phosphorus	Formation of bones and teeth; utilization of proteins, fats, and carbohydrates; nerve and muscle function	Meat, fish, poultry, milk and milk products, nuts, eggs
Iron	Allows red blood cells to carry oxygen	Liver and other organ meats, egg yolks, green leafy vegetables, breads and cereals
Iodine	Thyroid gland function, growth, and metabolism	Iodized salt, seafood and shellfish, vegetables
Sodium	Fluid balance; nerve and muscle function	Almost all foods
Potassium	Nerve function; muscle contraction; heart function	Fruits, vegetables, cereals, coffee, meats

FACTORS THAT AFFECT EATING AND NUTRITION

Nutrition and eating habits are influenced by many factors. Some habits begin during infancy and continue throughout life. Others develop later.

Culture

Dietary practices are greatly influenced by culture. The foods available in the region of a particular ethnic group also influence diet. Rice and tea are common in the diets of Chinese, Japanese, Korean, and other peoples of the Far East. Hispanic people like spicy foods such as tacos, tamales, and burritos. They also prefer rice, beans, and corn. Italians are known for spaghetti, lasagna, and other pastas. Scandinavians have a lot of fish in their diet. Americans enjoy foods from the meat group, fast foods, and processed foods (canned, packaged, and frozen foods).

Culture also influences food preparation. Frying, baking, smoking, or roasting food, or eating raw food, are influenced by culture. So is the use of sauces and spices.

Religion

Many religious beliefs involve dietary practices. Some religions have rules for selecting, preparing, and eating food. Some religions require days of fasting. During a fast, all or certain foods are avoided. Members of a religious group may not follow every dietary practice of their faith. Others follow all dietary teachings. You need to respect the resident's religious dietary practices. The right to personal choice must be protected. List 15-4 summarizes dietary practices of the major religious groups.

Finances

Cost of food is a major factor in a person's food choices. People with limited incomes, such as the elderly, usually buy cheaper carbohydrate foods. Therefore their diets lack protein and certain vitamins and minerals.

List 15-4

Religion and Dietary Practices

Religion	Dietary practice
Adventist (Seventh Day Adventist)	Coffee, tea, and alcohol are not allowed; beverages with caffeine (colas) are not allowed; some groups forbid the eating of meat
Baptist	Some groups forbid coffee, tea, and alcohol
Christian Scientist	Alcohol and coffee are not allowed
Church of Jesus Christ of Latter Day Saints (Mormon)	Alcohol and hot drinks, such as coffee and tea, are not allowed; meat is not forbidden, but members are encouraged to eat meat infrequently
Greek Orthodox Church	Wednesdays, Fridays, and Lent are days of fasting; meat and dairy products are usually avoided during days of fast
Islamic (Muslim or Moslem)	All pork and pork products are forbidden; alcohol is not allowed except for medical reasons
Judaism (Jewish faith)	Foods must be kosher (prepared according to Jewish law); meat of kosher animals (cows, goats, and sheep) can be eaten; chickens, ducks, and geese are kosher fowls; kosher fish have scales and fins, such as tuna, sardines, carp, and salmon; shellfish cannot be eaten; milk, milk products, and eggs from kosher animals and fowl are acceptable; milk and milk products cannot be eaten with or immediately after eating meat; milk and milk products can be eaten 6 hours after eating meat; milk and milk products can be part of the same meal with meat—they are served separately and before the meat; kosher foods cannot be prepared in utensils used to prepare nonkosher foods; breads, cakes, cookies, noodles, and alcoholic beverages are not consumed during Passover
Roman Catholic	Fasting for 1 hour before receiving Holy Communion; fasting from meat on Ash Wednesday and Good Friday—some may continue to fast from meat on Fridays

Appetite

Appetite relates to the desire for food. Hunger is an unpleasant feeling caused by the lack of food. Hunger causes a person to seek food and eat until the appetite is satisfied. Food aromas and thoughts also can stimulate the appetite. However, loss of appetite, known as **anorexia,** can occur. Illness, medications, unpleasant thoughts or sights, anxiety, fear, and depression are among the causes of anorexia. Elderly persons may have loss of appetite from decreased senses of taste and smell.

Personal Choice

The like or dislike of particular foods is an individual matter. Food preferences begin in childhood. They are influenced by the kinds of food served in the home. As a child grows older, new foods are introduced through school and social activities. Many people decide whether they like or dislike a certain food by the way it looks, the way it is prepared, its smell, or recipe ingredients. Usually food preferences expand with age and social experiences.

Food choices also are influenced by body reactions. People usually avoid foods that cause allergic reactions, nausea, vomiting, diarrhea, indigestion, gas, or headaches.

Nursing facilities allow residents some choice in the foods served. Meals must be balanced. Residents are encouraged to choose food from the five food groups. They can make personal choices from food menus (Fig. 15-4). Some facilities involve resident groups in planning special meals. Holiday meals—Christmas, St. Patrick's Day, Easter, Fourth of July, Labor Day, and Thanksgiving—may be planned by residents. Such events as picnics and pizza parties also may be planned (Fig. 15-5). Remember, residents have the right to personal choice.

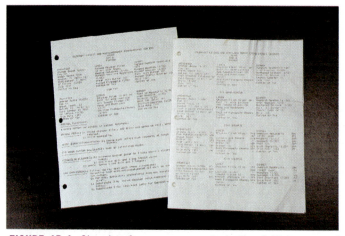

FIGURE 15-4 *Choosing from a menu protects the right to personal choice.*

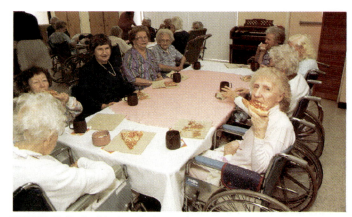

FIGURE 15-5 *Residents enjoying a pizza party.*

Illness

Appetite usually decreases during illness and recovery from injuries. Nutritional needs, however, are increased at these times. The body needs to fight infection, heal tissue, and replace lost blood cells. Nutrients lost through vomiting and diarrhea also must be replaced. Some diseases and medications cause a sore mouth, which makes eating painful. The loss of teeth also affects chewing. So do poor fitting dentures. Therefore foods that provide protein (the meat group) may be hard to chew.

SPECIAL DIETS

Doctors may order special diets. Such diets may be ordered because of a nutritional deficiency or a disease. They also may be ordered to eliminate or decrease certain substances in the diet or for weight control. The doctor, nurses, and dietitian work together to meet the resident's nutritional needs. They consider the need for dietary changes, personal choices, religion, culture, and eating problems.

Many residents do not need special diets. *General diet, regular diet,* and *house diet* are terms used in many facilities when there are no dietary restrictions or changes. Special or therapeutic diets may be ordered for residents with diabetes or diseases of the heart, kidneys, gallbladder, liver, stomach, or intestines. Residents with pressure sores or other wounds are likely to have high-protein diets. Added protein is needed for healing. Bran may be added to the diets of elderly or disabled persons. It provides fiber necessary for good bowel health. Some residents need special textured foods in their diets. Those with chewing or swallowing problems may need to have meat ground. Others need all foods pureed. Allergies, obesity, and other disorders also require therapeutic diets. List 15-5 summarizes the common therapeutic diets.

The sodium-restricted diet and diabetic diet are commonly ordered. You are likely to encounter these diets in nursing facilities.

Text continued on p. 340.

List 15-5

Common Therapeutic Diets

Diet	Description	Use	Foods allowed
Clear-liquid	Clear liquids that do not leave a residue; nonirritating and nongasforming	Postoperatively; for acute illness and nausea and vomiting	Water, tea, and coffee (without milk or cream); carbonated beverages; gelatin; clear fruit juices (apple, grape, and cranberry); fat-free clear broth; hard candy, sugar, and popsicles
Full-liquid	Foods that are liquid at room temperature or that melt at body temperature	Advance from clear-liquid diet; postoperatively, for stomach irritation, fever, and nausea and vomiting	All foods allowed on a clear-liquid diet; custard; eggnog; strained soups; strained fruit and vegetable juices; milk; creamed cereals; ice cream and sherbet
Soft	Semisolid foods that are easily digested	Advance from full-liquid diet; for chewing difficulties, gastrointestinal disorders, and infections	All liquids; eggs (not fried); boiled, baked, or roasted meat, fish, or poultry; mild cheeses (American, Swiss, cheddar, cream, and cottage); strained fruit juices; refined bread and crackers; cooked or pureed vegetables; cooked or canned fruit without skin or seeds; pudding; plain cakes
Low-residue	Food that leaves a small amount of residue in the colon	For diseases of the colon and diarrhea	Coffee, tea, milk, carbonated beverages, strained fruit juices; refined bread and crackers; creamed and refined cereal; rice; cottage and cream cheese; eggs (not fried); plain puddings and cakes; gelatin; custard; sherbet and ice cream; strained vegetable juices; canned or cooked fruit without skin or seed; potatoes (not fried); strained cooked vegetables; plain pasta
High-residue	Foods that increase the amount of residue in the colon to stimulate peristalsis	For constipation and colon disorders	All fruits and vegetables; whole wheat bread; whole grain cereals; fried foods; whole grain rice; milk, cream, butter, and cheese; meats
Bland	Foods that are mechanically and chemically nonirritating and low in roughage; foods served at moderate temperatures; strong spices and condiments are avoided	For ulcers, gallbladder disorders, and some intestinal disorders; postoperatively following abdominal surgery	Lean meats; white bread; creamed and refined cereals; cream or cottage cheese; gelatin, plain puddings, cakes, and cookies; eggs (not fried); butter and cream; canned fruits and vegetables without skin and seeds; strained fruit juices; potatoes (not fried); pastas and rice; strained or soft cooked carrots, peas, beets, spinach, squash, and asparagus tips; creamed soups from allowed vegetables; no fried foods are allowed

Continued.

Diet	Description	Use	Foods allowed
High-calorie	The number of calories is increased to approximately 4000; includes three full meals and between-meal snacks	For weight gain and some thyroid imbalances	Dietary increases in all foods
Low-calorie	The number of calories is reduced below the minimum daily requirements	For weight reduction	Foods low in fats and carbohydrates and lean meats; avoid butter, cream, rice, gravies, salad oils, noodles, cakes, pastries, carbonated and alcohlic beverages, candy, potato chips, and similar foods
High-iron	Foods that are high in iron	For anemia; following blood loss; for women during the reproductive years	Liver and other organ meats; lean meats; egg yolks; shellfish; dried fruits; dried beans; green leafy vegetables; lima beans; peanut butter; enriched breads and cereals
Low-fat (low cholesterol)	Protein and carbohydrates are increased with a limited amount of fat in the diet	For heart disease, gallbladder disease, disorders of fat digestion, and liver disease	Skim milk or buttermilk; cottage cheese (no other cheese are allowed); gelatin; sherbet; fruit; lean meat, poultry, and fish (baked, broiled, or roasted); fat-free broth; soups made with skim milk; margarine; rice, pasta, breads and cereals; vegetables; potatoes
High-protein	Protein is increased to aid and promote tissue healing	For burns, high fever, infection, and some liver diseases	Meat, milk, eggs, cheese, fish, poultry; breads and cereals; green leafy vegetables
Sodium-restricted	A specific amount of sodium is allowed; there are five basic levels of sodium restriction ranging from mild to severe	For heart disease, fluid retention, and some kidney diseases	Fruits and vegetables and unsalted butter are allowed; adding salt at the table is not allowed; highly salted foods and foods high in sodium are not allowed; the use of salt during cooking may be restricted
Diabetic	The amount of carbohydrates and number of calories are regulated; protein and fat are also regulated	For diabetes mellitus	Determined by nutritional and energy requirements

The Sodium-Restricted Diet

The average amount of sodium in the daily diet is 3000 to 5000 mg. The body needs only half this amount. Healthy people excrete excess sodium in the urine. Heart and kidney diseases, however, cause the body to retain the extra sodium.

Sodium-restricted diets are ordered for residents with heart disease. They also may be ordered for those with liver or kidney disease, hypertension (high blood pressure) or for those taking certain medications. Sodium causes the body to retain water. If there is too much sodium, the body retains more water. Body tissues swell with water, and there is excess fluid in the blood vessels. The increased fluid in the tissues and bloodstream forces the heart to work harder. In other words, the workload of the heart increases. With heart disease, the extra workload can cause serious complications or death. Restricting the amount of sodium in the diet decreases the amount of sodium in the body. The body retains less water. Less water in the tissues and blood vessels reduces the amount of work for the heart.

There are five levels of sodium-restricted diets. They range from mild to severe. The doctor orders the amount of restriction for the person. Some residents on sodium-restricted diets will return home. They need to know which foods are high and low in sodium. They also need to know how to calculate the amount of sodium in the diet. The nurse or dietitian will teach the resident and family about the diet.

1. *2000 to 3000 mg sodium diet.* This is called the low-salt or no added salt diet. Sodium restriction is "mild." A minimum amount of salt is used in cooking. Salt is not added to foods at the table. Highly salted foods and salty seasonings (e.g., ketchup, celery salt, garlic salt, chili sauce) are omitted from the diet. Canned and processed foods high in salt are not used. Ham, bacon, frankfurters, potato chips, olives, pickles, luncheon meats, and salted or smoked fish are omitted.

2. *1000 mg sodium diet.* Sodium restriction is "moderate." Food is cooked without salt. Foods high in sodium are omitted from the diet. Vegetables with a high amount of sodium are restricted in amount. Salt-free products, such as salt-free bread, are used. Diet planning is necessary.

3. *800 mg sodium diet.* Restrictions for the low-salt diet and the 1000 mg diet are followed. Diet planning is needed to further reduce the amount of sodium in the diet.

4. *500 mg sodium diet.* Sodium restriction is "strict." Restrictions for the less restricted diets are followed. Only fresh vegetables are allowed. Vegetables high in sodium are omitted, such as beets, carrots, celery, spinach, mustard greens, and saurkraut. Milk is limited to 2 cups per day, and only 1 egg per day is allowed. Meat is limited to 5 to 6 ounces per day. Diet planning is essential.

5. *250 mg sodium diet.* This diet is described as "severe." The diet is similar to the 500 mg sodium diet. However, regular whole and skim milk are eliminated. Low-sodium milk can be used instead.

The Diabetic Diet

The diabetic diet is ordered for persons with diabetes mellitus. *Diabetes mellitus* is a chronic disease in which there is a deficiency of insulin in the body (see Chapter 23). Insulin is produced and secreted by the pancreas and is needed for the body to use sugar. If there is not enough insulin, sugar builds up in the bloodstream rather than being used by body cells for energy. Diabetes usually is treated with oral medications or insulin therapy, diet, and exercise.

Carbohydrates are broken down into sugar during digestion. With the diabetic diet the amount of carbohydrates is controlled. The person takes in only the amount of carbohydrates needed by the body. Unneeded carbohydrates are eliminated from the diet so that the body does not have to use or store the excess. Therefore the diabetic diet involves the right amount and right kind of food for the person. The doctor determines how much carbohydrate, fat, protein, and calories a person needs. Age, sex, activity, and weight are considered in determining the person's diet.

The calories and nutrients allowed are divided among 3 meals and between-meal nourishments. The resident must eat only what is allowed and all that is allowed. This is important so that the resident does not get too much or too little carbohydrates. The American Diabetes Association has food lists with equal value in terms of nutrients and calories. These foods are grouped into 6 categories called "exchange lists" or "exchanges." They are milk, vegetables, fruits, bread, meat foods, and fat. Exchanges allow variety in menu planning. For example, a person may not want grapefruit. The dietitian or nurse helps the resident check the exchange list for fruits. The residents finds an orange more appealing. The resident notes that one small orange equals one-half grapefruit. Therefore the resident knows how much to eat. The nurse and dietitian help the resident and family learn how to use the exchange lists.

You must serve the resident's tray on time. The person with diabetes must eat at regular intervals to maintain a certain blood sugar level. You need to check the tray to determine what has been eaten. If all food has not been eaten, notify the nurse. A between-meal nourishment will be needed. The nourishment makes up for what was not eaten at the regular meal. The amount of insulin given also depends on the resident's daily food intake. You must inform the nurse of any change in a diabetic resident's eating habits.

OBRA DIETARY REQUIREMENTS

OBRA requires that residents have a well-balanced diet. The diet must be nourishing and must taste good. The nutritional and special dietary needs of each resident must be met.

Flavor and appearance of food are important. OBRA requires that residents be served appetizing food. That is, food should have an appealing aroma and be attractively served. Food also should be well-seasoned. It must not be too salty or too sweet. Temperature is important. OBRA requires that hot food be served hot and cold food served cold. Facilities have special food servers to keep food hot and cold as appropriate. Food should be served promptly in dining rooms. Residents who eat in their rooms need to have trays served promptly. Otherwise hot food will cool and cold food will warm. Survey teams (see Chapter 1) actually taste the food and measure the temperature to make sure the facility is meeting OBRA requirements.

OBRA also requires that food be prepared to meet the individual needs of each resident. Some residents need food cut, ground, or chopped. Others need special diets ordered by the doctor. Survey teams will check to make sure the resident is getting the special diet as ordered.

Each resident must receive at least three meals per day and a bedtime snack. The facility also must provide any special eating equipment and utensils that may be needed (Fig. 15-6). Hands, wrists, and arms may be affected by disease or injury. Special equipment may be needed so that the resident can eat independently. You must make sure that the resident uses needed equipment.

FLUID BALANCE

After oxygen, water is the most important physical need for survival. Death can result from inadequate water intake or from excessive fluid loss. Water enters the body through fluids and foods. Water is lost through the urine and feces. It also is lost through the skin, as perspiration, and through the lungs, with expiration. Fluid balance is important for health. There must be a balance between the amount of fluid taken in and the amount lost.

The amount of fluid taken in and the amount lost must be equal. If fluid intake exceeds fluid output (the amount lost), body tissues swell with water. This is called **edema.** Edema is common in persons with heart and kidney diseases. **Dehydration** is a decrease in the amount of water in body tissues. It results when fluid output exceeds intake. Inadequate fluid intake, vomiting, diarrhea, bleeding, excessive sweating, and increased urine production are common causes of dehydration.

Normal Requirements

An adult needs 1500 ml of water daily to survive. About 2000 to 2500 ml of fluid per day is required to maintain normal fluid balance. The water requirement increases with hot weather temperatures, exercise, fever, and illness. Excessive fluid loss also increases the water re-

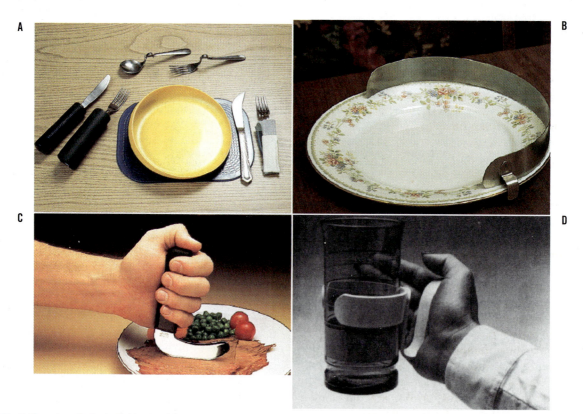

FIGURE 15-6 *Eating utensils for individuals with special needs. A, Note the curved fork, which fits over the hand. The rounded plate helps keep food on the plate. Special grips and swivel handles are helpful for some persons. B, Plate guards help keep food on the plate. C, Knives with rounded blades are rocked back and forth to cut food. They eliminate the need to have a fork in one hand and a knife in the other. D, Glass or cup holder. (Courtesy Bissell Healthcare Corp.; Fred Sammons, Inc.)*

quirement. Elderly persons may have a decreased sense of thirst. Their bodies need water, but they may not feel thirsty. You need to offer water often. Some residents will have special orders. The nurse will give you needed information.

Special Orders

The doctor may order the amount of fluid that a resident can have during a 24-hour period. This is done to maintain fluid balance. It may be necessary to *force fluids*. Force fluids means that the person needs to drink an increased amount of fluid. The force fluids order includes the specific amount of fluid to be ingested. When force fluids are ordered, a sign is placed above the bed. Records are kept of the amount taken in. The resident is given a variety of fluids allowed on the diet. Fluids must be kept within the person's reach and served at the correct temperature. Fluids are offered regularly to residents who cannot feed themselves.

The doctor may write an order to *restrict fluids*. Fluids are restricted to a specific amount. Water is offered in small amounts and in small containers. The water pitcher is removed from the room or kept out of sight. Like the force-fluids order, a sign is posted above the bed, and accurate intake records are kept. The resident needs to have frequent oral hygiene to help keep mucous membranes of the mouth moist.

Some residents can have **nothing by mouth.** They cannot eat or drink anything. **NPO** is the abbreviation for the Latin term *nil per os*, which means nothing by mouth. NPO often is prescribed before residents are to have some laboratory tests or x-ray procedures, as well as in the treatment of certain illnesses. Residents who are tube fed may be NPO. An NPO sign is posted above the bed. The water pitcher and glass are removed. Frequent oral hygiene is important, but the resident must not swallow any fluid. The NPO status begins at midnight before scheduled laboratory tests or x-ray examinations.

Intake and Output Records

The doctor or nurse may order that all of a resident's fluid intake and output (I&O) be measured. This order involves keeping records. I&O records are used to evaluate fluid balance and kidney function. They help in evaluating and planning medical treatment. They also are necessary when fluid intake must be forced or restricted.

All fluids taken by mouth are measured, and the amount is recorded. IV fluids and tube feedings also are measured. The obvious fluids are measured: water, milk, coffee, tea, juices, soups, and soft drinks. Soft and semisolid foods such as ice cream, sherbet, custard, pudding, creamed cereals, gelatin, and popsicles also are measured. Output includes urinary output, vomitus, diarrhea, and wound drainage.

Measuring Intake and Output

Intake and output are measured in milliliters (ml) or in cubic centimeters (cc). These metric system measurements are equal in amount. One ounce equals 30 ml. A pint is about 500 ml. There are about 1000 ml in a quart. You need to know the fluid capacity of the bowls, dishes, cups, pitchers, glasses, and other containers used to serve fluids. Most facilities have tables on the I&O record for use in measuring intake.

A container called a **graduate** is used to measure fluids. You will use it to measure leftover fluids, urine, vomitus, and drainage from suction (see Chapter 21). The graduate is like a measuring cup; it shows calibrations for amounts. Some graduates are marked in ounces and in milliliters or cubic centimeters (Fig. 15-7). Plastic urinals and emesis basins often are calibrated.

An I&O record is kept at the bedside. Whenever fluid is ingested or output measured, the amount is recorded in the correct column (Fig. 15-8, p. 344). The amounts are totaled at the end of the shift. The nurse records the amount in the resident's record. The resident's I&O also is communicated to the oncoming shift during the end-of-shift report. The nurse is responsible for recording any intake through IV therapy or tube feedings.

The purpose of measuring intake and output and how to help in the process are explained to the resident. Some residents measure and record their intake. The urinal, commode, bedpan, or specimen pan is used for urination. Remind the resident not to put toilet tissue into the container. Also remind the resident not to urinate in the toilet.

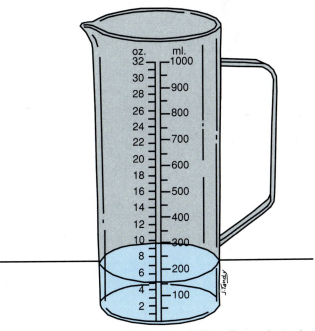

FIGURE 15-7 *A graduate calibrated in milliliters. The graduate shown is filled to 150 ml.*

DAILY INTAKE AND OUTPUT RECORD
(Bedside record)

Intake   Output

11-7

Time	Oral	IV		Time	Urine	Emesis	Drainage	

Total: _____   Total: _____

7-3

Time	Oral	IV		Time	Urine	Emesis	Drainage	

Total: _____   Total: _____

3-11

Time	Oral	IV		Time	Urine	Emesis	Drainage	

Total: _____   Total: _____

Water glass	= 150 ml	Milk carton	= 240 ml
Coffee pot	= 200 ml	Large paper cup	= 240 ml
Ice cream	= 60 ml	(like for eggnog,	
Coffee cup	= 120 ml	shakes, etc.)	
Soup bowl	= 180 ml	Jello per serving	= 120 ml

FIGURE 15-8 *An intake and output record.*

PROCEDURE

Measuring Intake and Output

1. Explain the procedure to the resident.

2. Collect the following:
   a. Intake and output (I&O) record
   b. Two I&O labels
   c. Graduate
   d. Disposable gloves

3. Place the I&O record at the bedside or on the room door (check facility policy).

4. Place one label in the bathroom. Place the other in the appropriate place near the bed.

5. Measure intake as follows:
   a. Pour liquid remaining in a container into the graduate.
   b. Measure the amount at eye level.
   c. Check the amount of the serving on the I&O record.
   d. Subtract the remaining amount from the full serving amount.
   e. Repeat steps 5a through 5d for each liquid.
   f. Add the amounts from 5e together. Record the amount and time on the I&O record.

6. Measure output as follows (wear gloves for this step):
   a. Pour fluid into the graduate.
   b. Measure the amount at eye level.
   c. Record the amount and time on the I&O record.
   d. Dispose of fluid in the toilet.
   e. Rinse and return the graduate to its proper place.
   f. Clean and rinse the bedpan, urinal, emesis basin, or other drainage container. Return it to its proper place.

7. Remove the gloves.

8. Wash your hands.

9. Report your observations to the nurse.

ASSISTING THE RESIDENT WITH FOODS AND FLUIDS

Weakness, illness, and confusion can affect a resident's appetite and ability to eat. So can unpleasant odors, sights, and sounds. Uncomfortable positions, the need for oral hygiene, or the need to use the bathroom also affect appetite. Residents vary in mental and physical abilities. Some are alert and oriented and enjoy being together for meals. Others like to eat in their rooms. Others are confused and noisy at mealtime. Some residents are incontinent or have other odor problems. Some are too weak or ill to be out of their rooms for meals. Because of these different situations, facilities have special dining and feeding programs.

In a *social dining* program, residents eat in a dining room. There are 4 or 6 persons at a table (Fig. 15-9). Tables have tablecloths or placemats. Food is served as in a restaurant. This program is for residents who are oriented and can feed themselves. Sometimes quietly confused

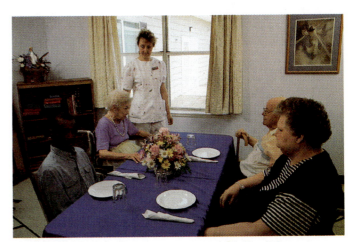

FIGURE 15-9 *Residents enjoy a pleasant meal in the dining room.*

residents are included if they can feed themselves and have good table manners.

Family dining is like social dining except that food is served differently. Food is placed in bowls and on platters. Residents serve themselves from these dishes as they would at home (Fig. 15-10).

Some facilities have *social feeder programs*. Circular or horseshoe-shaped dining tables are placed in a dining room. Residents who need to be fed are seated around these tables. Nursing assistants sit at the center of the tables and feed 4 to 8 residents (Fig. 15-11). The program has two advantages. Very confused residents can be with others at mealtime. Each nursing assistant can feed several residents at one time.

Residents must be comfortable. Their surroundings need to be free of unpleasant sights and odors at mealtime. Mealtime will be more pleasant if residents are properly prepared. Give oral care, and have residents urinate before going to their dining areas. Incontinent residents should be clean and dry. Mealtime enjoyment and comfort can be increased by removing unpleasant equipment from the room. Helping residents assume comfortable eating positions is also important.

PROCEDURE

Getting the Resident Ready for Meals

1. Explain to the resident that it is mealtime.

2. Wash your hands.

3. Collect the following:
   a. Equipment for oral hygiene
   b. Bedpan or urinal and toilet tissue
   c. Wash basin
   d. Soap
   e. Washcloth
   f. Towel
   g. Disposable gloves

4. Provide for privacy.

5. Assist with oral hygiene (use universal precautions). Be sure that dentures are in place if the resident uses them.

6. Offer the bedpan or urinal, or assist the resident to the bathroom. Make sure the incontinent resident is clean and dry. Use universal precautions for this step.

7. Help the resident wash the hands.

8. Do the following for residents who are bedfast:
   a. Raise the head of the bed to a comfortable sitting position.
   b. Position the overbed table in front of the resident. Make sure it is clean.
   c. Place the signal light within reach.
   d. Unscreen the resident.

9. Do the following for residents who eat in their rooms.
   a. Be sure the resident is comfortable in a chair or wheelchair.
   b. Remove items from the overbed table. Make sure it is clean.
   c. Position the overbed table in front of the resident. Adjust the height as needed.
   d. Place the signal light within reach.
   e. Unscreen the resident.

10. Assist residents in special dining programs to the correct dining area. Follow facility procedure for the dining programs.

11. Return to the room.

12. Clean and return equipment to its proper place. Use universal precautions.

13. Straighten the area. Eliminate unpleasant noise, odors, or equipment.

14. Wash your hands.

Serving Meal Trays

Meals are served in containers that keep foods hot or cold as appropriate. You will serve meal trays after preparing residents for the meals and assisting them to dining areas. Trays must be served promptly. Food must be at the desired temperature when the resident receives it. Trays are served last to residents who must be fed.

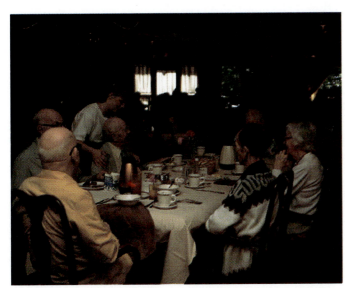

FIGURE 15-10 *These residents enjoy family dining. They serve themselves from bowls and platters of food.*

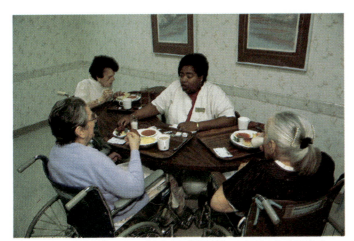

FIGURE 15-11 *Special dining tables are used for social feeder programs. The nursing assistant can feed several residents at one time. Residents can be in the company of others.*

PROCEDURE

Serving Meal Trays

1. Wash your hands.

2. Check items on the tray with the dietary card to make sure the tray is complete.

3. Identify the resident. Check the ID bracelet with the dietary card.

4. Have the resident in a sitting position if possible.

5. Place the tray on the overbed table within easy reach of the resident. Adjust table height as necessary.

6. Remove food covers. Open milk cartons and cereal boxes, cut meat, butter bread, etc., if indicated (Fig. 15-12).

7. Place the napkin and silverware within the resident's reach.

8. Measure and record intake if ordered. Note the amount and type of foods eaten.

9. Remove the tray.

10. Assist the resident with oral hygiene.

11. Clean any spills, and change soiled linen.

12. Help the resident return to bed if indicated.

13. Make sure the resident is comfortable and the signal light is within reach.

14. Raise or lower side rails as instructed by the nurse.

14. Wash your hands.

15. Report your observations to the nurse.

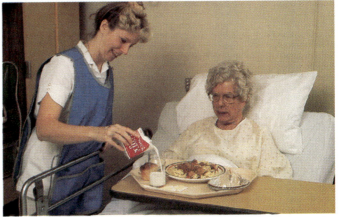

FIGURE 15-12 *The nursing assistant opens cartons and other containers for the resident.*

Feeding the Resident

Some residents cannot feed themselves. Weakness, paralysis, casts, confusion, and other limitations can make self-feeding impossible. These residents need to be fed. When feeding a resident, assume a comfortable position. Relax so the resident does not feel rushed. Many people pray before eating. Be sure to provide time and privacy for prayer. This shows respect and care for the resident. Ask the resident about the order in which to offer foods and fluids. Spoons are used to feed residents. They are less likely to cause injury. The spoon should be only one-third full. The portion can be easily chewed and swallowed.

Residents who cannot feed themselves may be angry, humiliated, and embarrassed at being dependent on others. Some may be depressed or resentful or may refuse to eat. Let these residents feed themselves as much as possible. Give them "finger foods" (bread, cookies, crackers) if they can manage them. If they are strong enough, let them hold milk or juice glasses (never hot drinks). Assist them to drink if necessary. Never exceed the limitations ordered by the doctor. Be supportive. Encourage them to keep trying even if food is spilled.

Many blind people are keenly aware of food aromas. However, they need to know what foods and fluids are on the tray. When feeding a blind resident, always tell the person what you are offering. If the blind person does not need to be fed, identify the foods and their location on the tray. Use the numbers on a clock to identify the location of foods (Fig. 15-13).

Meals provide social contact with others. You should engage the resident in pleasant conversation. However, give the resident enough time to chew and swallow food.

PROCEDURE

Feeding the Resident

1. Explain the procedure to the resident.
2. Wash your hands.
3. Position the resident in a comfortable sitting position.
4. Bring the tray into the room. Place it on the overbed table.
5. Identify the resident. Check the ID bracelet with the dietary card.
6. Drape a napkin across the resident's chest and underneath the chin. Use a clothing protector if available.
7. Prepare food for eating.
8. Tell the resident what foods are on the tray.
9. Serve foods in the order preferred by the resident. Alternate between solid and liquid foods. Use a spoon for safety (Fig. 15-14). Allow enough time for chewing. Do not rush the resident.
10. Use a straw for liquids if the resident cannot drink from a glass or cup. Have one straw for each liquid. Provide a short straw for weak residents.
11. Talk to the resident in a pleasant manner, even if the resident is confused or cannot speak.
12. Encourage him or her to eat as much as possible.
13. Wipe the resident's mouth with a napkin.
14. Note how much and which foods were eaten.
15. Measure and record intake if ordered.
16. Remove the tray.
17. Provide oral hygiene. (Use universal precautions.)
18. Position the resident in a comfortable position. Place the signal light within reach.
19. Raise or lower side rails as instructed by the nurse.
20. Wash your hands.
21. Report your observations to the nurse:
    a. The amount and kind of food eaten
    b. Resident complaints of nausea or **dysphagia** (difficulty or discomfort in swallowing)
22. Follow the facility procedure for residents in the social feeder program.

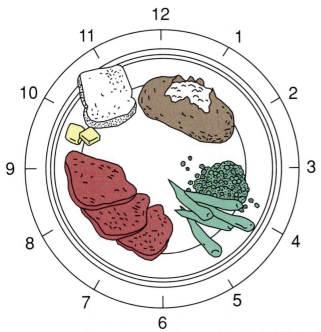

FIGURE 15-13 *The numbers on a clock are used to help the blind resident locate food on the tray.*

Between-Meal Nourishments

Many special diets involve between-meal nourishments. Commonly served nourishments are crackers, milk, juice, a milkshake, a piece of cake, wafers, a sandwich, gelatin, and custard. Nourishments are served as soon as they arrive on the nursing unit. Be sure to provide the necessary eating utensils, a straw, and napkin. Follow the same considerations and procedures described for serving meal trays and feeding residents.

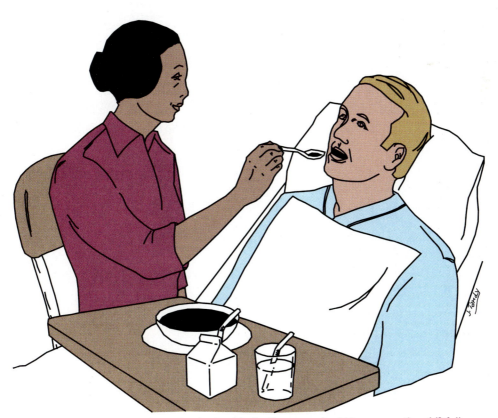

FIGURE 15-14 *A spoon is used to feed residents. The spoon should be no more than 1/3 full.*

Providing Drinking Water

Residents need fresh drinking water each shift. Fresh water also is given whenever the pitcher is empty. Before providing water, ask the nurse about any special orders such as NPO or restricted fluids. Some residents may not be allowed ice. Practice the rules of medical asepsis when passing drinking water.

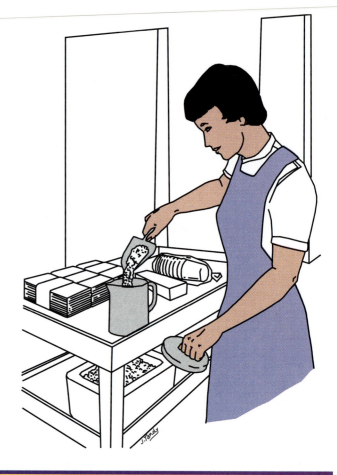

FIGURE 15-15 *The rules of medical asepsis are followed when drinking water is passed. The scoop does not touch any part of the water pitcher when ice is being added.*

PROCEDURE

Providing Drinking Water

1. Ask the nurse for a list of residents who have special fluid orders (e.g., NPO, fluid restriction, no ice).

2. Ask a co-worker to help you.

3. Wash your hands.

4. Collect the following:
   a. Cart for dirty pitchers, glasses, and trays
   b. Cart containing clean water pitchers, glasses, and trays
   c. Scoop for the ice machine
   d. Straws

5. Take the cart with the clean equipment to the ice machine. Use the scoop to put ice into the water pitchers (Fig. 15-15). Have your helper fill the pitchers with water.

6. Roll both carts to the area just outside a resident's room. Check the list to see if the resident has special orders.

7. Have your helper take the dirty pitcher, glass, and tray from the resident's room and place them on the empty cart.

8. Check the resident's ID bracelet, and call the resident by name.

9. Place the tray with the pitcher, glass, and straw on the overbed table. Make sure the resident can easily reach the items.

10. Fill the glass with fresh water.

11. Repeat steps 5 through 10 for each resident.

12. Return the cart with the dirty equipment to the kitchen to be washed.

13. Wash your hands.

Other Methods of Meeting Food and Fluid Needs

Many residents cannot eat or drink because of illness, surgery, or injury. Other methods must be used to meet their basic need for foods and fluids. These methods are ordered by the doctor. The nurse is responsible for carrying out the order.

Tube feedings. The doctor may order a nasogastric tube *(NG tube, Levine tube)*. The resident is fed through the tube. The nurse inserts the tube through the resident's nose into the stomach (Fig. 15-16). Commercial or blended fluids are passed through the tube into the stomach. The feeding is given at scheduled intervals using a syringe or funnel. Or it can be administered continuously using a special pump. **Gavage** is another term for a tube feeding.

A resident may have a gastrostomy. A **gastrostomy** is an opening (stomy) in the stomach (gastro). The opening is created surgically. A tube is inserted into the opening (Fig. 15-17). Commercial or blended foods are passed through the tube into the stomach.

A gastrostomy is indicated when food cannot pass normally from the mouth to the esophagus and into the stomach. Cancer of the head, neck, or esophagus may require a gastrostomy. The person cannot eat or drink fluids.

Persons with gastrostomies are NPO. The resident needs the same oral care as a resident with an NG tube (see Chapter 12). When giving care, do not pull on the tube. If it comes out, tell the nurse immediately. Also report any redness or drainage around the tube.

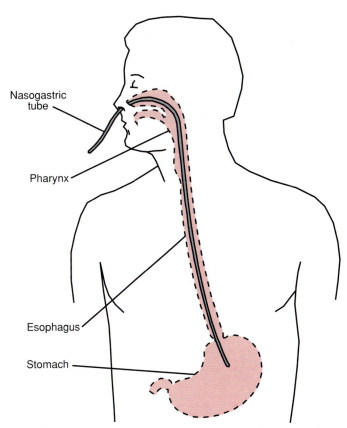

Nasogastric tube

Pharynx

Esophagus

Stomach

FIGURE 15-16 *A nasogastric tube is inserted through the nose into the stomach.*

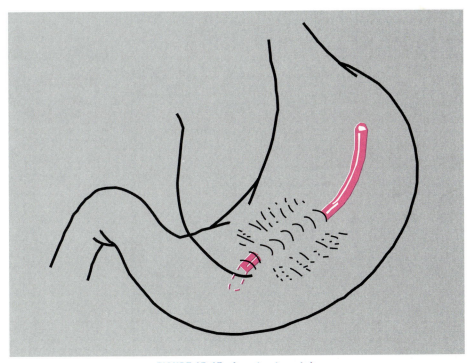

FIGURE 15-17 *A gastrostomy tube.*

351

Intravenous therapy. Many residents receive fluid through a needle inserted in a vein. Minerals and vitamins often are given in the same manner. The terms *IV* and *IV infusion* often are used in referring to **intravenous therapy.** Fluid is in a bottle or plastic bag. Clear IV tubing connects the container to the needle in a vein (Fig. 15-18). The amount of fluid given (infused) per hour is ordered by the doctor. The nurse is responsible for making suxre this amount is given. This is done by controlling the number of drops per minute (flow rate). Nursing assistants *never* are responsible for IV therapy or for regulating the flow rate.

Hyperalimentation. Hyperalimentation is the intravenous administration of a highly concentrated solution of proteins, carbohydrates, vitamins, and minerals. The solution is far more nutritious than a regular IV solution. Hyperalimentation is used for seriously ill and injured residents. These residents usually are in hospital-based long-term care units. Nursing assistants *never* are responsible for administering or regulating hyperalimentation solutions.

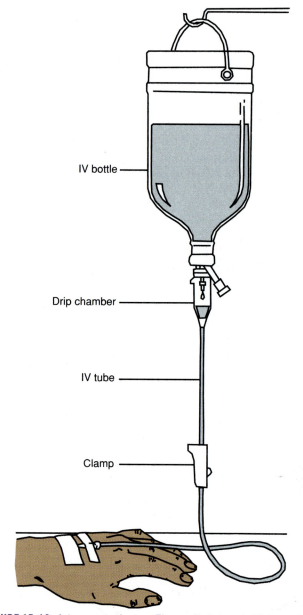

IV bottle

Drip chamber

IV tube

Clamp

FIGURE 15-18 *Intravenous therapy. The needle is inserted into a vein in the arm or hand. The needle is attached to the bottle by tubing.*

Quality OF LIFE

As explained in previous chapters, OBRA serves to promote the resident's quality of life. This includes the resident's health and safety. Nutrition and fluid balance are important for quality of life.

The resident's right to personal choice is important in meeting food and fluids needs. Everyone has a lifetime of food likes and dislikes. These do not change when a person enters a nursing facility. Food preferences may be based on religious practices or cultural background. The dietitian will work with the resident in planning healthy meals that include the resident's personal choices. Residents may tell you that they like or want certain foods. You need to share this information with the nurse.

Sometimes family and friends bring the resident food from home. This can help the resident's need for love and belonging. Sometimes it is very hard for the dietary department to provide all of the resident's food preferences. Residents usually are very pleased when family and friends bring favorite foods. Certain foods and food traditions are part of holidays. Holidays are more meaningful to residents when they can share in lifelong family traditions. Many families and friends bring residents food as holiday gifts. The nurse needs to know when food is brought to the resident. The food must not interfere with any special diet that may be ordered.

Some facilities have dining areas where residents can dine with guests. There the resident can have a family meal with a spouse, children, grandchildren, relatives, or friends. The dietary department provides the meal, or it may be brought by the family. Holidays, birthdays, anniversaries, and other special events can be celebrated (Fig. 15-19).

OBRA also requires that the resident's food be served correctly. Hot food must be hot; cold food must be cold. Mashed potatoes are not very appetizing if cold. You would not eat them, and the resident should not have to. Make sure meals are served promptly. There may be a time when there is an unavoidable delay in serving a tray. If so, get a new tray of food from the dietary department. Be sure tell the resident why the meal has been delayed. Make sure the resident is given any necessary assistance in eating. This includes providing any special equipment or eating utensils.

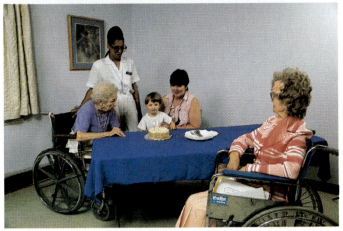

FIGURE 15-19 *A grandchild's birthday is celebrated in the nursing facility.*

SUMMARY

The need for foods and fluids is basic for health and survival. A well-balanced diet contains foods from the five lower levels of the Food Guide Pyramid. The diet provides the necessary amounts of proteins, carbohydrates, fats, vitamins, and minerals. Eating habits vary among individuals. They are affected by many factors, including religion and culture. When assisting a resident in meeting nutritional needs, you need to consider the factors that affect eating. Also try to make the meal as pleasant as possible for the person.

Fluid balance is essential for health and life. The amount of fluid taken into the body must equal the amount lost. Fluid is lost through the urine, feces, skin, and lungs. You will assist doctors and nurses in evaluating a person's fluid balance by keeping accurate I&O records when directed to do so.

Residents depend on nursing staff members to meet part or all of their food and fluid needs. Even residents who do most of their own care rely on the nursing team to serve meals. They also need nourishments served and fresh drinking water. Some residents have special dining programs. Some need to be fed. You need to remember that meals are a time for enjoyment and socializing. The person who is refreshed and comfortable will enjoy the meal even more.

Review QUESTIONS

Circle the *best* answer.

1. Nutrition is
   a. Fats, proteins, carbohydrates, vitamins, and minerals
   b. The many processes involved in the ingestion, digestion, absorption, and use of food and fluids by the body
   c. The four basic food groups
   d. The balance between fluids taken in and lost by the body

2. The Food Guide Pyramid has
   a. Three food groups   c. Five food groups
   b. Four food groups   d. Six food groups

3. The Food Guide Pyramid encourages
   a. A low-fat diet   c. A low-fiber diet
   b. A high-fat diet   d. A low-nutrient diet

4. How many daily servings of breads, cereals, rice, and pasta are recommended?
   a. 6 to 11   c. 2 to 4
   b. 3 to 5   d. 2 to 3

5. How many vegetable servings are recommended per day?
   a. 6 to 11   c. 2 to 4
   b. 3 to 5   d. 2 to 3

6. How many servings from the milk, yogurt, and cheese group are recommended per day?
   a. 6 to 11   c. 2 to 4
   b. 3 to 5   d. 2 to 3

7. How many daily servings of the meat group are recommended?
   a. 6 to 11   c. 2 to 4
   b. 3 to 5   d. 2 to 3

8. Which food group contains the most fat?
   a. Breads, cereals, rice, and pasta
   b. Fruits
   c. Milk, yogurt, and cheese
   d. Meat, poultry, fish, dry beans, eggs, and nuts

9. Fats, oils, and sweets
   a. Should be used in moderate amounts
   b. Are low in calories
   c. Should be used sparingly
   d. Have great nutritional value

10. Protein is needed for
    a. Tissue growth and repair
    b. Energy as well as fiber for elimination
    c. Body heat and protecting organs from injury
    d. Improving the taste of food

11. Which provide the most protein?
    a. Butter and cream
    c. Meats and fish
    b. Tomatoes and potatoes
    d. Corn and lettuce

12. Eating and nutrition are affected by
    a. A person's cultural background and religious practices
    b. Personal preferences and the way food is prepared
    c. The amount of money available to buy food
    d. All of the above

13. Sodium-restricted diets usually are *not* ordered for residents with
    a. Diabetes mellitus
    c. Kidney disease
    b. Heart disease
    d. Liver disease

14. Mrs. Ronan is on a sodium-restricted diet. She asks you to bring some salt for her chicken. You should bring her the salt.
    a. True
    b. False

15. The diabetic diet controls the amount of
    a. Water
    c. Carbohydrates
    b. Sodium
    d. Nutrients

16. Diet planning for the diabetic diet involves
    a. Calculating the amount of sodium
    b. Exchange lists
    c. Measuring fluid intake
    d. Giving insulin with meals

17. OBRA requires that
    a. Hot foods be served hot; cold foods be served cold
    b. Foods smell good
    c. Foods taste good
    d. All of the above

18. OBRA requires
    a. Two regular meals
    b. Three regular meals
    c. Three regular meals and a bedtime snack
    d. Four regular meals

19. Adult fluid requirements for normal fluid balance are about
    a. 1000 to 1500 ml daily
    b. 1500 to 2000 ml daily
    c. 2000 to 2500 ml daily
    d. 2500 to 3000 ml daily

20. A resident is NPO. You should
    a. Provide a variety of fluids
    b. Offer fluids in small amounts and small containers
    c. Remove the water pitcher and glass
    d. Prevent the resident from having oral hygiene

21. Which are *not* counted as liquid foods?
    a. Coffee, tea, juices, and soft drinks
    b. Butter, sauces, and melted cheese
    c. Ice cream, sherbet, custard, and pudding
    d. Jell-o, popsicles, and creamed cereals

22. Residents in dining rooms serve themselves from bowls and platters on their table. This is a
    a. Social dining program
    b. Family dining program
    c. Social feeder program
    d. Serve-yourself dining program

23. Which is *false?*
    a. Residents should be asked if they want to pray before eating.
    b. A fork is used to feed a resident.
    c. The resident should be asked the order in which foods should be served.
    d. You should engage the resident in a pleasant conversation.

24. Which is *false?*
    a. Between-meal nourishments must be served promptly.
    b. You are never responsible for IV therapy.
    c. You are never responsible for hyperalimentation.
    d. You can insert an NG tube and give a tube feeding.

25. Which is important for the resident's quality of life?
    a. Personal choice in foods
    b. Dining with family and friends
    c. Having family and friends bring favorite foods from home
    d. All of the above

Answers

1. b	8. d	15. c	22. b
2. d	9. c	16. b	23. b
3. a	10. a	17. d	24. d
4. a	11. c	18. c	25. d
5. b	12. d	19. c	
6. d	13. a	20. c	
7. d	14. b	21. b	

16

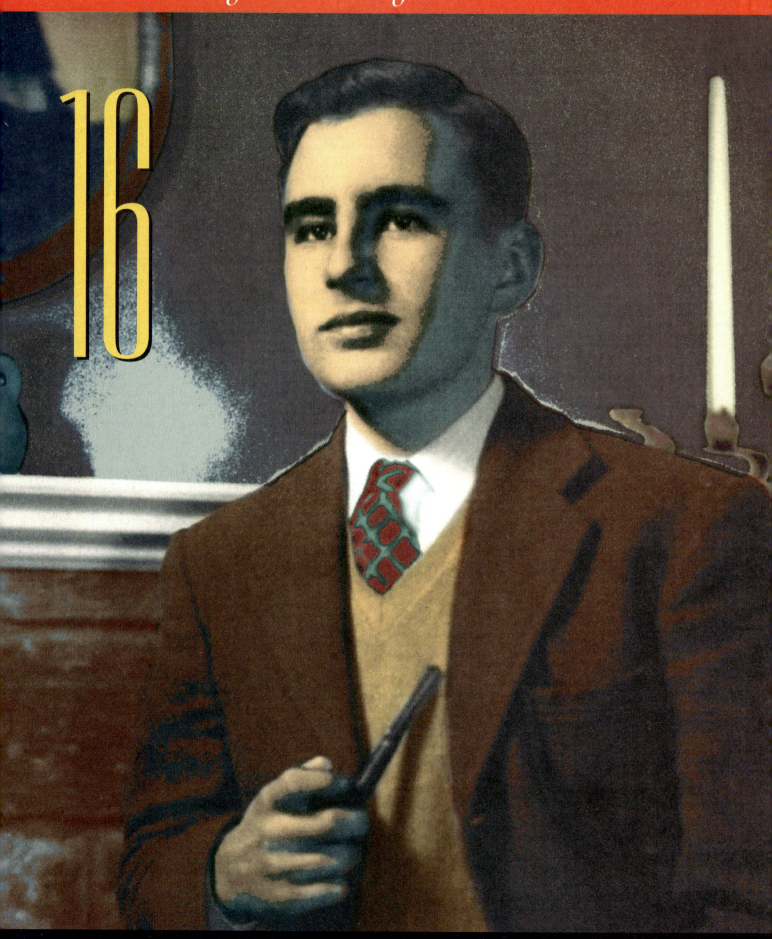

What You Will LEARN

- The key terms listed in this chapter

- Why vital signs are measured

- Factors that can affect vital signs

- Normal ranges of oral, rectal, and axillary body temperatures

- When to take oral, rectal, and axillary temperatures

- Sites for taking a pulse

- Normal pulse ranges of the different age-groups

- How to describe normal respirations

- Normal ranges for adult blood pressures

- Differences between mercury and aneroid sphygmomanometers

- Practices to be followed in measuring blood pressure

- How to perform the procedures described in this chapter

apical-radial pulse
Taking the apical and radial pulse at the same time; two workers are needed

apnea
The lack of or absence *(a)* of breathing *(pnea)*

blood pressure
The amount of force exerted against the walls of an artery by the blood

body temperature
The amount of heat in the body, which is a balance between the amount of heat produced and the amount lost by the body

bradypnea
Slow *(brady)* breathing *(pnea)*; the respiratory rate is less than 10 respirations per minute

Cheyne-Stokes
A pattern of breathing in which respirations gradually increase in rate and depth and then become shallow and slow; breathing may stop (apnea) for 10 to 20 seconds

diastole
The period of heart muscle relaxation

diastolic pressure
The pressure in the arteries when the heart is at rest

dyspnea
Difficult, labored, or painful *(dys)* breathing *(pnea)*

hypertension
Persistent blood pressure measurements above the normal systolic (140 mm Hg) or diastolic (90 mm Hg) pressures; in elderly persons, persistent blood pressure measurements above 160 mm Hg systolic or 95 mm Hg diastolic

hyperventilation
Respirations that are rapid *(hyper)* and deeper than normal

hypotension
A condition in which the systolic blood pressure is below 90 mm Hg and the diastolic pressure is below 60 mm Hg

hypoventilation
Respirations that are slow *(hypo)*, shallow, and sometimes irregular

pulse
The beat of the heart felt at an artery as a wave of blood passes through the artery

pulse deficit
The difference between the apical and radial pulse rates

pulse rate
The number of heartbeats or pulses felt in 1 minute

respiration
The act of breathing air into (inhalation) and out of (exhalation) the lungs

sphygmomanometer
The instrument used to measure blood pressure; it has a cuff (applied to the upper arm) and a measuring device

stethoscope
An instrument used to listen to the sounds produced by the heart, lungs, and other body organs

systole
The period of heart muscle contraction

systolic pressure
The amount of force it takes to pump blood out of the heart into the arterial circulation

tachypnea
Rapid *(tachy)* breathing *(pnea)*; the respiratory rate usually is greater than 24 respirations per minute

vital signs
Temperature, pulse, respirations, and blood pressure

I worry about my blood pressure. It's high sometimes. But Don lets me rest awhile before he takes it. He says that will give a better reading. ∼

Vital signs reflect the function of three body processes necessary for life: breathing, heart function, and regulation of body temperature. The four **vital signs** of body function are temperature, pulse, respirations, and blood pressure.

Nursing assistants often measure vital signs. Accuracy is absolutely essential. You must be accurate in measuring, reporting, and recording vital signs.

MEASURING AND REPORTING VITAL SIGNS

Vital signs are measured to detect changes in normal body function. They also are used to determine a resident's response to treatment. Life-threatening situations can be recognized. A person's temperature, pulse, and respirations (TPR) and blood pressure (BP) will vary within certain limits during a 24-hour period. Many factors affect vital signs. They include sleep, activity, eating, weather, noise, exercise, medications, fear, anxiety, and illness.

Vital signs are measured during routine physical examinations. They also are measured when a person is admitted to a health care facility. Usually patients in hospitals have vital signs measured at least four times a day. So do persons in hospital-based skilled nursing units. Nursing facility residents do not have vital signs measured as often. Vital signs may be measured daily or weekly. Residents with acute illnesses, however, may need their vital signs measured several times a day. The nurse will tell you when to measure vital signs. The doctor or nurse compares each measurement with previous ones. Unless orders state otherwise, vital signs are taken with the resident at rest. The person should be in a comfortable lying or sitting position.

Vital signs reflect even minor changes in a person's condition. They must be measured accurately. If unsure of your measurements, promptly ask a nurse to take them again. Vital signs also must be accurately reported and recorded. Immediately report any vital sign that is changed from a previous measurement. Vital signs above or below the normal range also must be reported immediately.

Facilities have different methods for recording vital signs. The nurse will tell you where to record them. In addition to recording them, report changed or abnormal vital signs to the nurse immediately.

BODY TEMPERATURE

Body temperature is the amount of heat in the body. It is a balance between the amount of heat produced and the amount lost by the body. Heat is produced as food is used for energy. It is lost through the skin, breathing, urine, and feces. Body temperature remains fairly stable. It normally is lower in the morning and higher in the afternoon and evening. Factors that affect body temperature include age, weather, exercise, pregnancy, the menstrual cycle, emotions, and illness.

Normal Body Temperature

The Fahrenheit (F) and centigrade, or Celsius (C), scales are used to measure temperature. Common sites for measuring body temperature are the mouth, rectum, and axilla (underarm). Ears also can be used. Normal body temperature is 98.6° F (37° C) when measured orally. The normal rectal temperature is one degree higher, or 99.6° F (37.5° C). The average axillary temperature is 97.6° F (36.5° C). Body temperature usually stays within a certain normal range. Normal ranges of body temperature for adults are as follows:

Oral—97.6° to 99.6° F (36.5° to 37.5° C)
Rectal—98.6° to 100.6° F (37.0° to 38.1° C)
Axillary—96.6° to 98.6° F (36.0° to 37.0° C)

Types of Thermometers

A thermometer is used to measure temperature. The glass thermometer is familiar to most people. Other kinds also will be described.

Glass thermometers. The glass thermometer (clinical thermometer) is a hollow glass tube with a bulb filled with mercury. The mercury expands and rises in the tube when heated by the body. The mercury contracts and moves down the tube when cooled.

There are three types of glass thermometers. Each has a different bulb or tip (Fig. 16-1). Long- or slender-tip thermometers are used for oral and axillary temperatures. So are stubby and pear-shaped tip thermometers. Rectal thermometers have stubby tips that are color-coded in red. Glass thermometers are available in Fahrenheit and centigrade scales. Some have both scales.

Text continued on p. 361.

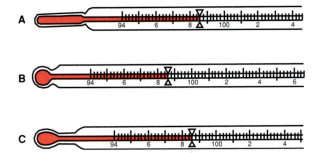

FIGURE 16-1 *Types of glass thermometers. **A,** The long or slender tip. **B,** The stubby tip (rectal thermometer). **C,** The pear-shaped tip.*

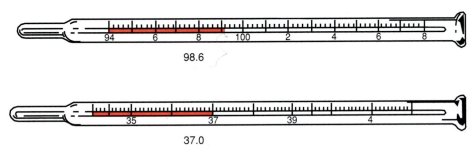

98.6

37.0

FIGURE 16-2 ***A,** Fahrenheit thermometer. The mercury level is at 98.6° F. **B,** Centigrade thermometer. The mercury level is at 37.0° C.*

List 16-1

Fahrenheit and Centigrade Equivalents

Fahrenheit	Centigrade
95.0	35.0
95.9	35.5
96.8	36.0
97.7	36.5
98.6	37.0
99.5	37.5
100.4	38.0
101.3	38.5
102.2	39.0
103.1	39.5
104.0	40.0
104.9	40.5
105.8	41.0
106.7	41.5
107.6	42.0
108.5	42.5
109.4	43.0
110.3	43.5

How to read a glass thermometer. Fahrenheit thermometers have long and short lines. Every other long line is marked in an even degree from 94° to 108° F. Short lines indicate 0.2 (two tenths) of a degree (Fig. 16-2, *A*). Centigrade thermometers also have long and short lines. Each long line means one degree from 34° to 42° C. Each short line means 0.1 (one tenth) of a degree (Fig. 16-2, *B*). List 16-1 shows equivalent values for Fahrenheit and centigrade scales.

Using a glass thermometer. The thermometer is inserted into the mouth or rectum or under the axilla. Each area has many microorganisms. Thus residents have their own thermometers to prevent the spread of microbes and infection. Thermometers are disinfected after use. They often are stored in a disinfectant solution between uses. Before being used again, a thermometer is rinsed under cold running water and wiped with a tissue to remove the disinfectant.

PROCEDURE

How to Read a Glass Thermometer

1. Make sure you have good lighting.

2. Hold the thermometer at the stem with your thumb and fingertips (Fig. 16-3).

3. Bring the thermometer to eye level (Fig. 16-4).

4. Rotate the thermometer until you see both the numbers and the long and short lines at the same time.

5. Note that each long line measures 1 degree and each small line measures 0.2 degrees on a Fahrenheit ther-

mometer. Each small line measures 0.1 degrees on a centigrade thermometer (see Fig. 16-2, p. 359).

6. Turn the thermometer back and forth slowly until the silver (or red) mercury line is seen.

7. Read the thermometer to the nearest degree (long line). Read the nearest tenth of a degree (short line)—an even number on a Fahrenheit thermometer.

8. Record the resident's name and temperature.

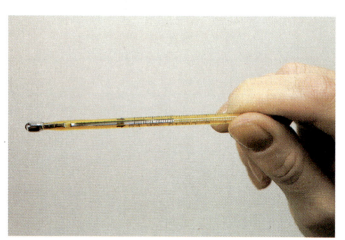

FIGURE 16-3 *The thermometer is held at the stem with the thumb and fingertips.*

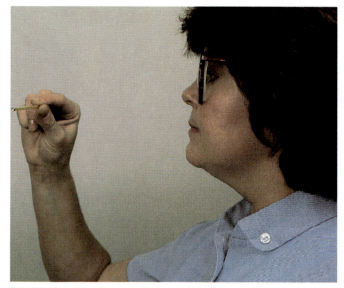

FIGURE 16-4 *The thermometer is read at eye level.*

Cleaning methods vary among facilities. The thermometer usually is wiped first with a tissue to remove mucus or feces. It is wiped from the stem to the bulb end with a twisting motion (Fig. 16-5). Then it is washed in cold soapy water. Hot water is not used. It causes the mercury to expand so much that the thermometer could break. After they are cleaned, thermometers are rinsed under cold running water. They are stored in a case or a container filled with disinfectant.

Many facilities use plastic covers for thermometers (Fig. 16-6). A cover is used once and discarded. The thermometer is inserted into a cover and the temperature is taken. The cover is removed to read the thermometer. The thermometer is then inserted into a clean cover and is ready for use. Disinfection and cleaning are not necessary because the thermometer never touches the resident.

Before taking a temperature, you must shake the thermometer down to move the mercury into the bulb. The thermometer is checked for breaks or chips that could cause injury.

There is no agreement on how long glass thermometers should be left in place. Time lines are given in the procedures for oral, rectal, and axillary temperatures. However, you need to follow facility policies when measuring temperatures.

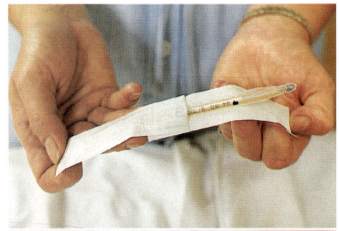

A

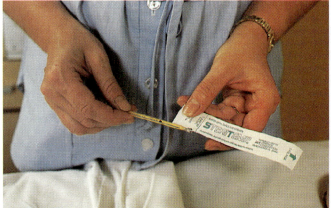

B

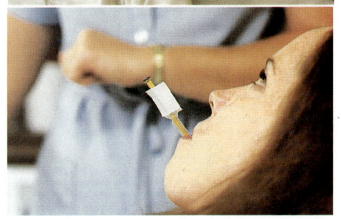

C

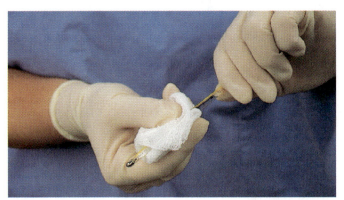

FIGURE 16-5 *The thermometer is wiped from the stem to the bulb end. A twisting motion is used.*

FIGURE 16-6 *A, The glass thermometer and plastic cover. B, The thermometer is inserted into a plastic cover. C, The resident's temperature is taken with the thermometer in the plastic cover.*

PROCEDURE

How to Use a Glass Thermometer

1. Collect a thermometer and tissues.

2. Wash your hands.

3. Hold the thermometer at the stem.

4. Rinse the thermometer under cold running water if it has been soaking in a disinfectant. Dry it from the stem to the bulb end with tissues.

5. Shake down the thermometer. Mercury must be below the lines and numbers.
   a. Hold the thermometer at the stem.
   b. Stand away from walls, tables, or other hard surfaces to avoid breaking the thermometer.
   c. Flex and snap your wrist until the mercury is shaken down (Fig. 16-7).

6. Take the temperature. Read the thermometer and record the temperature.

7. Shake down the thermometer again.

8. Wipe the thermometer with tissues from the stem to the bulb. Use a twisting motion. Clean it if plastic protective covers are not used.

9. Place the thermometer in a disinfectant solution or in a plastic cover.

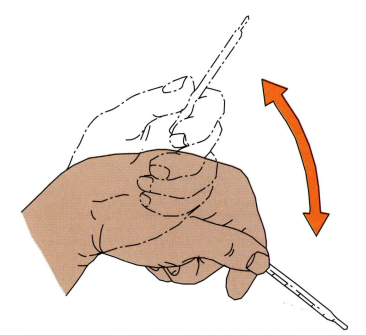

FIGURE 16-7 *The wrist is snapped to shake down the thermometer.*

Electronic thermometers. Electronic thermometers are portable and battery-operated (Fig. 16-8). Temperatures are measured in 2 to 60 seconds. The temperature is displayed on the front of the thermometer. The hand-held unit is kept in a battery charger when not in use.

Electronic thermometers have oral and rectal probes. Rectal probes are color-coded in red. A disposable cover or sheath covers the probe. Disposable probe covers are used only once and then discarded.

Electronic thermometers are expensive. However, they have several advantages. Disposable probe covers reduce the possibility of spreading infection. The temperature is measured rapidly, and the temperature display is easily read.

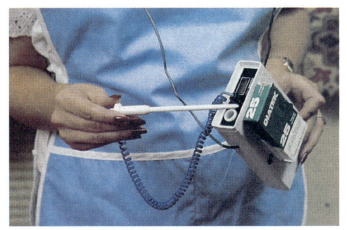

FIGURE 16-8 *An electronic thermometer.*

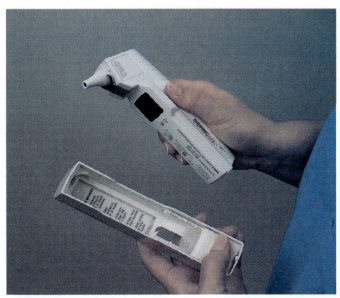

FIGURE 16-10 *Tympanic membrane sensor is portable. It is kept on its charging unit when not in use. (Courtesy of Thermoscan, Inc., San Diego, CA.)*

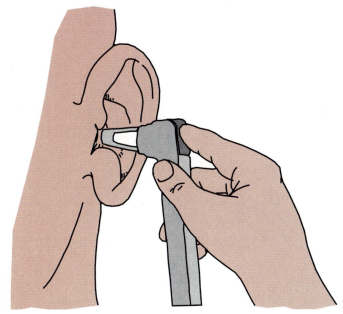

FIGURE 16-9 *Tympanic membrane sensor measures body temperature. A probe is inserted into the ear canal.*

Tympanic membrane sensors. A tympanic membrane sensor is inserted into the ear canal (Fig. 16-9). It measures the temperature at the tympanic membrane (eardrum). The eardrum and the hypothalamus share the same blood supply. The hypothalamus is in the brain and is the structure that regulates body temperature (see Fig. 5-13, p. 74). Therefore the eardrum is considered to be an accurate site for temperature measurement.

Tympanic membrane sensors (Fig. 16-10) measure temperatures in less than 2 seconds. The sensors are like electronic thermometers. They are portable and battery-operated. The measurement is displayed on the front unit. When not in use, they are kept in charging units. Disposable probe covers are used to cover the ear probe.

Disposable oral thermometers. Disposable oral thermometers (see p. 366.) have small chemical dots. The dots change color when heated by the body. Each dot must be heated to a certain temperature before it changes color. These thermometers are used only once. They measure the temperature in about 45 seconds.

Temperature-sensitive tape. Temperature-sensitive tape changes color in response to body heat. The tape is applied to the forehead or abdomen. It indicates if the temperature is normal or above normal. The exact body temperature is not measured. The color changes in about 15 seconds.

Taking Oral Temperatures

Oral temperatures usually are taken on older children and adults. Drinking and eating hot or cold foods or fluids, smoking, and chewing gum cause inaccurate measurements. If the resident has engaged in these activities, wait 15 minutes. A glass thermometer must remain in place 2 to 3 minutes for an accurate measurement.

Temperatures are not taken orally if the resident:
1. Is unconscious
2. Has had surgery or an injury to the face, neck, nose, or mouth
3. Breathes through the mouth instead of the nose
4. Has a nasogastric tube
5. Is delirious, restless, confused, or disoriented
6. Is paralyzed on one side of the body
7. Has a sore mouth

Taking an Oral Temperature With a Glass Thermometer

1. Explain the procedure to the resident. Ask him or her not to eat, drink, smoke, or chew gum for 15 minutes.

2. Collect the following:
   a. Oral thermometer and holder
   b. Tissues
   c. Plastic covers (if used)

3. Wash your hands.

4. Identify the resident. Check the ID bracelet and call the resident by name.

5. Provide for privacy.

6. Rinse the thermometer in cold water if it was soaking in disinfectant. Dry it with tissues.

7. Check the thermometer for breaks or chips.

8. Shake down the thermometer.

9. Place a plastic cover on the thermometer.

10. Ask the resident to moisten his or her lips.

11. Place the bulb end of the thermometer under the resident's tongue (Fig. 16-11).

12. Ask the resident to close his or her lips around the thermometer to hold it in place.

13. Leave the thermometer in place for 2 to 3 minutes.

14. Grasp the stem of the thermometer. Remove it from the resident's mouth.

15. Use tissues to remove the plastic cover. Wipe the thermometer with tissues from the stem to the bulb if no cover was used. Wipe with a twisting motion.

16. Read the thermometer.

17. Record the resident's name and temperature.

18. Shake down the thermometer.

19. Rinse and wash the thermometer.

20. Place the thermometer in the holder with disinfectant or in a plastic cover.

21. Make sure the resident is comfortable and the signal light is within reach.

22. Unscreen the resident.

23. Wash your hands.

24. Report any abnormal temperature to the nurse. Record the measurement in the proper place.

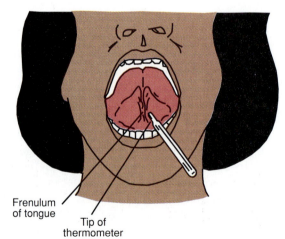

Frenulum of tongue

Tip of thermometer

FIGURE 16-11 *The thermometer is positioned at the base of the tongue next to the frenulum.*

364

PROCEDURE

Taking an Oral Temperature With an Electronic Thermometer

1. Explain the procedure to the resident. Ask him or her not to eat, drink, smoke, or chew gum for 15 minutes.

2. Collect the following:
   a. Electronic thermometer
   b. Oral probe (usually blue)
   c. Disposable probe covers

3. Plug the oral probe into the thermometer.

4. Wash your hands.

5. Identify the resident. Check the ID bracelet and call the resident by name.

6. Provide for privacy.

7. Insert the probe into a probe cover.

8. Ask the resident to open the mouth and raise the tongue.

9. Place the covered probe at the base of the tongue on either side (Fig. 16-12).

10. Ask the resident to lower the tongue and close the mouth.

11. Hold the probe in place.

12. Read the temperature on the display. A tone or flashing or steady light indicates the temperature has been measured.

13. Remove the probe from the resident's mouth. Press the eject button to discard the probe cover.

14. Record the resident's name and temperature.

15. Return the probe to the holder.

16. Make sure the resident is comfortable and the signal light is within reach.

17. Unscreen the resident.

18. Return the thermometer to the charging unit.

19. Wash your hands.

20. Report any abnormal temperature to the nurse. Record the measurement in the proper place.

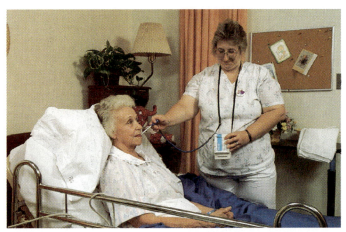

FIGURE 16-12 *The covered probe of the electronic thermometer is inserted under the tongue. The unit is carried in the hand with the carrying strap around the neck.*

PROCEDURE

Taking an Oral Temperature With a Disposable Thermometer

1. Explain the procedure to the resident. Ask him or her not to eat, drink, smoke, or chew gum for 15 minutes.

2. Get a disposable thermometer.

3. Wash your hands.

4. Identify the resident. Check the ID bracelet and call the resident by name.

5. Provide for privacy.

6. Remove the wrapper from the thermometer.

7. Ask the resident to open the mouth and raise the tongue.

8. Place the thermometer at the base of the tongue on either side.

9. Ask the resident to lower the tongue and close the mouth.

10. Leave the thermometer in place for 45 seconds.

11. Remove the thermometer and read the last colored dot. (Fig. 16-13.)

12. Record the resident's name and temperature.

13. Dispose of the thermometer.

14. Make sure the resident is comfortable and the signal light is within reach.

15. Unscreen the resident.

16. Wash your hands.

17. Report any abnormal temperature to the nurse. Record the measurement in the proper place.

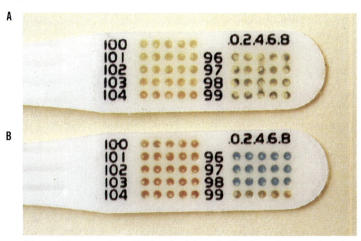

FIGURE 16-13 *A, Disposable oral thermometer with chemical dots. B, The dots change color when the temperature is taken.*

Taking Rectal Temperatures

Rectal temperatures are taken when oral methods cannot be used (see p. 363). Rectal temperatures are not taken if the resident has diarrhea, fecal impaction, a rectal disorder or injury, or severe heart disease or has had recent rectal surgery. Check with the nurse before taking a rectal temperature.

The rectal thermometer is lubricated for easy insertion and prevention of tissue injury. It is held in place so that it is not lost into the rectum or broken. A glass thermometer must remain in the rectum for 2 minutes for an accurate measurement.

PROCEDURE

Taking a Rectal Temperature With a Glass Thermometer

1. Explain the procedure to the resident.
2. Collect the following:
   a. Rectal thermometer and holder
   b. Toilet tissue
   c. Plastic covers (if used)
   d. Disposable gloves
   e. Water-soluble lubricant
3. Wash your hands.
4. Identify the resident. Check the ID bracelet and call the resident by name.
5. Provide for privacy.
6. Rinse the thermometer in cold water if it has been soaking in disinfectant. Dry it with tissues.
7. Check the thermometer for breaks or chips.
8. Shake down the thermometer.
9. Place a plastic cover on the thermometer.
10. Position the resident in the Sims' or side-lying position.
11. Put on the gloves.
12. Put a small amount of lubricant on a tissue. Lubricate the bulb end of the thermometer.
13. Fold back top linens to expose the anal area.
14. Raise the resident's upper buttock to expose the anus (Fig. 16-14, p. 368).
15. Insert the thermometer 1 inch into the rectum.
16. Hold it in place for 2 minutes (Fig. 16-15, p. 368).
17. Remove the thermometer.
18. Remove the plastic cover. Wipe the thermometer with tissues from stem to the bulb end if no cover was used. Wipe with a twisting motion.
19. Place the used toilet tissue on a paper towel or several thicknesses of toilet tissue. Place the thermometer on clean toilet tissue.
20. Wipe the anal area to remove excess lubricant and any feces. Cover the resident.
21. Discard soiled toilet tissue into the toilet.
22. Remove the gloves.
23. Read the thermometer. Record the resident's name and temperature. Write "R" to indicate a rectal temperature.
24. Make sure the resident is comfortable and the signal light is within reach.
25. Shake down the thermometer.
26. Rinse and wash the thermometer.
27. Place the thermometer in the holder with disinfectant or in a plastic cover.
28. Unscreen the resident.
29. Wash your hands.
30. Report any abnormal temperature to the nurse. Record the measurement with an "R" in the proper place.

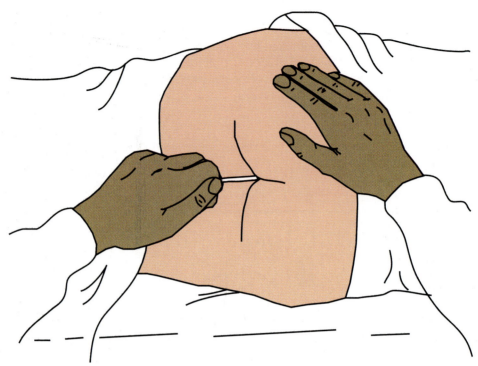

FIGURE 16-14 *The rectal temperature is taken with the resident in Sims' position. The buttock is raised to expose the anus.*

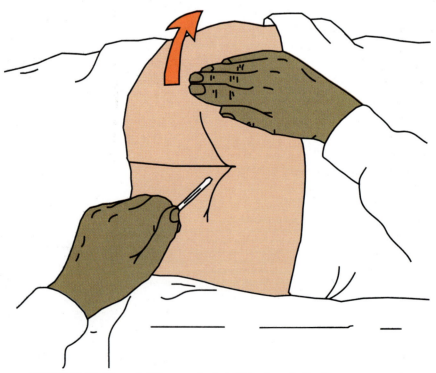

FIGURE 16-15 *The rectal thermometer is held in place during the measurement.*

PROCEDURE

Taking a Rectal Temperature With an Electronic Thermometer

1. Explain the procedure to the resident.
2. Collect the following:
   a. Electronic thermometer
   b. Rectal probe (usually red)
   c. Disposable probe covers
   d. Toilet tissue
   e. Water-soluble lubricant
   f. Disposable gloves
3. Plug the rectal probe into the thermometer.
4. Wash your hands.
5. Identify the resident. Check the ID bracelet and call the resident by name.
6. Provide for privacy.
7. Position the resident in a Sims' or side-lying position.
8. Put on the gloves.
9. Put a small amount of lubricant on some toilet tissue.
10. Insert the probe into a probe cover.
11. Lubricate the end of the covered probe.
12. Fold back top linens to expose the resident's anal area.
13. Raise the upper buttock to expose the anus.
14. Insert the covered probe ½ inch into the rectum.
15. Hold the probe in place until you hear a tone or see a flashing or steady light.
16. Read the temperature on the display.
17. Remove the probe from the rectum.
18. Press the eject button to discard the probe cover. Return the probe to the holder.
19. Wipe the anal area with toilet tissue to remove excess lubricant and any feces. Cover the resident.
20. Discard used toilet tissue into the toilet.
21. Remove the gloves.
22. Record the resident's name and temperature with an "R" (for a rectal temperature).
23. Make sure the resident is comfortable and the signal light is within reach.
24. Unscreen the resident.
25. Return the thermometer to the charging unit.
26. Wash your hands.
27. Report any abnormal temperature to the nurse. Record the measurement with an "R" in the proper place.

Taking Axillary Temperatures

Axillary temperatures are less reliable than oral or rectal temperatures. They are used when the temperature cannot be measured orally or rectally. This site is not used right after the axilla has been bathed. The axilla should be dry for the measurement. The thermometer must be held in place to keep it in position. A glass thermometer is held in place for 9 minutes for a reliable measurement.

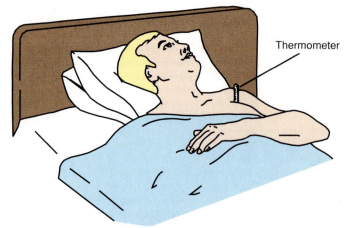
Thermometer

FIGURE 16-16 *The thermometer is held in place in the axilla by bringing the resident's arm over the chest.*

PROCEDURE

Taking an Axillary Temperature With a Glass Thermometer

1. Explain the procedure to the resident.
2. Collect the following:
   a. Oral glass thermometer and holder
   b. Plastic covers if used
   c. Tissues
   d. Towel
3. Wash your hands.
4. Identify the resident. Check the ID bracelet and call the resident by name.
5. Provide for privacy.
6. Rinse the thermometer in cold water if it has been soaking in disinfectant. Dry it with tissues.
7. Check the thermometer for breaks or chips.
8. Shake down the thermometer.
9. Place a plastic cover on the thermometer.
10. Help the resident remove an arm from the sleeve of the gown. Do not expose the resident.
11. Dry the axilla with the towel.
12. Place the bulb end of the thermometer in the center of the axilla.
13. Ask the resident to place the arm over the chest to hold the thermometer in place (Fig. 16-16). Hold it and the arm in place if the resident cannot help.
14. Leave the thermometer in place for 9 minutes.
15. Remove the thermometer from the plastic cover. Wipe it with tissues from the stem to the bulb end if a cover was not used. Wipe with a twisting motion.
16. Read the thermometer.
17. Record the resident's name and temperature with an "A" (for axillary temperature).
18. Help the resident put the gown back on.
19. Make sure the resident is comfortable and the signal light is within reach.
20. Shake down the thermometer.
21. Rinse and wash the thermometer. Place it in the holder with disinfectant or in a plastic cover.
22. Unscreen the resident.
23. Place the towel in the linen hamper.
24. Wash your hands.
25. Report any abnormal temperature to the nurse. Record the measurement with an "A" in the proper place.

Taking an Axillary Temperature With an Electronic Thermometer

1. Explain the procedure to the resident.

2. Collect the following:
   a. Electronic thermometer
   b. Oral probe (usually blue)
   c. Disposable probe covers
   d. Towel

3. Plug the oral probe into the thermometer.

4. Wash your hands.

5. Identify the resident. Check the ID bracelet and call the resident by name.

6. Provide for privacy.

7. Help the resident remove an arm from the gown. Do not expose the resident.

8. Dry the axilla with the towel.

9. Insert the probe into a probe cover.

10. Place the covered probe in the axilla. Place the resident's arm over the chest. Hold the probe in place until you hear a tone or see a steady or flashing light.

11. Remove the probe. Read the temperature.

12. Record the resident's name and temperature with an "A" (for an axillary temperature).

13. Press the eject button and discard the probe cover. Return the probe to the holder.

14. Help the resident put the gown back on.

15. Make sure the resident is in a comfortable position and the signal light is within reach.

16. Unscreen the resident.

17. Place the towel in the linen hamper.

18. Return the thermometer to the charging unit.

19. Wash your hands.

20. Report any abnormal temperature to the nurse. Record the measurement with an "A" in the proper place.

PULSE

The **pulse** is the beat of the heart felt at an artery as a wave of blood passes through the artery. A pulse can be felt every time the heart beats.

Sites for Taking a Pulse

The pulse can be taken at many sites (Fig. 16-17). Pulses are easy to feel at these sites. The arteries are close to the body's surface and lie over a bone. The radial site is used the most. It is easily accessible and can be taken without disturbing or exposing the resident.

The temporal, carotid, brachial, radial, femoral, and popliteal arteries and the dorsal artery of the foot are present on both sides of the body. The apical pulse is felt over the apex of the heart. It is taken with a stethoscope.

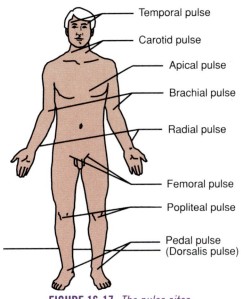

FIGURE 16-17 *The pulse sites.*

- Temporal pulse
- Carotid pulse
- Apical pulse
- Brachial pulse
- Radial pulse
- Femoral pulse
- Popliteal pulse
- Pedal pulse (Dorsalis pulse)

Using a Stethoscope

A **stethoscope** is an instrument used to listen to the sounds produced by the heart, lungs, and other body organs. It amplifies the sounds so they can be heard easily. The parts of a stethoscope are shown in Fig. 16-18. Earpieces should fit snugly to block out external noise. However, they should not cause pain or ear discomfort.

Stethoscopes are shared by doctors and the nursing team. Care must be taken in the use of stethoscopes because they come in contact with many residents and workers. The earpieces and diaphragm are cleaned before and after use. Cleaning prevents the spread of microorganisms.

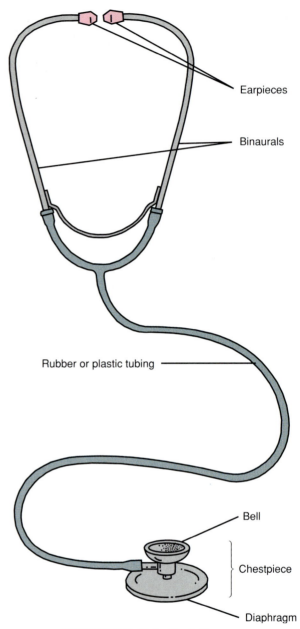

Earpieces

Binaurals

Rubber or plastic tubing

Bell

Chestpiece

Diaphragm

FIGURE 16-18 *Parts of a stethoscope.*

PROCEDURE

How to Use a Stethoscope

1. Collect the following:
    a. A stethoscope with diaphragm
    b. Alcohol wipes

2. Wash your hands.

3. Wipe the earpieces and diaphragm with alcohol wipes.

4. Warm the diaphragm in your hand (Fig. 16-19).

5. Place the earpiece tips in your ears so that the bend of the tips points forward.

6. Place the diaphragm over the artery. Hold the diaphragm in place as in Fig. 16-20.

7. Do not let anything touch the tubing.

8. Ask the resident to be quiet during the procedure.

9. Wipe the earpiece tips and diaphragm with alcohol wipes when the procedure is completed.

10. Return the stethoscope to its proper place.

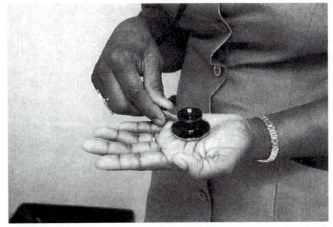

FIGURE 16-19 *The diaphragm of the stethoscope is warmed in the palm of the hand.*

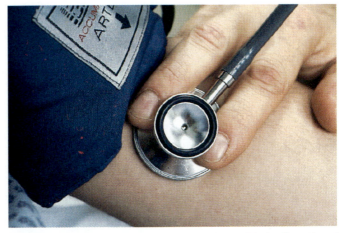

FIGURE 16-20 *The stethoscope is held in place with the fingertips of the index and middle fingers.*

Pulse Rate

The **pulse rate** is the number of heartbeats or pulses felt in 1 minute. The rate is affected by many factors. They include age, elevated body temperature (fever), exercise, fear, anger, anxiety, excitement, heat, position, and pain. These and other factors cause the heart to beat faster. Some medications increase the pulse rate. Others slow down the pulse.

The adult pulse rate is between 60 and 100 beats per minute. A rate less than 60 or greater than 100 is considered abnormal. Abnormal rates must be reported to the nurse immediately.

Rhythm and Force of the Pulse

When taking a pulse, pay attention to its rhythm and force. The rhythm should be regular. That is, a pulse should be felt in a pattern. The same time interval should occur between beats (Fig. 16-21, *A*). An irregular pulse occurs when the beats are unevenly spaced or beats are skipped (Fig. 16-21, *B*). The force of the pulse relates to its strength. A forceful pulse is easy to feel and is described as strong, full, or bounding. Hard to feel pulses often are described as weak, thready, or feeble.

Electronic blood pressure equipment (see p. 380) also counts pulses. The pulse rate is displayed along with the blood pressure. No information is given, however, about the rhythm and force of the pulse. If electronic blood pressure equipment is used, you still must feel the pulse to determine rhythm and force.

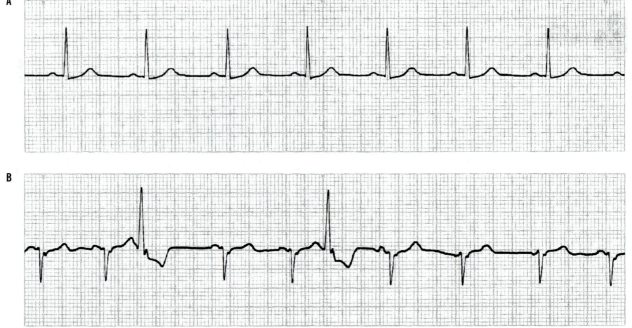

FIGURE 16-21 *A, The electrocardiogram shows a regular pulse. The beats occur at regular intervals. **B**, The beats in this electrocardiogram occur at irregular intervals. (From Huszar RJ: Basic dysrhythmias: interpretation and management, ed 2, St Louis, 1993, Mosby–Year Book.)*

Taking a Radial Pulse

The radial pulse is used for routine vital signs. The pulse is felt by placing the first three fingers of one hand against the radial artery. The radial artery is on the thumb side of the wrist (Fig. 16-22). Do not use your thumb to take a pulse. The thumb has a pulse of its own. The pulse in your thumb could be mistaken for the resident's pulse. The pulse is counted for 30 seconds. The number is multiplied by 2 for the number of beats per minute. If the pulse is irregular, it is counted for 1 full minute.

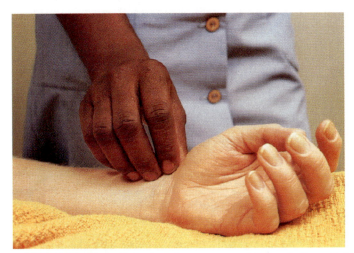

FIGURE 16-22 *The middle three fingers are used to locate the radial pulse on the thumb side of the wrist.*

PROCEDURE

Taking a Radial Pulse

1. Wash your hands.
2. Identify the resident. Check the ID bracelet and call the resident by name.
3. Explain the procedure to the resident.
4. Provide for privacy.
5. Have the resident sit or lie down.
6. Locate the radial pulse with your middle three fingers (see Fig. 16-22).
7. Note if the pulse is strong or weak; regular or irregular.
8. Count the pulse for 30 seconds. Multiply the number of beats by 2.
9. Count the pulse for 1 minute if it is irregular.
10. Record the resident's name and pulse. Make a note about the its strength and if it was regular or irregular.
11. Make sure the resident is comfortable and the signal light is within reach.
12. Unscreen the resident.
13. Wash your hands.
14. Report the following to the nurse:
    a. A pulse rate less than 60 or greater than 100 beats per minute must be reported immediately
    b. Whether the pulse is regular or irregular
    c. The pulse rate
    d. The strength of the pulse (strong, full, bounding; or weak, thready, feeble)
15. Record the pulse rate in the proper place.

Taking an Apical Pulse

The apical pulse is taken with a stethoscope. Apical pulses are taken on residents who have heart diseases or who are taking medications that affect the heart. The apical pulse is on the left side of the chest slightly below the nipple (Fig. 16-23). The apical pulse is counted for 1 full minute.

The heartbeat normally sounds like a "lub-dub." Each "lub-dub" is counted as one beat. Do not count the "lub" as one beat and the "dub" as another.

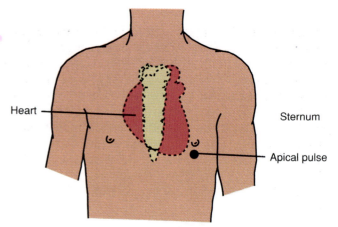

Heart — Sternum — Apical pulse

FIGURE 16-23 *The apical pulse is located 2 to 3 inches to the left of the sternum (breast bone) and below the left nipple.*

PROCEDURE

Taking an Apical Pulse

1. Collect the following:
   a. Stethoscope with diaphragm
   b. Alcohol wipes

2. Wash your hands.

3. Identify the resident. Check the ID bracelet and call the resident by name.

4. Explain the procedure to the resident.

5. Provide for privacy.

6. Wipe the earpieces and diaphragm with alcohol wipes.

7. Have the resident sit or lie down.

8. Warm the diaphragm in your palm.

9. Expose the nipple area of the left chest.

10. Place the earpiece in your ears.

11. Locate the apical pulse. Place the diaphragm 2 to 3 inches to the left of the breastbone and below the left nipple (see Fig. 16-23).

12. Count the pulse for 1 full minute. Note if it is regular or irregular.

13. Cover the resident. Remove the earpieces.

14. Record the resident's name and pulse. Note whether the pulse was regular or irregular.

15. Make sure the resident is comfortable and the signal light is within reach.

16. Unscreen the resident.

17. Clean the earpieces and diaphragm of the stethoscope with alcohol wipes.

18. Return the stethoscope to its proper place.

19. Wash your hands.

20. Report the following to the nurse:
    a. A pulse rate less than 60 or greater than 100 beats per minute is reported immediately
    b. Whether the pulse was regular or irregular
    c. The pulse rate
    d. Any unusual heart sounds

21. Record the pulse rate in the proper place with an "Ap" to indicate apical pulse.

Taking an Apical-Radial Pulse

The apical and radial pulse rates should be equal. Sometimes heart contractions are not strong enough to create pulses in the radial artery. This may occur in residents with heart disease. The radial pulse may be less than the apical pulse. To see if there is a difference between the apical and radial rates, the pulses are taken at the same time by two workers. This is called an **apical-radial pulse.** The **pulse deficit** is the difference between the apical and radial pulse rates. To find the pulse deficit, subtract the radial rate from the apical rate. The apical pulse is never less than the radial pulse rate.

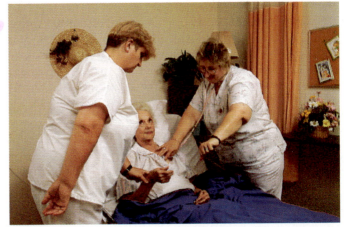

FIGURE 16-24 *Two nursing assistants take an apical-radial pulse. One nursing assistant takes the apical pulse, and the other takes the radial pulse.*

PROCEDURE

Taking an Apical-Radial Pulse

1. Ask a nurse or another nursing assistant to help you.
2. Collect the following:
   a. Stethoscope with diaphragm
   b. Alcohol wipes
3. Wash your hands.
4. Identify the resident. Check the ID bracelet and call the resident by name.
5. Explain the procedure to the resident.
6. Provide for privacy.
7. Wipe the earpieces and diaphragm with alcohol wipes.
8. Have the resident sit or lie down.
9. Warm the diaphragm in your palm.
10. Expose the nipple area of the left side of the chest.
11. Place the earpieces in your ears.
12. Find the apical pulse. Have your helper find the radial pulse (Fig. 16-24).
13. Give the signal to begin counting.
14. Count the pulse for 1 full minute.
15. Give the signal to stop counting.
16. Cover the resident. Remove the earpieces.
17. Record the resident's name and the apical and radial pulses. Subtract the radial pulse from the apical pulse for the pulse deficit. Note whether the pulse was regular or irregular.
18. Make sure the resident is comfortable and the signal light is within reach.
19. Unscreen the resident.
20. Clean the earpieces and diaphragm with alcohol wipes.
21. Return the stethoscope to its proper place.
22. Wash your hands.
23. Report the following to the nurse:
    a. An apical pulse rate less than 60 or greater than 100 beats per minute is reported immediately
    b. The apical and radial pulse rates
    c. The pulse deficit
    d. Whether the pulse was regular or irregular
    e. Any unusual heart sounds
24. Record the pulses in the proper place. Indicate that an apical-radial pulse was taken.

RESPIRATIONS

Respiration is the act of breathing air into the lungs (inhalation) and out of the lungs (exhalation). Oxygen is taken into the lungs during inhalation. Carbon dioxide is moved out of the lungs during exhalation. Each respiration involves one inhalation and one exhalation. The chest rises during inhalation and falls during exhalation.

Healthy adults have 14 to 20 respirations per minute. The respiratory rate is affected by many of the factors that affect body temperature and pulse. Heart and respiratory diseases usually cause an increased number of respirations per minute.

Abnormal Respirations

Normal respirations occur between 14 and 20 times per minute in the adult. They are quiet, effortless, and regular. Both sides of the chest rise and fall equally. You should know the following abnormal respiratory patterns:

1. **Tachypnea**—rapid *(tachy)* breathing *(pnea);* the respiratory rate usually is greater than 24 respirations per minute
2. **Bradypnea**—slow *(brady)* breathing *(pnea);* the respiratory rate is less than 10 respirations per minute
3. **Apnea**—the lack or absence *(a)* of breathing *(pnea)*
4. **Hypoventilation**—respirations that are slow *(hypo)*, shallow, and sometimes irregular
5. **Hyperventilation**—respirations that are rapid *(hyper)* and deeper than normal
6. **Dyspnea**—difficult, labored, or painful *(dys)* breathing *(pnea)*
7. **Cheyne-Stokes**—a breathing pattern in which respirations gradually increase in rate and depth and then become shallow and slow; breathing may stop *(apnea)* for 10 to 20 seconds

Counting Respirations

Respirations are counted when the resident is at rest. The resident should be positioned so you can see the chest rise and fall. The depth and rate of breathing can be voluntarily controlled to a certain extent. People tend to change breathing patterns when they know their respirations are being counted. Therefore the resident should not know that respirations are being counted.

Respirations are counted right after taking a pulse. The fingers or stethoscope stay over the pulse site. The resident thinks the pulse is still being taken. Respirations are counted by watching the rise and fall of the chest. They are counted for 30 seconds. The number is multiplied by 2 for the total number of respirations in 1 minute. If an abnormal pattern is noted, the respirations are counted for 1 full minute.

PROCEDURE

Counting the Resident's Respirations

1. Continue to hold the resident's wrist after taking the radial pulse. Keep the stethoscope in place if an apical pulse was taken.
2. Do *not* tell the resident you are counting respirations.
3. Begin counting when you see the chest rise. Count each rise and fall of the chest as 1 respiration.
4. Observe if respirations are regular and if both sides of the chest rise equally. Also note the depth of respirations and if the resident has any pain or difficulty in breathing.
5. Count respirations for 30 seconds. Multiply the number by 2.
6. Count the respirations for 1 full minute if they are abnormal or irregular.
7. Record the resident's name, respiratory rate, and other observations.
8. Make sure the resident is comfortable and the signal light is within reach.
9. Wash your hands.
10. Report the following to the nurse:
    a. The respiratory rate
    b. Equality and depth of respirations
    c. If the respirations were regular or irregular
    d. If the resident experienced pain or difficulty in breathing
    e. Any respiratory noises
    f. Any abnormal respiratory patterns
11. Record the respiratory rate in the proper place.

BLOOD PRESSURE

Blood pressure is the amount of force exerted against the walls of an artery by the blood. Blood pressure is controlled by the force of heart contractions, the amount of blood pumped with each heartbeat, and how easily the blood flows through the blood vessels. The period of heart muscle contraction is called **systole.** The period of heart muscle relaxation is called **diastole.**

Both systolic and diastolic pressures are measured. The **systolic pressure** is the higher pressure. It represents the amount of force needed to pump blood out of the heart into the arterial circulation. The **diastolic pressure** is the lower pressure. It reflects the pressure in the arteries when the heart is at rest. Blood pressure is measured in millimeters (mm) of mercury (Hg). The systolic pressure is recorded over the diastolic pressure. For example, a resident has a systolic pressure of 120 mm Hg and a diastolic pressure of 80 mm Hg. This is written as 120/80 mm Hg.

Factors That Affect Blood Pressure

Blood pressure is affected by many factors and can change from minute to minute. Age, sex, the amount of blood in the system, and emotions affect blood pressure. So do pain, exercise, body size, and medications. Because it can vary so easily, there are normal ranges for blood pressure. Systolic pressures between 100 and 140 mm Hg are considered normal for adults. Normal diastolic pressures are between 60 and 90 mm Hg. The pressure of elderly persons may be higher but still normal. A systolic pressure between 100 and 160 mm Hg is normal for the elderly. So is a diastolic pressure of 60 to 95 mm Hg.

Persistent measurements above the normal systolic and diastolic pressures are considered abnormal. This condition is called **hypertension.** Report any elevated systolic or diastolic pressure immediately. Also report immediately systolic pressures below 90 mm Hg and diastolic pressures below 60 mm Hg. This is called **hypotension.** Some people normally have low blood pressures. In most people, however, hypotension means a serious condition that can lead to death if not corrected.

Equipment

A stethoscope and a sphygmomanometer are used to measure blood pressure. The **sphygmomanometer** (blood pressure cuff) consists of a cuff and a measuring device. There are three types of sphygmomanometers: aneroid (Fig. 16-25, *A*), mercury (Fig. 16-25, *B*), and electronic (Fig. 16-26, p. 380). The aneroid type has a round dial and a needle that points to the calibrations. The aneroid manometer is small and easy to carry. The mercury manometer is more accurate than the aneroid type. The mercury type has a column of mercury within

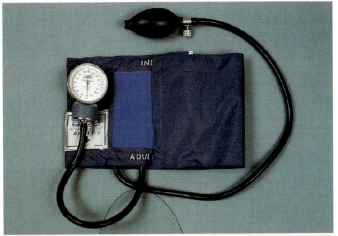

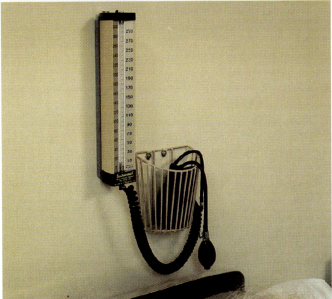

FIGURE 16-25 *A, Aneroid manometer and cuff. B, Mercury manometer and cuff.*

a calibrated tube. Hospital-based skilled nursing units may have wall-mounted mercury sphygmomanometers.

The blood pressure cuff is wrapped around the upper arm. Tubing connects the cuff to the manometer. Another tube connects the cuff to a small hand-held bulb. A valve on the bulb is turned to allow the cuff to inflate as the bulb is squeezed. The inflated cuff causes pressure over the brachial artery. The valve is turned in the opposite direction for cuff deflation. Blood pressure is measured as the cuff is deflated.

Sounds are produced as blood flows through the arteries. The stethoscope is used by the nursing assistant to listen to the sounds in the brachial artery as the cuff is deflated. Stethoscopes are not needed with electronic sphygmomanometers.

There are many types of electronic sphygmomanometers (Fig. 16-26). The systolic and diastolic pressures are displayed on the front of the instrument. The pulse usually is displayed also. The cuff automatically inflates and deflates on some models. Others have only automatic deflation. If electronic blood pressure equipment is used where you work, you need to learn how to use it. Ask the nurse to show you what to do. The manufacturer's instructions also will help.

Measuring Blood Pressure

Blood pressure normally is measured in the brachial artery. Use the following guidelines when measuring blood pressure.

1. Do not take blood pressure on an arm with an IV infusion or a cast, or on an injured arm. If a resident has had breast surgery, blood pressure is *not* taken on that side.
2. Let the resident rest about 15 minutes before the blood pressure is measured.
3. The cuff is applied to the bare upper arm, not over clothing. Clothing can affect the measurement.
4. The diaphragm of the stethoscope is placed firmly over the artery. The entire diaphragm must be in contact with the skin.
5. The room should be quiet so that the blood pressure can be heard. Talking, television, radio, and sounds from the hallway can interfere with an accurate measurement.
6. The sphygmomanometer must be clearly visible.
7. The radial artery is located and the cuff is inflated. When the radial pulse is no longer felt, the cuff is inflated an additional 30 mm Hg. This prevents cuff inflation to an unnecessarily high pressure, which is painful to the resident.
8. The point at which the radial pulse is no longer felt is where you should expect to hear the first blood pressure sound. The first sound is the systolic pressure. The point where the sound disappears is the diastolic pressure.

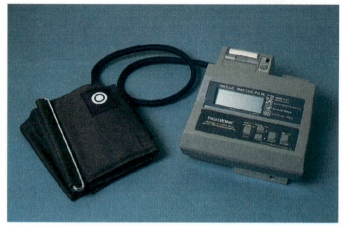

FIGURE 16-26 *Electronic sphygmomanometer.*

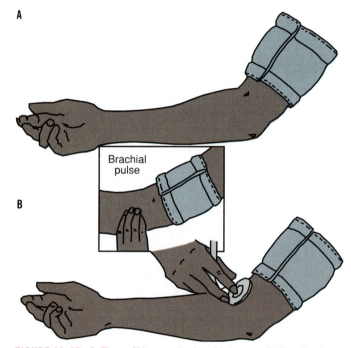

Brachial pulse

FIGURE 16-27 *A,* The cuff is over the brachial artery. *B,* The diaphragm of the stethoscope is over the brachial artery.

PROCEDURE

Measuring Blood Pressure

1. Collect the following:
   a. Sphygmomanometer (blood pressure cuff)
   b. Stethoscope
   c. Alcohol wipes

2. Wash your hands.

3. Identify the resident. Check the ID bracelet and call the resident by name.

4. Explain the procedure to the resident.

5. Provide for privacy.

6. Wipe the stethoscope earpieces and diaphragm with alcohol wipes.

7. Have the resident sit or lie down.

8. Position the resident's arm so that it is level with the heart. The palm should be up.

9. Stand no more than 3 feet away from the sphygmomanometer. A mercury model should be vertical, on a flat surface, and at eye level. The aneroid type should be directly in front of you.

10. Expose the upper arm.

11. Squeeze the cuff to expel any remaining air. Close the valve on the bulb.

12. Find the brachial artery at the inner aspect of the elbow.

13. Place the arrow marking on the cuff over the brachial artery (Fig. 16-27, *A*). Wrap the cuff around the person's upper arm at least 1 inch above the elbow. It should be even and snug.

14. Place the stethoscope earpieces in your ears.

15. Find the radial artery. Inflate the cuff until you can no longer feel the radial pulse. Inflate the cuff 30 mm Hg beyond the point at which you last felt the pulse.

16. Position the diaphragm over the brachial artery (Fig. 16-27, *B*).

17. Deflate the cuff at an even rate of 2 to 4 millimeters per second. Turn the valve counterclockwise to deflate the cuff.

18. Note the point on the scale where you hear the first sound. This is the systolic reading. It should be near the point where the radial pulse disappeared.

19. Continue to deflate the cuff. Note the point where the sound disappears for the diastolic reading.

20. Deflate the cuff completely. Remove it from the resident's arm. Remove the stethoscope.

21. Record the resident's name and blood pressure.

22. Return the cuff to the case or wall holder.

23. Make sure the resident is comfortable and the signal light is within reach.

24. Unscreen the resident.

25. Clean the earpieces and diaphragm with alcohol wipes.

26. Return equipment to its proper place.

27. Wash your hands.

28. Report the blood pressure. Record it in the proper place.

Quality OF LIFE

You must protect the resident's right to privacy when measuring vital signs. Privacy must be provided during the procedures. This is especially important if you are taking axillary or rectal temperatures and apical pulses. The resident must not be exposed unnecessarily.

You also need to keep resident information confidential. Vital signs are just as private as other resident information. Share this information only with the nurse. Refer questions from family and visitors to the nurse.

The right to personal choice is important. Unless orders note otherwise, vital signs can be measured with the resident sitting or lying down. Let the resident choose the position. The resident also may prefer that you use the right or left arm for pulses and blood pressures. Use the arm the resident prefers if it is safe to do so (see p. 380).

SUMMARY

Temperature, pulse, respirations, and blood pressure give valuable information about a person's state of health or illness. Vital signs can vary within certain normal ranges. Changes above or below the normal range mean a disorder or serious illness. Vital signs can change in response to the slightest change in body functions.

Measuring vital signs is an important part of your job.

These signs must be accurately measured. Any abnormal measurements must be immediately reported to the nurse. They could signal serious threats to the resident's life. Clear and accurate recording of vital signs is equally important. Doctors and nurses use them to decide on treatment and to evaluate care.

Review QUESTIONS

Circle the *best* answer.

1. Which statement is *false?*
   a. The vital signs are temperature, pulse, respirations, and blood pressure.
   b. Vital signs detect changes in normal body function.
   c. Vital signs change only when a person is ill.
   d. Sleep, exercise, medications, emotions, and noise can affect vital signs.

2. Which should you report immediately?
   a. An oral temperature of 98.4° F
   b. A rectal temperature of 101.6° F
   c. An axillary temperature of 97.6° F
   d. An oral temperature of 99.0° F

3. Electronic thermometers measure temperatures in
   a. 2 to 60 seconds
   b. 45 seconds
   c. 3 to 4 minutes
   d. 9 minutes

4. Do not take a rectal temperature when the resident
   a. Is unconscious
   b. Is confused
   c. Has a nasogastric tube
   d. Has had rectal surgery

5. Which usually is used to take a pulse?
   a. The radial pulse
   b. The apical-radial pulse
   c. The apical pulse
   d. The brachial pulse

6. Which should be reported immediately?
   a. A resident has a pulse of 120 beats per minute.
   b. A resident has a pulse of 62 beats per minute.
   c. A resident has a pulse of 80 beats per minute.
   d. All of the above

7. Which statement about apical-radial pulses is *true?*
   a. The pulse can be taken by one person.
   b. The radial pulse can be greater than the apical pulse.
   c. The apical pulse can be greater than the radial pulse.
   d. The apical and radial pulses are always equal.

8. Normal respirations are
   a. Between 14 and 20 per minute
   b. Quiet and effortless
   c. Regular, with both sides of the chest rising and falling equally
   d. All of the above

9. Difficult, painful, or labored breathing is known as
   a. Tachypnea
   b. Bradypnea
   c. Apnea
   d. Dyspnea

10. Respirations usually are counted
    a. After taking the temperature
    b. After taking the pulse
    c. Before taking the pulse
    d. After taking the blood pressure

11. Which blood pressure is normal in an adult?
    a. 98/54 mm Hg
    b. 210/100 mm Hg
    c. 130/82 mm Hg
    d. 162/100 mm Hg

12. When taking a blood pressure, do all of the following *except*
    a. Take the blood pressure in the arm with an IV infusion
    b. Apply the cuff to a bare upper arm
    c. Turn off the television and radio
    d. Locate the brachial artery

13. Which is the systolic blood pressure?
    a. The point at which the pulse is no longer felt
    b. The point where the first sound is heard
    c. The point where the last sound is heard
    d. The point 30 mm Hg above where the pulse was felt

14. Vital signs are considered confidential information.
    a. True
    b. False

Answers

1. c	5. a	9. d	13. b
2. b	6. a	10. b	14. a
3. a	7. c	11. c	
4. d	8. d	12. a	

17

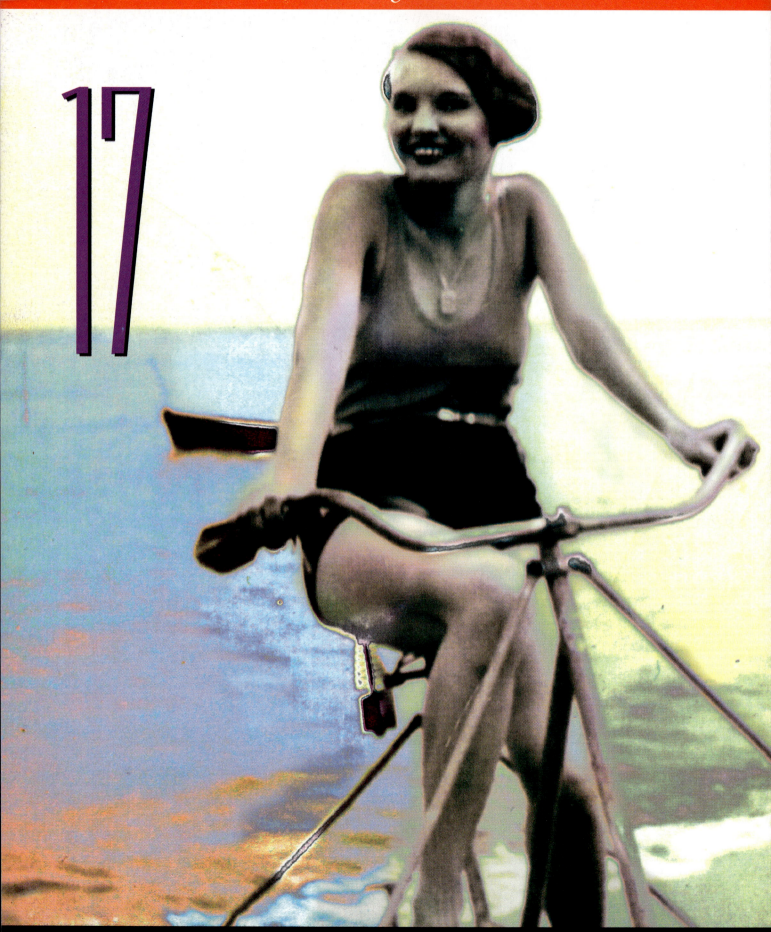

What You Will LEARN

- The key terms listed in this chapter

- The purpose of bed rest

- The complications of bed rest

- How to prevent muscle atrophy and contractures

- What devices are used to support and maintain the body in alignment

- The uses of a trapeze

- The purpose of range-of-motion exercises

- How to perform range-of-motion exercises

- How to help a resident walk

- How to help a falling resident

- Four types of walking aids

abduction
Moving a body part away from the body

adduction
Moving a body part toward the body

ambulation
The act of walking

atrophy
A decrease in size or a wasting away of tissue

contracture
The abnormal shortening of a muscle

deconditioning
The loss of muscle strength as a result of inactivity

dorsiflexion
Bending backward

extension
Straightening of a body part

external rotation
Turning the joint outward

flexion
Bending a body part

footdrop
Permanent plantar flexion

hyperextension
Excessive straightening of a body part

internal rotation
Turning the joint inward

plantar flexion
The foot is bent; footdrop

pronation
Turning downward

range-of-motion (ROM)
The movement of a joint to the extent possible without causing pain

rotation
turning the joint

supination
Turning upward

Being active is important for physical and mental well-being. Ideally, we can move about without help from others. Unfortunately, aging, illness, surgery, and injury can result in weakness and can limit activity. Depression may cause people to limit their activity. Some people feel tired and weak. They may sit or lie down frequently. For others, bed rest is prescribed for long periods. Inactivity, whether minimal or severe, can affect the normal function of every body system.

Deconditioning is the loss of muscle strength from inactivity. Elderly persons become deconditioned quickly when they are inactive. The nursing team is responsible for promoting exercise and activity for all residents. Each resident needs to be as active as physically possible. The nurse will tell you about each resident's activity level and what exercises to perform. To effectively assist in promoting exercise and activity, you need to understand certain concepts. You need to understand bed rest and how to prevent the complications of bed rest. You need to know how to help residents exercise and remain active. You also need to know how to help deconditioned residents regain their strength.

BED REST

Bed rest has many meanings. It varies among facilities, nursing personnel, and doctors. The person on bed rest may be allowed to take part in activities of daily living (ADL). Bathing, oral hygiene, hair care, and feeding may be allowed. "Strict" or "absolute" bed rest may be ordered. If so, everything is done for the resident. ADL are not allowed. Strict bed rest rarely is seen in nursing facilities. Residents are encouraged to do as much for themselves as possible. Some residents, however, cannot help themselves.

Bed rest may be ordered by the doctor because of a person's health problems. It also may be a nursing measure because of a change in the resident's condition. You must know what activities are allowed for each person. The Kardex and the resident's care plan will have this information. Be sure to check with the nurse if you have any questions.

The Complications of Bed Rest

Bed rest has many useful purposes. The person can rest rather than move about as usual. Pain is reduced and healing promoted. However, bed rest and the lack of exercise and activity can cause serious complications. Pres-

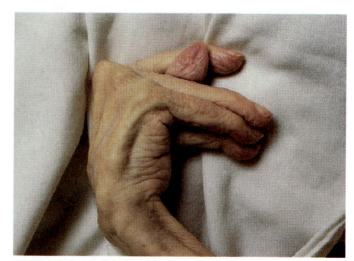

FIGURE 17-1 *A contracture.*

sure sores, constipation, and fecal impaction can occur. So can blood clots, urinary tract infections, and pneumonia (infection of the lung). Contractures, muscle atrophy, and deconditioning are other complications.

A **contracture** is the abnormal shortening of a muscle. The contracted muscle is fixed into position (Fig. 17-1), is permanently deformed, and cannot be stretched. The person is permanently deformed and disabled. Contractures must be prevented. Some residents already have contractures when admitted to the facility. **Atrophy** is the decrease in size or wasting away of tissue. Muscle atrophy is a decrease in size or wasting away of muscle (Fig. 17-2). Some degree of muscle atrophy is part of normal aging. Contractures and severe muscle atrophy must be prevented so that normal body movement can occur.

Deconditioning can begin in elderly persons after only 24 hours of bed rest or inactivity. This lose of muscle strength increases the risk for falls. Falls can result in serious injury or death.

Preventing the Complications of Bed Rest

The complications of bed rest can be prevented by good nursing care. You have an important role in preventing contractures, muscle atrophy, and deconditioning. Positioning residents in good body alignment is essential. Performing range-of-motion exercises is another important preventive measure.

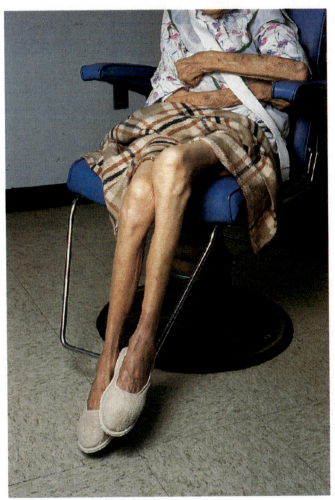

FIGURE 17-2 *Muscle atrophy.*

Positioning. Body alignment and positioning the resident in bed were discussed in Chapter 9. In addition to positioning the person in good alignment, supportive devices may be needed. They support and maintain the resident in a certain position.

Bed boards. Bed boards are placed under the mattress. They keep the resident in better alignment by preventing the mattress from sagging (Fig. 17-3). Bed boards usually are made of plywood and are covered with material. There are two sections. One is for the head of the bed and the other for the foot. The two sections allow the head of the bed to be raised.

Footboards. A footboard (Fig. 17-4) is placed at the foot of the mattress to prevent **plantar flexion (foot-drop).** In plantar flexion the foot (plantar) is bent (flexion). The footboard is positioned so that the soles of the feet are flush against the footboard. The feet are in good alignment as in the standing position. The footboard can also be used as a bed cradle to keep top linens off the feet.

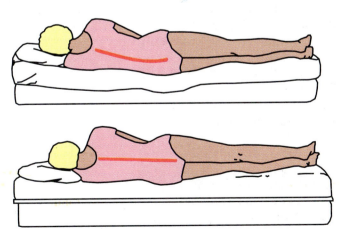

FIGURE 17-3 *A, Mattress sagging without bed boards. B, Bed boards are placed under the mattress. No sagging occurs.*

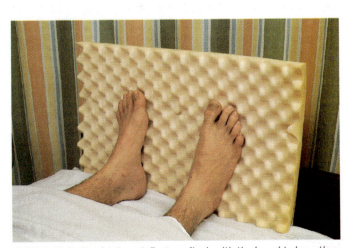

FIGURE 17-4 *The footboard. Feet are flush with the board to keep them in normal alignment.*

Trochanter rolls. Trochanter rolls (Fig. 17-5) prevent the hips and legs from turning outward (external rotation). Bath blankets are used for trochanter rolls. The blanket is folded to the desired length and rolled up. The loose end is placed under the resident from the hip to the knee. Then the roll is tucked alongside the body. Pillows or sandbags also can be used to keep the hips and knees in alignment.

Handrolls. The person can grasp a handroll to prevent contractures of the thumb, fingers, and wrist. Commercial handrolls are common (Fig. 17-6). One can be made by rolling up a washcloth (see Fig. 7-15, p. 123). Finger cushions prevent the hand from closing completely (Fig. 17-7). Foam rubber sponges, rubber balls, and special palm cones (Fig. 17-8) also may be used.

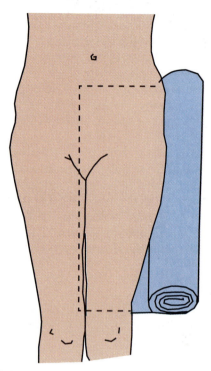

FIGURE 17-5 *Trochanter roll made from a bath blanket. It extends from the hip to the knee.*

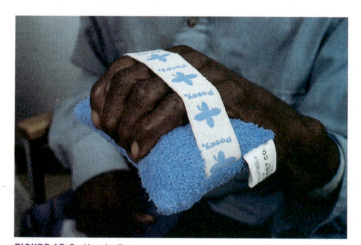

FIGURE 17-6 *Handroll.*

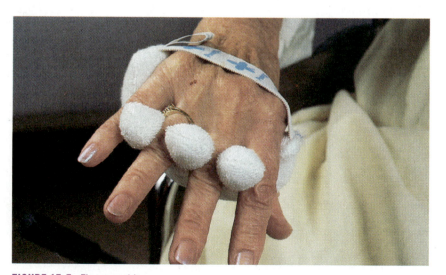

FIGURE 17-7 *Finger cushion.*

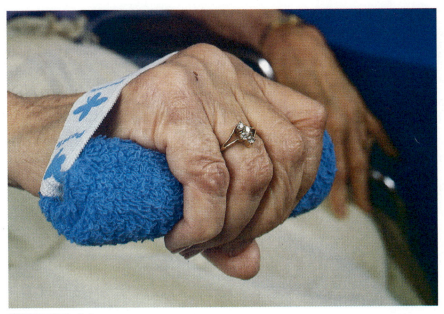

FIGURE 17-8 *Palm cone.*

Bed cradles. The weight of linens on the foot can cause footdrop and pressure sores. A bed cradle (see Fig. 12-53, p. 278) often is used to keep top linens off the feet.

Exercise. Exercise helps prevent contractures, muscle atrophy, deconditioning, and other complications of bed rest. Some exercise occurs with activities of daily living and with turning and moving in bed without assistance. Additional exercises, however, are needed for muscles and joints. These may include range-of-motion exercises, sitting in a chair for brief periods, or walking short distances with assistance.

Trapeze. A trapeze or trapeze bar is a swinging bar suspended from an overbed frame. The resident grasps the bar with both hands to lift the trunk off the bed. The trapeze also is used to move up and turn in bed. If allowed, it can be used for pulling exercises to strengthen arm muscles.

Range-of-motion exercises. The movement of a joint to the extent possible without causing pain is the **range-of-motion (ROM)** of that joint. Range-of-motion exercises involve exercising the joints through their complete range-of-motion. These exercises may be active, passive, or active-assistive. *Active* range-of-motion exercises are done by the person. *Passive* exercises involve having another person move the joints through their range of motion. *Active-assistive* range of motion means that the person does the exercises with some assistance from another person.

The following movements relate to range-of-motion exercises:

1. **Abduction**—moving a body part away from the body
2. **Adduction**—moving a body part toward the body
3. **Extension**—straightening a body part
4. **Flexion**—bending a body part
5. **Hyperextension**—the excessive straightening of a body part
6. **Dorsiflexion**—bending backward
7. **Rotation**—turning the joint
8. **Internal rotation**—turning the joint inward
9. **External rotation**—turning the joint outward
10. **Pronation**—turning downward
11. **Supination**—turning upward

Range-of-motion exercises usually are part of morning care. Residents on bed rest may require more frequent range-of-motion exercises. So may those who have loss of mobility resulting from a stroke or injury. Therefore the doctor or nurse may order more frequent range-of-motion exercises. The nurse will tell you which joints to exercise, the frequency of the exercises, and if the exercises are to be active, passive, or active-assistive.

General rules. Range-of-motion exercises can cause injury if not performed properly. The following rules are practiced when you are performing or assisting with range-of-motion exercises.

1. Exercise only the joints that the nurse tells you to exercise.
2. Expose only the body part being exercised.
3. Use good body mechanics.
4. Support the extremity being exercised.
5. Move the joint slowly, smoothly, and gently.
6. Do not force a joint beyond its present range-of-motion or to the point of pain.

PROCEDURE

Performing Range-of-Motion Exercises

1. Identify the resident. Check the ID bracelet and call the resident by name.

2. Explain the procedure to the resident.

3. Wash your hands.

4. Obtain a bath blanket.

5. Provide for privacy.

6. Raise the bed to the best level for good body mechanics.

7. Lower the side rail.

8. Position the resident supine and in good alignment.

9. Cover the resident with a bath blanket. Fan-fold top linens to the foot of the bed.

10. Exercise the neck (Fig. 17-9).
    a. Place your hands over the resident's ears to support the head.
    b. Flexion—bring the head forward so the chin touches the chest.
    c. Extension—straighten the head.
    d. Hyperextension—bring the head backward until the chin is up.
    e. Rotation—turn the head from side to side.
    f. Lateral flexion—move the head to the right and to the left.
    g. Repeat flexion, extension, hyperextension, rotation, and lateral flexion 5 to 6 times.

11. Exercise the shoulder (Fig. 17-10).
    a. Grasp the wrist with one hand and the elbow with the other.
    b. Flexion—raise the arm straight in front and over the head.
    c. Extension—bring the arm down to the side.
    d. Hyperextension—move the arm behind the body. (This step can be done if the person is standing or sitting in a straight-back chair.)
    e. Abduction—move the straight arm away from the side of the body.
    f. Adduction—move the straight arm to the side of the body.
    g. Internal rotation—bend the elbow and place it at the same level as the shoulder. Move the forearm down toward the body.
    h. External rotation—move the forearm toward the head.
    i. Repeat flexion, extension, hyperextension, abduction, adduction, and internal and external rotation 5 to 6 times.

12. Exercise the elbow (Fig. 17-11).
    a. Grasp the resident's wrist with one hand and the elbow with the other.
    b. Flexion—bend the arm so that the same-side shoulder is touched.
    c. Extension—straighten the arm.
    d. Repeat flexion and extension 5 to 6 times.

13. Exercise the forearm (Fig. 17-12).
    a. Pronation—turn the hand so the palm is down.
    b. Supination—turn the hand so the palm is up.
    c. Repeat pronation and supination 5 to 6 times.

14. Exercise the wrist (Fig. 17-13).
    a. Hold the wrist with both of your hands.
    b. Flexion—bend the hand down.
    c. Extension—straighten the hand.
    d. Hyperextension—bend the hand back.
    e. Radial flexion—turn the hand toward the thumb.
    f. Ulnar flexion—turn the hand toward the little finger.
    g. Repeat flexion, extension, hyperextension, and radial and ulnar flexion 5 to 6 times.

15. Exercise the thumb (Fig. 17-14).
    a. Hold the resident's hand with one hand and the thumb with your other hand.
    b. Abduction—move the thumb out from the inner part of the index finger.
    c. Adduction—move the thumb back next to the index finger.

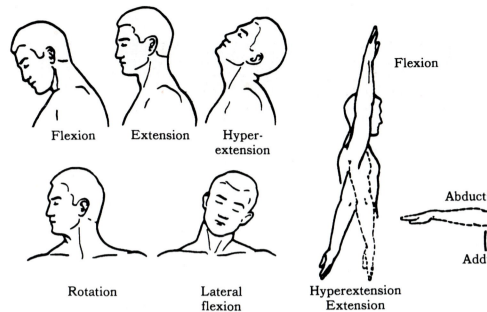

FIGURE 17-9 *Range-of-motion exercises for the neck.*

Flexion   Extension   Hyper-extension

Rotation   Lateral flexion

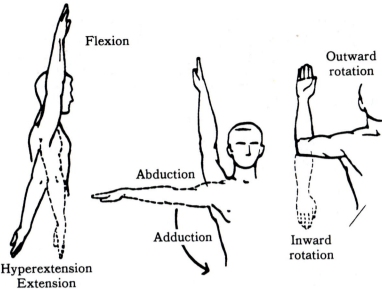

Flexion

Outward rotation

Abduction

Adduction

Inward rotation

Hyperextension Extension

FIGURE 17-10 *Range-of-motion exercises for the shoulder.*

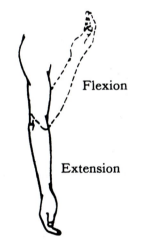

Flexion

Extension

FIGURE 17-11 *Range-of-motion exercises for the elbow.*

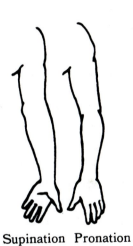

Supination   Pronation

FIGURE 17-12 *Range-of-motion exercises for the forearm.*

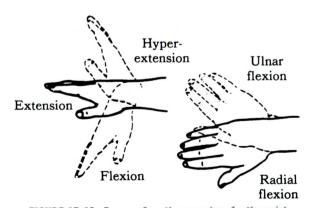

Hyper-extension

Ulnar flexion

Extension

Flexion

Radial flexion

FIGURE 17-13 *Range-of-motion exercises for the wrist.*

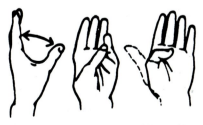

Abduction Adduction   Opposition to little finger   Extension Flexion

FIGURE 17-14 *Range-of-motion exercises for the thumb.*

Continued.

391

d. Opposition—touch each fingertip with the thumb.

e. Flexion—bend the thumb into the hand.

f. Extension—move the thumb out to the side of the fingers.

g. Repeat flexion, extension, abduction, adduction, and opposition 5 to 6 times.

16. Exercise the fingers (Fig. 17-15).

a. Abduction—spread the fingers and the thumb apart.

b. Adduction—bring the fingers and thumb together.

c. Extension—straighten the fingers so that the fingers, hand, and arm are straight.

d. Flexion—make a fist.

e. Repeat abduction, adduction, extension, and flexion 5 to 6 times.

17. Exercise the hip (Fig. 17-16).

a. Place one hand under the resident's knee and the other under the ankle to support the leg.

b. Flexion—raise the leg.

c. Extension—straighten the leg.

d. Abduction—move the leg away from the body.

e. Adduction—move the leg toward the other leg.

f. Internal rotation—turn the leg inward.

g. External rotation—turn the leg outward.

h. Repeat flexion, extension, abduction, adduction, and inward and outward rotation 5 to 6 times.

18. Exercise the knee (Fig. 17-17).

a. Place one hand under the knee and the other under the ankle to support the leg.

b. Flexion—bend the leg.

c. Extension—straighten the leg.

d. Repeat flexion and extension of the knee 5 to 6 times

19. Exercise the ankle (Fig. 17-18).

a. Place one hand under the foot and the other under the ankle to support the part.

b. Dorsiflexion—pull the foot forward and push down on the heel at the same time.

c. Plantar flexion—turn the foot down or point the toes.

d. Repeat dorsal flexion and plantar flexion 5 to 6 times.

20. Exercise the foot (Fig. 17-19).

a. Pronation—turn the outside of the foot up and the inside down.

b. Supination—turn the inside of the foot up and the outside down.

c. Repeat pronation and supination 5 to 6 times.

21. Exercise the toes (Fig. 17-20).

a. Flexion—curl the toes.

b. Extension—straighten the toes.

c. Abduction—pull the toes together.

d. Repeat flexion, extension, abduction, and adduction 5 to 6 times.

22. Cover the leg and raise the side rail.

23. Go to the other side and lower the side rail.

24. Repeat steps 11 through 22.

25. Make sure the resident is comfortable.

26. Return top linens to their proper position. Remove the bath blanket.

27. Lower the bed to its lowest level.

28. Raise or lower side rails as instructed by the nurse.

29. Place the signal light within reach.

30. Unscreen the resident.

31. Return the bath blanket to its proper place.

32. Wash your hands.

33. Report the following to the nurse:

a. The time the exercises were performed

b. The joints that were exercised

c. The number of times the exercises were performed on each joint

d. Any complaints of pain or signs of stiffness or spasm

e. The degree to which the resident participated in the exercises

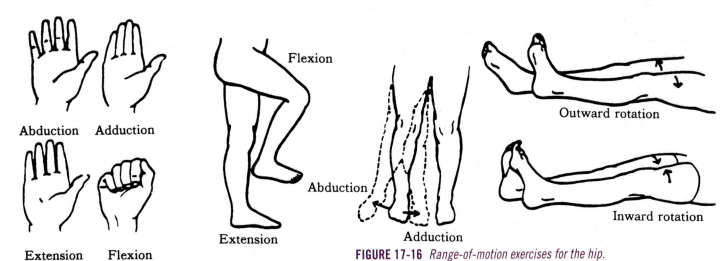

Abduction   Adduction

Extension   Flexion

FIGURE 17-15 *Range-of-motion exercises for the fingers.*

FIGURE 17-16 *Range-of-motion exercises for the hip.*

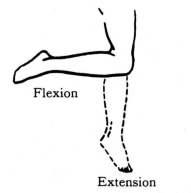

FIGURE 17-17 *Range-of-motion exercises for the knee.*

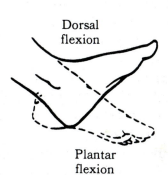

FIGURE 17-18 *Range-of-motion exercises for the ankle.*

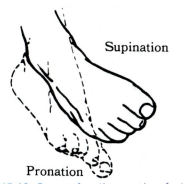

FIGURE 17-19 *Range-of-motion exercises for the foot.*

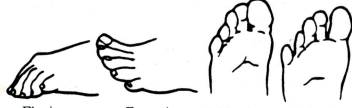

FIGURE 17-20 *Range-of-motion exercises for the toes.*

AMBULATION

Many residents cannot walk without assistance. However, they must walk regularly to prevent deconditioning. Some will become independent in walking. Others will always need help. Residents on bed rest need to increase activity slowly. Activity is increased in steps. First the resident dangles (sits on the side of the bed). The next step is to sit in a bedside chair. Next the resident walks about in the room and then in the hallway. **Ambulation,** the act of walking, should pose few problems if compli-

cations have been prevented. Deconditioning, contractures, and muscle atrophy are prevented by proper positioning and exercise.

Residents may be weak and unsteady from inactivity, illness, or injury. You need to help them begin to walk after bed rest or illness. Use a transfer (gait or safety) belt if the person is weak or unsteady. For additional support, the resident can use the handrails along the wall. Some residents in wheelchairs can walk with assistance. They should be ambulated at least once per shift.

PROCEDURE

Helping the Resident to Walk

1. Explain the procedure to the resident.

2. Wash your hands.

3. Collect the following:
   a. Robe and shoes if the resident has been in bed
   b. Paper or sheet to protect bottom linens
   c. Transfer (gait or safety) belt

4. Identify the resident. Check the ID bracelet and call the resident by name.

5. Provide for privacy.

6. Move furniture if necessary to allow moving space for you and the resident.

7. Put the bed in the lowest position. Lock the bed wheels.

8. Fan-fold top linens to the foot of the bed.

9. Place the paper or sheet under the feet. This protects the bottom sheet from the shoes. Put the shoes on the resident.

10. Help the resident to dangle (see *Helping the Resident to Sit on the Side of the Bed*, p. 178).

11. Help the resident put on the robe.

12. Apply the transfer belt (see *Applying a Transfer [Gait] Belt*, p. 180).

13. Assist the resident to a standing position.
    a. Stand facing the resident.
    b. Grasp the transfer belt at each side.

   c. Brace your knees against the resident's knees. Block his or her feet with your feet (see Fig. 9-24).
   d. Pull the resident up into a standing position as you straighten your knees (see Fig. 9-26).

14. Stand at the resident's side while he or she gains balance. Do not let go of the transfer belt. Grasp the belt at the side and back.

15. Encourage the resident to stand erect with the head up and back straight.

16. Assist the resident to walk. Walk at his or her side, and support the resident with the transfer belt (Fig. 17-21).

17. Encourage the resident to walk normally. Ask him or her to allow the heel of the foot to strike the floor first. Discourage shuffling, sliding, or walking on tiptoes.

18. Walk the required distance if the resident can tolerate the activity. Do not rush him or her.

19. Help the resident return to bed.
    a. Have the resident stand at the side of the bed.
    b. Pivot him or her a quarter turn. The backs of the knees should touch the bed.
    c. Grasp the sides of the transfer belt.
    d. Lower the resident onto the bed as you bend your knees. Remove the transfer belt and robe.
    e. Help the resident lie down (see *Helping the Resident to Sit on the Side of the Bed*, p. 178).

20. Lower the head of the bed. Help the resident to the center of the bed.

21. Remove the shoes and the paper or sheet used to protect the bottom sheet.

22. Make sure the resident is comfortable. Return top linens to their proper position.

23. Make sure the signal light is within reach.

24. Raise or lower side rails as instructed by the nurse.

25. Return robe and shoes to their proper place.

26. Move the furniture back to its proper location.

27. Unscreen the resident.

28. Wash your hands.

29. Report the following to the nurse:
    a. How well the resident tolerated the activity
    b. The distance walked

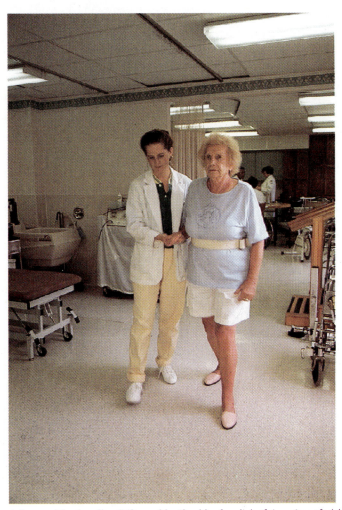

FIGURE 17-21 *The nursing assistant walks at the resident's side. A gait (safety or transfer) belt is used for safety.*

The Falling Resident

Sometimes residents begin to fall when standing or walking. They may become weak, lightheaded, or dizzy. Fainting may occur. Falling may be due to slipping or sliding because of spills, waxed floors, throw rugs, or improper shoes (see Chapter 7). When a resident is falling, there is a tendency to try to prevent the fall. However, trying to prevent a fall could cause greater harm. Twisting and straining to stop the fall could result in injuries to you and the resident. Falls commonly result in head injuries. Balance is lost as a person is falling. If you try to prevent the fall, you could lose your balance. Thus both you and the resident could fall or cause the other person to fall.

If a resident begins to fall, ease him or her to the floor. This lets you control the direction of the fall. You also can protect the resident's head. Do not move the resident once he or she is on the floor. The nurse needs to check the resident before he or she is moved.

PROCEDURE

Helping the Falling Resident

1. Stand with your feet apart. Keep your back straight.

2. Bring the resident close to your body as quickly as possible. Use the gait belt if one is worn. If not, wrap your arms around the resident's waist or hold the resident under the arms (Fig. 17-22).

3. Move your leg so the resident's buttocks rest on it (Fig. 17-23). Move the leg nearest to the resident.

4. Lower the resident to the floor. Let him or her slide down your leg to the floor (Fig. 17-24). Bend at your hips and knees as you do this.

5. Call a nurse to check the resident.

6. Help the nurse return the resident to bed. Get other co-workers to help if necessary.

7. Report the following to the nurse:
   a. How the fall occurred
   b. Any resident complaints before the fall
   c. The amount of assistance needed by the resident while walking

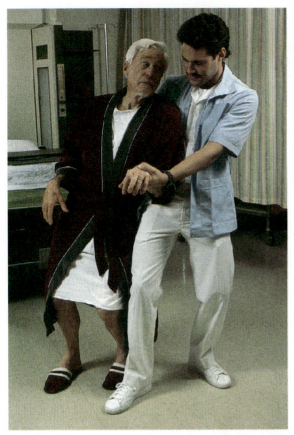

FIGURE 17-22 *Support the falling resident by holding the resident under the arms.*

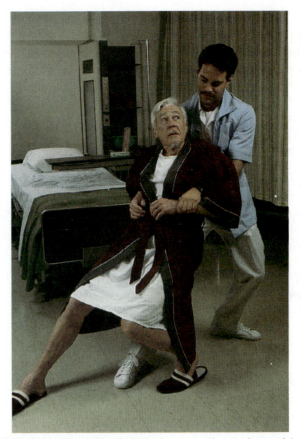

FIGURE 17-23 *The resident's buttocks are on the nursing assistant's leg.*

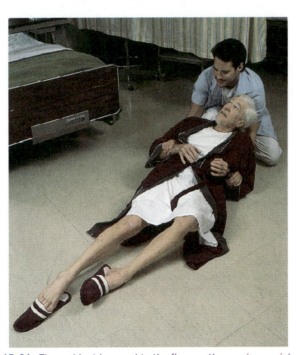

FIGURE 17-24 *The resident is eased to the floor on the nursing assistant's leg.*

Walking Aids

Walking aids support the body. Elderly residents often need walkers or canes for safety while they walk. Walking aids are ordered by the doctor, physical therapist, or nurse. The need may be temporary or permanent. The type ordered depends on the person's physical condition, the amount of support needed, and the type of disability. The physical therapist or nurse teaches the resident to use the walking aid.

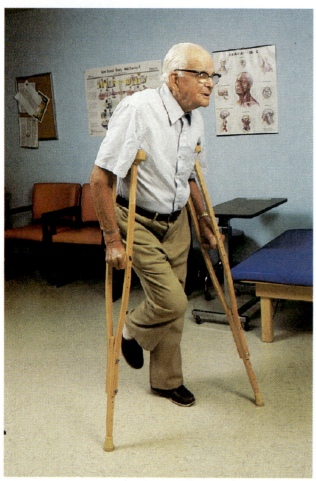

FIGURE 17-25 *A resident using crutches.*

Crutches. Crutches (Fig. 17-25) are used when the person cannot use one leg or when one or both legs need to gain strength. Some residents with permanent leg weakness are able to use crutches. Crutches are not often ordered for elderly persons, but they may be used by younger residents.

Safety must be considered when crutches are used. The person on crutches is at risk of falling. Although crutches provide support, certain safety measures must be followed.

1. The crutches must fit. The resident is measured and fitted with crutches by the nurse or physical therapist. If they do not fit properly, the resident may fall and suffer further injury. The person also is at risk for back pain, nerve damage, and injuries to the underarms and palms.
2. Crutch tips must be attached to the crutches. They must not be worn down or wet.
3. Crutches are checked for flaws. Wooden crutches must be checked for cracks and aluminum crutches for bends. Bolts on both types must be tight.
4. Street shoes are worn. They should be flat with non-skid soles.
5. Clothes must fit well. Loose clothing may get caught between the crutches and underarms. Loose clothing also can hang forward and block the resident's view of the feet and crutch tips.
6. Safety rules to prevent falls must be followed (see Chapter 7).

Canes. Canes are used when there is weakness on one side of the body. They help provide balance and support. There are single-tipped canes and canes with three point and four point canes (Fig. 17-26). A cane is held on the strong side of the body. (If the left leg is weak, the cane is held in the right hand.) Three-point and four-point canes give more support than single-tipped canes. However, they are harder to move.

The tip of the cane should be about 6 to 10 inches (15 to 25 cm) to the side of the foot. The grip is level with the hip (Fig. 17-27). When the resident walks, the cane is moved first. The cane is moved forward about 12 inches (Fig. 17-28, *A*). The weak leg (opposite the cane) is then moved forward even with the cane (Fig. 17-28, *B*). Then the strong leg is brought forward and ahead of the cane and weak leg (Fig. 17-28, *C*). (For Fig. 17-28, *A-C*, see p. 400.)

Walkers. A walker is a four-point walking aid (Fig. 17-29, p. 401). It gives more support than a cane. Many elderly persons feel safer and more secure with a walker than with a cane. There are many kinds of walkers. The standard walker is picked up and moved about 6 inches in front of the resident. The resident then moves the right and then the left foot up to the walker (Fig. 17-30, p. 401).

Text continued on p. 402.

A   B   C

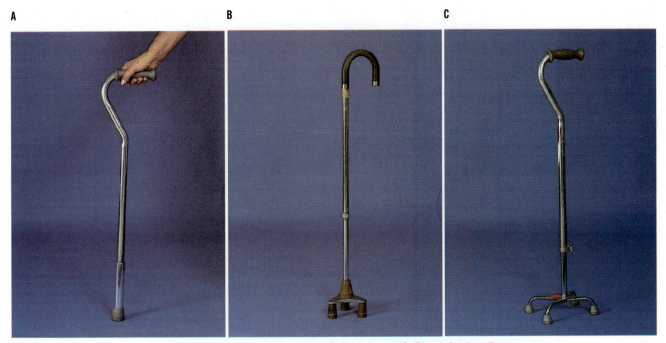

FIGURE 17-26 *A, Single-tipped cane. B, Tripod cane. C, Four-point (quad) cane.*

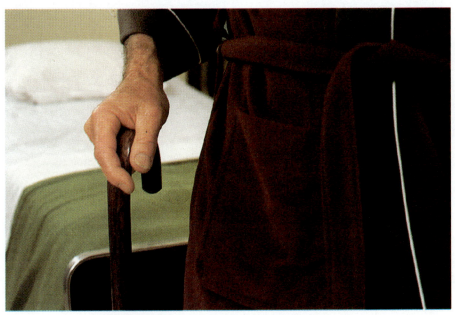

FIGURE 17-27 *The cane grip is held level with the hip.*

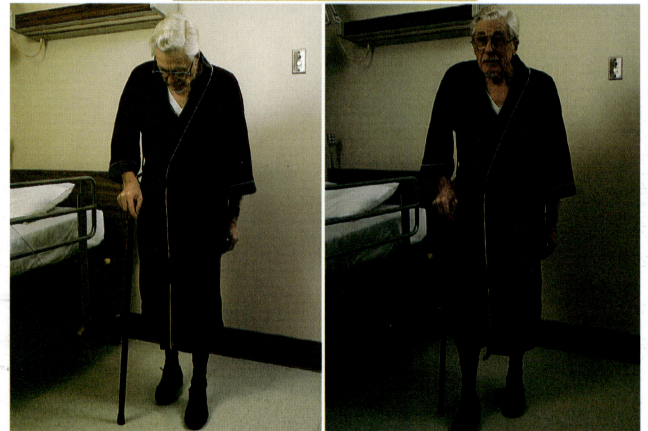

FIGURE 17-28 *Walking with a cane. **A,** The cane is moved forward about 1 foot. **B,** The leg opposite the cane (weak leg) is brought forward even with the cane. **C,** The leg on the cane side (strong leg) is moved ahead of the cane and the weak leg.*

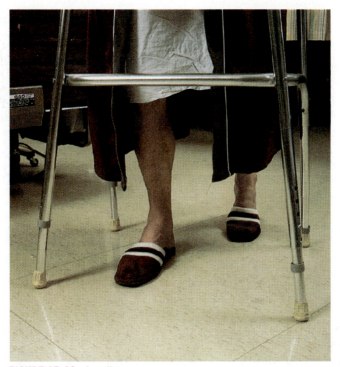

FIGURE 17-29 *A walker.*

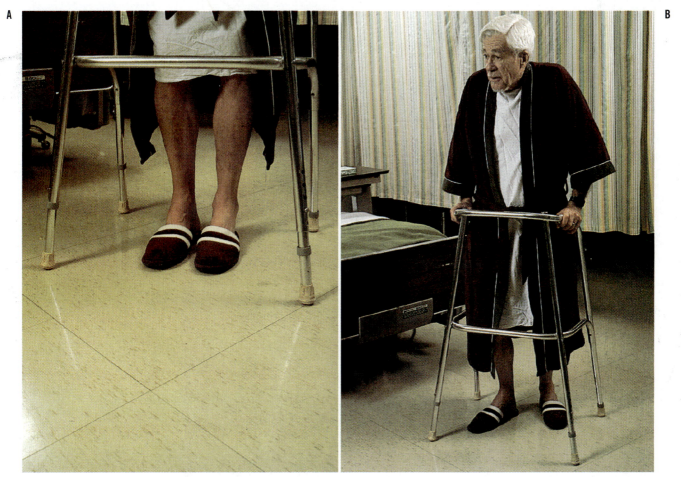

FIGURE 17-30 *Walking with a walker.* ***A,*** *The walker is moved about 6 inches in front of the resident.* ***B,*** *Both feet are moved up to the walker.*

You may see the elderly use wheeled walkers (Fig. 17-31). A wheeled walker has wheels on the front legs and rubber tips on the back legs. This walker is used by residents who cannot pick up a standard walker. The resident pushes the walker ahead about 6 inches and then walks up to it. The rubber tips on the back legs prevent the walker from moving while the resident is walking.

Baskets, pouches, and trays can be attached to the walker (Fig. 17-32). These attachments allow residents to carry needed items rather than rely on others to do so. This allows them greater independence. The attachment also keeps the hands free to grip the walker.

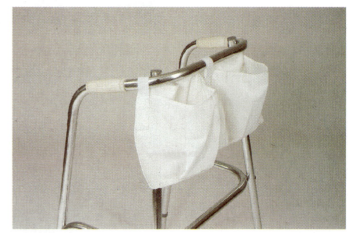

FIGURE 17-32 *The pouch is a walker attachment.*

Braces. Braces support weak body parts. They also are used to prevent or correct deformities or to prevent movement of a joint. Metal, plastic, or leather is used for braces. A brace is applied over the ankle, knee, or back (Fig. 17-33). An ankle-foot orthosis (AFO) is positioned in the shoe (Fig. 17-34). Then the foot is inserted. The device is secured in place with Velcro. This type of brace frequently is used by stroke victims. Bony points under the brace must be protected. Otherwise skin breakdown can occur. You must check the skin before applying a brace. Report any skin breakdown immediately to the nurse.

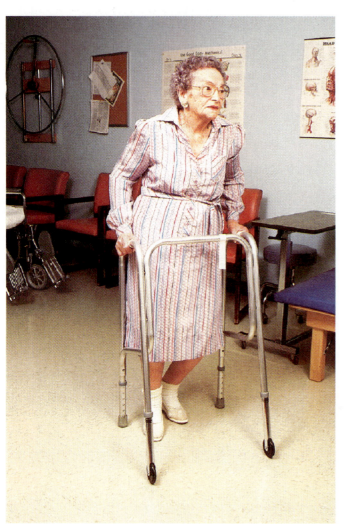

FIGURE 17-31 *An elderly woman using a wheeled walker.*

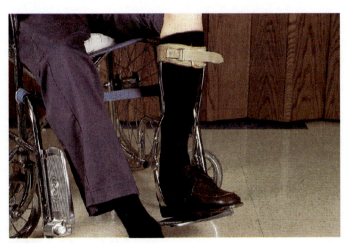

FIGURE 17-33 *A leg brace.*

RECREATIONAL ACTIVITIES

Recreational activities are important for elderly persons, both physically and psychologically. Joints and muscles are exercised, and circulation is stimulated. Recreational activities also provide social opportunities and are mentally stimulating.

Exercise groups, art and writing classes, bingo, dances, community outings (shopping, museums, concerts), movies, and live entertainment often are arranged by nursing facilities. Some facilities have family cookouts, gardening activities, and pets for the residents to care for. Grade school and high school students often provide entertainment or visit certain residents they have "adopted."

Some residents need to be reminded to attend activities. Others may need help getting to activities or taking part in them. You need to know the daily activity schedule so that you can provide assistance as necessary.

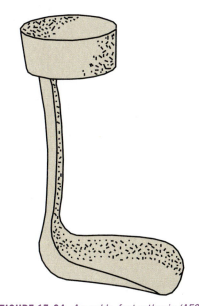

FIGURE 17-34 *An ankle-foot orthosis (AFO).*

Quality OF LIFE

OBRA requires activity programs for residents. As explained in Chapter 1, activities must meet the interests and physical, mental, and psychosocial needs of each resident. The resident's right to personal choice must be protected. That is, the resident is allowed to choose which activities to take part in. The resident must not be forced to take part in an activity that is of no interest to him or her. Remember, OBRA requires that activities promote physical, intellectual, social, and emotional well-being. Well-being is promoted when the resident attends activities of personal choice.

New ideas for activities always are welcome. Residents may share ideas with you or tell you about favorite pastimes. Or you may have ideas of your own. Be sure to share these with the health care team. They can be passed onto the resident group responsi-ble for planning activities. Remember, OBRA also requires that residents be allowed to participate in resident groups.

The rights to privacy and personal choice must be protected when exercising residents. Make sure the resident's privacy is protected when performing range-of-motion exercises. Also make sure that residents are properly clothed when walking in hallways. The resident's body must not be exposed.

Personal choice in ambulating is to be encouraged. The person may want to walk outside. The person may prefer to walk in the morning, afternoon, or evening. The resident may want to wait until a family member arrives or leaves. The resident should be allowed to make such decisions whenever safe and possible. Be sure to get the nurse's approval.

SUMMARY

Exercise and activity are necessary for physical and mental well-being. Complications from lack of activity or exercise can occur when a person is confined to bed. You will position and exercise residents. Such measures prevent muscle atrophy, contractures, and deconditioning. Muscle atrophy and deconditioning can make walking difficult. Contractures cause loss of function and movement of the body part. A leg contracture may make normal walking impossible. Supportive devices and range-of-motion exercises also help prevent deconditioning, muscle atrophy, and contractures.

Residents who can walk are encouraged to ambulate after illness, injury, or surgery. These residents need to walk every day. Weak residents need some assistance at first. Other residents may always need assistance. Some persons need walking aids on a permanent or temporary basis. Crutches, canes, walkers, or braces may be ordered.

Review QUESTIONS

Circle the *best* answer.

1. Which statement about bed rest is *false?*
   a. Persons on bed rest are never allowed to take part in activities of daily living.
   b. Bed rest helps red[...] [...] to healing.
   c. Complications of bed [...] sores, constipation [...] clots, urinary infe[...]
   d. Contractures and [...]

2. A contracture is
   a. The loss of musc[...] [...] tivity
   b. The abnormal sh[...] [...] of a musc[...]
   c. A decrease in si[...] [...]
   d. All of the above

3. Which helps to prev[...]
   a. Bed boards
   b. A footboard

4. Which prevents the [...]
   a. Bed boards
   b. A footboard

5. A trapeze can be u[...]
   a. Lift the trunk [...]
   b. Move up or tu[...]
   c. Strengthen arm[...]
   d. All of the abo[...]

6. Passive range-of-[...] by
   a. The resident
   b. A member of the health care team
   c. The resident, with the help of another
   d. The resident, with the use of a trapeze

7. To safely perform range-of-motion exercises, you should do all of the following *except*
   a. Support the extremity being exercised
   b. Move the joint slowly, smoothly, and gently
   c. Force the joint through full range-of-motion
   d. Exercise only the joints indicated by the nurse

8. Flexion involves
   a. Bending the body part
   b. Straightening the body part
   c. Moving the body part toward the body
   d. Moving the body part away from the body

9. Which statement about ambulation is *false?*
   a. A transfer belt is used if the resident is weak or unsteady.
   b. The resident should shuffle or slide the feet.
   c. Walking aids may be permanent or temporary.
   d. Crutches, canes, walkers, and braces are common walking aids.

10. A single-tipped cane is used
    a. At waist level
    b. On the strong side
    c. On the weak side
    d. On either side

11. You are getting a resident ready to crutch walk. You should do all of the following *except*
    a. Check the crutch tips
    b. Have the resident wear street shoes
    c. Get any pair of crutches from physical therapy
    d. Tighten the bolts on the crutches

Circle *T* if the answer is true and *F* if the answer is false.

T F 12. A single-tipped cane and a four-point cane give equal support.

T F 13. When the resident uses a cane, the feet are moved first.

T F 14. A walker is moved in front of the resident. Then the feet are moved.

T F 15. You feel a resident falling. You should try to prevent the fall.

T F 16. A resident has a brace. Bony areas must be protected from skin breakdown.

T F 17. Recreational activities exercise only muscles and joints.

T F 18. OBRA requires activity programs for residents.

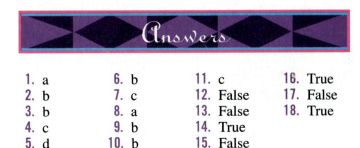

Answers

1. a	6. b	11. c	16. True
2. b	7. c	12. False	17. False
3. b	8. a	13. False	18. True
4. c	9. b	14. True	
5. d	10. b	15. False	

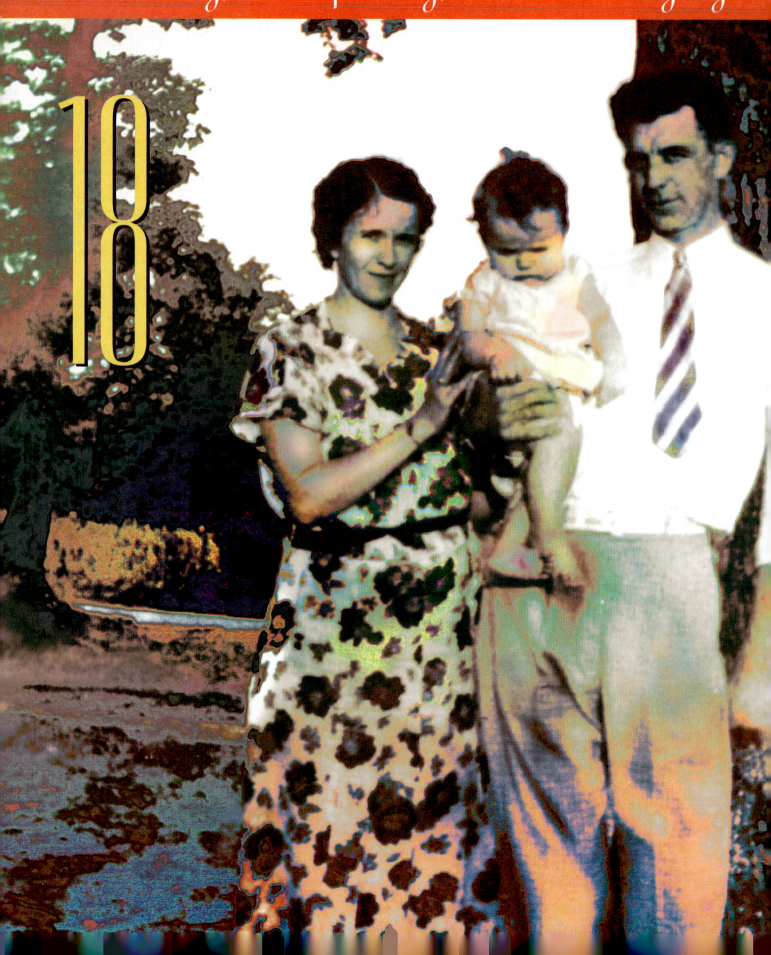

10

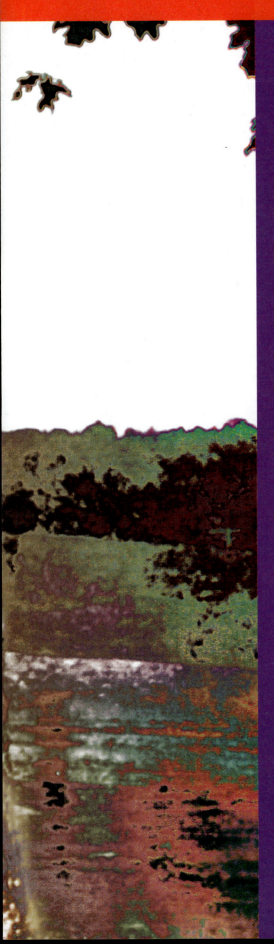

What You Will

LEARN

- The key terms listed in this chapter

- The admission process followed by the business office

- Ways to help the resident feel comfortable in the facility

- How to admit a resident to the nursing unit

- How to weigh and measure residents

- How to handle the resident's clothing and valuables

- Why a person may be transferred to another nursing unit within the facility

- How to prepare a resident for discharge

- How to perform the procedures described in this chapter

admission
Official entry of a person into a facility or nursing unit

discharge
Official departure of a resident from a facility

transfer
Moving a resident from one room, nursing unit, or facility to another

I cried so hard when I had to come here. So did my wife. She couldn't give me the care I need. But she visits every day. And the staff has been very kind. ❧

Admission to a nursing facility causes anxiety and fear. Residents and families may be unfamiliar with nursing facilities. There are fears of never returning home. Some residents know they will not return home. There also are concerns about the care: who will be giving the care, and how will it be given? Residents do not know what is expected of them. They worry about getting meals, where the bathroom is, and how to get help. They may be frightened by the strange sights and sounds of the facility. They do not know either the staff members or other residents. They will be without family and friends. They leave behind their homes and possessions.

Residents may have similar concerns if they are transferred to another nursing unit within the facility. Discharge usually is a happy time. However, it may cause other concerns. The resident may be going to another health care facility or may need home care.

Admission, transfer, and discharge are critical events for both residents and families. All persons involved need to feel comfortable and secure. You must function competently and efficiently and be sensitive to their fears and concerns. You must show courtesy, kindness, and respect.

ADMISSIONS

The admission process begins in the business office. **Admission** is the official entry of a person into the facility. A member of the health care team conducts the initial admitting procedures. Many facilities now have admission coordinators. They make sure the resident's admission is as simple and easy as possible. Often admission procedures are completed 2 or 3 days before the admission. Identifying information is obtained from the resident or a family member. This includes the person's full name, age, date of birth, doctor's name, Social Security number, and religion. The information is recorded on the admission record.

The nursing staff is notified of the admission and room assignment before the resident arrives. Some residents arrive by ambulance or wheelchair van. They are taken directly to their rooms by the attendants. Residents may arrive by private car. A nurse or nursing assistant takes them to their rooms. Some new residents may want to have a family member with them. The family also may go to the room with the new resident. This is a critical and emotional time for the resident and family. They should not be separated until they are comfortable doing so. Remember, the facility is now the person's home.

Admitting papers and a general consent for treatment need to be signed. They should be signed by the resident. If the resident is not mentally competent, they are signed by the responsible family member. This can be done before or after the resident is taken to his or her room. Sometimes these procedures are completed a day or two before the resident is admitted.

At some time after admission, a photograph is taken or the person is given an ID bracelet. This is used to identify the resident (see Chapter 7).

Preparing the Room

The room needs to be ready for the new resident. This usually is your responsibility. Fig. 18-1 shows a room ready for a resident's arrival.

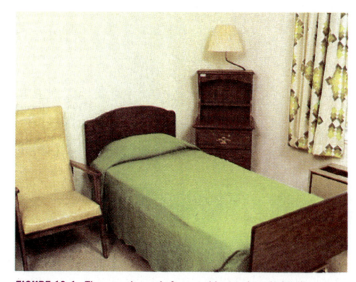

FIGURE 18-1 *The room is ready for a resident to be admitted.*

Preparing the Resident's Room

1. Know which room and bed to prepare. Find out if the resident will arrive by wheelchair or stretcher.

2. Wash your hands.

3. Collect the following:
   a. Personal-care items: bath basin, pitcher, glass, bedpan, and urinal (for a male resident)
   b. Admission checklist
   c. Sphygmomanometer
   d. Stethoscope
   e. Gown or pajamas, towel, and washcloth
   f. IV pole if needed

4. For the resident arriving by stretcher:
   a. Open the bed as for a surgical bed (see Chapter 11, p. 219).
   b. Raise the bed to its highest level.

5. For the ambulatory or wheelchair resident:
   a. Leave the bed closed.
   b. Lower the bed to its lowest level.

6. Attach the signal light to the bed linens.

7. Place the sphygmomanometer, stethoscope, and admission checklist on the overbed table.

8. Place the gown or pajamas, towel, washcloth, and personal-care items in the bedside stand.

9. Place the water pitcher and glass on the bedside stand or overbed table.

10. Wash your hands.

Admitting the Resident

The resident usually is greeted and escorted to the room by the nurse. However, you may be given this responsibility if the resident is in no apparent discomfort or distress. The admission record will give you the resident's name. When you greet the resident, call him or her by name. Use an appropriate title of address (Miss, Ms., Mrs., Mr.) and the person's last name. Do not call the resident by the first name. Introduce yourself by name and title. Also introduce yourself to family members (Fig. 18-2).

The resident needs to feel physically and mentally comfortable, safe, and secure. Avoid rushing into admission procedures. Rather, treat the resident and family as if they are guests in your home. Offer them a cup of coffee, tea, or other beverage. Visit with them awhile, and tell them some of the many good things about the facility. This is a good time to introduce the person's roommate. You also can introduce the person to other residents in nearby rooms. You might write down their names for the new resident. Remembering names given during introductions is hard for many people. It is important that when the family does leave, the resident will know others. He or she will not be left in the awkward position of not knowing anyone. In addition, other residents can be a source of great comfort and support to the new resident. They understand, better than any member

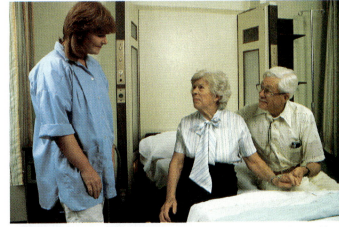

FIGURE 18-2 *The nursing assistant introduces herself to the resident and family member.*

of the health care team, what it is like to be admitted to a nursing facility.

Remember, this is the resident's home. You need to help the resident make his or her room as homelike as possible. You can help the resident unpack. Perhaps the resident needs help hanging clothes and putting things in drawers. Maybe the resident wants to hang a picture or display photographs. This is a time to show caring and compassion. You must do all that you can to help the person feel safe, comfortable, and secure.

After you have helped the resident adjust to the facility, an admission checklist needs to be completed. The resident's vital signs, weight, and height are measured. The resident is oriented to the room and told about the nursing unit and the facility. The nurse will explain the resident's rights to the person and family. They will be given a booklet explaining these rights.

PROCEDURE

Admitting the Resident—Admission Checklist

1. Wash your hands.

2. Prepare the room.

3. Greet the resident by name. Ask if he or she prefers a certain name.

4. Introduce yourself to the resident and relatives or friends who may be present. Explain that you are a nursing assistant and that you assist the nurses in giving care.

5. Introduce the resident to the roommate.

6. Call for a nurse immediately if the resident complains of any severe pain or appears to be in distress.

7. Proceed if the resident's condition does not present an immediate or serious problem.

8. Provide for privacy. Elderly residents may want family members or friends to stay with them. They should always stay in the room if the resident is confused. The resident may not mind if they leave the room for a brief period. Tell them how long you will need and where they can wait comfortably.

9. Help the person put on a gown or pajamas if he or she will be in bed. Assist him or her into bed if indicated. Raise or lower side rails as instructed by the nurse.

10. Make sure the resident is comfortable. He or she should be in bed or a chair or wheelchair as directed by the nurse.

11. Hang clothes in the closet. Place personal items in the bedside stand and dresser drawers.

12. Complete the admission checklist (Fig. 18-3).

13. Complete a clothing and valuables list. (p. 415).

14. Explain activity limitations that have been ordered.

15. Orient the resident to the new environment.
    a. Give names of the head nurse and the team leader.
    b. Identify and explain the purpose of equipment in the bedside stand.
    c. Demonstrate use of the call system (Fig. 18-4, p. 412).
    d. Show the resident where the bathroom is.
    e. Explain how telephone calls are made (pay telephone or room telephone).
    f. Explain visiting hours and policies.
    g. Explain the location of the nurses' station, lounge, dining room, and other areas.
    h. Identify resident services: newspaper, library, activities, educational programs, religious services, and others.
    i. Identify other staff members involved with the resident: housekeeping, dietary, activities, students, physical therapy, and others.
    j. Explain when meals and nourishments are served.

16. Fill the water pitcher if oral fluids are allowed.

17. Place the signal light and overbed table within reach. Place other items in reach as requested by the resident.

18. Make sure the bed is in its lowest position. Unscreen the resident.

19. Clean any used equipment. Discard used disposable items.

20. Provide a denture container if needed. Label it with the resident's name and room number.

21. Report your observations to the nurse. If the resident is agitated, restless, or wandering, do not leave the resident alone. Have a family member or another nursing assistant stay with him or her while you report your observations to the nurse.

Date: _____   Time: _____   Introduced: Self _____   Roommate _____

Admitted per: Wheelchair _____   Cart _____   Ambulatory _____   Carried by _____

Age: _____   Sex: M _____   F _____

Condition on admission:

Ambulatory ☐	Feeds self ☐	Admitted by ambulance ☐	Alert ☐
Semiambulatory ☐	Requires help with feeding ☐	From hospital ☐	Forgetful ☐
Chairridden ☐	Continent ☐	From home ☐	Confused ☐
Bedridden ☐	Incontinent ☐	From nursing home ☐	

State of consciousness: Alert _____   Confused _____   Semiconscious _____   Unconscious _____

Emotional state: Calm _____   Nervous _____   Fearful _____   Angry _____   Depressed _____

Pain: No _____   Yes _____   Where _____

Vital signs: BP _____   T _____   P _____   R _____   Ht _____   Wt _____

Glasses: Yes _____   No _____   Contact lenses: Yes _____   No _____   Hearing aid: Yes _____   No _____

Dentures: Yes _____   No _____   Artificial limb: Yes _____   No _____

Artificial eye: Yes _____   No _____   Right _____   Left _____   Pacemaker: Yes _____   No _____

Orientation to environment:

Call light _____   Emergency light _____   Bed controls _____   Bedside stand _____   Closet _____

Drawers _____   Bathroom _____   Mealtime _____   Visiting hours _____

Information obtained from: Patient _____   Spouse _____   Parent: M _____   F _____   Other _____

Other observations and comments: _____

_____

Show all body marks: scars, bruises, cuts, decubiti, ulcers, and discolorations (birth marks should not be shown).

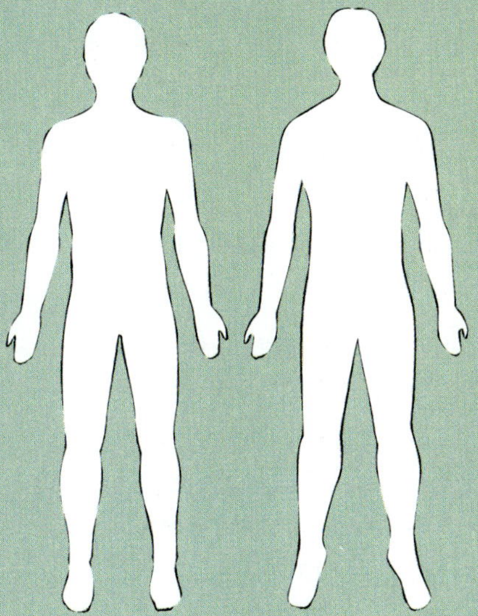

Signed _____

FIGURE 18-3 *Admission checklist.*

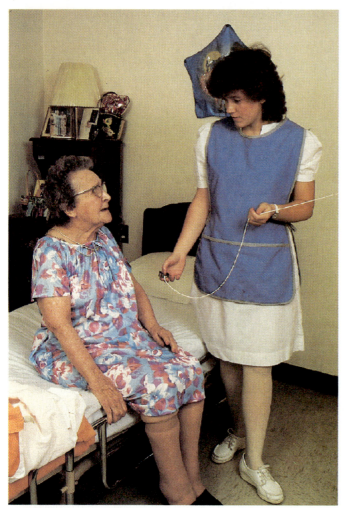

FIGURE 18-4 *The resident is shown how to use the call system.*

Measuring height and weight. Height and weight are measured on admission. The person wears only a gown or pajamas. Shoes or slippers add weight. They also cause inaccurate height measurement. Residents who are fully dressed on admission may be weighed and measured at bedtime. The resident should urinate before being weighed. A full bladder can affect the weight measurement.

There are standing, chair, and lift scales (Fig. 18-5). Chair and lift scales are used for persons who cannot stand. You need to follow the manufacturer's instructions when using chair or lift scales.

A B C

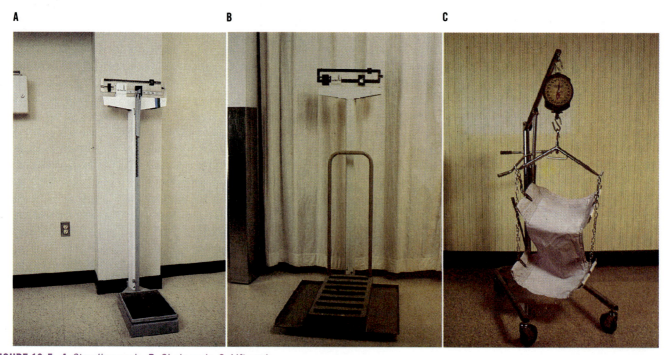

FIGURE 18-5 *A, Standing scale. B, Chair scale. C, Lift scale.*

PROCEDURE

Measuring Height and Weight

1. Explain the procedure to the resident.

2. Ask the resident to urinate (see Chapter 13).

3. Wash your hands.

4. Collect the following:
   a. Scale (standing, chair, wheelchair, or lift scale)
   b. Paper towels

5. Identify the resident. Check the ID bracelet and call the resident by name.

6. Provide for privacy.

7. Standing scale.
   a. Raise the height-measurement rod.
   b. Place the paper towels on the scale platform.
   c. Ask the resident to remove the robe and slippers. Assist if necessary.
   d. Help the resident stand on the scale platform with the arms to the sides.
   e. Move the weights until the balance pointer is in the middle (Fig. 18-6, p. 414).
   f. Record the name and weight.
   g. Have the resident stand as straight as possible.
   h. Lower the height measurement rod until it rests on the resident's head.
   i. Record the height.

8. Chair scale.
   a. Help the resident transfer from the wheelchair to the chair scale (see *Transferring the Resident to a Chair or Wheelchair,* p. 177).
   b. Place the resident's feet on the foot platform (Fig. 18-7, p. 414).

   c. Move the weights until the balance pointer is in the middle.
   d. Record the weight.

9. Lift scale.
   a. Attach the sling and chains to the lift.
   b. Place both weights on zero.
   c. Level and balance the scale according to the manufacturer's instructions.
   d. Remove the sling from the scale.
   e. Place the resident on the sling and attach it to the lift. Raise the resident about 4 inches off the bed (see *Using a Mechanical Lift,* p. 182).
   f. Move the weights until the balance pointer is in the middle.
   g. Record the weight.
   h. Lower the resident to the bed.
   i. Remove the sling.

10. Help the resident put on robe and slippers or clothing if he or she will be up. Or help him or her back to bed.

11. Make sure the resident is comfortable and the signal light is within reach.

12. Raise or lower side rails as instructed by the nurse.

13. Unscreen the resident.

14. Return the scale to its proper place.

15. Wash your hands.

16. Report the height and weight to the nurse. Record the measurements in the proper place.

413

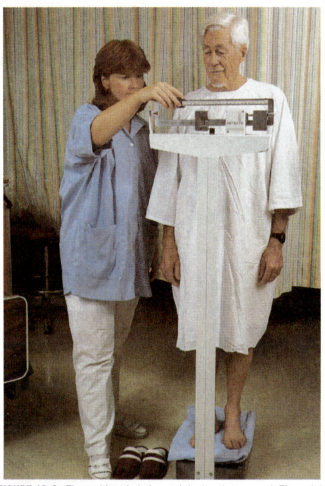

FIGURE 18-6 *The resident is being weighed and measured. The weight is read when the balance pointer is in the middle.*

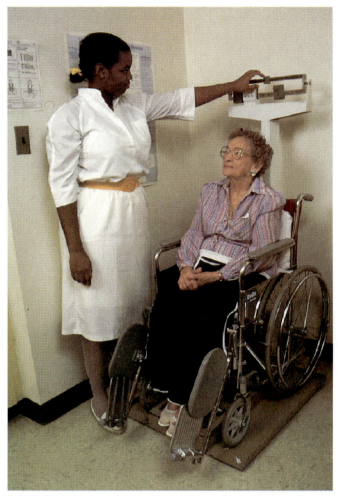

FIGURE 18-7 *The nursing assistant places the resident on the chair scale with the feet on the foot platform.*

Measuring Height: the Wheelchair or Bed Resident

1. Explain the procedure to the resident.

2. Wash your hands.

3. Collect a measuring tape and ruler.

4. Get a helper.

5. Provide for privacy.

6. Position the resident supine if this position is allowed.

7. Have your helper hold the end of the measuring tape at the resident's heel.

8. Pull the measuring tape alongside the resident's body until it extends past the head.

9. Place the ruler flat across the top of the head. It should extend from the resident's head to the measuring tape. Make sure the ruler is level (Fig. 18-8).

10. Record the height.

11. Make sure the resident is comfortable. Assist him or her back to the wheelchair if appropriate.

12. Raise or lower side rails as instructed by the nurse if the resident stays in bed.

13. Place the signal light within reach. Unscreen the resident.

14. Return equipment to its proper location.

15. Wash your hands.

16. Report the height to the nurse. Record the measurement in the proper place.

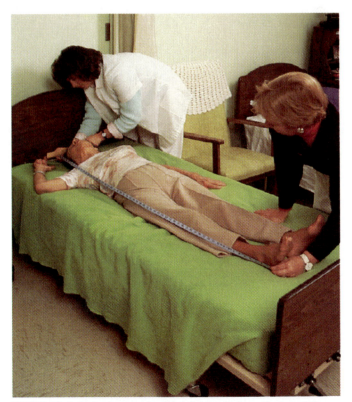

FIGURE 18-8 *Ruler is placed so that it extends from the top of the resident's head to the measuring tape.*

Clothing and valuables. A list is made of the resident's clothing and valuables. Valuables, including money and jewelry, must be kept in a safe place. They may be sent home with a family member. A clothing list is completed by the staff member admitting the resident. Each item is identified and described on the list. The staff member and resident both sign the completed list. If the resident cannot sign, it is signed by a family member.

A valuables envelope is used for money and jewelry. Each piece of jewelry is listed and described on the envelope. It is placed in the envelope while the resident watches. Money is counted with the resident before being put in the envelope. The envelope is sealed and signed like the clothing checklist. The envelope is given to the nurse. The nurse takes the envelope to the safe or sends it home with the family.

Some valuables are kept at the bedside. These include dentures, eyeglasses, contact lenses, watches, electric shavers, clocks, and radios. Valuables kept at the bedside are listed in the resident's record. Also include wheelchairs, walkers, canes, crutches, or other special equipment brought from home. Some residents keep money for newspapers, telephone calls, and vending machines. The amount of money kept by the resident is noted in the resident's record.

TRANSFERS

A resident may be transferred to another room or nursing unit. A **transfer** is moving a resident from one room, nursing unit, or facility to another. Transfers usually are related to changes in condition. Residents may be transferred to hospitals. Some may transfer to hospice units. A resident may request a room change. Room changes may be necessary if roommates do not get along.

Reasons for the transfer are explained by the doctor or nurse. The family and business office are notified. You may assist in the transfer or carry out the entire procedure. The resident usually is transported by wheelchair or stretcher. Sometimes the bed is used.

DISCHARGES

Discharges usually are planned in advance. **Discharge** is the official departure of the resident from the facility. This is usually a happy time if the resident is going home. Some residents are discharged to a hospital or to another nursing facility. Others need home care. These residents may have fears and concerns. The doctor, nurse, dietitian, social worker, and other health care team members plan the resident's discharge. They teach the resident and family about diet, exercise, and medications. They also teach the resident and family how to perform care procedures or give treatments. They arrange for special home care and therapy. A doctor's appointment may be given.

You will help the resident dress and pack belongings. You also will transport the resident out of the facility.

PROCEDURE

Transferring the Resident to Another Nursing Unit

1. Find out where the resident is going. Find out if the bed, a wheelchair, or stretched will be used.

2. Explain the procedure to the resident.

3. Get a stretcher or wheelchair, bath blanket, and a utility cart if needed.

4. Wash your hands.

5. Identify the resident. Check the ID bracelet with the transfer slip and call the resident by name.

6. Put the resident's personal belongings and bedside equipment on the utility cart.

7. Assist the resident to the wheelchair or stretcher (see *Transferring the Resident to a Wheelchair,* p. 177, or *Moving the Resident onto a Stretcher,* p. 185). Cover the resident with a bath blanket.

8. Transport the resident to the assigned place.

9. Introduce the resident to the receiving nurse.

10. Help the nurse transfer the resident from the wheelchair or stretcher into bed. Help position the resident.

11. Bring the resident's personal belongings and equipment to the new room. Help put them away.

12. Report the following to the receiving nurse:
    a. How the resident tolerated the transfer
    b. That a nurse will bring the resident's chart, care plan, Kardex, and medications

13. Return the wheelchair or stretcher and utility cart to the storage area.

14. Wash your hands.

15. Strip the bed, clean the unit, and make a closed bed. (This may be done by the housekeeping department in some facilities.)

The nurse will tell you when to begin the discharge procedure. The doctor must write a discharge order before the resident can leave. The nurse tells you when the person may leave and how to transport him or her. Usually a wheelchair is used. Some facilities allow the person to walk if able. Occasionally a resident leaves by ambulance. Ambulance attendants bring the stretcher to the room.

The resident or family needs to make arrangements for payment at the business office. Sometimes financial arrangements are made on admission or before discharge.

A resident may wish to leave the facility without the doctor's permission. You must notify the nurse immediately if the resident expresses the wish or intent to leave. This situation is handled by the nurse.

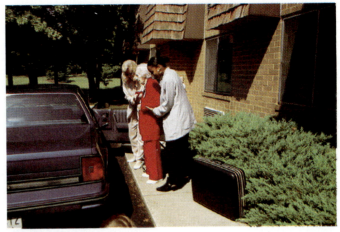

FIGURE 18-9 *Resident is being discharged.*

PROCEDURE

Discharging the Resident

1. Make sure the resident is to be discharged. Find out if transportation arrangements have been made.

2. Explain the procedure to the resident.

3. Wash your hands.

4. Identify the resident. Check the ID bracelet with the discharge slip and call the resident by name.

5. Provide for privacy.

6. Help the resident dress if assistance is needed (see *Dressing the Resident*, p. 272).

7. Help the resident pack. Check all drawers and closets to make sure all items are collected.

8. Check off the clothing list. Ask the resident or responsible party to sign the form indicating that all clothing has been returned.

9. Tell the nurse that the resident is ready for the final visit. The nurse:
   a. Gives prescriptions written by the doctor
   b. Provides discharge instructions
   c. Secures valuables from the safe

10. Get a wheelchair and a utility cart for the resident's belongings. Ask a co-worker to help you.

12. Assist the resident into the wheelchair (see *Transferring the Resident to a Wheelchair*, p. 177).

13. Take the resident to the exit area. Lock the wheels of the wheelchair. Help the resident out of the wheelchair and into the car (Fig. 18-9).

14. Help put the belongings into the car.

15. Return the wheelchair and utility cart to the storage area.

16. Wash your hands.

17. Strip the bed, clean the resident unit, and make a closed bed. (This may be the done by the housekeeping department in some facilities.)

Quality OF LIFE

First impressions always are important. You have only one chance to make a good first impression. The resident's and family's first impression of the facility is important in helping the resident feel safe, comfortable, and secure. You must treat residents in a manner that protects their dignity and self-esteem. You must be kind, respectful, thoughtful, and caring. Think of how you would want to be treated or how you would want a loved one treated.

The resident's rights are important from the beginning. The nurse will explain these rights to the resident and family. You must always respect the resident's rights. Residents should be allowed the right of personal choice in deciding when and where to put personal belongings. What may be unimportant to you is precious to them. Residents probably have brought some treasured belongings. They may be all residents will ever see of home. The person's property must be handled carefully and with respect.

The first hours and days in the facility may be very lonely and difficult. Be sure to check on new residents often. Introduce them to other residents. You also should encourage them to take part in activities. Be sure to explain all procedures and what the various sounds mean. You may need to repeat the same information often. Remember, the person is in a new place and is receiving all kinds of new information. It may take awhile to remember things. The resident will feel safer and more secure if he or she knows what is happening and why.

SUMMARY

Admission to a nursing facility usually is a disturbing time for the resident and family. Transfers also can cause fear and apprehension. Discharge usually is a happy and pleasant event. However, it may cause worries and concerns if more care and treatment are needed. You can help the resident and family cope with these events. Be courteous, caring, efficient, and competent. Also be sensitive to the resident's and the family's fears and concerns. The person's property and valuables must be handled carefully and with respect. They must be kept in a safe place and protected from loss or damage. Always treat the resident and family the way you would like your loved ones to be treated. Remember always to protect the resident's rights and to promote quality of life for the resident.

Review QUESTIONS

Circle *T* if the answer is true and *F* if the answer is false.

T F **1.** Identifying information is obtained when the resident arrives on the nursing unit.

T F **2.** Residents who arrive by ambulance are taken to their rooms by the attendants.

T F **3.** The resident should be greeted by name when being admitted.

T F **4.** The admission checklist must be completed as soon as the resident arrives in his or her room.

T F **5.** You are responsible for explaining the resident's rights to the resident and family.

T F **6.** A resident complains of pain. You should report the complaint after the admission checklist has been completed.

T F **7.** You are not responsible for orienting the resident to the new environment.

T F **8.** A robe and slippers are worn when the resident is weighed and measured.

T F **9.** A tape measure is used to measure the height of ambulatory residents.

T F **10.** A list is made of clothing and valuables during the admission process.

T F **11.** The resident's condition may require that the person be transferred to another nursing unit within the facility.

T F **12.** A doctor's order is required for discharge from the nursing facility.

T F **13.** You are responsible for instructing the resident about diet and medications.

T F **14.** Starting with admission, the resident's rights must be protected.

Answers

1. False
2. True
3. True
4. False
5. False
6. False
7. False
8. False
9. False
10. True
11. True
12. True
13. False
14. True

19

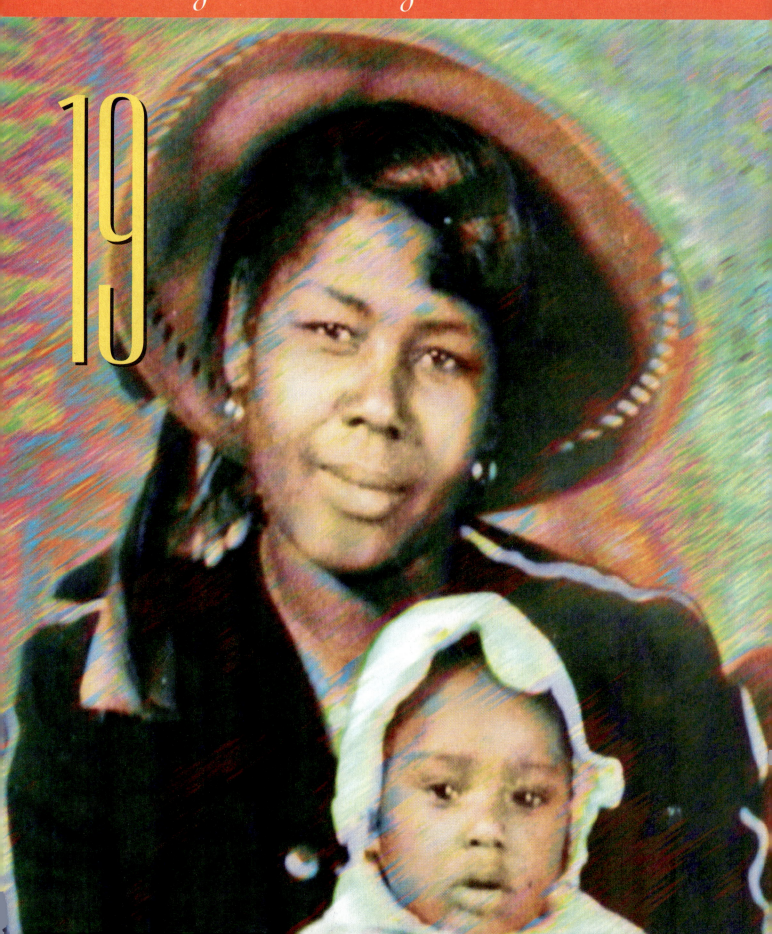

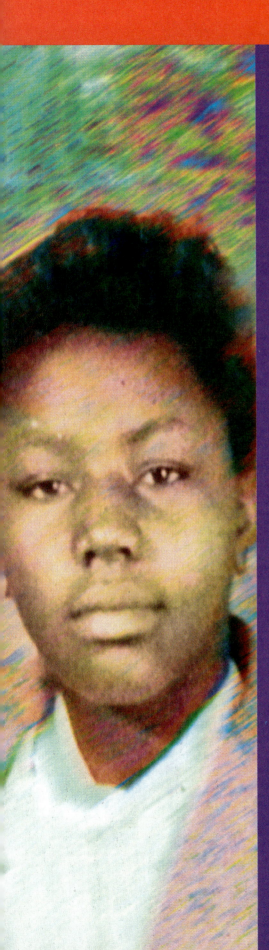

What You Will LEARN

- The key terms listed in this chapter

- Your responsibilities in assisting with the physical examination

- Equipment used for a physical examination

- How to prepare the resident for an examination

- Four examination positions

- How to drape the resident for each examination position

- How to prepare the resident for an examination

- Rules for assisting with a physical examination

- Your responsibilities after the physical examination

- How to promote quality of life for the person having a physical examination

dorsal recumbent position
The supine or back-lying examination position; legs are together

horizontal recumbent position
The dorsal recumbent position

knee-chest position
The resident kneels and rests the body on the knees and chest; the head is turned to one side, arms are above the head or flexed at the elbows, back is straight, and the body is flexed about 90 degrees at the hips

laryngeal mirror
Instrument used to examine the mouth, teeth, and throat

lithotomy position
Resident is in a back-lying position, hips are at the edge of the examination table, knees are flexed, hips are externally rotated, and feet are in stirrups

nasal speculum
Instrument used to examine the inside of the nose

ophthalmoscope
Lighted instrument used to examine the internal structures of the eye

otoscope
Lighted instrument used to examine the external ear and the eardrum (tympanic membrane)

percussion hammer
Instrument used to tap body parts to test reflexes

tuning fork
Instrument used to test hearing

vaginal speculum
Instrument used to open the vagina so that it and the cervix can be examined

Physical examinations usually are performed by doctors. Nurses also are learning how to perform physical examinations. In long-term care, physical exams are done to promote health and to diagnose disease. Each resident has a physical exam at least yearly. You may be asked to assist the doctor or nurse with an exam.

RESPONSIBILITIES OF THE NURSING ASSISTANT

Your responsibilities depend on facility policies and procedures. The examiner's preferences also affect what you will do. You may perform some or all of these functions.

1. Collect linens to be used during the procedure. This includes linens for draping the resident.
2. Collect equipment used for the examination.
3. Prepare the examination room or resident unit for the exam.
4. Make sure there is adequate lighting.
5. Measure the resident's vital signs, height, and weight.
6. Position and drape the resident for the examination.
7. Hand equipment and instruments to the examiner.
8. Label specimen containers.
9. Dispose of soiled linen and discard used disposable items. Clean reusable equipment after the exam.
10. Help the resident dress or to a comfortable position after the exam.

EQUIPMENT

Some equipment and supplies used for examination are used for resident care. You may recognize other instruments used by the examiner. Some probably were used when you were examined. You need to know the instruments shown in Fig. 19-1 on p. 424.

The **ophthalmoscope** is a lighted instrument used to examine the internal structures of the eye. The otoscope also is lighted. It is used to examine the external ear and the eardrum (tympanic membrane). Some scopes have interchangeable parts and can be changed into an ophthalmoscope or otoscope. The **percussion hammer** is used to tap body parts to test reflexes. The **vaginal speculum** is used to open the vagina so that it and the cervix can be examined. The **nasal speculum** is used to examine the inside of the nose. A **tuning fork** is vibrated to test hearing. The **laryngeal mirror** is needed to examine the mouth, teeth, and throat.

Some facilities have examination trays. If not, the necessary items are collected. The items listed in *Preparing the Resident for the Examination* usually are used for an examination. They are arranged on a tray or table for the examiner.

PREPARING THE RESIDENT

The physical examination is an anxious time for many residents. There also are fears about finding diseases and disorders. Residents may be confused and fearful about what the examiner is going to do. Other factors can add to the person's anxiety. These include unfamiliar surroundings, discomfort, embarrassment, fear of exposure, and unfamiliarity with the procedure. You must be sensitive to the person's feelings and concerns. The resident needs to be prepared physically and psychologically for the examination. Under OBRA, the resident has the right to know who will do the exam, why it is being done, and what to expect. The doctor or nurse explains these things to the resident.

Usually all clothes are removed for a complete physical examination. The resident is covered with a drape. The drape may be a disposable paper drape, a bath blanket, a sheet, or a drawsheet. A bath blanket provides greater warmth. Sometimes a hospital gown is worn. It helps reduce feelings of nakedness and fears of exposure. Explain to the resident that the amount of exposure during the exam is minimal. Some exposure, however, is necessary to examine the body. Only the body part being examined is exposed. You must screen the resident and close the door to the room. This further protects the person's right to privacy.

Residents are asked to urinate before the examination. The bladder must be empty so the examiner can feel the abdominal organs. A full urinary bladder can alter the normal position and shape of the organs. It also can cause discomfort, especially when the abdominal organs are being felt. If a urine specimen is needed, it is obtained at this time. Explain how to collect the specimen and label the container properly (see Chapter 13).

Warmth is major concern during the examination. The resident, especially if ill or elderly, should be protected from chilling. An extra bath blanket should be nearby. Measures also are taken to prevent drafts.

The examiner may want height, weight, and vital signs measured. Obtain these before the examiner begins. Record them on the examination form. Then position and drape the resident for the exam.

PROCEDURE

Preparing the Resident for the Examination

1. Explain the procedure to the resident.

2. Wash your hands.

3. Assemble the following items on a tray at the bedside or in the examination room:
   a. Flashlight
   b. Blood pressure cuff
   c. Stethoscope
   d. Thermometer
   e. Tongue depressors (blades)
   f. Laryngeal mirror
   g. Ophthalmoscope
   h. Otoscope
   i. Nasal speculum
   j. Percussion (reflex) hammer
   k. Tuning fork
   l. Tape measure
   m. Disposable gloves
   n. Water-soluble lubricant
   o. Vaginal speculum
   p. Cotton-tipped applicators
   q. Specimen containers and labels
   r. Disposable bag
   s. Emesis basin
   t. Towel
   u. Bath blanket
   v. Tissues
   w. Drape (sheet, bath blanket, drawsheet, or disposable drape)
   x. Paper towels
   y. Cotton balls
   z. Disposable bed protector
   aa. Eye chart (Snellen chart)
   bb. Slides
   cc. Gown
   dd. Alcohol wipes
   ee. Wastebasket
   ff. Container for soiled instruments
   gg. Marking pencils or pens

4. Identify the resident. Check the ID bracelet and call the resident by name.

5. Provide for privacy.

6. Help the resident put on a hospital gown.

7. Ask the resident to urinate. If he or she is not ambulatory, offer the bedpan or urinal. Use universal precautions when emptying and cleaning the bedpan or urinal.

8. Transport the resident to the examination room. Help him or her onto the examination table. Have the resident use a stool if necessary. Omit this step if the exam will be done in the resident's room.

9. Position the resident as directed (see pp. 424-425). Raise the bed to its highest level.

10. Drape the resident. Untie the gown.

11. Place a bed protector under the buttocks.

12. Arrange for adequate lighting.

13. Put the signal light on for the nurse or examiner. Do not leave the resident unattended.

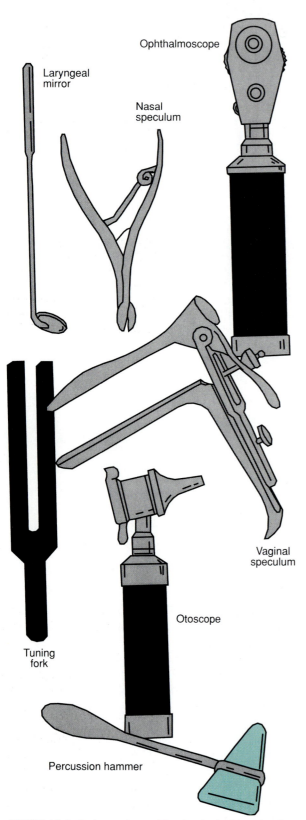

Ophthalmoscope

Laryngeal mirror

Nasal speculum

Vaginal speculum

Otoscope

Tuning fork

Percussion hammer

FIGURE 19-1 *Instruments used for the physical examination.*

Positioning and Draping

A special position may be required. Some examining positions (Fig. 19-2) are uncomfortable and may be embarrassing. The examiner decides how to position the resident. Explain the need for the position to the resident and how it is assumed. Also explain how draping is done to prevent exposure. The person needs to know how long he or she will have to stay in the position. You may need to help the resident assume and maintain the position.

The **dorsal recumbent (horizontal recumbent)** or supine position usually is used to examine the abdomen, chest, and breasts. The resident is supine with the legs together. If the perineal area is examined, the knees are flexed and hips externally rotated (see Fig. 19-2, *A*). The resident is draped as for perineal care (see *Giving Female Perineal Care*, p. 256).

The **lithotomy position** (see Fig. 19-2, *B*) is used to examine the vagina. The resident lies on her back, and her hips are brought to the edge of the examination table. The knees are flexed and hips externally rotated. Feet are supported in stirrups. The woman is draped as for the dorsal recumbent position. Some facilities provide socks to cover the feet and calves. Some elderly women cannot assume this position. The examiner will tell you how to position the resident.

The **knee-chest position** (see Fig. 19-2, *C*) is used to examine the rectum and sometimes the vagina. The resident kneels on the bed or examination table. Then the person rests his or her body on the knees and chest. The head is turned to one side. Arms are above the head or flexed at the elbows. The back is straight and the body is flexed about 90 degrees at the hips. The resident wears a gown and sometimes socks. The drape is applied in a diamond shape to cover the back, buttocks, and thighs. This position rarely is used for elderly persons. They usually assume the side-lying position.

The **Sims' position** (see Fig. 19-2, *D*) can be used to examine the rectum or vagina. Chapter 9 described the Sims' position (see p. 192). The drape is applied in a diamond shape. The corner near the examiner is folded back to expose the rectum or vagina.

ASSISTING WITH THE EXAMINATION

You may be responsible for preparing, positioning, and draping the resident. You also may be asked to assist the doctor or nurse during the exam. Follow these rules when assisting with the examination.

1. Wash your hands before and after the examination.
2. Provide for privacy throughout the examination. This is done by screening, closing doors, and draping. Expose only the body part being examined.
3. Assist the resident in assuming positions as directed by the examiner.
4. Place instruments and equipment near the examiner.

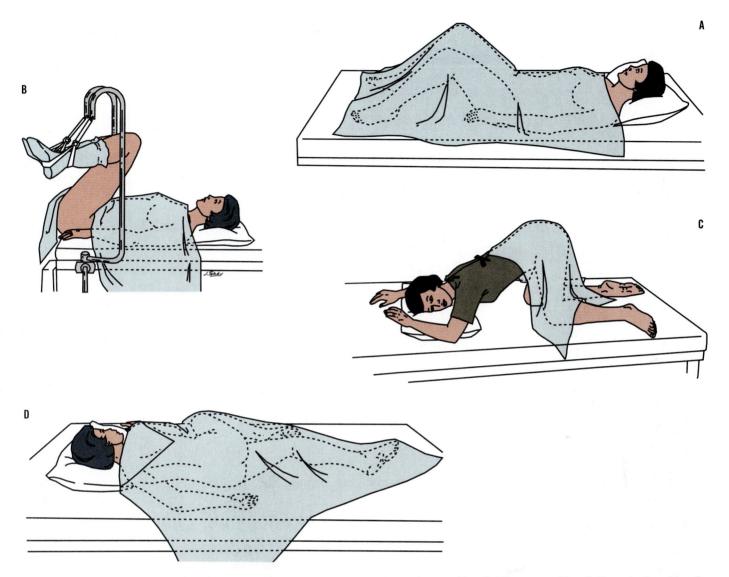

FIGURE 19-2 *Positioning and draping for the physical examination.* **A,** *Dorsal recumbent position.* **B,** *Lithotomy position.* **C,** *Knee-chest position.* **D,** *Sims' position.*

5. Stay in the room during the examination of a woman (unless you are a male). When a woman is examined by a man, another woman is in attendance. This is for the legal protection of the woman and the male examiner. A female attendant also adds to the person's psychological comfort.
6. Protect the resident from falling.
7. Reassure the resident. Touch is important. Hold a hand or place your hand on a shoulder. Assure the resident that you will not leave.
8. Anticipate the examiner's need for equipment.

After the Examination

The resident is taken back to the room after the examination. If the resident will be out of bed, help him or her dress. Lubricant is used for vaginal and rectal examination. The area is wiped or cleaned before the resident dresses or returns to the room.

Used disposable items are put in a bag or waste container. Examples are bed protectors, paper drapes, tongue blades, applicators, and cotton balls. These items are replaced so the tray is ready for the next examination. Reusable equipment is cleaned and returned to the tray. These include otoscope and ophthalmoscope tips, speculums, and the stethoscope. The examination table is covered with a clean drawsheet or paper. All specimens are labeled and taken to a designated area. The resident's unit or examination room should be neat and orderly after the exam. Soiled linens are put in the linen bag.

Quality OF LIFE

OBRA requires that residents be cared for in a way that promotes their dignity, self-esteem, and physical, mental, and social well-being. The resident wears only a gown for the examination. An uncomfortable position may be required. Private body parts (breasts, vagina, penis, and rectum) may be examined. The person may have fears about who will perform the exam and how it will be done. There may also be fears about what why the exam is needed. Is the person dying? Will cancer be found? Will surgery be needed? Will more medicine be needed? Will an illness or a disorder be found? All these factors affect the person's dignity, self-esteem, and well-being.

The resident's quality of life must be promoted. First, the resident has the right to personal choice. The doctor or nurse is responsible for informing the resident about the examination. Reasons for the exam are given. The resident is told who will do the examination and when it will be done. The procedure is explained. The resident's consent must be given. The resident may want a different examiner. Or the resident may want a family member present. Some residents may want the exam results explained with a family member present. All of these are part of the resident's right to personal choice.

The right to privacy and confidentiality is very important. The resident must be protected from exposure. Only those involved in the examination have the right to see the resident's body. They are the examiner and the examiner's assistant. The resident must give consent for others to be present. Proper draping and screening are important during the exam. Only the body part being examined is exposed. If assisting with the examination, you must help keep the resident covered.

Confidentiality also is important. Only staff members involved in the resident's care need to know the reason for the examination and the results. To give good care, the health care team needs to know. The doctor or nurse will share the results with those who need to know. Family members also will be told. Other residents and visitors, however, do not need to know. The resident can share the information if he or she wants to.

The examination environment is important for the resident's quality of life. The person needs to feel safe and secure. The resident must be protected from falls and other injuries. Remember, the resident will wear only a hospital gown. The person must be kept warm and free from chills and drafts. The resident also must feel covered and protected from exposure.

Safety and security also relate to mental well-being. Knowing why the exam is needed and how it will be done helps the person feel safe and secure. The presence of a friendly staff member is important. The person assisting with the exam should be someone the resident feels comfortable with. Touch and reassuring words also help the person feel safe and secure. The doctor needs to tell the resident the results as soon as possible. Otherwise the resident will continue to worry and be fearful. Worries and fears do not help the person feel safe and secure.

SUMMARY

Physical examinations can be frightening. Residents may be confused or fear exposure. Examinations may cause discomfort, especially for the elderly, ill, or injured person. You may be asked to prepare residents for examinations. Collecting and arranging supplies and equipment sometimes are done by nursing assistants. You may be asked to assist with the exam. Be aware of the resident's feelings, fears, and sources of discomfort during the examination. Use touch whenever possible. This is essential for the resident's physical and psychological comfort. You must function efficiently and competently. This allows the exam to be performed smoothly and in a reasonable length of time.

Review QUESTIONS

Circle the *best* answer.

1. The otoscope is used to
   a. Examine the internal structures of the eye
   b. Examine the external ear and the eardrum
   c. Test reflexes
   d. Open the vagina

2. You are preparing the resident for the physical examination. You should do the following *except*
   a. Have the resident urinate
   b. Ask the resident to undress
   c. Drape the resident
   d. Go tell the nurse the resident is ready

3. Which part of the exam can you perform?
   a. Examination of the eyes and ears
   b. Inspection of the mouth, teeth, and throat
   c. Measurement of height, weight, and vital signs
   d. Observation of the perineum and rectum

4. A resident is supine with the hips flexed and externally rotated. The feet are in stirrups. This is the
   a. Dorsal recumbent position
   b. Lithotomy position
   c. Knee-chest position
   d. Sims' position

5. You are to assist with the physical examination. Which statement is *false?*
   a. Handwashing is done before and after the examination.
   b. Instruments are placed close to the examiner.
   c. The female nursing assistant leaves the room when a woman is being examined.
   d. The resident's privacy is protected by screening, closing the door, and draping.

6. Which statement is *true?*
   a. You can explain the reason for the exam to the resident.
   b. The resident must be safe from injury during the exam.
   c. You can tell the family the results of the exam.
   d. All of the above

7. Proper screening and draping are important for
   a. The right to privacy
   b. Safety and security
   c. Quality of life
   d. All of the above

Answers

1. b	3. c	5. c	7. d
2. d	4. b	6. b	

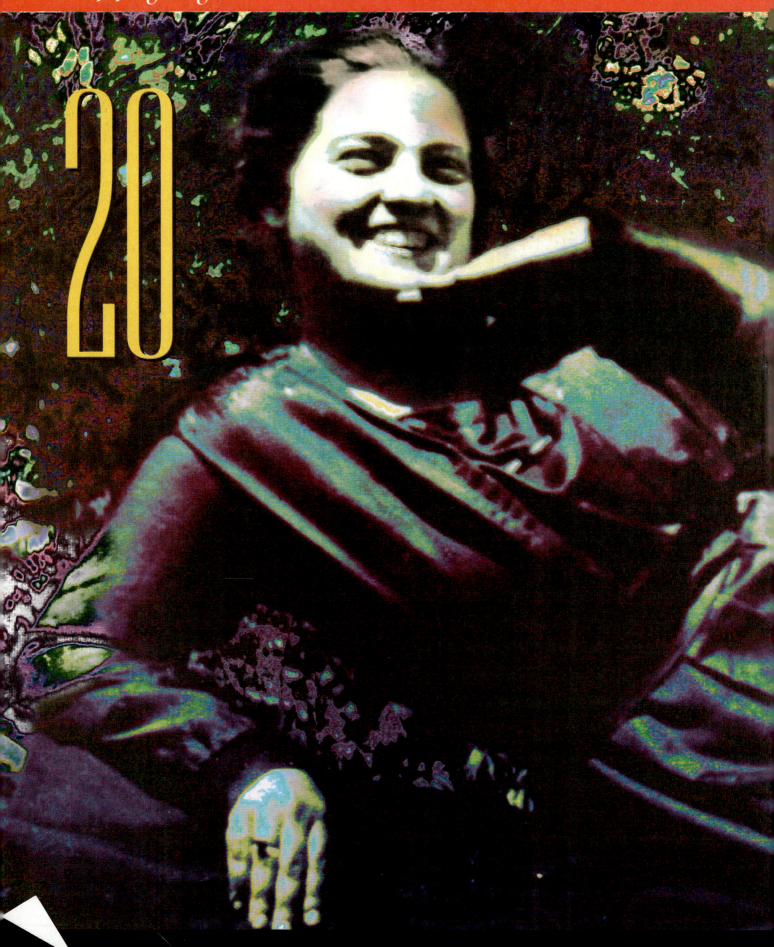

20

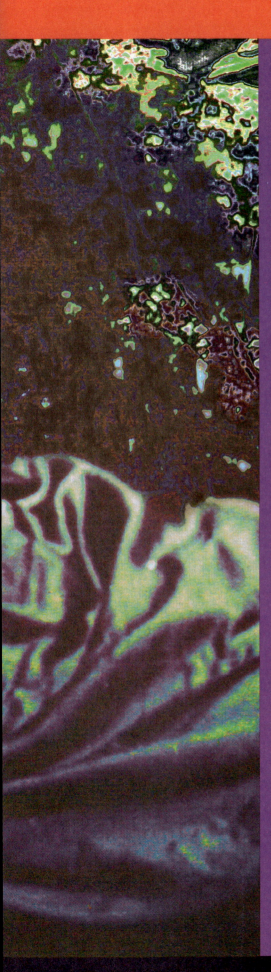

What You Will L E A R N

- The key terms listed in this chapter

- The purposes, effects, and complications of heat applications

- The persons at risk for complications from heat applications

- Differences between moist and dry heat applications

- Rules for the application of heat

- The purposes, effects, and complications of cold applications

- The persons at risk for complications from cold applications

- Differences between moist and dry cold applications

- Rules related to the application of cold

- How to promote quality of life during heat and cold applications

- How to perform the procedures described in this chapter

constrict
To narrow

cyanosis
Bluish discoloration of the skin

dilate
To expand or to open wider

Those cold applications give me the chills and make me have to go to the bathroom. So I ask to go to the bathroom first. And Jean makes sure I have my robe on and covers me with my afghan.

Heat and cold applications are ordered by doctors. They promote healing and comfort and reduce tissue swelling. Heat and cold have opposite effects on the body. Serious injury can occur if safety precautions are not taken.

In some facilities, heat and cold applications are done by the nurse. These applications are complex and more advanced nursing functions because severe injuries and changes in body function can easily result. The risks are greater than those for other procedures. Some facilities allow nursing assistants to apply heat and cold under the direction of a nurse. You are advised to perform these procedures only if you have a thorough understanding of their purpose, effects, and complications. Review the procedure with a nurse beforehand. A nurse should closely supervise your work and the effects of the procedure on the resident.

HEAT APPLICATIONS

Heat applications usually are small and can be applied to almost any body part. "Local heat application" means that heat is applied to a part of the body. Heat has many therapeutic effects. It relieves pain, relaxes muscles, promotes healing, and reduces swelling.

Effects

When applied to the skin, heat causes blood vessels in that area to dilate. **Dilate** means to expand or open wider (Fig. 20-1, *B*). More blood flows through the vessels. Tissues get more oxygen and nutrients for healing. There is faster removal of toxic (poisonous) substances and waste products. Excess fluid is removed from the area more rapidly. The skin feels warm and appears reddened in the area of the heat. These effects result from increased blood flow.

Complications

Complications can occur from heat applications. High temperatures can cause burns. Pain, excessive redness, and blisters are danger signs. Report these to the nurse immediately. You also need to observe for pale skin. When heat is applied for a long time, blood vessels **constrict** or narrow (see Fig. 20-1, *C*). Blood flow decreases when vessels constrict. This reduces the amount of blood flow to tissues. Decreased blood supply causes tissue damage and makes the skin look pale.

Elderly and fair-skinned persons are at greater risk for complications. Their skin is very delicate, fragile, and easily burned. Complications also may occur in those who have difficulty sensing (feeling) heat or pain. Many factors can interfere with sensation. They include circulatory disorders, central nervous system damage, aging, and loss of consciousness. Persons with diabetes are especially at risk. Confused residents or those receiving strong pain medication also may have decreased sensation.

Moist and Dry Applications

Moist or dry heat applications may be ordered. A *moist heat application* means that water is in contact with the skin. Water is a good conductor of heat. Therefore the effects of heat are greater and faster than with a dry application. Heat penetrates deeper with a moist application. There is less drying of the skin. To prevent injury, the temperature of moist heat applications is lower than those of dry heat applications.

Water is not in contact with the skin with *dry heat applications*. Dry heat has advantages. The application stays at the desired temperature longer. Heat is not lost through evaporation as with moist applications. The risk of burns is less because dry heat does not penetrate as deeply as moist heat. Also, water, which conducts heat, is not involved. Higher temperatures are used with dry heat to achieve the desired effect. Therefore burns are still a risk.

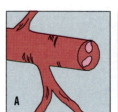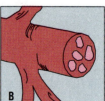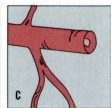

FIGURE 20-1 *A, Blood vessel under normal conditions. **B**, Dilated blood vessel. **C**, Constricted blood vessel.*

430

General Rules

Residents must be protected from injury during local heat applications. Some residents cannot protect themselves. They need special attention. The following rules are practiced to prevent burns and the other complications.

1. Know how to operate the equipment used in the procedure. Be sure to follow the manufacturer's instructions.
2. Use a bath thermometer to measure the temperature of moist heat applications.
3. Follow facility policies for the temperature ranges for heat applications.
4. Know the different temperature ranges for warm, hot, and very hot applications. The following ranges are guidelines:

    Warm—93° to 98° F (33.8° to 37° C)
    Hot—98° to 105° F (37° to 40.5° C)
    Very hot—105° to 115° F (40.5° to 46.1° C)

5. Ask the nurse what the temperature of the application should be. Lower temperatures usually are used for persons at risk.
6. Cover dry heat applications before applying them to the skin. Flannel covers usually are used.
7. Observe the resident's skin closely for signs of complications. Immediately report any such signs (pain, redness, blisters, pale skin) or resident complaints of pain or burning.
8. Do not let the resident increase the temperature of the application.
9. Know how long to leave the application in place. Carefully watch the time.
10. Follow the rules of electrical safety when using electrical appliances to apply heat.
11. Expose only the body part where the heat is to be applied. Provide for the resident's privacy.
12. Place the signal light within the resident's reach.

Hot Compresses and Packs

Hot compresses and packs are moist heat applications. Washcloths, small towels, or gauze dressings are used. Compresses are applied to small areas. Packs are applied to large body areas. Sterile or nonsterile compresses and packs may be ordered. Sterile applications are used for open wounds and areas with breaks in the skin. The nurse applies sterile hot compresses or packs.

Nonsterile applications are used for intact skin. The compress or pack is moistened in a basin of hot water. It is then wrung out and applied to the body part. The application is removed after 20 minutes.

PROCEDURE

Applying Hot Compresses

1. Explain the procedure to the resident.
2. Wash your hands.
3. Collect the following:
    a. Basin
    b. Bath thermometer
    c. Small towel, washcloth, or gauze squares
    d. Plastic wrap (if ordered)
    e. Ties, tape, or rolled gauze
    f. Bath towel
    g. Waterproof bed protector
    h. Aquathermia pad (if ordered)
4. Identify the resident. Check the ID bracelet and call the resident by name.
5. Provide for privacy.
6. Place the bed protector under the body part.
7. Fill the basin ½ to ⅔ full with water. Water temperature should be 105° to 115° F (40.5° to 46.1° C).
8. Place the compress in the water.
9. Wring out the compress (Fig. 20-2, p. 432).
10. Apply the compress. Note the time.
11. Cover the compress quickly with the plastic wrap (if ordered). Then cover with the bath towel as in Fig. 20-2.
12. Apply an aquathermia pad over the towel (if ordered). See *Applying an Aquathermia Pad*, p. 439.

Continued.

431

Applying Hot Compresses—cont'd

13. Secure the towel in place with ties, tape, or rolled gauze.

14. Place the signal light within reach. Raise or lower side rails as instructed by the nurse.

15. Check the area every 5 minutes. Check for redness and complaints of pain, discomfort, or numbness. Remove the compress if any occur. Tell the nurse immediately.

16. Change the compress if cooling occurs.

17. Remove the compress after 20 minutes. Pat the area dry with a towel. (Lower the side rail if up.)

18. Make sure the resident is comfortable and unscreened. Place the signal light within reach.

19. Raise or lower side rails as instructed by the nurse.

20. Clean equipment. Discard disposable equipment. Put used linen in the hamper.

21. Wash your hands.

22. Report the following to the nurse:
    a. Time, site, and length of the application
    b. Resident's response
    c. Your observations of the skin

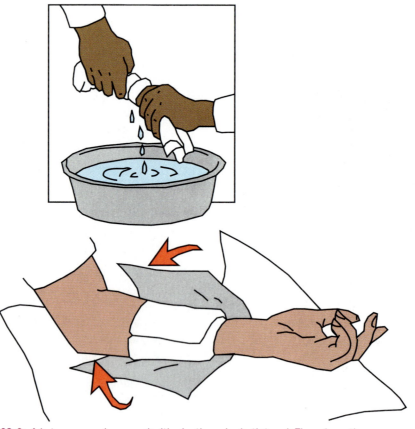

FIGURE 20-2 *A hot compress is covered with plastic and a bath towel. These keep the compress warm.*

Commercial Compresses

Commercial compresses are premoistened and packaged in foil. They are heated under an ultraviolet light for 10 minutes and then applied. The ultraviolet light may be kept in the "clean" utility room, treatment room, medication room, or the resident's room.

Commercial compresses are sterile. Sometimes they are ordered for nonsterile compresses. Nurses may decide that they are necessary in certain situations. Commercial compresses are costly and should be used only when necessary.

PROCEDURE

Applying Commercial Compresses

1. Explain the procedure to the resident.

2. Wash your hands.

3. Collect the following:
   a. Commercial compress
   b. Ultraviolet light
   c. Towel
   d. Ties, tape, or rolled gauze
   e. Waterproof bed protector
   f. Aquathermia pad (if ordered)

4. Place the compress under the ultraviolet light for 10 minutes.

5. Identify the resident. Check the ID bracelet and call the resident by name.

6. Provide for privacy.

7. Place the bed protector under the body part.

8. Open the foil-wrapped compress.

9. Apply the compress quickly with the foil wrap. Cover with the towel.

10. Secure the towel in place with ties, tape, or rolled gauze.

11. Apply the aquathermia pad over the towel (if ordered). See *Applying an Aquathermia Pad,* p. 439.

12. Place the signal light within reach. Raise or lower side rails as instructed by the nurse.

13. Check the area every 5 minutes for redness and for resident complaints of pain, discomfort, or numbness. Remove the compress if any occur. Tell the nurse immediately.

14. Change the compress if it cools. An aquathermia pad may be ordered to keep the compress warm.

15. Remove the compress after 20 minutes. Pat the area dry with the towel. (Lower the side rail if up).

16. Make sure the resident is comfortable and unscreened. Place the signal light within reach.

17. Raise or lower side rails as instructed by the nurse.

18. Clean equipment. Discard disposable equipment. Put used linen in the hamper.

19. Wash your hands.

20. Report the following to the nurse:
    a. The time, site, and length of the application
    b. The resident's response
    c. Your observations of the skin

Hot Soaks

A hot soak involves putting the body part into a container of water. This method usually is used for smaller body parts, such as a hand, lower arm, foot, and lower leg (Fig. 20-3). Large areas (torso, arm, leg) may need to be soaked. A tub is used for a large area. The soak usually lasts 15 to 20 minutes. Resident comfort and good alignment are maintained during the hot soak.

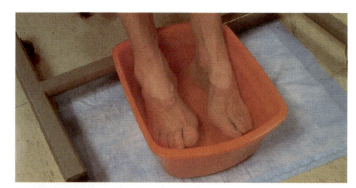

FIGURE 20-3 *The hot soak.*

PROCEDURE

Applying Hot Soaks

1. Explain the procedure to the resident.

2. Wash your hands.

3. Collect the following:
   a. Small basin or an arm or foot bath
   b. Bath thermometer
   c. Bath blanket
   d. Waterproof pads

4. Identify the resident. Check the ID bracelet and call the resident by name.

5. Provide for privacy.

6. Assist the resident to a comfortable position for the treatment. Place the signal light within reach.

7. Place a waterproof pad under the area.

8. Fill the container ½ full with water. Water temperature should be 105° to 110° F (40.5° to 43.3° C).

9. Expose the area without unnecessary exposure of the resident.

10. Place the part into the water. Pad the edge of the container with a towel if needed. Note the time.

11. Cover the resident with a bath blanket for extra warmth.

12. Check the area every 5 minutes for redness and for resident complaints of pain, discomfort, or numbness. Remove the part from the soak if any occur. Wrap the part in a towel and tell the nurse immediately.

13. Check water temperature every 5 minutes. Change water as necessary. Wrap the part in a towel while changing water.

14. Remove the part from the water in 15 to 20 minutes. Pat dry with a towel.

15. Make sure the resident is comfortable and unscreened. Place the signal light within reach.

16. Raise or lower side rails as instructed by the nurse.

17. Clean and return equipment to its proper place. Discard disposable equipment. Put soiled linen in the hamper.

18. Wash your hands.

19. Report the following to the nurse:
    a. The time the procedure began
    b. The site that was soaked
    c. The length of the treatment
    d. The resident's response
    e. Your observations of the skin

A

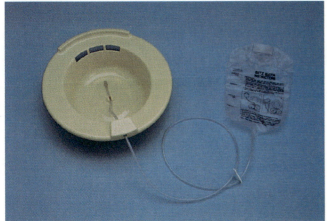

B

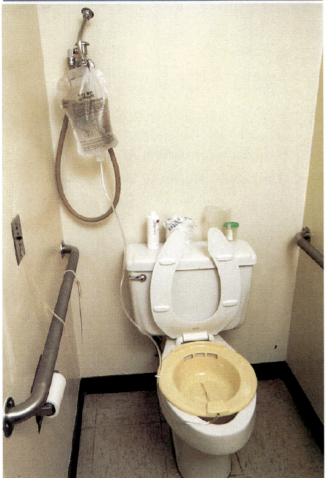

FIGURE 20-4 *A, Disposable sitz bath. B, Disposable sitz bath fits onto the toilet seat.*

The Sitz Bath

The sitz bath (hip bath) involves immersing the pelvic area in warm or hot water for 20 minutes. It can be used to clean a perineal wound, relieve pain, increase circulation, or stimulate voiding.

The disposable plastic sitz bath fits onto the toilet seat (Fig. 20-4). It can be used in the home or health care facility. A sitz tub is a built-in fixture with a deep seat. The seat is filled with water (Fig. 20-5). A portable sitz chair is similar. Sometimes a bathtub is used. The knees are flexed for these sitz baths (built-in, portable, and bathtub) to keep the legs out of the water.

The sitz bath increases the blood flow to the pelvic area. Therefore less blood flows to other body parts. As a result the resident may become weak or feel faint. The relaxing effect of the treatment may cause drowsiness. Observe the resident frequently for signs of weakness, faintness, or fatigue. Also take precautions to keep the resident safe from injury.

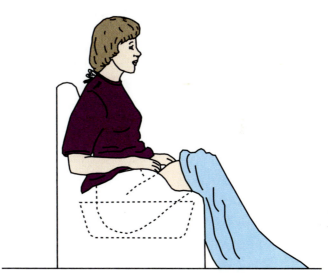

FIGURE 20-5 *The built-in sitz bath.*

PROCEDURE

Assisting the Resident in Taking a Sitz Bath

1. Explain the procedure to the resident.

2. Wash your hands.

3. Collect the following:
   a. Portable sitz bath or disposable sitz bath
   b. Wheelchair if the resident will use a built-in sitz bath or bathtub
   c. Bath thermometer
   d. Large water container
   e. Two bath blankets
   f. Footstool if the resident is short
   g. Bath towels
   h. Disinfectant solution

4. Identify the resident. Check the ID bracelet and call the resident by name.

5. Provide for privacy.

6. Do one of the following.
   a. Position the portable sitz bath at the bedside or in the bathroom.
   b. Place the disposable sitz bath on the toilet seat.
   c. Assist the resident into the wheelchair. Transport the person to the built-in sitz bath or tub room.

7. Fill the sitz bath ⅔ full with water. Water temperature should be:
   a. 100° to 104° F (37.7° to 40° C) if used to clean the perineum
   b. 105° to 110° F (40.5° to 43.3° C) if used to increase circulation

8. Lock the wheels of the portable unit.

9. Use bath towels to pad metal parts that will be in contact with the resident.

10. Raise the gown or clothing and secure it above the waist. Remove pants.

11. Help the resident sit in the sitz bath. If the tub is used, see *Assisting the Resident With a Tub Bath,* on p. 250.

12. Place one bath blanket around the resident's shoulders. Place another over the legs for warmth.

13. Provide a footstool for the resident if there is pressure under the knees.

14. Make sure the signal light is within reach and the resident is comfortable.

15. Stay with the resident who is weak, unsteady, or confused.

16. Check the resident every 5 minutes for complaints of weakness, faintness, and drowsiness. If any occur, get assistance to help the resident back to bed.

17. Help the resident out of the sitz bath after 20 minutes.

18. Assist the resident in drying and dressing.

19. Assist the resident back to bed or chair. Make sure he or she is comfortable, unscreened, and that the signal light is within reach.

20. Raise or lower side rails as instructed by the nurse.

21. Clean the sitz bath or tub with disinfectant.

22. Return reusable equipment to its proper place. Discard used linens in the hamper.

23. Wash your hands.

24. Report the following to the nurse:
    a. The time the sitz bath started and ended
    b. The resident's response
    c. The water temperature
    d. Any other observations

Heat Lamps

Dry heat can be applied with a heat lamp. A gooseneck lamp (Fig. 20-6) is used. The gooseneck is flexible. The lamp is placed at various distances from the body part. The distance between the lamp and the body part is determined by the bulb wattage. The lamp is checked for breakage and bulb wattage. The lamp is warmed up before the treatment. Do not cover it with linens. Heat from the lamp could burn the linen and cause a fire.

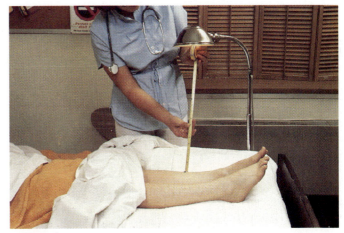

FIGURE 20-6 *Gooseneck lamp.*

PROCEDURE

Applying a Heat Lamp

1. Explain the procedure to the resident.

2. Wash your hands.

3. Collect the following:
   a. Gooseneck lamp
   b. Bath blanket
   c. Yardstick or tape measure

4. Identify the resident. Check the ID bracelet and call the resident by name.

5. Provide for privacy.

6. Plug in the lamp and let it warm up.

7. Cover the resident with a bath blanket. Fan-fold top linens to the foot of the bed.

8. Expose the body part.

9. Position the lamp a safe distance from the resident. Use the following guidelines:
   a. 25-watt bulb—14 inches
   b. 40-watt bulb—18 inches
   c. 60-watt bulb—24 inches

10. Note the time of application.

11. Measure the distance from the lamp to the resident. Use a tape measure or yardstick (Fig. 20-7, p. 438).

12. Check the resident every 5 minutes. Stay with confused or restless residents. Check for redness or blistering or resident complaints of discomfort. Discontinue the treatment if any occur. Tell the nurse immediately.

13. Cover body parts not being treated.

14. Remove the lamp after 20 minutes. (Lower the side rail if up.)

15. Return top linens. Remove the bath blanket.

16. Make sure the resident is comfortable and unscreened. Place the signal light within reach.

17. Raise or lower side rails as instructed by the nurse.

18. Clean the lamp according to facility policy. Return it and other supplies to their proper location.

19. Wash your hands.

20. Report the following to the nurse:
    a. Time the treatment started and ended
    b. The site of application
    c. Bulb wattage and the distance between the bulb and the resident
    d. The resident's response
    e. Any other observations

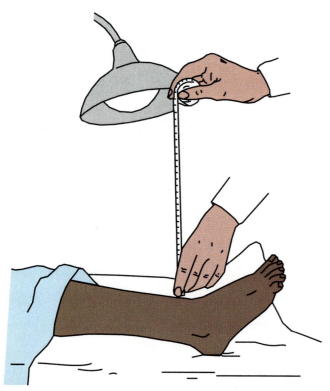

FIGURE 20-7 *The distance between the heat lamp and the resident is measured.*

The Aquathermia Pad

The aquathermia pad is an electric heating pad. It is different from heating pads sold in stores. Those sold in stores have electric coils made of wire. Aquathermia pads have tubes that are filled with water. A heating unit at the bedside also is filled with water. The water (aqua) is heated (thermia) and flows to the pad through a connecting hose (Fig. 20-8). Another hose returns water to the heating unit. The water is reheated and flows back into the pad. Distilled water is used in the heating unit.

The heating unit is kept level with the pad and connecting hoses. Water must be able to flow freely. Hoses should be free of kinks and air bubbles. The temperature is set at 105° F (40.5° C) with a key provided by the manufacturer. After it is set, the key is removed. This prevents the resident, a visitor, or other staff member from changing the temperature. The temperature may be preset in the central supply room. The key is then kept in the central supply room.

The aquathermia pad is an electrical device. Equipment-related accidents must be prevented.

1. The cord is checked for fraying.
2. A three-pronged plug is used to ground the device.
3. The cord is kept out of the way of traffic.
4. The heating unit must be placed on an uncluttered and even surface. This prevents it from being knocked over or knocked off the surface.
5. Ties, tape, or rolled gauze is used to secure the pad in place. Pins are not used. They can puncture the pad and cause leaking.
6. A flannel cover is used to insulate the pad. It also absorbs perspiration.
7. The pad is not placed under the resident or a body part. The weight of the body or body part exerts pressure against the pad and mattress. This prevents the escape of heat. Burns can result if heat cannot escape.

PROCEDURE

Applying an Aquathermia Pad

1. Explain the procedure to the resident.

2. Wash your hands.

3. Collect the following:
   a. Aquathermia pad and heating unit
   b. Distilled water
   c. Flannel cover
   d. Ties, tape, or rolled gauze

4. Identify the resident. Check the ID bracelet and call the resident by name.

5. Provide for privacy.

6. Fill the heating unit ⅔ full with distilled water.

7. Remove air bubbles. Place the pad and tubing below the level of the heating unit. Then tilt the unit from side to side.

8. Set the temperature with the key. The nurse will tell you what the temperature should be (usually 105° F or 40.5° C).

9. Place the pad into the flannel cover.

10. Plug in the unit. Let the water warm to the desired temperature.

11. Set the heating unit on the bedside stand. Keep the pad and connecting hoses level with the heating unit. Hoses must be free of kinks.

12. Apply the pad to the part. Note the time.

13. Secure the pad in place with ties, tape, or rolled gauze. Do not use pins.

14. Unscreen the resident. Place the signal light within reach.

15. Raise or lower side rails as instructed by the nurse.

16. Check the skin for redness, swelling, and blisters. Ask about pain, discomfort, or decreased sensation. Remove the pad if any of these occur. Tell the nurse immediately.

17. Remove the pad at the specified time. (Lower the side rail if up.)

18. Make sure the resident is comfortable and unscreened. Place the signal light within reach.

19. Raise or lower side rails as instructed by the nurse.

20. Clean and return equipment to its proper place.

21. Wash your hands.

22. Report the following to the nurse:
    a. The time of application and when it was removed
    b. The site of the application
    c. The temperature of the aquathermia pad
    d. The resident's response
    e. Any other observations

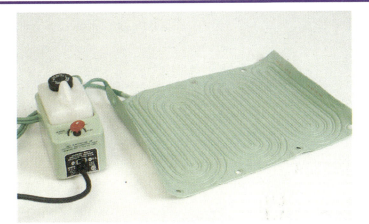

FIGURE 20-8 *The aquathermia pad and heating unit.*

COLD APPLICATIONS

Cold applications reduce pain and prevent swelling. They also decrease circulation and cool the body when fever is present. Remember, heat and cold have opposite effects on body function.

Effects

When cold is applied to the skin, blood vessels constrict (see Fig. 20-1, *C,* p. 430). Blood flow decreases. Less oxygen and nutrients are carried to the tissues. Tissue metabolism also decreases. As a result, fewer toxic substances and waste products are produced. Cold applications are useful after injuries. The decreased circulation reduces the amount of bleeding. Tissue swelling also is reduced. Cold has a numbing effect on the skin. This helps reduce or relieve pain in the part. The skin appears pale and feels cool in the area of the cold because of decreased blood flow.

Complications

Complications can occur from local cold applications. They include pain, burns and blisters, and cyanosis. **Cyanosis** is a bluish discoloration of the skin. Burns and blisters tend to occur from intense cold. They also occur when dry cold applications are in direct contact with the skin. When cold is applied for a long period of time, blood vessels tend to dilate. Blood flow increases. Therefore the prolonged application of cold has the same effects as local heat applications.

Elderly and fair-skinned persons have very fragile skin. Therefore they are at high risk for complications from local cold applications.

Moist and Dry Applications

Cold applications can be moist or dry. The ice bag is a dry cold application. The cold compress and cool water bath are moist applications. Moist cold applications penetrate deeper than dry applications. Therefore moist applications do not have to be as cold as dry applications.

General Rules

Residents must be protected from injuries that can result from cold applications. The general rules for the application of heat apply for cold applications, with the following exceptions.

1. Know the different temperature ranges for cool, cold, and very cold applications. The following ranges are guidelines:
   Cool—65° to 80° F (18.3° to 26.6° C)
   Cold—59° to 65° F (15° to 18.3° C)
   Very cold—59° F and below (15° C and below)
2. Do not let the resident lower the temperature of the application.
3. Report resident complaints of numbness, pain, or burning to the nurse immediately. Also report blisters or burns; pale, white, or gray skin; cyanosis; and shivering.

Ice Bags

An ice bag is a dry cold application. The bag is filled with crushed ice or ice chips. Crushed ice is better than ice cubes. The smaller pieces of crushed ice allow easier molding of the bag to the body part. There is less air space between crushed ice. The result is more even cooling. The ice bag is placed in a flannel cover before being applied. If the cover becomes moist, remove it and apply a dry one. Ice bags are applied for 30 minutes. If it is to be reapplied, wait 1 hour. This gives tissues time to recover from the cold.

Ice collars are applied to the neck. Some facilities have commercial ice bags that are refrozen for reuse. They are filled with a special solution and kept in a freezer until needed. Flannel covers are needed with ice collars or commercial ice bags.

PROCEDURE

Applying an Ice Bag or Collar

1. Explain the procedure to the resident.

2. Wash your hands.

3. Collect the following:
   a. Ice bag or collar
   b. Crushed ice or ice chips
   c. Flannel cover
   d. Paper towels

4. Fill the ice bag with water. Put in the stopper. Turn the bag upside down to check for leaks.

5. Empty the bag.

6. Fill the bag ½ to ⅔ full with the crushed ice or ice chips (Fig. 20-9).

7. Remove excess air. Bend, twist, or squeeze the bag, or press it against a firm surface.

8. Place the cap or stopper on securely.

9. Dry the bag with the paper towels.

10. Place the bag in the flannel cover.

11. Identify the resident. Check the ID bracelet and call the resident by name.

12. Provide for privacy.

13. Apply the ice bag to the part.

14. Place the signal light within reach. Raise or lower side rails as instructed by the nurse.

15. Check the skin every 10 minutes for blisters; pale, white, or gray skin; cyanosis; and shivering. Ask about numbness, pain, or burning. Remove the bag if any occur. Tell the nurse immediately.

16. Remove the bag after 30 minutes. (Lower the side rail if up.)

17. Make sure the resident is comfortable and unscreened. Place the signal light within reach.

18. Raise or lower side rails as instructed by the nurse.

19. Clean equipment. Discard the flannel cover in the linen hamper.

20. Wash your hands.

21. Report to the nurse:
    a. The time, site, and length of the application
    b. The resident's response
    c. Your observations of the skin

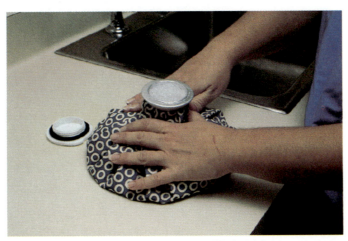

FIGURE 20-9 *The ice bag is filled with ice.*

Disposable Cold Packs

Disposable cold packs are dry cold applications. They are used only once and then discarded. They come in various sizes to fit different body parts. Some have an outer covering so the pack can be applied directly to the skin. If not, use a flannel cover. The cold pack is left in place no longer than 30 minutes.

PROCEDURE

Applying Disposable Cold Packs

1. Explain the procedure to the resident.

2. Wash your hands.

3. Collect the following:
   a. Disposable cold pack
   b. Flannel cover
   c. Ties, tape, or rolled gauze

4. Identify the resident. Check the ID bracelet and call the resident by name.

5. Provide for privacy.

6. Squeeze, knead, or strike the cold pack as directed by the manufacturer. This causes a chemical reaction that releases cold.

7. Cover the pack with the flannel cover.

8. Apply the cold pack. Secure it in place with ties, tape, or rolled gauze. Note the time.

9. Place the signal light within reach. Raise or lower side rails as instructed by the nurse.

10. Check the skin every 10 minutes. Check for blisters; pale, white, or gray skin; cyanosis; and shivering. Ask the resident about pain, numbness, or burning. Remove the pack if any occur. Tell the nurse immediately.

11. Remove the bag after 30 minutes. (Lower the side rail if up.)

12. Make sure the resident is comfortable and unscreened. Place the signal light within reach.

13. Raise or lower side rails as instructed by the nurse.

14. Discard the pack and other disposable equipment.

15. Wash your hands.

16. Report to the nurse:
    a. The time, site, and length of the application
    b. The resident's response
    c. Your observations of the skin

Cold Compresses

Applying cold compresses is similar to applying hot compresses. The cold compress is a moist cold application. It may be sterile or nonsterile. The nurse applies sterile cold compresses. Sterile compresses are ordered for open wounds or breaks in the skin. Moist cold compresses are left in place for no more than 20 minutes.

PROCEDURE

Applying Cold Compresses

1. Explain the procedure to the resident

2. Wash your hands.

3. Collect the following:
   a. Large basin with ice
   b. Small basin with cold water
   c. Gauze squares, washcloths, or small towels
   d. Waterproof pad
   e. Bath towel

4. Identify the resident. Check the ID bracelet and call the resident by name.

5. Provide for privacy.

6. Place the small basin with cold water into the large basin with ice.

7. Place the compresses into the cold water.

8. Place a waterproof pad under the part. Expose the area.

9. Wring out the compress.

10. Apply the cold compress to the part. Note the time.

11. Check the area every 5 minutes. Check for blisters; pale, white, or gray skin; cyanosis; or shivering. Ask about numbness, pain, or burning. Remove the compress if any occur. Tell the nurse immediately.

12. Change the compress when it becomes warm. Usually compresses are changed every 5 minutes.

13. Remove the compress after 20 minutes.

14. Pat the area dry with the bath towel.

15. Make sure the resident is comfortable and unscreened. Place the signal light within reach.

16. Raise or lower side rails as instructed by the nurse.

17. Clean equipment. Discard used linen in the linen hamper.

18. Wash your hands.

19. Report to the nurse:
    a. The time, site, and length of the application
    b. The resident's response
    c. Your observations of the skin

Cool Water Baths

The cool water bath is used to reduce body temperature when there is a high fever. A doctor's order is required. At first the cool water bath causes vasoconstriction, chilling, and shivering. These reactions to cold cause the body temperature to increase. As the body adjusts to the cold, body temperature decreases. The bath should last for 25 to 30 minutes to give the body time to adjust to the cold.

Vital signs are taken before, during, and after the procedure. Ice bags or moist cold compresses may be ordered to help lower the body temperature. They are applied to the forehead, axillae, and groin areas. The nurse also may request that cold applications be placed on each side of the neck. Cool water baths rarely are given to elderly residents.

PROCEDURE

Giving a Cool Water Bath

1. Explain the procedure to the resident.

2. Wash your hands.

3. Collect the following:
   a. Bath basin
   b. Bath thermometer
   c. Six ice bags or disposable ice packs (if ordered)
   d. Bath blanket
   e. Two or more bath towels
   f. Two or more washcloths
   g. Thermometer for body temperature
   h. Linen bag
   i. Sphygmomanometer and stethoscope
   j. Ice chips
   k. Six flannel covers for ice bags (if ordered)

4. Identify the resident. Check the ID bracelet and call the resident by name.

5. Provide for privacy.

6. Measure and record the vital signs. Note the time.

7. Raise the bed to the best level for good body mechanics. Lower the side rail.

8. Place the bath blanket over the top linens. Remove top linens.

9. Remove the gown without exposing the resident. Raise the side rail.

10. Prepare the ice bags or packs for application (if ordered). Place them in the flannel covers.

11. Lower the side rail. Move the resident to the side of the bed near you.

12. Apply the ice bags or packs to the resident's forehead, axillae, and groin. Place one on each side of the neck if requested by the nurse (Fig. 20-10). Apply the ice bags or packs only if ordered.

13. Raise the side rail.

14. Fill the wash basin ⅔ full with cool water. Measure the water temperature. Temperature should be 98.6° F (37° C). Add ice chips to cool the water if necessary.

15. Place washcloths in the water. Alternate use of washcloths during the procedure. Make sure no ice chips stick to them.

16. Lower the side rail.

17. Place a towel under the far arm.

18. Sponge the arm for about 5 minutes using long, slow, and gentle strokes. Pat dry; do not rub dry.

19. Repeat steps 17 and 18 for the near arm.

20. Place the bath towel lengthwise over the resident's chest and abdomen. Fan-fold the bath blanket to the pubic area.

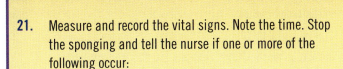

21. Measure and record the vital signs. Note the time. Stop the sponging and tell the nurse if one or more of the following occur:
    a. Body temperature is reduced to normal or slightly over normal
    b. Shivering
    c. Cyanosis
    d. Other signs and symptoms of cold. Check the skin under the ice bags. Tell the nurse about signs of complications.

22. Place a towel under the far leg.

23. Sponge the leg with long, slow, and gentle strokes for 5 minutes. Pat the leg dry, cover, and remove the bath towel.

24. Repeat steps 22 and 23 for the near leg.

25. Help the resident turn away from you.

26. Place a bath towel on the bed along the length of the resident's back and buttocks.

27. Sponge the back and buttocks with long, slow, gentle strokes for 5 minutes. Pat dry. Remove the towel.

28. Position the resident supine in the center of the bed.

29. Remove the ice packs.

30. Measure and record the vital signs. Note the time.

31. Put a clean gown on the resident. Make the bed. Change any damp or soiled linen.

32. Make sure the resident is comfortable and the bed is in the lowest position. Place the signal light within reach. Unscreen the resident.

33. Raise or lower side rails as instructed by the nurse.

34. Clean and return equipment to its proper place.

35. Take soiled linen and disposable items to the "dirty" utility room.

36. Measure vital signs 30 minutes after the procedure.

37. Wash your hands.

38. Report the following to the nurse:
    a. The time the procedure was started and completed
    b. Vital signs taken before, during, and after the procedure, and those taken 30 minutes after the procedure
    c. How the resident tolerated the procedure
    d. Condition of the skin under the applications
    e. Other signs and symptoms

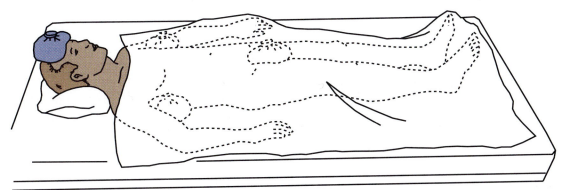

FIGURE 20-10 *Ice bags may be ordered for the cool water bath to help cool the body. The nurse may ask that they be applied to the forehead, axillae, and groin. Sometimes they are applied to the side of the neck.*

Quality OF LIFE

Heat and cold applications are ordered to promote healing and comfort and to reduce tissue swelling. Residents who need these applications have some injury or disorder. A resident may worry about why the heat or cold application is needed. You can promote the resident's quality of life by trying to understand the resident's concern. Be kind, caring, and patient. Refer any questions about the need for the application to the nurse. Remember, the resident has the right to personal choice. This means that the resident has the right to be involved in planning care. To do so, the resident must know why the application is needed.

Also remember to explain procedures to residents. What is familiar to you may not be so to them. Also, residents can plan if they know what will be done. A person may want to make a phone call or finish an activity before the treatment. Or a person may want the treatment done by a certain time—for example, before visitors arrive, before a favorite TV program, or before a scheduled activity. Having residents help plan when treatments will be done protects their right to personal choice.

The right to privacy also must be protected. Protecting privacy shows respect for the person. It also protects the person's dignity. Remember, only the body part involved in the procedure must be exposed. Unnecessary exposure violates the resident's right to privacy. It also can affect comfort if there is unnecessary chilling.

You can promote quality of life by making sure the resident's environment is safe and comfortable. Heat and cold applications take between 20 and 30 minutes. Therefore the resident will not be free to move about during this time. Encourage the resident to use the toilet, commode, urinal, or bedpan before the procedure. Make sure the room is free of unpleasant equipment or odors. Needed items must be within the resident's reach. These include the signal light, water, books or magazines, needlework, telephone, and other items requested by the resident. Be sure to check the resident often. You are responsible for the resident's safety.

SUMMARY

Heat and cold applications often are ordered by the doctor. They have opposite effects on blood flow. Both, however, are used for healing, comfort, and tissue swelling. Extreme care must be taken to make sure the right temperature is used. The heat or cold must be applied properly. Close observation of the resident also is necessary. Complications can occur quickly. Of all the complications, burns are the most serious.

You may not be allowed to apply heat or cold. Only RNs or LPNs may be allowed to do so. If you do apply heat and cold, extreme care must be taken. Dangers to the resident are severe. Therefore greater knowledge and judgment are needed. Review the purpose and steps of the procedure with a nurse. Request that a nurse closely supervise the procedure and its effects on the resident. The resident's safety and quality of life are the most important considerations.

Circle the *best* answer.

1. Which is *not* an effect of local heat applications?
   a. Pain relief
   b. Muscle relaxation
   c. Healing
   d. Decreased blood flow

2. The major complication of local heat applications is
   a. Infection
   b. Burns
   c. Chilling
   d. Decubiti

3. Who has the greatest risk of complications from local heat applications?
   a. A 25-year-old man
   b. A teenager
   c. A 40-year-old woman
   d. An 80-year-old woman

4. These statements are about moist heat applications. Which is *false?*
   a. Water is in contact with the skin.
   b. The effects are less than with a dry heat application.
   c. Heat penetrates more deeply than with a dry heat application.
   d. The temperature of the application is lower than that of a dry heat application.

5. A hot application usually is between
   a. 65° and 80° F
   b. 93° and 98° F
   c. 98° and 105° F
   d. 105° and 115° F

6. An extremity is in a basin of hot water. This is a
   a. Hot compress
   b. Hot pack
   c. Hot soak
   d. Sitz bath

7. These statements are about sitz baths. Which is *false?*
   a. The pelvic area is in warm or hot water for 20 minutes.
   b. The resident may become weak or faint during the bath.
   c. Sitz baths last 25 to 30 minutes.
   d. Sitz baths can be used to clean the perineum, relieve pain, increase circulation, or stimulate voiding.

8. You are applying a heat lamp. You should do the following *except*
   a. Cover the lamp with bed linens
   b. Let the lamp warm up before starting the procedure
   c. Check the bulb wattage
   d. Measure the distance between the bulb and the resident's body

9. These statements are about aquathermia pads. Which is *false?*
   a. The aquathermia pad is a dry heat application.
   b. The temperature of the aquathermia pad usually is set at 105° F.
   c. Electrical safety precautions must be practiced.

   d. Pins are used to secure the aquathermia pad in place.

10. Local cold applications are used to
    a. Reduce pain, prevent swelling, and decrease circulation
    b. Dilate blood vessels
    c. Prevent infection and the spread of microbes
    d. All of the above

11. Which is *not* a complication of local cold applications?
    a. Pain
    b. Burns and blisters
    c. Cyanosis
    d. Infection

12. Which is a dry cold application?
    a. The ice bag
    b. The cold compress
    c. The cool water bath
    d. All of the above

13. Before applying an ice bag
    a. The bag is placed in a freezer
    b. The temperature of the bag is measured
    c. The bag is placed in a flannel cover
    d. The resident is asked to void

14. Moist cold compresses are left in place no longer than
    a. 20 minutes
    b. 30 minutes
    c. 45 minutes
    d. 60 minutes

15. The cool water bath is ordered to
    a. Reduce swelling
    b. Relieve pain
    c. Decrease circulation
    d. Lower body temperature

16. The cool water bath should last
    a. 15 to 20 minutes
    b. 25 to 30 minutes
    c. 45 to 50 minutes
    d. 60 minutes or longer

17. A resident asks to read a book during a hot soak. You should allow this activity.
    a. True
    b. False

18. A resident asks to have a heat application before her son arrives. This is an example of the
    a. Right to privacy
    b. Right to personal choice
    c. Right to participate in resident and family groups
    d. Right to be free from restraint

1. d	6. c	11. d	16. b
2. b	7. c	12. a	17. a
3. d	8. a	13. c	18. b
4. b	9. d	14. a	
5. c	10. a	15. d	

21

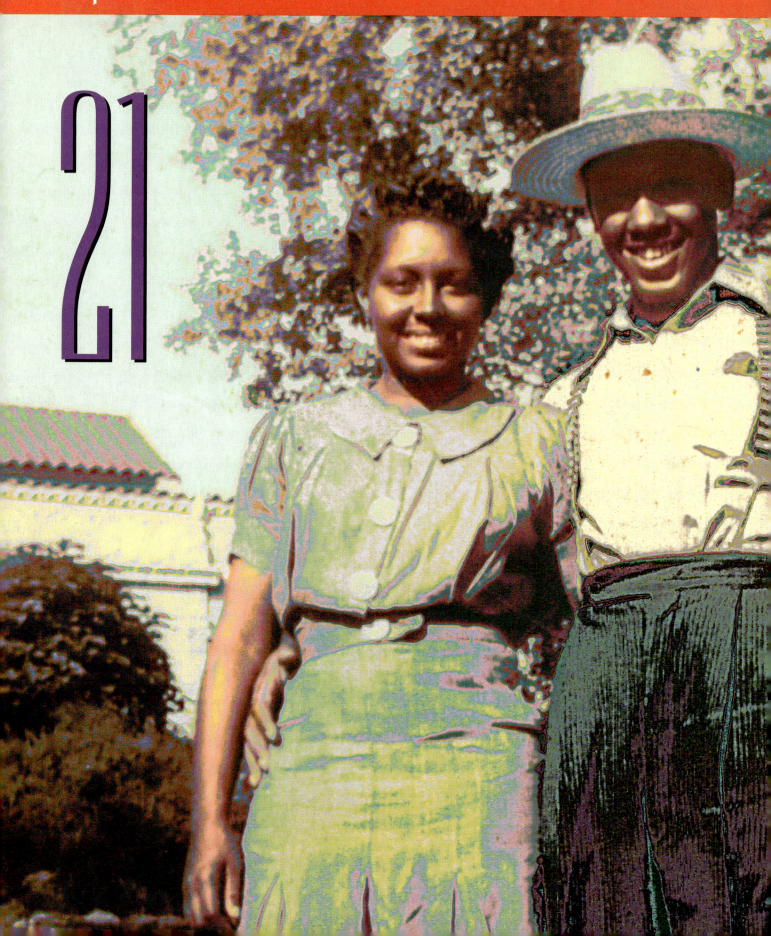

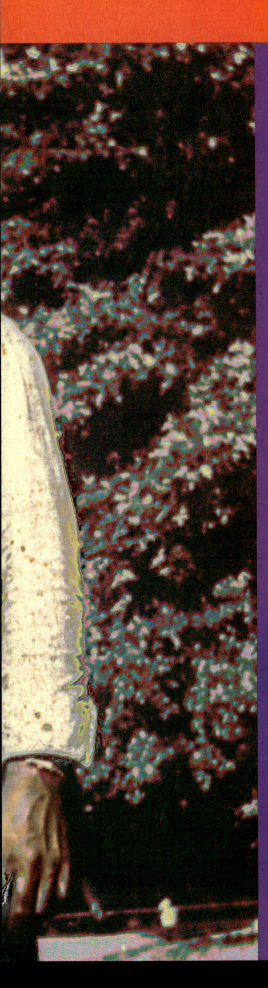

What You Will LEARN

- The key terms listed in this chapter

- Safety measures for caring for residents with IV infusions

- Common routes and reasons for suctioning

- Rules related to suctioning

- The purpose of oxygen therapy

- Oxygen sources and devices used to administer oxygen

- Rules related to oxygen therapy

- How to collect sputum specimens

- Why coughing and deep breathing exercises are done

- The purpose of support stockings and bandages

- The purposes of vaginal irrigations

- How to promote quality of life for residents who require special procedures

- How to perform the procedures in this chapter

atelectasis
A collapse of a portion of the lung

embolus
A blood clot that travels through the vascular system until it lodges in a distant blood vessel

pneumonia
An inflammation of the lung

sputum
Mucus secreted by the lungs, bronchi, and trachea during respiratory illnesses or disorders

suction
The process of withdrawing or sucking up fluids

thrombus
A blood clot

I need to wear elastic stockings. They go on so much easier when put on before I get out of bed.

RNs and LPNs are responsible for most of the topics and procedures in this chapter. Complex principles are involved, and there are great risks to the resident. Nursing assistants usually learn very basic knowledge about biology, body structure and function, and diseases. More knowledge and practice are needed to safely perform the procedures in this chapter. Nursing assistant courses usually are not long enough to include content from this chapter.

IV therapy, suctioning, and oxygen therapy are *never* your responsibility. However, you may be asked to collect a sputum specimen, give a vaginal irrigation, or apply elastic bandages or elastic stockings. These procedures are performed only if you thoroughly understand them. You must understand the purpose, procedure, and complications that may result. The procedure is reviewed with the nurse. The nurse closely supervises the procedure and its effect on the resident.

THE RESIDENT WITH AN INTRAVENOUS INFUSION

An intravenous (IV) infusion is the administration of fluid through a needle within a vein. Nursing assistants are never responsible for IV therapy. However, you may care for residents with IV infusions. You must give safe care. Therefore you need a basic understanding of the purposes of IV therapy. You also must know the measures taken to assist the resident and the nurse.

Purposes

Intravenous infusions are ordered by doctors. IVs provide needed fluids to residents unable to take fluids by mouth. Minerals and vitamins lost because of illness or injury can be replaced through IVs. IVs also are used to provide sugar for energy and to administer medications and blood. The doctor orders the amount and type of IV solution to be given.

Safety Measures

RNs start and maintain IV infusions. To start an IV, a needle is inserted into the vein. Then IV tubing is connected from the IV bottle (or bag) to the needle. RNs regulate the flow rate (number of drops per minute). They change IV bottles or bags, tubing, and dressings applied at insertion sites. Some states allow LPNs to perform these duties. Blood or IV medications ordered by the doctor, however, are given by RNs.

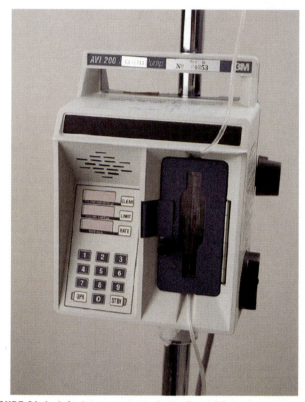

FIGURE 21-1 *Infusion pump controls the flow of fluid through tubing.*

You need to know two parts of the IV infusion (see Fig. 15-18). One is the drip chamber. Fluid drips from the bottle into the drip chamber. You can tell if the fluid is flowing by looking at the chamber. If no fluid is dripping, tell the nurse immediately. The second part is the clamp on the tubing. The RN uses the clamp to regulate the flow rate. *Never change the position of the clamp.*

Infusion pumps may be used to regulate IV flow rates (Fig. 21-1). The IV tubing fits into the pump. The nurse sets the flow rate on the pump. An alarm sounds if the flow is stopped for any reason. If the alarm sounds, tell the nurse immediately. Never adjust the pump in any way.

You are never responsible for starting or maintaining IV infusions. Nor do you regulate flow rates or change bottles, tubing, or dressings. Nursing assistants never administer blood or medications. You may assist residents with IVs to meet their personal hygiene and activity needs. Care must be taken to maintain the position of the IV needle when you assist a resident. If the needle is

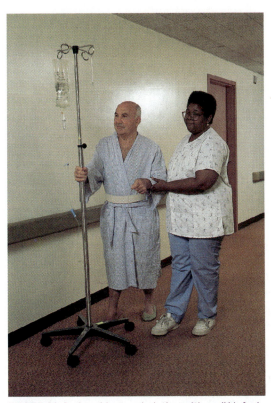

FIGURE 21-2 *A resident ambulating with an IV infusion.*

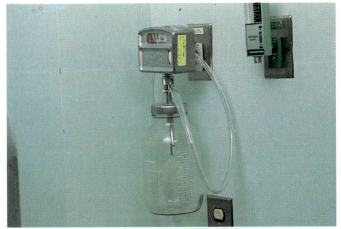

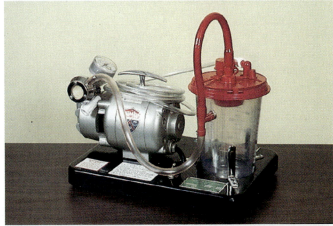

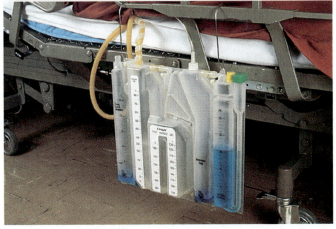

FIGURE 21-3 *A, Wall suction. B, Suction machine. C, Disposable suction apparatus.*

moved, it may come out of the vein. Fluid may flow into the tissues (infiltration), or solution flow may stop. Sometimes a nurse has to splint or restrain the extremity to prevent movement of the part. This helps keep the needle from moving. Safety measures for the use of restraints must be followed (see Chapter 7). When changing a gown, be careful not to move the needle (see *Changing the Gown of a Resident With an IV*, p. 274).

The IV bottle, tubing, and needle must be protected when the resident ambulates. Portable IV standards can be rolled alongside the ambulating resident (Fig. 21-2). Infusion pumps are attached to the standard and run on batteries when the resident is ambulating. The resident also needs help turning and repositioning in bed. The bottle is moved to the side of the bed on which the resident is lying. Always allow enough slack in the tubing. The needle will dislodge if pressure is exerted by the tubing.

SUCTIONING

Injury and illness often cause secretions to collect in body parts. Common areas are the upper airway, stomach, and surgical wounds. Secretions need to be removed for the resident's recovery and well-being. Suction is ordered by the doctor to remove excess secretions. **Suction** is the process of withdrawing or sucking up fluid (secretions). A tube is connected to a wall suction outlet or a suction machine (Fig. 21-3). The other end of the tube is inserted into the body part. Secretions are withdrawn through the tube (or catheter) into a collecting container.

Nursing assistants are never responsible for inserting tubes or for suctioning residents. However, you may care for residents who need suctioning.

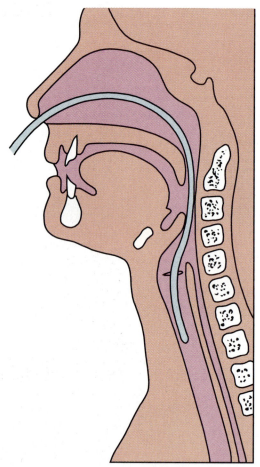

FIGURE 21-4 *A suction catheter inserted through the resident's nose into the trachea. Tubing connects the catheter to wall suction.*

Upper Airway Suctioning

The airway must be clear of secretions for normal breathing. Secretions may collect in the upper airway during certain illnesses. Some residents cannot remove them by coughing. The upper airway needs to be suctioned to remove the secretions. A nurse inserts the suction catheter through the resident's mouth or nose into the trachea whenever suctioning is needed (Fig. 21-4). The suction catheter is removed after the procedure. Certain signs and symptoms indicate the need for suctioning. They are tachypnea, dyspnea, moist sounding respirations or gurgling, restlessness, or cyanosis. The signs and symptoms must be reported to the nurse immediately.

Wound Suctioning

After surgery, it may be necessary to suction blood and other drainage from a wound. A drain or catheter is inserted during surgery and attached to a suction source. Residents may be admitted from a hospital with a suction apparatus in place.

Nasogastric Suctioning

Food and fluid may be given through a nasogastric (NG) tube (see Chapter 15). The tube also can be used to suction stomach contents and to keep the stomach empty. Gastrointestinal injuries, illnesses, and surgeries often require NG suctioning. The nurse inserts the tube through the resident's nose, the esophagus, and into the stomach (see Fig. 15-16, p. 351). The tube is connected to a suction source. The NG tube is left in place until the doctor orders its removal.

The NG tube can be very irritating to the nose and mouth. Most people breathe through their mouths when an NG tube is in place. Residents are also NPO when the tube is attached to suction. Frequent oral hygiene is necessary. The lips and oral mucous membranes can become dry and may crack. A bad taste in the mouth and mouth odor may occur. The nose also must be kept clean. Pressure and friction from the tube can irritate the nostril. Nasal secretions may harden and form crusts. The tube should not cause pressure on the nose.

General Rules

Suctioning is not a common procedure in nursing facilities. There may be times, however, when it is needed. You must assist the nurse in giving safe care. The resident is protected from harm during suctioning. The suction tubing or catheter and the suction source are handled carefully. You need to practice the following safety rules:

1. Never perform suctioning on a resident.
2. Make sure the resident is not lying on the catheter or tubing.
3. Make sure the catheter or tubing is not kinked.
4. Never turn off the suction source.
5. Do not raise the drainage container above the insertion site.
6. Do not empty the drainage container.
7. Do not disconnect any part of the suction system.
8. Report bright red drainage or an increase in the amount of blood to the nurse immediately.
9. Observe the amount and appearance of drainage in the container. Report your observations to the nurse at regular intervals. Report unusual observations immediately.
10. Make sure there is enough slack in the tubing. There should not be any pull or pressure at the insertion site.

OXYGEN THERAPY

Oxygen is a tasteless, odorless, and colorless gas. Oxygen is needed for survival. Death occurs within 4 minutes if a person stops breathing. Serious health problems develop if a person's oxygen supply is inadequate. During illness the amount of oxygen carried in the blood may be below normal levels. If so, the doctor may order supplemental oxygen. Acutely ill residents, those with respiratory disorders, and those with heart disease often need supplemental oxygen.

Oxygen is a drug. The doctor orders the amount of oxygen to be administered and whether it is to be given continuously or intermittently (periodically). The device used to give the oxygen also is ordered. You are never responsible for administering oxygen. However, you may care for residents receiving oxygen therapy. You need to know how to give safe and effective care to these residents.

Devices Used to Administer Oxygen

Oxygen is supplied through wall outlets, oxygen tanks, and air concentrators. With the wall outlet (Fig. 21-5), oxygen is piped into resident units. Each unit is connected to a centrally located oxygen supply.

Oxygen tanks are portable (Fig. 21-6). Large tanks are brought to the bedside when oxygen is not available through wall outlets. Small oxygen tanks are used by some ambulatory or wheelchair residents who need continuous oxygen. They use the small tanks when they walk or use a wheelchair (Fig. 21-7). Small tanks also are

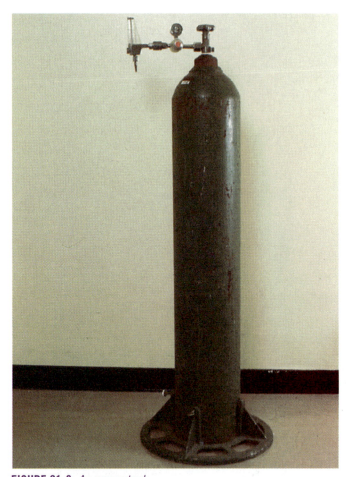

FIGURE 21-6 *An oxygen tank.*

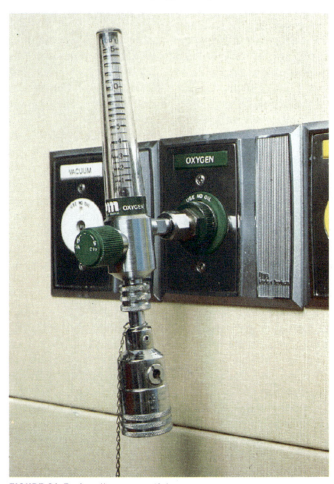

FIGURE 21-5 *A wall oxygen outlet.*

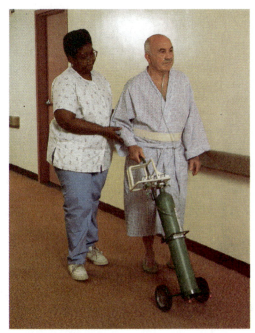

FIGURE 21-7 *A resident uses a portable oxygen tank during ambulation.*

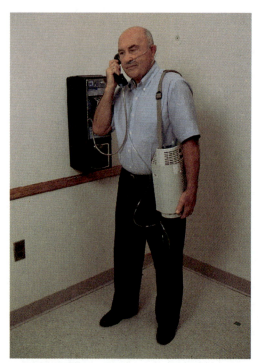

FIGURE 21-8 *A resident uses an oxygen "walker."*

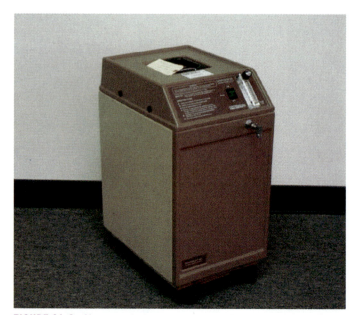

FIGURE 21-9 *Air concentrator.*

used during transfers within the facility. The oxygen "walker" is another type of portable oxygen container. It can be carried on a shoulder strap or hung on the back of a wheelchair (Fig. 21-8). These "walkers" are filled by the nursing staff from a liquid oxygen storage tank. Liquid oxygen is very cold and can cause severe burns. Be sure to receive instructions from the nurse before filling an oxygen "walker."

Air concentrators may be used instead of oxygen tanks (Fig. 21-9). The air concentrator is a machine that removes oxygen from the air. Like the oxygen tank, it is brought to the resident's bedside. The oxygen provided by the concentrator is the same as that in the tank.

There are several devices used to administer oxygen. The *nasal catheter* (Fig. 21-10, *A*) is inserted by a doctor, nurse, or respiratory therapist. It is inserted through the resident's nose until it can be seen in the back of the throat. The nasal catheter can be uncomfortable. Residents with nasogastric tubes and those with nasal catheters have similar needs. Frequent oral hygiene and nasal care must be given.

Nasal cannulas (Fig. 21-10, *B*) are the most common devices for administering oxygen. They are simple to use. Two prongs project from the tubing and are inserted a short distance into the nostrils. The resident can eat and talk with a cannula in place. Nasal irritation is possible if the prongs are too tight.

A *face mask* (Fig. 21-10, *C*) covers the nose and mouth. There are small holes in the sides of the mask.

They allow for the escape of carbon dioxide during exhalation and the entry of room air during inhalation. The mask is removed for eating and drinking. A nasal cannula usually is used during meals. Care of the resident with a face mask includes keeping the face clean and dry. This helps prevent irritation from the mask.

Residents may experience fright and feelings of suffocation with face masks. Talking can be difficult. The nurse is with the resident when the face mask is first used. The nurse explains its purpose and reassures the person that oxygen is being delivered. The resident may be frightened for awhile. You may be asked to stay with the resident if he or she is frightened. Remind the resident about the purpose of the mask. Speak clearly and calmly.

General Rules

The nurse and the respiratory therapist start and maintain oxygen therapy. You need to practice the following safety precautions related to oxygen therapy:
1. Post "NO SMOKING" signs, and follow safety precautions related to fire and the use of oxygen (see Chapter 7).
2. Never remove the device (cannula, catheter, or mask) used to administer oxygen.
3. Never shut off the flow of oxygen from the source.
4. Give oral hygiene as directed by the nurse.
5. Make sure connecting tubing is taped or pinned to the resident's clothing or gown.

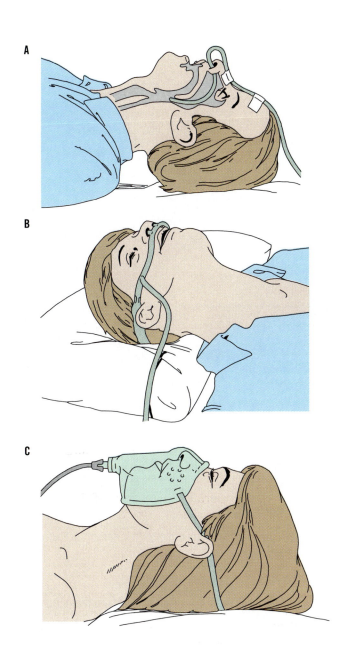

FIGURE 21-10 *A, Nasal catheter. B, Nasal cannula. C, Oxygen face mask.*

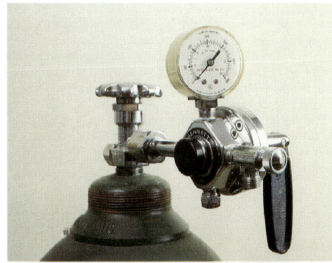

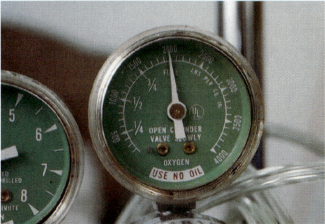

FIGURE 21-11 *A, Gauge on an oxygen tank. B, Fill level on the oxygen walker.*

6. Make sure there are no kinks in the tubing.
7. Make sure the resident is not lying or sitting on any part of the tubing.
8. Report signs and symptoms of respiratory distress or abnormal breathing patterns to the nurse immediately (see Chapter 16).
9. Observe the gauge on the tank or the fill level on the oxygen walker. Make sure there is enough oxygen (Fig. 21-11).
10. Notify the nurse immediately if the alarm sounds on the air concentrator. The alarm means that the unit is not working properly.

COLLECTING SPUTUM SPECIMENS

Respiratory disorders cause the lungs, bronchi, and trachea to secrete mucus. This mucous secretion is called **sputum** when it is expectorated (expelled) through the mouth. Do not confuse sputum and saliva. Saliva is a thin, clear liquid produced by the salivary glands in the mouth. Saliva often is called "spit."

Sputum specimens are studied for the presence of blood, microorganisms, and abnormal cells. The resident needs to cough up the sputum from the bronchi and trachea. Coughing and raising sputum can be very painful and difficult. It usually is easier to collect a specimen in the early morning. The resident tends to cough up secretions after awakening. Let the resident rinse his or her mouth with water before collecting the specimen. Rinsing decreases the amount of saliva and removes food particles. Mouthwash is not used before collecting a sputum specimen. It can destroy some microorganisms that may be present.

Collecting a sputum specimen can embarrass the resident. Other residents may be upset or nauseated by the coughing and expectorating sounds. The appearance of sputum also can be disagreeable to the resident and others. For these reasons the resident is allowed privacy during the procedure. The specimen container should be immediately covered and placed in a paper bag. Some facilities have paper-covered sputum containers that conceal the contents. Be sure to follow universal precautions when collecting sputum specimens. The blood-borne pathogen standard is also followed.

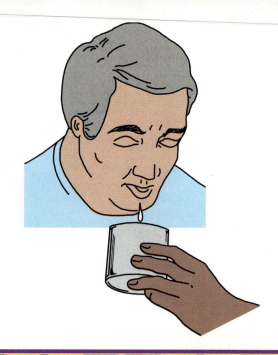

FIGURE 21-12 *The resident expectorates directly into the center of the specimen container.*

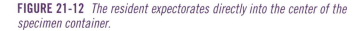

PROCEDURE

Collecting a Sputum Specimen

1. Explain the procedure to the resident.

2. Wash your hands.

3. Collect the following:
   a. Sputum specimen container with cover
   b. Tissues
   c. Label
   d. Laboratory requisition slip
   e. Paper bag
   f. Disposable gloves

4. Write the requested information on the label. Put it on the container.

5. Identify the resident. Check the ID bracelet and call the resident by name.

6. Provide for privacy. Let the resident use the bathroom to obtain the specimen if able.

7. Ask the resident to rinse the mouth with clear water.

8. Put on the gloves.

9. Have the resident hold the container if able. Only the outside of the container is touched. Hold the container if the resident cannot do so.

10. Ask the resident to cover the mouth and nose with tissues when coughing.

11. Ask him or her to take 2 or 3 deep breaths and cough up the sputum.

12. Have the resident expectorate directly into the container (Fig. 21-12). Sputum should not touch the outside of the container.

13. Collect 1 to 2 tablespoons of sputum unless directed to collect more.

14. Put the lid on the container immediately.

15. Place the container in the paper bag. Attach the requisition slip to the bag.

16. Make sure the resident is comfortable and unscreened.

17. Take the bag to the designated area.

18. Remove the gloves and wash your hands.

19. Report the following to the nurse:
   a. The time the specimen was collected
   b. The amount of sputum collected
   c. How easily the resident raised the sputum
   d. The consistency and appearance of the sputum (thick, clear, white, green, yellow, brown, or blood-tinged)
   e. Any other observations

into a part of the lung, and that part of the lung collapses. Coughing and deep breathing exercises help prevent these complications. Mucus is removed by coughing. Deep breathing promotes the movement of air into most parts of the lung. These exercises also may be ordered for residents with respiratory disorders.

Residents may have pain when doing the exercises after surgery. This is especially true after chest and abdominal surgeries. Others may find the exercises tiring. Even so, coughing and deep breathing are necessary to prevent complications.

The frequency of coughing and deep breathing exercises varies. Some doctors order the exercises every 2 hours while the resident is awake. Others want coughing and deep breathing exercises done 4 times a day. The nurse tells you when coughing and deep breathing exercises need to be done. You also will be told how many deep breaths and coughs the resident needs to do. Remember that coughing and deep breathing exercises are done only when directed by the nurse.

PROCEDURE

Coughing and Deep Breathing Exercises

1. Explain the procedure to the resident.

2. Identify the resident. Check the ID bracelet and call the resident by name.

3. Provide for privacy.

4. Help the resident to a comfortable position. Semi-Fowler's position is preferred.

5. Have the resident deep breathe.
   a. Have the resident place the hands over the rib cage (Fig. 21-13, p. 458).
   b. Ask the resident to exhale. Explain that he or she should exhale until the ribs move as far down as possible.
   c. Have the resident take a deep breath. It should be as deep as possible. Remind him or her to inhale through the nose.
   d. Ask the resident to hold the breath for 3 to 5 seconds.
   e. Ask the resident to exhale slowly through pursed lips (Fig. 21-14, p. 458). He or she should exhale until the ribs move as far down as possible.

f. Repeat this step four more times or as ordered.

6. Ask the resident to cough:
   a. Ask the resident to interlace the fingers over the incision (Fig. 21-15, *A*). Or have the resident hold a small pillow or folded towel over the area (Fig. 21-15, *B*). Figure 21-15, A & B is on p. 458.
   b. Have the resident take in a deep breath as in step 5.
   c. Ask the resident to cough strongly twice with the mouth open. Repeat as ordered.

7. Assist the resident to a comfortable position.

8. Raise or lower side rails as instructed by the nurse.

9. Place the signal light within reach.

10. Unscreen the resident.

11. Report your observations to the nurse:
    a. The number of times the resident coughed and deep breathed
    b. How the resident tolerated the procedure

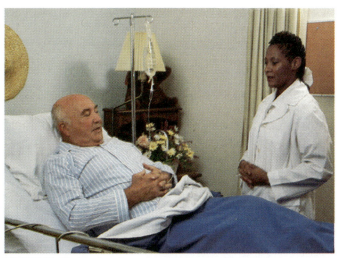

FIGURE 21-13 *The hands are placed over the rib cage for deep breathing.*

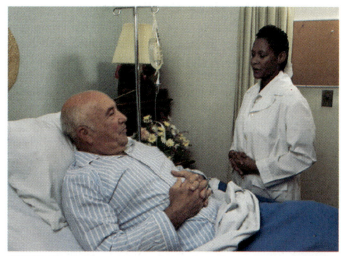

FIGURE 21-14 *The resident exhales through pursed lips during the deep breathing exercise.*

A

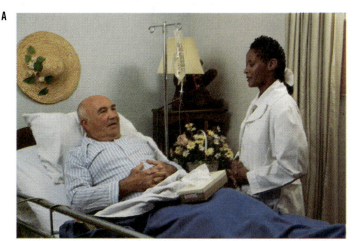

B

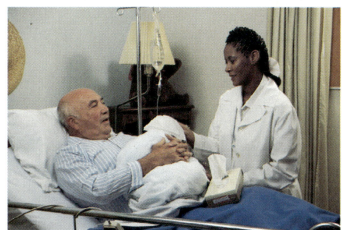

FIGURE 21-15 *The incision is supported for the coughing exercise.* **A,** *The resident interlaces the fingers over the incisional area.* **B,** *A small pillow can be held over the incision.*

SUPPORT STOCKINGS AND BANDAGES

Support stockings and bandages are applied to extremities. They promote comfort and circulation and provide support and pressure. They also promote healing and prevent injury. They must be applied properly. Incorrect application can cause severe discomfort, skin irritation, and circulatory complications.

Elastic Stockings

Elastic stockings often are ordered for persons with heart disease and circulatory disorders. They also are indicated for residents on bed rest. These persons are at risk for developing blood clots **(thrombi).** A blood clot is called a **thrombus.**

Blood clots can form if blood flow is sluggish. They are more likely to form in deep leg veins (Fig. 21-16, *A*, p. 460). A thrombus can break loose and travel through the blood-stream. It then becomes an embolus. An **embolus** is a blood clot that travels through the vascular system until it lodges in a distant vessel (Fig. 21-16, *B*, p. 460). An embolus from a vein eventually lodges in the lungs (pulmonary embolus). A pulmonary embolus can cause severe respiratory problems and death.

Elastic stockings are also known as antiembolism stockings or antiembolic (AE) stockings. They help prevent the development of thrombi. The elastic exerts pressure on the veins, promoting venous blood flow to the heart.

Stockings come in a many sizes. Thigh-high or knee-high lengths are available. The nurse measures the resident to determine the proper size. The stockings are removed at least twice a day. They are applied before the resident gets out of bed.

PROCEDURE

Applying Elastic Stockings

1. Explain the procedure to the resident.

2. Wash your hands.

3. Obtain elastic stockings in the correct size.

4. Identify the resident. Check the ID bracelet and call the resident by name.

5. Provide for privacy.

6. Raise the bed to the best position for good body mechanics.

7. Lower the side rail if up.

8. Position the resident supine.

9. Expose the legs. Fan-fold top linens toward the resident.

10. Turn the stocking inside-out down to the heel (Fig. 21-17, *A*, p. 460).

11. Slip the foot of the stocking over the toes, foot, and heel (Fig. 21-17, *B*, p. 460).

12. Grasp the stocking top. Slip it over the foot and heel, and pull it up the leg. It turns right side–out as it is pulled up. The stocking should be even and snug (Fig. 21-17, *C*, p. 460).

13. Make sure the stocking is not twisted and has no creases or wrinkles.

14. Repeat steps 10 through 13 for the other leg.

15. Return top linens to their proper position.

16. Help the resident to a comfortable position.

17. Lower the bed to its lowest position.

18. Raise or lower side rails as instructed by the nurse.

19. Place the signal light within reach.

20. Unscreen the resident.

21. Wash your hands.

22. Tell the nurse that the stockings have been applied.

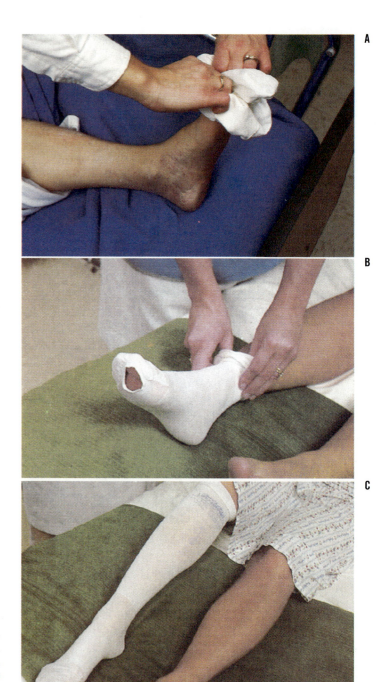

A

B

C

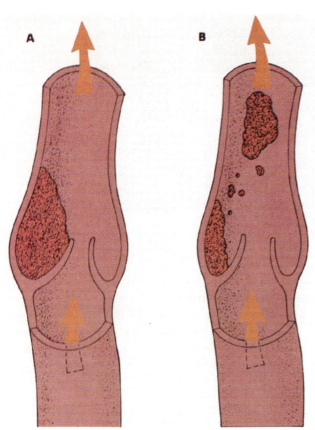

FIGURE 21-16 **A,** *A blood clot is attached to the wall of a vein. The arrows show the direction of blood flow.* **B,** *Part of the thrombus has broken off and has become an embolus. The embolus will travel in the bloodstream until it lodges in a distant vessel. (Modified from Phipps WJ et al: Medical-surgical nursing: concepts and clinical practice, ed 4, St Louis, 1991, Mosby–Year Book.)*

FIGURE 21-17 **A,** *The stocking is turned inside-out down to the heel and is ready for application.* **B,** *The stocking is pulled up over the toes, foot, and heel.* **C,** *The stocking is pulled up over the leg.*

Elastic Bandages

Elastic bandages have the same purposes as elastic stockings. They also provide support and reduce swelling from injuries. In addition, they can be used to hold dressings in place. Elastic bandages may be ordered for persons with varicose veins. Varicose veins are veins under the skin that have become dilated (wide) and bulging (Fig. 21-18, p. 462). The bandage is applied from the lower (distal) part of the extremity to the top (proximal) part. The nurse will tell you what area to bandage. Some facilities do not let nursing assistants apply elastic bandages. Make sure that you know the facility's policy.

General rules. You need to follow these rules when applying elastic bandages:
1. Obtain the elastic bandage in the proper length and width.
2. Make sure the extremity is in good alignment.
3. Face the resident during the procedure.
4. Leave fingers or toes exposed if possible. This allows the circulation to be checked.
5. Apply the bandage with firm, even pressure.
6. Check the color and temperature of the extremity every hour.
7. Reapply a loose, wrinkled, moist, or soiled bandage.

PROCEDURE

Applying Elastic Bandages

1. Explain the procedure to the resident.
2. Wash your hands.
3. Collect the following:
   a. Elastic bandage as determined by the nurse
   b. Tape, metal clips, or safety pins
4. Identify the resident. Check the ID bracelet and call the resident by name.
5. Provide for privacy.
6. Raise the bed to the best level for good body mechanics.
7. Help the resident to a comfortable position. Expose the part to be bandaged.
8. Make sure the area is clean and dry.
9. Hold the bandage so that the roll is up and the loose end is on the bottom (Fig. 21-19, *A*, p. 462).
10. Apply the bandage to the smallest part of the wrist, foot, ankle, or knee.
11. Make two circular turns around the part (Fig. 21-19, *B*, p. 462).
12. Make overlapping spiral turns in an upward direction. Each turn overlaps about 2/3 of the previous turn (Fig. 21-19, *C*, p. 462).
13. Apply the bandage smoothly with firm, even pressure. The bandage should not be tight.
14. Pin, tape, or clip the end of the bandage to hold it in place. Make sure the pin or clip is not under the part.
15. Check the fingers or toes for coldness or cyanosis. Also check for complaints of pain, numbness, or tingling. Remove the bandage if any are noted. Report your observations to the nurse.
16. Make sure the resident is comfortable and the signal light is within reach.
17. Lower the bed.
18. Raise or lower side rails as instructed by the nurse.
19. Unscreen the resident.
20. Wash your hands.
21. Report the following to the nurse:
    a. The time the bandage was applied
    b. The site of the application
    c. Any other observations

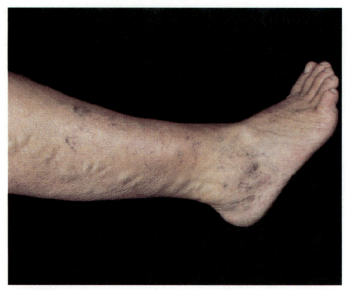

FIGURE 21-18 *Varicose veins are large and bulge under the skin.*

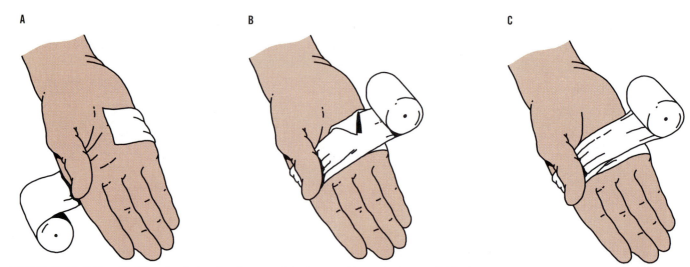

A **B** **C**

FIGURE 21-19 *A,*The roll of the elastic bandage is up, and the loose end is on the bottom. *B,* The bandage is applied to the smallest part with two circular turns. *C,*The bandage is applied with spiral turns in an upward direction. (Redrawn from Parcel GS, Rinear CE: Basic emergency care of the sick and injured, ed 4, St Louis, 1990, Mosby–Year Book.)

THE VAGINAL IRRIGATION

A vaginal irrigation (douche) is the introduction of a fluid into the vagina and the immediate return of the fluid. Vaginal douches are ordered by doctors to relieve pain and inflammation. They may be done to clean the vagina because of discharge. Medications and heat and cold can be applied with a vaginal irrigation. You should not perform the procedure if heat, cold, or a medication is being applied.

Vaginal irrigations are not done during menstruation. Normally douching is not necessary. Vaginal secretions cleanse the vagina naturally and protect it from infection.

A disposable kit is used. It has a container, connecting tubing, and nozzle. The nozzle is plastic. It is checked for chips and cracks that could cause vaginal injury. The resident is positioned on her back for the procedure. The nozzle is gently inserted backward and upward (Fig. 21-20, pp. 464-465). This follows the angle of the vagina when the resident is in the back-lying position.

PROCEDURE

Giving a Vaginal Irrigation

1. Explain the procedure to the resident.
2. Wash your hands.
3. Collect the following:
   a. Disposable vaginal irrigation kit
   b. 1000 ml of the irrigation solution
   c. Bath thermometer
   d. Bath blanket
   e. Bedpan
   f. Toilet tissue
   g. Waterproof pad
   h. Disposable gloves
   i. IV pole
   j. Water pitcher
   k. Equipment for perineal care
4. Identify the resident. Check the ID bracelet and call the resident by name.
5. Provide for privacy.
6. Have the resident urinate. Help her to the bathroom or offer the bedpan. Her bladder should be empty for the procedure.
7. Raise the bed to the best level for good body mechanics. Provide the bedpan if the resident will be using it.
8. Put on the gloves and empty the bedpan. Measure and record output if appropriate. Clean the bedpan and bring it back to the bedside.
9. Remove the gloves and wash your hands.
10. Warm the solution. It should be body temperature or 105° F (40.5° C) as directed by the nurse. If the solution has been prepared by central supply, set the container in a basin of hot water. Let it warm.
11. Do the following to warm a tap-water solution.
    a. Fill the pitcher with 1000 ml of warm water.
    b. Measure the temperature of the water.
    c. Adjust the water accordingly.
12. Cover the resident with a bath blanket. Fan-fold top linens to the foot of the bed.
13. Help the resident assume a back-lying position. Drape her as for perineal care.
14. Place the waterproof pad under her buttocks.
15. Put on gloves.
16. Provide perineal care (see *Giving Female Perineal Care*, p. 256).
17. Position the resident on the bedpan.
18. Clamp the irrigation tubing. Pour the solution into the irrigation container.
19. Hang the irrigation container from the IV pole. It should be 12 inches above the level of the vagina.
20. Position the nozzle over the vulva. Unclamp the tubing. Let some solution run over the perineal area.
21. Insert the nozzle 3 to 4 inches into the vagina (see Fig. 21-20). Rotate the nozzle gently during the procedure.

Continued.

Giving a Vaginal Irrigation—cont'd

22. Clamp the tubing when the container is empty. Remove the nozzle.

23. Place the tubing in the irrigation container.

24. Help the resident sit up on the bedpan if able. This allows the rest of the solution to drain from the vagina.

25. Help the resident lie down again.

26. Remove the bedpan. Dry the perineal area with toilet tissue.

27. Take the bedpan to the bathroom. Clean and return it to its proper place.

28. Remove the waterproof pad.

29. Discard disposable supplies.

30. Change any damp linen. Remove the gloves.

31. Help the resident to a comfortable position.

32. Return top linens to their proper position. Remove the bath blanket.

33. Lower the bed to its lowest position. Make sure the signal light is within reach.

34. Raise or lower side rails as instructed by the nurse.

35. Unscreen the resident.

36. Wash your hands.

37. Report the following to the nurse:
    a. The time the irrigation was given
    b. The amount, type, and temperature of the solution
    c. The resident's response
    d. The character of the returned solution
    e. Any other observations

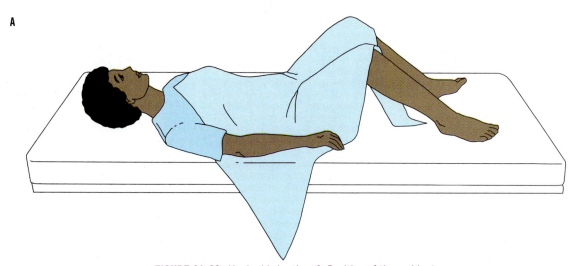

FIGURE 21-20 *Vaginal irrigation.* **A,** *Position of the resident.*

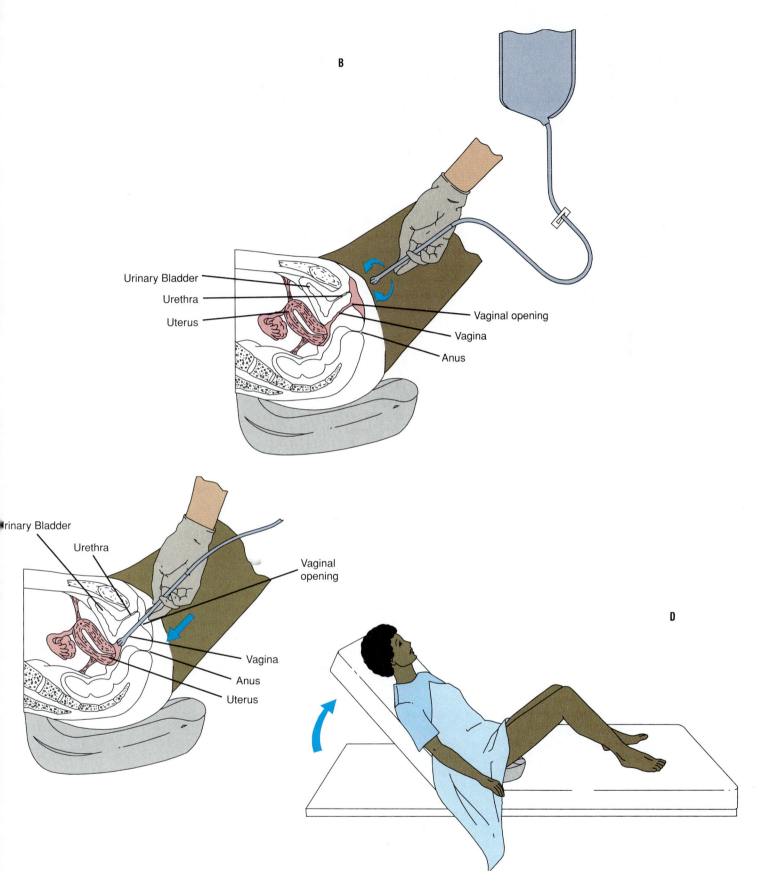

FIGURE 21-20 **B,** *Solution is used to cleanse the vulva.* **C,** *Solution flows into the vagina through a nozzle that has been inserted 3 to 4 inches.* **D,** *Elevating the head of the bed allows the solution to drain from the vagina. (Modified from Dison N:* Clinical nursing techniques, *ed 4, 1979, Mosby–Year Book.)*

Quality OF LIFE

The procedures in this chapter are complex. Serious complications can occur if incorrect care is given. You may be assigned to care for residents who need suctioning or IV therapy or oxygen therapy. You must provide safe care. A safe environment promotes quality of life for the resident. Be sure to follow the safety measures for IV therapy. The rules for suctioning and oxygen therapy also must be followed.

The right to privacy is very important when sputum specimens are collected and when vaginal irrigations are given. Both procedures can be embarrassing for residents. You must do all that you can to provide privacy. Merely pulling the privacy curtain is not enough. If possible, schedule the procedure when the roommate is out of the room. Be sure to close doors and window shades, blinds, or curtains. Proper draping is very important for the resident having a vaginal irrigation. The resident raising a sputum specimen should be allowed to do so in private if able.

OBRA also protects residents from all forms of abuse. Remember, abuse can be physical, verbal, financial, mental, or sexual. Involuntary seclusion is also abuse. Vaginal irrigations require touching and exposure of the genital area. The genital area also is a sexual area. The resident must be protected from sexual abuse. You also must protect yourself from being accused of sexually abusing the resident. Remember, some people do not like to be touched. The purpose of touch can be taken in the wrong way. Culture, religion, and personal values and beliefs can affect the meaning of touch. You must perform the procedure in a competent and professional manner. Be sure to explain the procedure to the resident and get the resident's consent to proceed. You also must protect the resident's privacy. Exposure of the resident could be viewed as a form of sexual abuse. How you communicate with the resident also deserves attention. You must be careful what you say and do. Some words have different meanings to different people. Your non-verbal communication is important. Following the principles of communication (see Chapter 4) should protect both the resident and yourself.

The right to personal choice must be protected. Sputum specimens usually are collected when the resident awakens. Elastic stockings are applied before the resident gets out of bed. Personal choice can be allowed, however, for coughing and deep breathing exercises and the vaginal irrigation. The resident should be involved in planning when these procedures will be done.

SUMMARY

You are never responsible for intravenous therapy, suctioning, or oxygen therapy. You may, however, care for residents receiving these therapies. You need to have a sound, basic understanding of their purposes and general safety rules. Resident safety must never be overlooked. Careful observation of the resident is necessary. You must promptly report observations and resident complaints. The side effects and complications of some treatments and procedures can be severe. Every sign, symptom, or resident complaint is important.

Finally, you need to know your own limitations. Do not perform any procedure that you do not understand or with which you are unfamiliar. Remember your legal and ethical responsibilities. *You have the right to say no.* You should not do anything that is beyond your legal scope, preparation, and skill level.

Review QUESTIONS

Circle the *best* answer.

1. A resident has an IV infusion. You should
   a. Add a new bottle if necessary
   b. See if fluid is dripping in the drip chamber
   c. Regulate the flow rate with the clamp
   d. Change the tubing daily

2. These statements are about suctioning the upper airway. You can
   a. Suction the resident whenever necessary
   b. Set up the suction system
   c. Observe for signs and symptoms that indicate a need for suction
   d. Turn on the suction source

3. Which device is the simplest and most commonly used to administer oxygen?
   a. Nasal catheter
   b. Nasal cannula
   c. Face mask
   d. IV therapy

4. A resident is receiving supplemental oxygen. You should do the following *except*
   a. Follow the safety measures related to fire and the use of oxygen
   b. Remove the administration device for meals
   c. Give oral hygiene as directed by the nurse
   d. Make sure there are no kinks in the tubing

5. You are to collect a sputum specimen. Which is *false*?
   a. An early morning specimen is best.
   b. Provide for the resident's privacy.
   c. Have the resident use mouthwash before raising the sputum.
   d. The sputum is expectorated directly into the specimen container.

6. Coughing and deep breathing exercises prevent
   a. Bleeding
   b. A pulmonary embolus
   c. Respiratory complications
   d. Pain and discomfort

7. Elastic stockings are worn to
   a. Prevent blood clots
   b. Hold dressings in place
   c. Reduce swelling
   d. All of the above

8. When applying an elastic bandage
   a. The extremity must be in good alignment
   b. The fingers or toes are covered if possible
   c. It is applied from the largest to smallest part of the extremity
   d. It is applied from the upper to the lower part of the extremity

9. You are to give a vaginal irrigation. You should do the following *except*
   a. Ask the resident to void before the procedure
   b. Warm the solution to body temperature or to 105° F
   c. Check the nozzle for chips or cracks
   d. Hang the container 18 to 24 inches above the vagina

10. The resident receiving a vaginal irrigation must be protected from
    a. Thrombi
    b. Emboli
    c. Sexual abuse
    d. All of the above

Answers

1. b	4. b	7. d	10. c
2. c	5. c	8. a	
3. b	6. c	9. d	

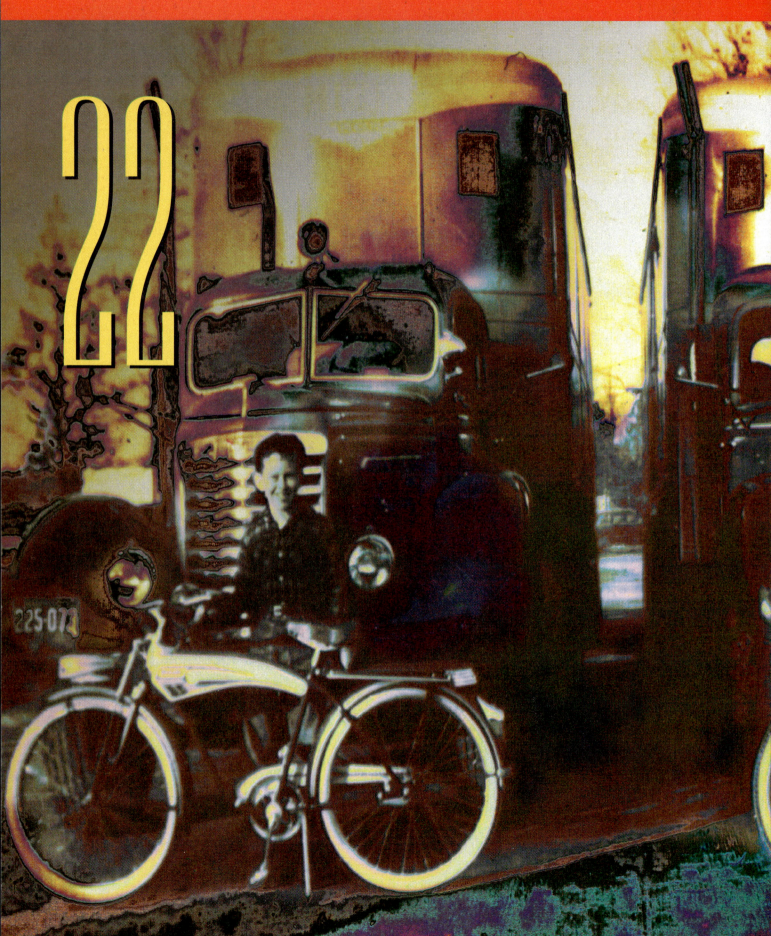

22

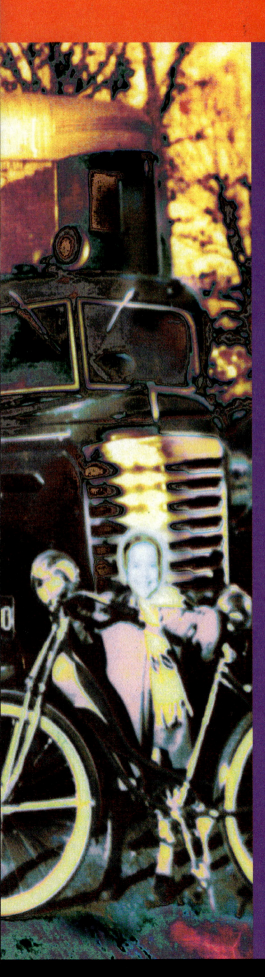

What You Will

L E A R N

- The key terms listed in this chapter

- What rehabilitation means in terms of the whole person

- The complications that need to be prevented for successful rehabilitation

- Ways to help disabled persons perform activities of daily living

- The psychological reactions that are common during rehabilitation

- The members of the rehabilitation team

- Common rehabilitation services

- Your responsibilities as a nursing assistant in rehabilitation

- How to promote quality of life during rehabilitation

activities of daily living (ADL)
Those self-care activities a person performs daily to remain independent and to function in society

prosthesis
An artificial replacement for a missing body part

rehabilitation
The process of restoring the disabled person to the highest possible level of physical, psychological, social, and economic functioning

I get frustrated sometimes that I can't do as much as I used to. Then the staff reminds me of how far I've come. They used to have to completely dress and bathe me. Now I can do most of that myself.

Disease, injury, and surgery can cause loss of body function or loss of a body part. Birth injuries and birth defects also can affect functioning. Often there is loss of more than one function. The loss may be temporary or permanent. Everyday activities such as eating, bathing, dressing, and walking may be difficult or seem impossible. The disabled person may be totally or partially dependent on others to meet basic needs. The degree of disability affects how much function is possible.

Health care is increasingly concerned with preventing and reducing the degree of disability. The person also is helped to adjust to the disability. **Rehabilitation is the process of restoring the disabled person to the highest possible level of physical, psychological, social, and economic functioning.**

Persons admitted to nursing facilities often have physical disabilities. Some have been hospitalized or restricted to bed rest with acute illnesses. They are weak and cannot perform activities of daily living. Restorative care helps them regain their strength and independence. Others have progressive illnesses—they become more and more disabled. Rehabilitation helps these residents maintain their highest level of functioning. Still others have suffered strokes, fractures, amputations, or other injuries. Rehabilitation programs help them to regain their former level of functioning or to live with the disability if it is permanent. Often these persons go home or to other levels of care. You will work with different types of rehabilitation programs.

REHABILITATION AND THE WHOLE PERSON

Rehabilitation involves the whole person. A physical illness or injury always has some psychological and social effect. Physical disabilities have similar effects. Suppose you wake up one morning and cannot move one side of your body. Would you be afraid, angry, or depressed? How would you get around in your home and care for yourself? How would you care for your family? How would you shop or visit friends or family? How would you support yourself? What work could you do?

Rehabilitation helps a person adjust physically, psychologically, socially, and economically. Abilities are emphasized, not the disability. However, complications that can cause further disability need to be prevented. Therefore rehabilitation begins when the person first enters the health care facility. Rehabilitation usually starts at a hospital. Transfer to a nursing facility may be required.

Physical Considerations

Rehabilitation begins by preventing complications. Complications can occur from bed rest, prolonged illness, or recovery from injury. Contractures, pressure sores, and bowel and bladder problems must be prevented. Measures to prevent contractures and pressure sores include good alignment, frequent turning and repositioning, range-of-motion exercises, and supportive devices (see Chapters 9 and 17). Good skin care is very important in preventing pressure sores (see Chapter 12).

Bladder training was described in Chapter 13. The bladder training program depends on the person's physical problems, capabilities, and needs. The nurse will explain the person's program. The rules to follow also will be explained.

Bowel training was described in Chapter 14. It involves gaining control of bowel movements and developing a regular pattern of elimination. Fecal impaction, constipation, and anal incontinence are prevented.

A major goal of rehabilitation is for the person to be able to perform self-care activities. **Activities of daily living (ADL)** refer to self-care activities. The person performs these activities daily to remain independent and to function in society. ADL include bathing, dressing, oral hygiene, eating, bowel and bladder elimination, and moving about. A person's ability to perform activities of daily living and the need for self-help devices are evaluated.

The hands, wrists, and arms may be affected by disease or injury. Self-help devices may be needed for various activities. Equipment usually can be changed or made to meet the person's needs. Special eating utensils may be required. Glass holders, plate guards, and silverware with curved handles or cuffs (Fig. 22-1) are avail-

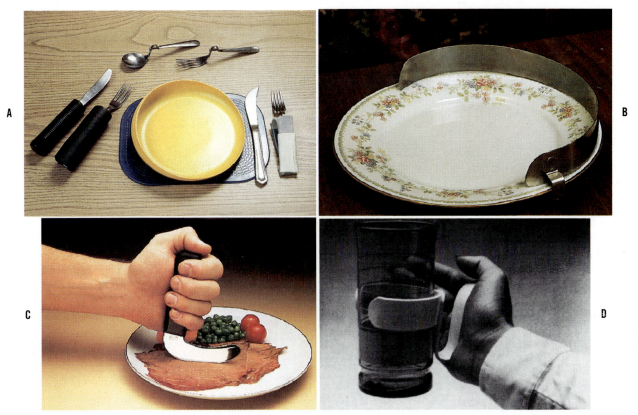

FIGURE 22-1 *Eating utensils for persons with special needs.* ***A,*** *Note the cuffed fork, which fits over the hand. The rounded plate helps keep food on the plate. Special grips and swivel handles are helpful for some individuals.* ***B,*** *Plate guards help keep food on the plate.* ***C,*** *Knives with rounded blades are rocked back and forth to cut food. They eliminate the need to have a fork in one hand and a knife in the other.* ***D,*** *Glass or cup holder.* (***B*** *to* ***D,*** *Courtesy Bissell Healthcare Corp/Fred Sammons, Inc. From Hoeman SP:* Rehabilitation/restorative care in the community, *St Louis, 1990, Mosby–Year Book.)*

able. Some devices are attached to special splints (Fig. 22-2). Electric toothbrushes are helpful if the person cannot perform back-and-forth motions necessary for brushing teeth. Longer handles can be attached to combs, brushes, and sponges (Fig. 22-3, p. 472). Self-help devices also are available for cooking, dressing, writing, dialing telephones, and many other activities (Fig. 22-4, pp. 472-473).

Some persons have lower extremity involvement. They may have to learn how to walk with a supportive device or how to use a wheelchair. If walking is possible, the person may be taught to use crutches or a walker, cane, or brace (Fig. 22-5, p. 474). Both legs may be paralyzed or amputated. If so, a wheelchair is necessary. Persons paralyzed on one side of the body also may need wheelchairs. If possible, the person is taught how to transfer from the bed to the wheelchair without assistance. Other transfers will be taught. These include

Text continued on p. 474.

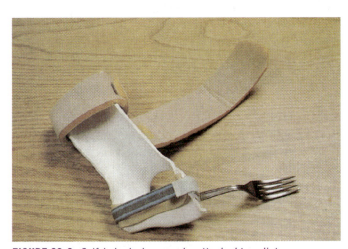

FIGURE 22-2 *Self-help devices can be attached to splints.*

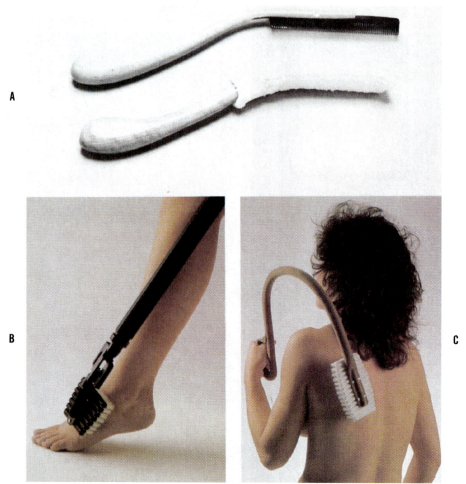

FIGURE 22-3 *A, A long-handled comb for hair care.* *B, The brush has a long handle for bathing.* *C, This brush has a curved handle. (Courtesy Lumex, Inc. From Hoeman SP*: Rehabilitation/restorative care in the community, *St Louis, 1990, Mosby–Year Book.)*

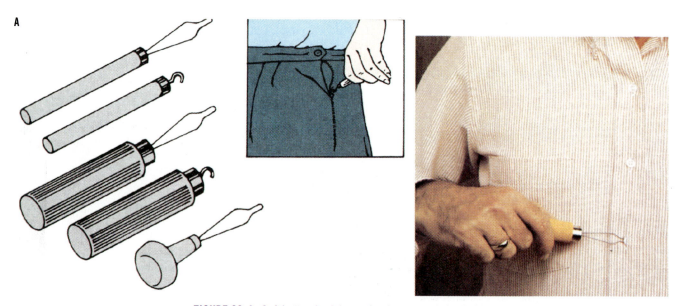

FIGURE 22-4 *A, A button hook is used to button and zip clothing.*

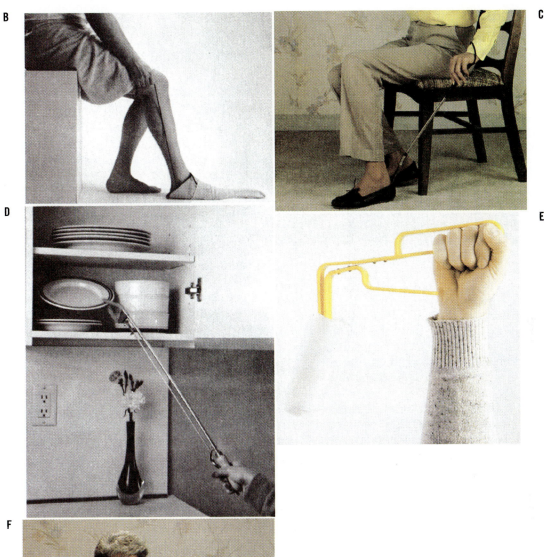

FIGURE 22-4, *B, A sock puller is used to put on socks and stockings. **C,** A long-handled shoe horn is for putting on shoes. **D,** Reachers are helpful for those in wheelchairs. **E,** A toilet paper holder is used for wiping. **F,** The telephone holder is for those who cannot hold a phone. (**A,** Courtesy Lumex, Inc; **B,** to **F,** courtesy Bissell Healthcare Corp/Fred Sammons, Inc. From Hoeman SP: Rehabilitation/restorative care in the community, St Louis, 1990, Mosby–Year Book.)*

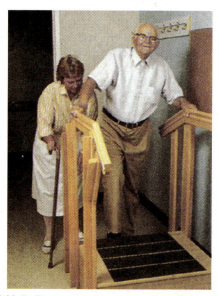

FIGURE 22-5 *The resident learns to walk in physical therapy.*

transfers to and from the toilet, bathtub, and chairs and in and out of cars (Fig. 22-6).

The resident with a missing body part may be fitted with a prosthesis. A **prosthesis** is an artificial replacement for the missing part. A person usually can be fitted with an artificial arm or leg and taught how to use the prosthesis (Fig. 22-7, p. 477). Artificial eyes are available. There are breast prostheses for women who have had a breast removed. Modern technology will provide even better prostheses. The goal is to have a prosthesis that closely resembles the missing part in function and appearance.

Difficulty swallowing (dysphagia) may occur after a stroke. When possible, these residents are taught special exercises to improve swallowing. Some may never swallow again. These persons will be fed through a gastrostomy tube (see Chapter 15 p. 351). Stroke victims may have *aphasia* (difficulty speaking). Speech therapy or special devices (see Chapter 4) can help them communicate.

Psychological and Social Considerations

Self-esteem and relationships with others often are affected by a disability. Changes in body appearance and function may cause a person to feel unwhole, useless, unattractive, unclean, or undesirable to others. In the early stages of rehabilitation, the person may refuse to acknowledge the disability. The person also may expect therapy to correct the disability. He or she may be depressed, angry, and hostile.

Successful rehabilitation depends on the person's attitude, acceptance of limitations, and motivation. The person must focus on remaining abilities. Discouragement and frustration are common feelings. Progress may be slow or efforts unsuccessful. Elderly persons may have greater difficulty with rehabilitation than do younger people. They often are weak and tire easily. Their progress may be slower, with fewer successes. Each new task to be learned is a reminder of the disability. Old fears and emotions may recur. Residents need to be reminded of the *progress* they have made. They need help in accepting their disabilities and limitations. Support, reassurance, encouragement, and sensitivity from the health care team are necessary.

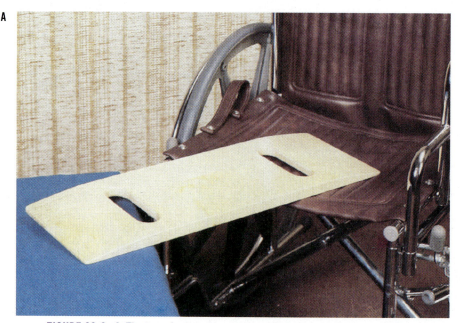

FIGURE 22-6 *A, The transfer board is used to transfer from one seat to another.*

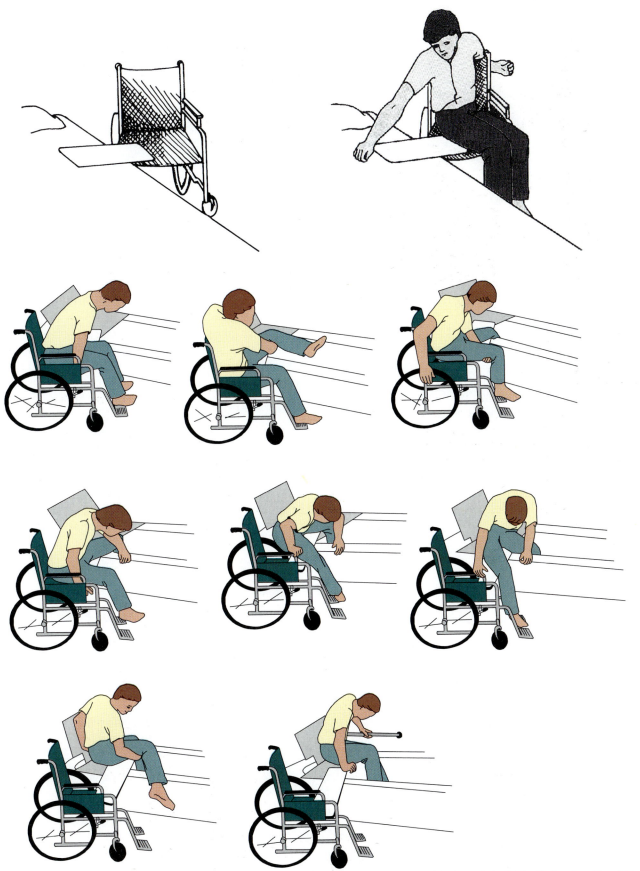

FIGURE 22-6, _B,_ _The resident transfers from the wheelchair to the bed._ **_C,_** _A transfer from the wheelchair to the bathtub._ **(_A,_** _Courtesy Bissell Health-care Corp/Fred Sammons, Inc. From Hoeman SP:_ Rehabilitation/restorative care in the community, _St Louis, 1990, Mosby–Year Book.)_

Continued.

D

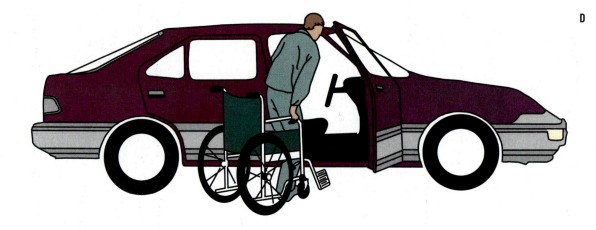

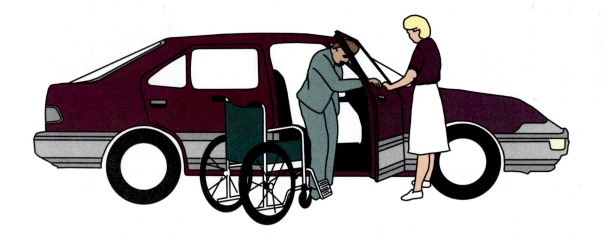

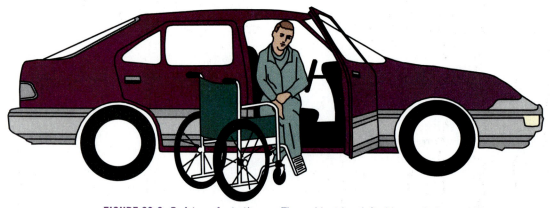

FIGURE 22-6, *D*, *A transfer to the car. The resident has left side paralysis.*

A 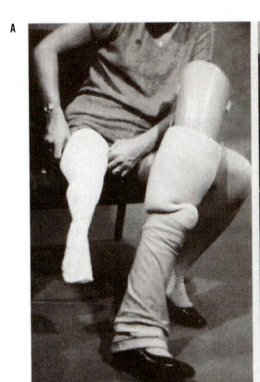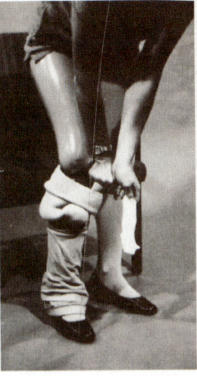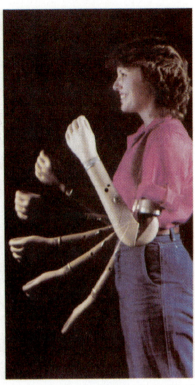 B

FIGURE 22-7 **A,** *Leg prosthesis.* **B,** *Arm prothesis.* (**A,** *Courtesy Otto Bock Orthopedic Industry, Inc.* **B,** *Courtesy Motion Control, Salt Lake City, Utah.* **A** *and* **B** *from Hoeman SP: Rehabilitation/restorative care in the community, St Louis, 1990, Mosby–Year Book.)*

THE REHABILITATION TEAM

Rehabilitation requires a team effort. The team consists of the resident, the doctor, the nursing team, other health care team members, and the family. All help the disabled person become independent. A physical therapist, occupational therapist, psychiatrist, psychologist, speech therapist, social worker, cleric, and dietitian may all be involved (Fig. 22-8).

The team meets regularly to discuss and evaluate the person's progress. Goals are set for the person. Changes in the rehabilitation plan are made when indicated. Often the disabled person and family are included in the meetings.

REHABILITATION SERVICES

Rehabilitation begins when the person first requires health care. This usually involves hospital care. Depending on the person's needs and problems, the process may be continued. The person may need more care in a nursing facility. Some individuals are transferred to rehabilitation centers, which have many specialized services. There are centers for the blind, deaf, mentally retarded, physically disabled, those with speech problems, and the mentally ill. Home care agencies and adult day care centers also provide rehabilitation services.

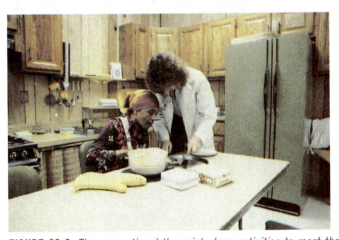

FIGURE 22-8 *The occupational therapist plans activities to meet the needs and interest of the disabled person.*

OBRA Requirements

OBRA requires that nursing facilities provide rehabilitation services. The services may be provided by facility staff members. If not, the facility must obtain the service from another source. For example, a facility may not employ a physical therapist. Instead, the facility obtains the service from a local hospital. OBRA rules state that rehabilitation services required by a resident's comprehensive care plan must be provided. If a resident requires physical therapy, it must be provided. If a resident requires occupational therapy, it must be provided. If a resident requires speech therapy, it must be provided. Such rehabilitation services require a doctor's order.

RESPONSIBILITIES OF THE NURSING ASSISTANT

Nursing assistants are key members of the rehabilitation team. The procedures and care measures you have learned will be part of the care given to a disabled person. Safety, communication, legal, and ethical considerations apply in rehabilitation. The many rules described throughout this book apply regardless of the type of disability.

As a part of the rehabilitation team, you need to practice the following points:

1. Follow the instructions and directions given by the nurse very carefully.
2. Report early signs and symptoms of complications such as pressure sores, contractures, and bowel and bladder problems.
3. Keep the person in good alignment at all times (see Chapter 9).
4. Practice measures to prevent pressure sores (see Chapter 12).
5. Turn and reposition the person as directed.
6. Perform range-of-motion exercises as instructed. Do them as often as stated by the nurse or resident's care plan.
7. Encourage the person to perform as many activities of daily living as possible and to the extent possible. Allow time for the person to complete the tasks.
8. Give praise when even a little progress is made.
9. Provide emotional support and reassurance.
10. Practice the techniques developed by other members of the rehabilitation team when assisting the person.
11. Know how to apply self-care devices used by the person.
12. Try to understand and appreciate the person's situation, feelings, and concerns.
13. Do not pity or give the person sympathy.
14. Concentrate on the person's abilities, not the disabilities.
15. Remember that muscles will atrophy if not used.
16. Practice the task that the person must perform. This will help you guide and direct the individual.
17. Know how to use and operate any special equipment that is part of the person's rehabilitation program.
18. Convey an attitude of hopefulness to the individual.

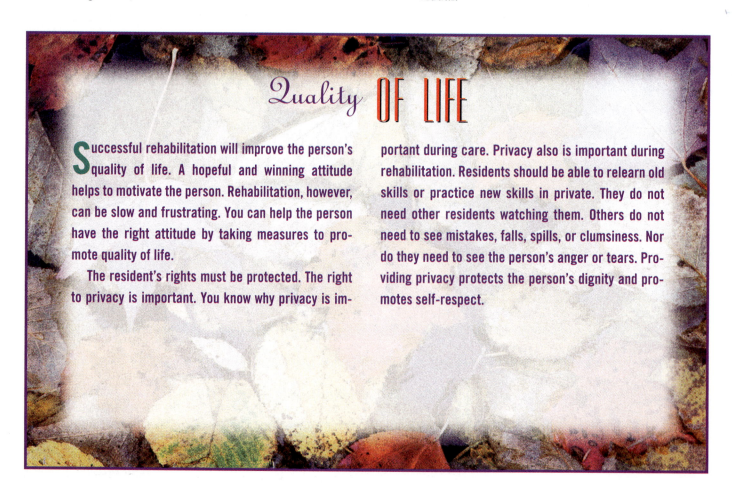

Quality OF LIFE

Successful rehabilitation will improve the person's quality of life. A hopeful and winning attitude helps to motivate the person. Rehabilitation, however, can be slow and frustrating. You can help the person have the right attitude by taking measures to promote quality of life.

The resident's rights must be protected. The right to privacy is important. You know why privacy is important during care. Privacy also is important during rehabilitation. Residents should be able to relearn old skills or practice new skills in private. They do not need other residents watching them. Others do not need to see mistakes, falls, spills, or clumsiness. Nor do they need to see the person's anger or tears. Providing privacy protects the person's dignity and promotes self-respect.

The right to personal choice gives the resident control. Being unable to control body movements or functions is very frustrating. Residents should be allowed and encouraged to control the other aspects of their lives to the extent possible. Personal choice has been discussed throughout this book. You need to allow personal choice whenever possible. Residents who are sad and depressed may not want to make personal choices. You need to encourage them to do so. Making personal choices will help residents feel in control of those things that affect them.

The resident is part of the rehabilitation team. The team plans and evaluates the person's rehabilitation program. Being part of the team allows the resident personal choice in planning care.

The resident has the right to be free from abuse and mistreatment. Rehabilitation can be a very slow process. Sometimes improvement is not seen for weeks. Learning how to use an assistive device can be a painfully slow process. Learning to speak again after a stroke can take a long time. So can learning how to dress when there is paralysis on one side. These are just a few examples of the skills that may be part of rehabilitation. What seems so simple to you can be very hard for the person. Repeated explanations and demonstrations may have no or little results. You may become impatient and short-tempered with the resident. Or you may see such behavior from other team members or the family. You must protect the resident from physical and mental abuse and mistreatment. No one can shout, scream, or yell at the person. Nor can they hit or strike the resident. The resident cannot be called names. Unkind remarks must not be made. You need to report signs of abuse or mistreatment to the nurse.

You must learn to deal with your own anger and frustration. Remember that the resident wants to have function and control of body movements. The person does not choose loss of function. If the process is frustrating to you, just think how the resident must feel. Discuss your feelings with the nurse. The nurse can suggest ways to help you control your feelings. Perhaps you can be reassigned to other residents for a while.

Taking part in resident activities promotes quality of life. The resident should be encouraged to join in activities. The person may be concerned about how others view the disability. You need to provide support and reassurance. The person needs to know that other residents have disabilities. Residents are likely to be very supportive and understanding because of their own disabilities. Allow personal choice in activities. Residents usually choose those of interest and those that are the least threatening.

The resident's environment is important for quality of life. It must be safe and must meet the person's needs. Adjustments may be needed because of disabilities. Location of the overbed table or the bedside stand may need to be changed. The resident may need a special chair. If the signal light cannot be used, another way is needed to communicate with the staff. These and other adjustments are recommended by nurses, occupational and physical therapists, and other team members. They will explain the need and purpose to the resident and family.

SUMMARY

Rehabilitation is part of your job as a nursing assistant. It can be challenging and rewarding for the health care team. Patience, understanding, and sensitivity are needed when working with the disabled person. This is especially true when the disabled person is elderly. Progress may be slow and hard to see. The person may be frustrated and discouraged. You must give support, encouragement, and praise when needed. The disabled person does not need pity or sympathy.

Emphasizing abilities is important. So is preventing disabling complications. Contractures, decubitus ulcers, and bowel and bladder problems must be prevented. Therefore good nursing care is necessary. In addition to helping to prevent complications, you need to observe the techniques taught to the disabled person. This lets you guide the person more effectively during care. If the person has to perform tasks in different ways for different staff members, frustration takes the place of progress. Finally, remember that the more the person can do alone, the better the person's quality of life.

Review QUESTIONS

Circle the *best* answer.

1. Rehabilitation is concerned with
   a. Physical disabilities
   b. Physical capabilities
   c. The whole person
   d. Psychological and social functioning

2. Physical rehabilitation begins with the prevention of
   a. Anger, frustration, and depression
   b. Contractures, decubiti, and bowel and bladder problems
   c. Illness and injury
   d. Loss of self-esteem

3. Mr. Williams has paralysis of both legs. Activities of daily living should be
   a. Done by Mr. Williams to the extent possible
   b. Done by the nursing assistant
   c. Postponed until he regains use of his legs
   d. Supervised by the physical therapist

4. Which reaction may be experienced by the disabled individual?
   a. Feelings of being undesirable or unattractive
   b. Anger and hostility
   c. Depression
   d. All of the above

5. The rehabilitation team consists of the resident and
   a. The nursing team
   b. The doctor
   c. Various members of the health care team
   d. The family

6. The nursing assistant
   a. Plans the rehabilitation program
   b. Supplies prostheses
   c. Gives praise when even slight progress is made
   d. Does as much as possible for the disabled person

7. Which statement is *false?*
   a. Sympathy and pity help the person adjust to the disability.
   b. You should know how to apply self-care devices.
   c. You should know how to use equipment used in the person's care.
   d. Hopefulness needs to be conveyed to the person.

8. A resident requires speech therapy after a stroke. Therapy should be provided in private.
   a. True
   b. False

9. Mr. Lund is in physical therapy to learn how to use a walker. He asks to have music played. You should
   a. Tell him music is not allowed
   b. Choose some music
   c. Let the resident choose some music
   d. Ask the resident group in charge of activities to choose some music

10. You tell Mr. Lund that he cannot have dessert unless he does his exercises. This is abuse and mistreatment of the resident.
    a. True
    b. False

11. Mr. Lund does not want to attend a concert scheduled at the facility. This is his right to
    a. Personal choice
    b. Privacy
    c. Be free from abuse and neglect
    d. All of the above

12. Mr. Angelo is paralyzed on the right side. The signal light has been placed on the right side. You move it to the left side. You have promoted his quality of life by
    a. Protecting him from abuse and mistreatment
    b. Allowing personal choice
    c. Providing a safe environment
    d. All of the above

Answers

1. c	4. a	7. a	10. a
2. b	5. c	8. a	11. a
3. b	6. c	9. c	12. c

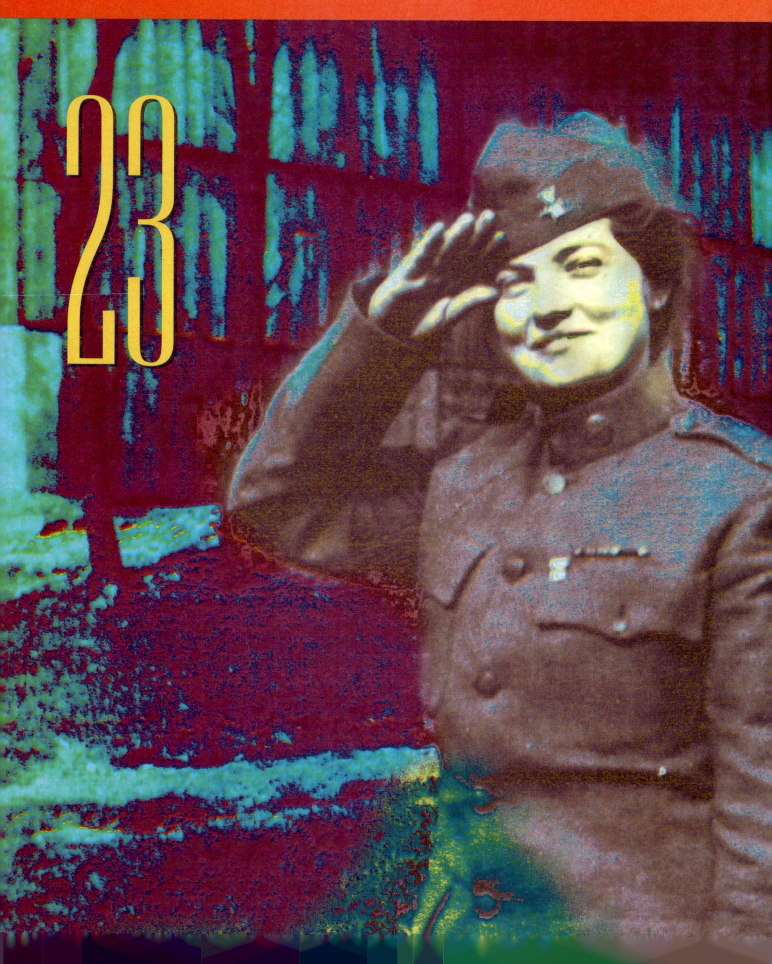

23

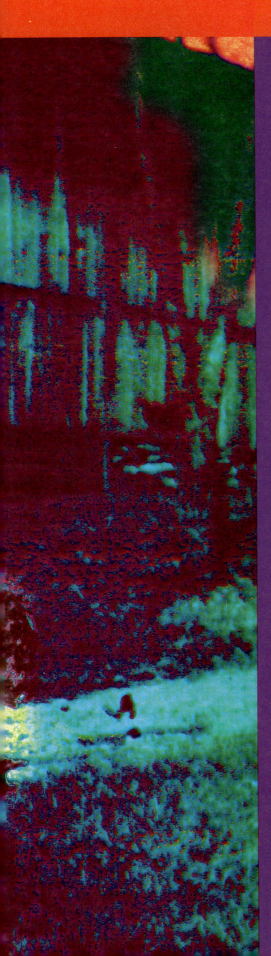

Key TERMS

What You Will LEARN

- The key terms listed in this chapter
- Seven warning signs of cancer and three cancer treatments
- How to maintain joint function in arthritis
- How to care for residents in casts
- The care required by residents with hip pinnings
- The care required by persons with osteoporosis
- Why loss of a limb requires a major psychological adjustment
- The signs and symptoms and care required by a person after a cerebrovascular accident
- Differences between Parkinson's disease and multiple sclerosis
- The effects of head and spinal cord injuries and the care required
- How to communicate with the hearing impaired person
- Differences between glaucoma and cataract
- How to care for a blind person
- The care required by persons with chronic obstructive lung disease and pneumonia
- The signs, symptoms, complications, and treatment of hypertension
- The care required by persons with angina pectoris, myocardial infarction, and congestive heart failure
- The signs, symptoms, and complications of diabetes mellitus
- The signs and symptoms and care required by persons with hepatitis and AIDS

alopecia
Loss of hair

amputation
The removal of all or part of an extremity

aphasia
The inability (a) to speak (phasia)

arthritis
Joint (arthro) inflammation (itis)

arthroplasty
The surgical treatment *(plasty)* of a joint *(arthro)*

benign tumor
A tumor that grows slowly and within a localized area; it does not usually cause death

closed fracture
The bone is broken but the skin is intact; a simple fracture

compound fracture
The bone is broken and has come through the skin; open fracture

fracture
A broken bone

gangrene
A condition in which there is death of tissue; tissues become black, cold, and shriveled

malignant tumor
A tumor that grows rapidly and invades other tissues; causes death if untreated

metastasis
The spread of cancer to other body parts

stomatitis
Inflammation (itis) of the mouth (stomat)

stroke
A cerebral vascular accident (CVA); blood supply to a part of the brain is suddenly interrupted

tumor
A new growth of abnormal cells; tumors can be benign or malignant

I get winded very easily. I have to stop and catch my breath at some point during almost everything I do. It just takes me longer to accomplish things.

This chapter gives basic information about common health problems seen in nursing facilities. Having this information makes required care more meaningful. If more information is needed, ask a nurse for additional explanations.

A review of Chapter 5 (Body Structure and Function) will be helpful in studying this chapter.

CANCER

Cancer is a new growth of abnormal cells. The growth is called a **tumor.** Tumors can be benign or malignant (Fig. 23-1). **Benign tumors** grow slowly within localized areas. They are not cancerous. Benign tumors usually do not cause death. **Malignant tumors** are cancerous. They grow rapidly and invade other tissues (Fig. 23-2). They cause death if not treated and controlled. The spread of cancer to other parts of the body is called **metastasis** (Fig. 23-3). Metastasis occurs if the cancer is not treated and controlled. Cancer can occur in almost any part of the body. The most common sites are the lungs, colon and rectum, breast, prostate, and uterus.

The exact causes of cancer are not known. Certain factors, however, contribute to its development. These include a family history of cancer, exposure to radiation or certain chemicals, smoking, alcohol, and viruses. Chronic exposure to sunlight and high-fat diets are other factors.

Cancer can be treated and controlled with early detection. The American Cancer Society has identified seven early warning signs of cancer:

1. A change in bowel or bladder habits
2. A sore that does not heal
3. Unusual bleeding or discharge from a body opening
4. A lump or thickening in the breast or elsewhere in the body
5. Difficulty swallowing or indigestion
6. An obvious change in a wart or mole
7. Nagging cough or hoarseness

There are three major cancer treatments: surgery, radiation therapy, and chemotherapy. Treatment depends on the type of tumor, its location, and if it has spread. One treatment type or a combination of treatments may be used.

Surgery involves removing the malignant tissue. Surgery is performed to cure cancer or to relieve pain from advanced cancer. Some surgeries are very disfiguring. A nurse plans measures for any special needs of a resident.

Radiation therapy and chemotherapy are common after surgery. Radiation therapy destroys living cells. Its greatest effect is on immature cells that are not fully developed. Cancer cells are immature. X-rays are directed at the tumor. Cancer cells and normal cells are both exposed to radiation. Both are destroyed. Radiation therapy is used to cure certain cancers and also to control the growth of cancer cells. Pain can be relieved or prevented by controlling cell growth. Radiation therapy has side effects. "Radiation sickness" involves discomfort, nausea, and vomiting. Skin breakdown can occur in exposed areas. Special skin care procedures may be ordered.

Chemotherapy involves drugs that kill cells. Like radiation therapy, chemotherapy affects both normal cells and cancer cells. It is used to cure cancer or to control the rate of cell growth. Side effects can be severe. They are caused by the destruction of normal cells. The gastrointestinal tract is irritated. Nausea, vomiting, and diarrhea result. **Stomatitis,** an inflammation *(itis)* of the mouth *(stomat),* also may develop. Hair loss **(alopecia)** may occur. There is decreased production of blood cells. As a result the person is at risk for bleeding and infection. The heart, lungs, liver, kidney, and skin also may be affected.

Residents with cancer have many needs, such as:

1. Pain must be controlled.
2. Adequate rest and exercise are needed.
3. Fluid and nutritional status must be maintained.
4. Skin breakdown and bowel problems must be prevented.
5. Constipation is a side effect of pain medications.
6. Diarrhea can occur from chemotherapy.
7. Side effects from radiation therapy and chemotherapy must be dealt with.

Some persons are admitted to nursing facilities to regain strength after radiation or chemotherapy. Some residents are still having therapy. Still others need hospice or terminal care. The care given includes comfort and psychological support until they die.

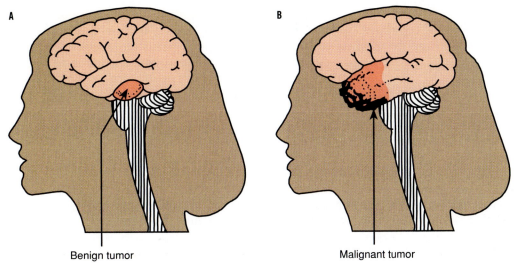

A

B

Benign tumor

Malignant tumor

FIGURE 23-1 *A, Benign tumors grow within a localized area. B, Malignant tumors invade other tissues.*

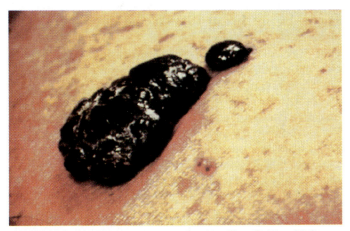

FIGURE 23-2 *A malignant tumor on the skin. (From Belcher AE: Cancer nursing, St. Louis, 1992, Mosby-Year Book.)*

The psychological and social needs of the person with cancer are great. The person may be angry, afraid, and depressed. He or she may be dealing with disfigurement from surgery. The person may feel unwhole, unattractive, or unclean. Both the resident and family members need much emotional support. The future may be uncertain. The possibility of death may be very real.

Put yourself in the person's position. How would you feel, and what would you want if you had cancer? Do not be afraid to talk to the resident. Avoiding the person because you are uncomfortable is one of the worst things you can do. Use touch to communicate you care. Listen to the person. Often the person needs to talk and have someone listen. Being there when the person needs you is important. You may not have to say anything. Just be there to listen and hold a hand.

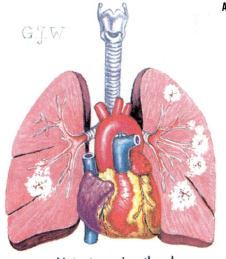

A

Metastases in other lung

B

Primary lesion

FIGURE 23-3 *A, A tumor in the lung. B, The tumor has metastasized to the other lung. (From Belcher AE: Cancer nursing, St. Louis, 1992, Mosby-Year Book.)*

MUSCULOSKELETAL DISORDERS

Musculoskeletal disorders are common. They affect the ability to move about. They are the result of disease or injury.

Arthritis

Arthritis means joint *(arth)* inflammation *(itis)*. It is the most common joint disease. Pain and decreased mobility occur in affected joints. There are two types of arthritis, osteoarthritis and rheumatoid arthritis.

Osteoarthritis. In *osteoarthritis,* the smooth surfaces of the joints break down (degenerate). It is common in people older than 60 years of age. Joint injury, however, can be a cause at any age. The spine, hips, and knees are commonly affected. These joints bear the weight of the body. Joints in the fingers and thumbs also can be affected. Symptoms are joint stiffness, pain, and limited range of motion. Cold weather and dampness seem to increase the symptoms.

Osteoarthritis has no cure. Treatment involves relieving pain and stiffness. Doctors often order aspirin. Aspirin relieves pain and reduces the joint inflammation. Local heat or cold applications also may be ordered. Persons with advanced disease may need help walking. A walking aid (cane, walker) may be needed. Measures to prevent falls are important. Assistance with ADL is given as necessary. Elevated toilet seats are helpful when there is limited range of motion in the hips.

Rheumatoid arthritis. Rheumatoid arthritis is a chronic disease. It can occur at any age. Connective tissue throughout the body is affected. The disease affects the heart, lungs, eyes, kidneys, and skin. The joints, however, are main targets. Smaller joints in the fingers, hands, and wrists are affected first (Fig. 23-4). Eventually, larger joints are involved. Severe inflammation causes very painful and swollen joints. The person probably will restrict movement because of severe pain.

Signs and symptoms are pain, redness, and swelling in the joint area; limitation of joint motion; fever; fatigue; and weight loss. As the disease progresses, more and more joints become involved. Changes in other organs eventually occur.

The three goals in treating rheumatoid arthritis are:
1. Maintaining joint motion
2. Controlling pain
3. Preventing deformities

The person needs a lot of rest. Bed rest may be ordered if several joints are involved and if fever is present. Turning and repositioning are done every 2 hours for those on bed rest. The person is positioned to prevent contractures. Eight to ten hours of sleep are needed each night. Morning and afternoon rest periods also are necessary. Rest is balanced with exercise. Range-of-motion exercises are done. Walking aids may be needed. Splints may be applied to the affected body parts. Safety measures to prevent falls are practiced.

Medications are ordered by the doctor for pain. Local heat or cold applications also may be ordered. A back massage is relaxing. Positioning to prevent deformities promotes comfort.

These residents need emotional support and reassurance. The disease is chronic. Death from other organ in-

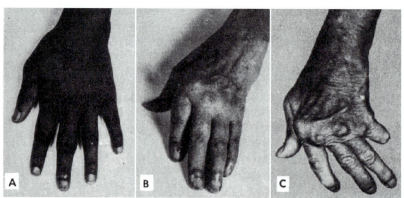

FIGURE 23-4 *Rheumatoid arthritis of the hand.* **A,** *Early stages.* **B,** *Moderate involvement.* **C,** *Advanced stage. (From Lewis SM, Collier IC:* Medical-surgical nursing: Assessment and management of clinical problems, *ed 3, St. Louis, 1992, Mosby-Year Book.)*

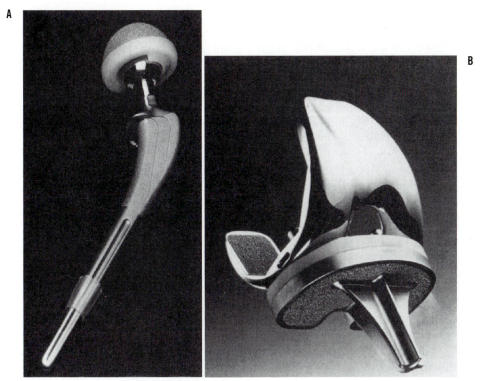

FIGURE 23-5 *A,* *Hip replacement prosthesis.* ***B,*** *Knee replacement prosthesis. (From Thompson, JM, et al:* Mosby's clinical nursing, *ed 3, St. Louis, 1993, Mosby-Year Book.)*

volvement is always possible. A good attitude is important for the resident. Residents should be as active as possible. The more residents can do for themselves, the better off they will be. A resident may need someone to talk to. You need to be a good listener when the resident needs to talk.

Total joint replacement. **Arthroplasty** is the surgical replacement *(plasty)* of a joint *(arthro).* Ankle, knee, hip, shoulder, wrist, finger, and toe joints can be replaced. The diseased joint is removed and replaced with a prosthesis (Fig. 23-5). The surgery is performed to relieve pain and to restore joint motion. You may care for residents who have had joint replacement surgery. The nurse will share the resident's care plan with you.

Fractures

A **fracture** is a broken bone. Tissues around the fracture—muscles, blood vessels, nerves, and tendons—usually are injured as well. Fractures may be open or closed (Fig. 23-6). A **closed fracture (simple fracture)** means the bone is broken but the skin is intact. An **open fracture (compound fracture)** means the broken bone has come through the skin.

Fractures are caused by falls and accidents. A bone

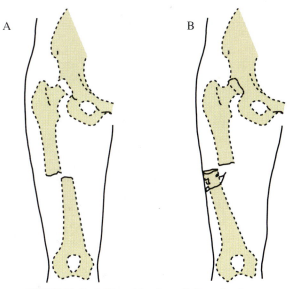

FIGURE 23-6 *A,* *Closed fracture.* ***B,*** *Open fracture.*

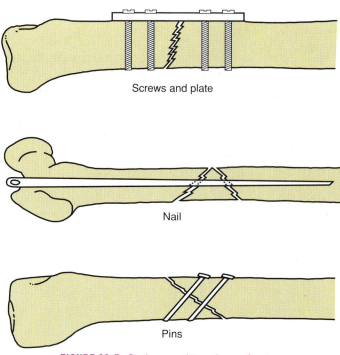

Screws and plate

Nail

Pins

FIGURE 23-7 *Devices used to reduce a fracture.*

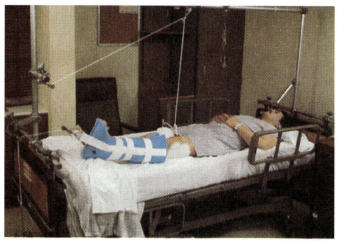

FIGURE 23-8 *Traction set up.*

disease called *osteoporosis* (see p. 494) also can cause fractures. Signs and symptoms of a fracture are pain, swelling, limitation of movement, deformity, bruising, and color changes at the fracture site. Bleeding also may occur.

The bone has to heal. The two bone ends are brought into normal position. This is called *reduction. Closed reduction* involves manipulating the bone back into place. The skin is not opened. *Open reduction* involves surgery. The bone is exposed and brought back into alignment. Nails, pins, screws, metal plates, or wires may be used to keep the bone in place (Fig. 23-7). After reduction, the fracture is immobilized. In other words, movement of the two bone ends is prevented. A cast or traction may be used to immobilize the bone. Traction involves pulling. Pull from two directions keeps the fractured bone in place (Fig. 23-8). Traction rarely is used in nursing facilities.

Cast care. Casts are made of fiberglass, plastic, or plaster of Paris. The cast covers all or part of an extremity (Fig. 23-9). Before the doctor applies the cast, the extremity is covered with stockinette. Material for plaster of Paris casts comes in rolls. The rolls are moistened and wrapped around the extremity. Plaster of Paris casts dry in 24 to 48 hours. A dry cast is odorless, white, and shiny. A wet cast is gray, cool, and has a musty smell.

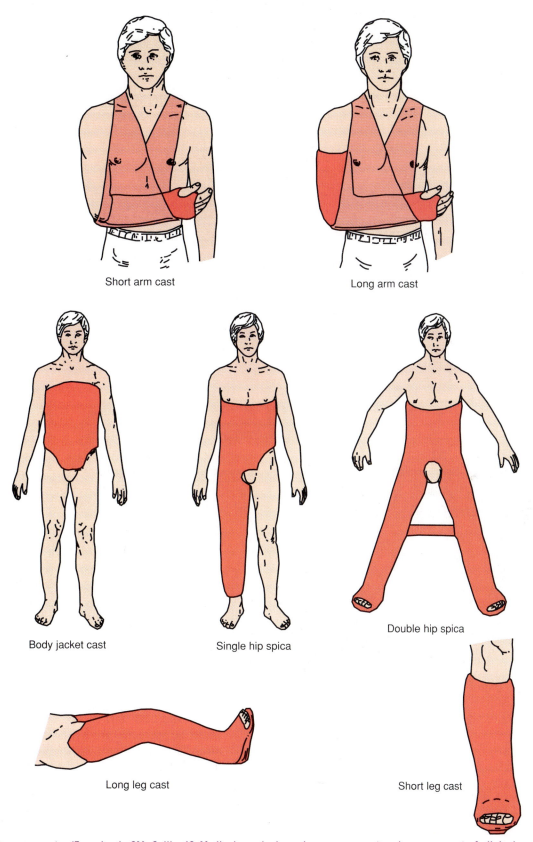

Short arm cast

Long arm cast

Body jacket cast

Single hip spica

Double hip spica

Long leg cast

Short leg cast

FIGURE 23-9 *Common casts. (From Lewis SM, Collier IC:* Medical-surgical nursing: assessment and management of clinical problems, *ed 3, St. Louis, 1992, Mosby-Year Book.)*

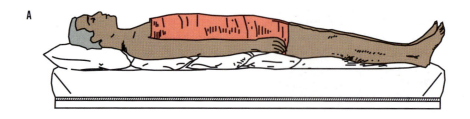

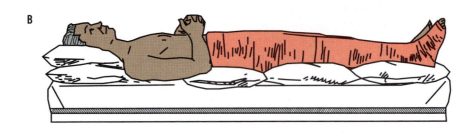

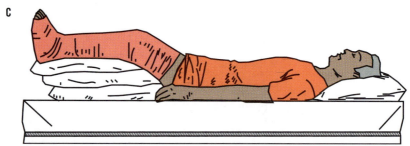

FIGURE 23-10 *Pillows support the entire length of the wet cast.* **A,** *Body cast.* **B,** *hip spica cast.* **C,** *Long-leg cast. (From Harkness Hood GH, Dincher, JR:* Total patient care: foundations and practice for adult health nursing, *ed 8, St. Louis, 1992, Mosby-Year Book.)*

The following rules apply to cast care:

1. Do not cover the cast with blankets, plastic, or other material. The cast gives off heat as it dries. Covers prevent heat from escaping. Burns can occur if heat cannot escape.
2. Turn the resident as directed by the nurse. All cast surfaces are exposed to the air at one time or another. Even drying is promoted by turning.
3. The cast must maintain its shape. It should not be placed on a hard surface while wet. A hard surface can cause the cast to flatten. Pillows are used to support the entire length of the cast (Fig. 23-10). When turning and positioning the person, support the cast with your palms (Fig. 23-11). Fingers can make dents in the cast. The dents can cause pressure areas and lead to skin breakdown.

4. Protect the person from rough edges of the cast. Cast edges can be covered with tape. This is called *petaling* (Fig. 23-12). If stockinette is used, the doctor pulls it up over the cast. The stockinette is then secured in place by using a roll of cast material.
5. Keep the cast dry. A wet cast loses its shape. It must be protected from moisture from the perineal area. The nurse may apply a waterproof material around the perineal area once the cast is dry.
6. Do not let the person insert anything into the cast. Itching often occurs under the cast and causes an intense desire to scratch. Skin can be broken by items used to scratch (pencils, hangers, knitting needles, back scratchers). Open areas under a cast can become infected. Items used to scratch can

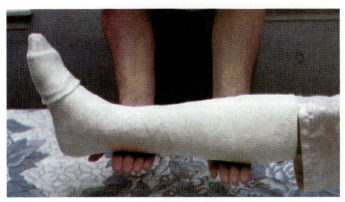

FIGURE 23-11 *The cast is supported with the palms during lifting.*

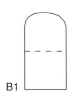
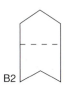

B1

B2

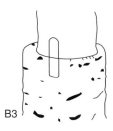

B

B3

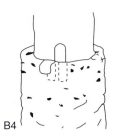

B4

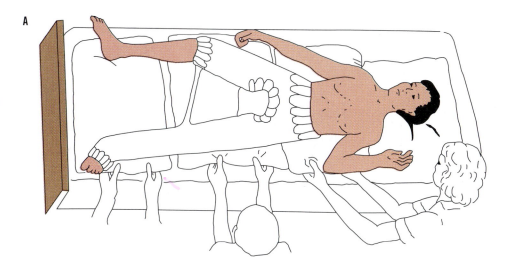

FIGURE 23-12 *A,* *The edges of the cast are petaled.* ***B,*** *Pieces of tape are used to make the petals. The petal is placed inside the cast and then brought over the edge.*

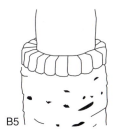

B5

cause wrinkles in the stockinette. The object can be lost into the cast. Both can cause pressure, which leads to skin breakdown.

7. A casted extremity is elevated on pillows. Elevating the body part reduces swelling.

8. Have enough help when turning and repositioning the resident. Some casts are heavy and awkward. Balance can be easily lost.

9. Lying on the injured side usually is not allowed. The nurse tells you how to position the resident.

10. Report these signs and symptoms immediately:
   a. Pain—a warning sign of pressure sores, poor circulation, or nerve damage.
   b. Swelling and a tight cast—blood flow to the part may be affected.
   c. Pale skin—reduced blood flow to the part.
   d. Cyanosis—reduced blood flow to the part.
   e. Odor—an infection may be present.
   f. Inability to move the fingers or toes—the cast may be causing pressure on a nerve.
   g. Numbness—the cast may be causing pressure on a nerve. Reduced blood flow may be another cause.
   h. Temperature changes—cool skin means poor circulation. Hot skin means inflammation.
   i. Drainage on or under the cast—there may be an infection under the cast.
   j. Chills, fever, nausea, and vomiting—there may be an infection under the cast.

491

Hip fractures. Fractured hips are common in elderly persons (Fig. 23-13). They are especially serious because healing is slower in older people. The person may have other disorders. These disorders and slow healing may complicate the person's condition and care. The risk for postoperative complications is great.

Open reduction usually is required. The fracture is fixed in position with a pin, nail, plate, screw, or prosthesis (Fig. 23-14). A cast may be used in some situations. Therefore, care of the resident with a cast may be required. The resident with a hip pinning also requires the following care:

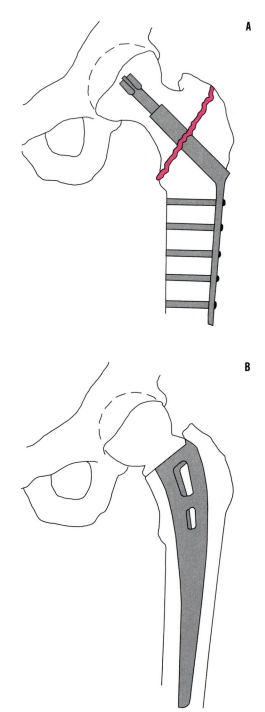

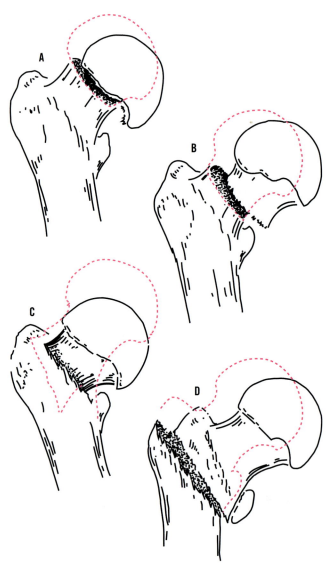

FIGURE 23-13 *Fractures of the hip. (From Long, BC, et al: Medical-surgical nursing: a nursing process approach, ed 3, St. Louis, 1993, Mosby-Year Book.)*

FIGURE 23-14 *A, Nail used to repair a hip fracture. B, Prosthesis used to repair a hip fracture. (From Long, BC, et al: Medical-surgical nursing: a nursing process approach, ed 3, St. Louis, 1993, Mosby-Year Book.)*

1. Give good skin care. Skin breakdown can occur rapidly.
2. Turn and reposition the resident as directed by the nurse. The doctor's orders for turning and positioning depend on the type of fracture and the surgery performed.
3. Keep the operated leg abducted at all times. The leg is abducted when the resident is supine, being turned, or in a side-lying position (Fig. 23-15, *A*). Abductor splints or pillows may be used as directed (Fig. 23-15, *B*).
4. Prevent external rotation of the hip (Fig. 23-16, p. 494). Use trochanter rolls or adduction splints as directed.

5. Provide a straight-backed chair with armrests when the resident is to be up. A low, soft chair is not used.
6. Place the chair on the unoperated side.
7. Assist the nurse in transferring the resident from the bed to the chair as directed.
8. Do not let the resident stand on the operated leg unless permitted by the doctor.
9. Support and elevate the leg as directed when the resident is in the chair.

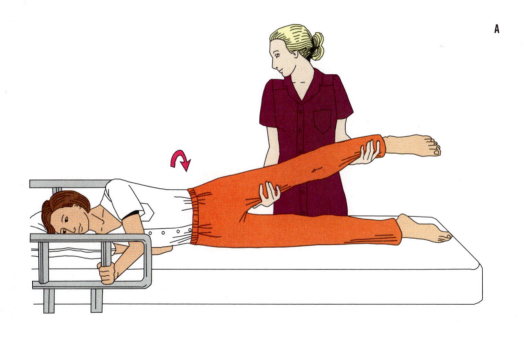

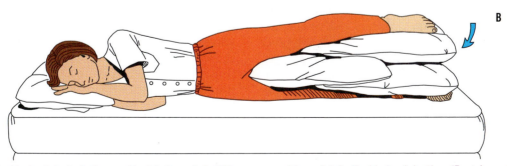

FIGURE 23-15 *A, The hip is abducted when resident is turned. B, Pillows are used to maintain the hip in abduction. (From Long, BC et al:* Medical-surgical nursing: a nursing process approach, *ed 3, St. Louis, 1993, Mosby-Year Book.)*

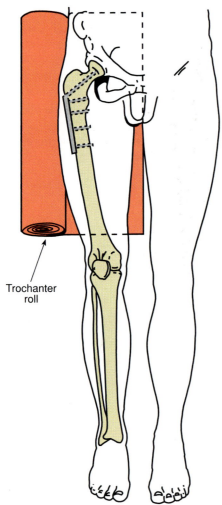

FIGURE 23-16 *A trochanter roll is used to prevent external rotation after a hip pinning.*

Osteoporosis

Osteoporosis is a bone disorder in which the bone *(osteo)* becomes porous and brittle *(porosis)*. The disorder is common in elderly persons. It is more common in women than in men. Women are at risk after menopause. Loss of the hormone estrogen seems to cause calcium loss from the bones of women. A dietary lack of calcium also is a major cause. Bed rest and immobility are other causes because they do not allow for proper bone use. For bone to form properly, it must be used to bear weight. If it is not, calcium is absorbed and the bone becomes porous and brittle.

Signs and symptoms include back pain, gradual loss of height, and stooped posture. Fractures are a major threat. Common sites are the spine, hips, and wrists. The loss of height is due to fractures of the vertebrae. Bones are so brittle that the slightest stress can cause a fracture.

Turning in bed or getting up from a chair can cause a fracture. Fractures are a great risk if the person falls or has an accident.

Osteoporosis is treated with calcium and vitamin supplements. The hormone estrogen may be given to women. Exercise, good posture, and a back brace or corset are important. Walking aids may be necessary. Bed rest is avoided. Caution is used when turning and positioning the resident. The resident must be protected from falls and accidents (see Chapter 7).

Loss of a Limb

An **amputation** is the removal of all or part of an extremity. Usually the part is removed surgically. Traumatic amputations, however, can occur from accidents. Amputations sometimes are performed for severe injuries, bone tumors, severe infections, and circulatory disorders.

Gangrene is a condition in which there is death of tissue. Infection, injuries, and circulatory disorders may result in gangrene. These conditions interfere with blood supply to the tissues. The tissues do not receive enough oxygen and nutrients. Poisonous substances and waste products build up in the affected tissues. Tissue death results. The tissue becomes black, cold, and shriveled (Fig. 23-17) and can eventually fall off. If untreated, gangrene spreads through the body and causes death.

All or part of an extremity may be amputated. Fingers, a hand, a forearm, or an entire arm may be removed. Toes, the foot, the lower leg, the upper leg, or the entire leg may be amputated. A below-the-knee amputation is called a BK (below the knee) or BKA (below-knee amputation). An above-the-knee amputation is called an AK (above the knee) or AKA (above-knee amputation).

Much psychological support is needed. A major psychological adjustment is necessary. The person's life is affected by the amputation. Appearance, activities of daily living, and moving about are just a few areas affected. Put yourself in the resident's position. How would you feel if you lost an arm or a leg, or even a finger?

Nurses are responsible for the postoperative care of the resident. At some point the resident probably will be fitted with a prosthesis. The stump must be conditioned for the prosthesis to fit properly. Stump conditioning involves shrinking and shaping the stump into a cone shape. Bandaging is used to shrink and shape the stump (Fig. 23-18). Exercises are ordered to strengthen the stump and the other limbs. Physical therapy is ordered to help the resident learn how to use the prosthesis (Fig. 23-19, p. 496). Occupational therapy is necessary if the person has to learn to perform ADL with the stump or prosthesis.

The resident may feel that the limb is still there or complain of pain in the amputated part. This is called

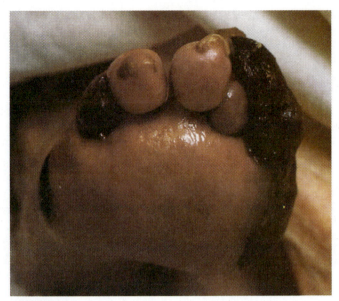

FIGURE 23-17 *Gangrene.*

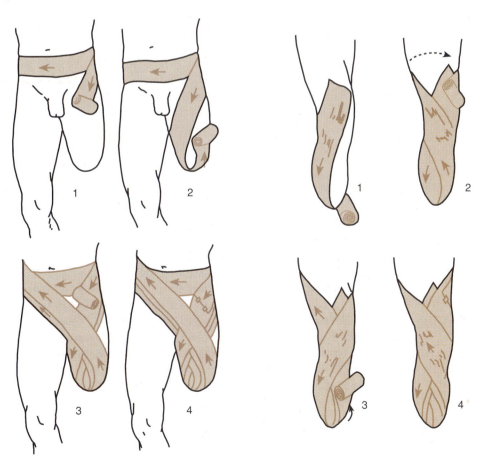

FIGURE 23-18 *An above-the-knee amputation is bandaged to shrink and shape the stump. (From Long, BC, et al:* Medical-surgical nursing: a nursing process approach, *ed 3, St. Louis, 1993, Mosby-Year Book.)*

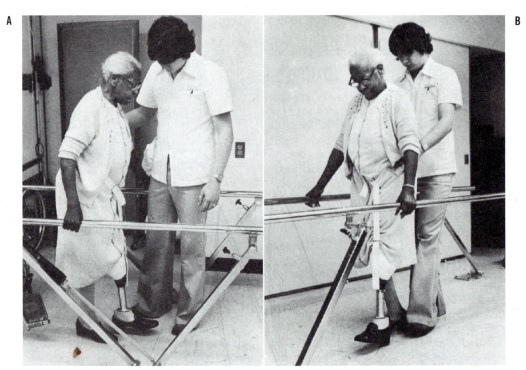

FIGURE 23-19 *A resident learns to use a leg prosthesis in physical therapy. (From Long, BC, et al:* Medical-surgical nursing: a nursing process approach, *ed 3, St. Louis, 1993, Mosby-Year Book.)*

phantom limb pain. The exact cause is unknown. However, it is a normal reaction. The sensation may be present only for a short time after surgery. Some persons, however, have phantom limb pain for several years.

NERVOUS SYSTEM DISORDERS

Nervous system disorders can affect mental and physical functioning. The ability to speak, understand, feel, see, hear, touch, think, control bowels and bladder, or move may be affected. There are many causes and types of nervous system disorders. The more common ones are described here.

Cerebrovascular Accident

A cerebrovascular accident (CVA) is commonly called a **stroke.** Blood supply to a part of the brain is suddenly interrupted. Brain damage occurs. The interruption can be due to the rupture of a blood vessel, which causes hemorrhage (excessive bleeding) into the brain. Or a blood clot can obstruct blood flow to a portion of the brain.

Stroke is more common among elderly persons. However, people in their 20s and 30s have had strokes. A common cause of stroke is hypertension (elevated blood pressure). Other risk factors include diabetes mellitus, obesity, birth control pills, a family history of stroke, hardening of the arteries, smoking, and stress.

Signs and symptoms vary. Sometimes there is a warning. The victim may be dizzy, have ringing in the ears, headache, weakness of one side of the body, nausea and vomiting, and memory loss. These symptoms also may indicate a *transient ischemic attack (TIA).* Transient means brief or temporary. A TIA may last a few minutes. Ischemic means a lack of blood supply to an organ or body part. Therefore a TIA is a temporary interruption of blood supply to a part of the brain. The person has the signs and symptoms of a stroke but recovers within hours. TIAs mean that the person is at risk for a stroke.

A stroke may occur suddenly. Unconsciousness, noisy breathing, elevated blood pressure, slow pulse, redness of the face, seizures, and paralysis on one side of the body (hemiplegia) may occur. The person may lose bowel and bladder control and the ability to speak. **Aphasia** is the inability *(a)* to speak *(phasia).*

Emergency care of the stroke victim is described in Chapter 26. If the person survives, some brain damage is likely. The functions lost depend on the area of brain damage (Fig. 23-20). Rehabilitation begins immediately. The person may be partially or totally dependent on others for care. Care of the resident is as follows:

1. The resident is positioned in the lateral position to prevent aspiration.

2. Coughing and deep breathing are encouraged.
3. The bed is kept in semi-Fowler's position.
4. Side rails are kept up except when giving care.
5. Turning and repositioning are done every 2 hours.
6. Elastic stockings usually are ordered to prevent blood clots in the legs.
7. Range-of-motion exercises are performed to prevent contractures.
8. A catheter or a bladder training program may be needed.
9. A bowel training program may be necessary.
10. Safety precautions are practiced.
11. Assistance is given in self-care activities. The person is encouraged to do as much as possible.
12. Methods are established for communicating with the resident. Magic slates, pencil and paper, a picture board, or other methods may be used.
13. Good skin care is given to prevent pressure sores.
14. Speech therapy, physical therapy, and occupational therapy may be ordered.
15. The comprehensive care plan is followed. Know what measures you are expected to carry out.
16. Emotional support and encouragement are given. Praise is given for the slightest accomplishment.

The resident with aphasia. Speech is controlled by the left side of the brain. Persons with right-sided hemiplegia also may have aphasia. There are two basic types of aphasia. *Expressive aphasia* relates to difficulty expressing or sending out thoughts. There are problems with speaking, spelling, counting, gesturing, or writing. The person may think one thing but say another. For example, the person thinks about food but asks for a newspaper. People are called the wrong names even when correct names are known. Or the person is able to think clearly but cannot speak. Some only produce sounds rather than words. The person may cry or swear for no apparent reason.

Receptive aphasia relates to receiving information. The person has trouble understanding what is being said or read. Everyday objects are not recognized. The person may have no idea what to do with a fork, toilet, water glass, television, telephone, or other items. The person may not recognize people. Remember, for communication to occur, the message sent must be received and correctly interpreted. The person with receptive aphasia simply cannot interpret the message received. The person with expressive aphasia cannot send messages.

Some people have both expressive and receptive aphasia. This is called *expressive-receptive aphasia.*

Persons with aphasia have many emotional needs. Frustration, depression, and anger are common. Communication is important for independent functioning and for relationships with others. Remember, the resident wants to communicate but cannot. You need to be patient and kind.

Parkinson's Disease

Parkinson's disease is a slow, progressive disorder. Degeneration of a part of the brain occurs. There is no cure. The disease usually occurs in elderly persons. Signs and symptoms are a masklike facial expression; tremors; pill-rolling movements of the fingers; a shuffling gait; stooped posture; stiff muscles; slow movements; slurred speech or monotone speech; and drooling. Mental function usually is not affected early in the disease process. As the disease progresses, confusion and forgetfulness may develop.

Drugs specific for Parkinson's disease are ordered by the doctor. Physical therapy also may be ordered. The resident may need help with eating and other self-care activities. Measures to promote normal bowel elimination are practiced. There is risk of constipation because of decreased activity and poor nutrition. Safety practices are carried out to protect the person from injury. Mental function may not be affected. Remember to treat and talk to the person as an adult.

Multiple Sclerosis

Multiple sclerosis (MS) is a progressive disease. The myelin sheath (which covers the nerves), the spinal cord, and the white matter in the brain are destroyed. As a result, nerve impulses cannot be sent to and from the brain in a normal manner.

Symptoms begin in young adulthood. The onset is gradual. There is blurred or double vision. Difficulty with balance and walking occur. Tremors, numbness and tingling, weakness, dizziness, urinary incontinence, bowel incontinence or constipation, behavior changes, and incoordination eventually occur. Signs and symptoms progressively worsen over several years. Blind-

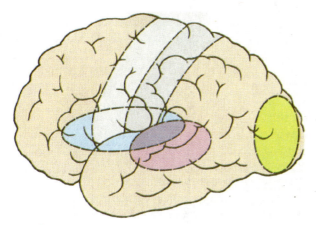

FIGURE 23-20 *Functions lost from a stroke depend on the area of brain damage.*

ness, contractures, paralysis of all extremities (quadriplegia), loss of bowel and bladder control, and respiratory muscle weakness are among the person's many problems. The person eventually is totally dependent on others for care.

There is no known cure. Residents are kept active as long as possible. They are allowed and encouraged to do as much for themselves as possible. Nursing care depends on the person's needs and condition. Skin care, personal hygiene, and range-of-motion exercises are important. Residents are protected from injury. Measures are taken to promote bowel and bladder elimination. Turning, positioning, coughing, and deep breathing also are important. Measures are planned to prevent the complications of bed rest. Complete bed rest is avoided whenever possible.

Head Injuries

The scalp, skull, and brain tissue can be injured. Sometimes injuries are minor. They may cause only a temporary loss of consciousness. Other injuries are more serious. Permanent brain damage or death may result. Brain tissue can be bruised or torn. Skull fractures can cause brain damage. Hemorrhage from head injuries can occur in the brain or surrounding structures.

Head injuries can be caused by falls, vehicle accidents, industrial accidents, and sports injuries. Other body parts may be injured also. Spinal cord injuries are likely. Birth injuries are another major cause of head trauma. Persons with head injuries are treated in emergency rooms and intensive care units. If a person survives a severe head injury, some permanent damage is likely. Paralysis, mental retardation, personality change, speech problems, breathing difficulties, and loss of bowel and bladder control may be permanent. Rehabilitation is required. Individuals may be admitted to nursing facilities for rehabilitation or for permanent placement. Nursing care depends on the resident's needs and remaining abilities. The comprehensive care plan outlines the resident's care.

Spinal Cord Injuries

Spinal cord injuries can cause permanent damage to the nervous system. These injuries usually occur from stab or bullet wounds, vehicle accidents, industrial accidents, falls, or sports injuries. Emergency and intensive care unit treatment is necessary. Transfer to a rehabilitation center or to a nursing facility for rehabilitation may be necessary. Some persons may require permanent placement.

The type of damage depends on the level of the injury. The higher the level of injury, the greater the loss of function (Fig. 23-21). If the injury is in the lumbar area, muscle function in the legs is lost. Injuries at the thoracic

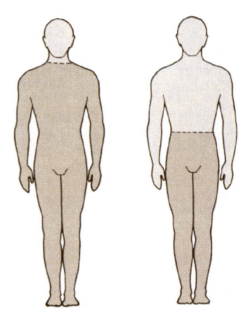

FIGURE 23-21 *The* shaded areas *indicate the areas of paralysis.*

level cause loss of muscle function below the chest. Those with injuries at the lumbar or thoracic levels are paraplegics. *Paraplegia* is paralysis of the legs. Cervical injuries may result in loss of function to the arms, chest, and all muscles below the chest. Persons with these injuries are quadriplegics. *Quadriplegia* is paralysis of the arms, legs, and trunk.

If the person survives, rehabilitation is necessary. The person's needs and the rehabilitation program depend on the functions lost and remaining abilities. The care plan outlines specific care measures. Emotional needs cannot be overlooked. These residents have severe emotional reactions to paralysis and loss of function. Paralyzed residents generally need the following care:

1. Protect the resident from injury. Falls and burns are major risks. Keep side rails up, the bed in low position, and the call light within reach. Bath water, heat applications, and food must be at the proper temperature.
2. Turn and reposition the person every 2 hours.
3. Give skin care and other measures to prevent pressure sores.
4. Maintain good alignment at all times. Pillows, trochanter rolls, footboards, and other devices are used as needed.
5. Carry out bowel and bladder training programs.
6. Perform range-of-motion exercises to maintain muscle function and prevent contractures. Other exercises may be ordered.
7. Assist with food and fluids as needed. The resident may have to be fed. Self-help devices may be needed.

8. Give emotional and psychological support. Psychiatrists or psychologists may be involved in the resident's care.

9. Physical therapy and occupational therapy may be ordered. They help the resident regain independent functioning to the extent possible.

Hearing Problems

Hearing losses range from slight impairment to complete deafness. Hearing is required for many functions. Learning to talk, speech, responding to others, safety, and awareness of surroundings all require hearing. Many people deny having difficulty hearing. This is because hearing loss usually is associated with aging.

Effects on the resident. A person may be unaware of gradual difficulty in hearing. Others may see changes in the person's behavior or attitude. They may not know that the changes are due to hearing problems. Symptoms and effects of hearing loss vary. They are not always obvious to the person or to others.

There are some obvious signs of hearing impairment. These include speaking too loudly, leaning forward to hear, and turning and cupping the better ear toward the speaker. The person may answer questions or respond inappropriately or often may ask for words to be repeated.

Psychological and social effects are less obvious. Persons with hearing problems are aware of their inappropriate responses in conversation or to questions. Therefore they tend to avoid social situations to avoid embarrassment. However, loneliness, boredom, and feelings of being left out often result. Only parts of conversations may be heard. Persons with hearing loss may become suspicious. They may think they are being talked about or think that others are talking softly on purpose. Elderly persons fear being labeled "senile" because of inappropriate responses. Some people try to control conversations so they do not have to respond or answer questions. Straining and working hard to hear can cause fatigue, frustration, and irritability.

Persons with hearing loss may develop speech problems. You hear yourself as you talk. How you pronounce words and your voice volume depend on how you hear yourself. Hearing loss may result in slurred speech and improper word pronunciation. Monotone speech and dropping word endings also may occur.

Communicating with the resident. Hearing-impaired persons may wear hearing aids or read lips. They also watch facial expressions, gestures, and body language to understand what is being said. Sign language may be necessary for the totally deaf. Some hearing-impaired persons have "hearing" dogs. The dogs alert the person to such things as ringing phones, door bells, sirens, or oncoming cars. Certain measures are used when communicating with the person. The following measures can help the person to hear or lip read:

1. Gain attention and alert the person to your presence in the room by lightly touching his or her arm. Do not startle or approach the person from behind.
2. Face the person directly when speaking. Do not turn or walk away from the person while you are talking.
3. Stand or sit in good light. Shadows and glares interfere with the person's ability to see your face clearly.
4. Speak clearly, distinctly, and slowly.
5. Speak in a normal tone of voice. Do not shout.
6. Do not cover your mouth, smoke, eat, or chew gum while talking. These actions affect mouth movements.
7. Stand or sit on the side of the better ear.
8. State the topic of conversation first.
9. Use short sentences and simple words.
10. Write out important names and words.
11. Keep conversation and discussions short to avoid tiring the person.
12. Repeat and rephrase statements as needed.
13. Be alert to the messages being sent by your facial expressions, gestures, and body language.
14. Reduce or eliminate background noises.

The person with a hearing impairment also may have speech problems. Understanding what the person is trying to say can be difficult. Do not assume that you understand what is being said. Do not pretend to understand to avoid embarrassing the person. Serious consequences can result if you assume or pretend to understand. The following guidelines will help you communicate with the speech-impaired person:

1. Listen and give the person your full attention.
2. Ask the person questions to which you know the answer. This helps you to become familiar with the person's speech.
3. Determine the subject being discussed. This helps you understand essential points.
4. Ask the person to repeat or rephrase statements if necessary.
5. Repeat what the person has said. Ask if you have understood correctly.
6. Ask the person to write down key words or the message.
7. Watch the person's lip movements.
8. Watch facial expressions, gestures, and body language for clues about what is being said.

Hearing aids. A *hearing aid* amplifies sound (Fig. 23-22, p. 500). It does not correct or cure the hearing problem. The person may hear better with a hearing aid. This is because the hearing aid makes sounds louder. Both background noise and speech are amplified. Noises must be minimized to help the person adjust to the hearing aid. Some hearing aids have a switch that dampens

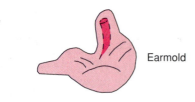

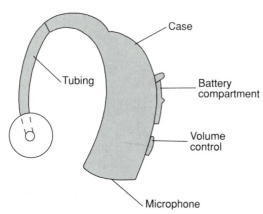

FIGURE 23-22 *Parts of a hearing aid. (From Long, BC, et al: Medical-surgical nursing: a nursing process approach, ed 3, St. Louis, 1993, Mosby-Year Book.)*

background noise. Remember, the hearing aid does not make speech clearer, only louder. Measures for communicating with the hearing-impaired person apply to those with hearing aids.

Hearing aids operate on batteries. There is an *on* and *off* switch. Some hearing aids have a setting for use with the telephone. Others also may have settings for decreasing background noise. Sometimes hearing aids do not seem to work properly. Several things must be checked. See if the instrument is on. Also check if the switch is in the proper setting. Check battery position. New batteries may be needed. The earpiece may need cleaning. The hearing aid may need repair.

Hearing aids are expensive. They must be handled carefully and cared for properly. Only removable earpieces can be washed. Make sure the opening in the earpiece is free of wax. Check with the nurse before cleaning a hearing aid. Remove the battery at night. This prolongs the life of the battery.

Vision Problems

Vision problems occur at all ages. Problems range from very mild vision loss to complete blindness. They may develop suddenly or gradually. One or both eyes may be affected. Surgery, eyeglasses, or contact lenses often are necessary.

Glaucoma. Glaucoma is an eye disease. Pressure within the eye is increased, which damages the retina and optic nerve. The result is visual loss with eventual blindness. The disease may be gradual or sudden in onset. Signs and symptoms include tunnel vision (Fig. 23-23), blurred vision, and blue-green halos around lights. With sudden onset there also is severe eye pain, nausea, and vomiting. Glaucoma is a major cause of blindness. Persons older than 40 years of age are at risk. The cause is unknown.

Treatment involves drug therapy and possibly surgery. The goal is to prevent further damage to the retina and optic nerve. Damage that has already occurred cannot be reversed.

Cataract. Cataract is an eye disorder in which the lens becomes cloudy (opaque). The cloudiness prevents light from entering the eye (Fig. 23-24). Gradual blurring and dimming of vision occurs. Sight eventually is lost. A cataract can occur in one or both eyes. Aging is the most common cause of cataracts. Surgery is the only treatment.

The resident may have to wear an eye shield or patch for several days after surgery. This protects the eye from injury. One or both eyes may be covered. Measures for the blind person are practiced when an eye shield is worn. Even if one shield is worn, there may be visual loss in the other eye from cataract formation or other causes.

A permanent lens implant usually is done during surgery (Fig. 23-25). The lens restores vision to near normal. The implant is held in place with a suture that is as fine as a human hair. The eye most be protected during healing. The following rules are important in caring for a resident with a new lens implant:

1. Keep the eye shield in place as directed. Some doctors allow the shield to be left off during the day if the person wears eyeglasses. The shield is worn for sleep, including napping.
2. Remind the person not to bend from the waist. Bending increases the pressure in the eye and can cause the suture to break.
3. Do not shampoo or shower the resident without a doctor's order.
4. Remind the resident not to pick up items weighing more than 5 pounds. Lifting increases eye pressure.
5. Take care not to bump the eye.
6. Report the following to the nurse immediately:
   a. Increasing pain after the first 24 hours following surgery
   b. Drainage from the eye
7. Remind the resident to sleep on the unaffected side. This prevents pressure on the eye.

Text continued on p. 502.

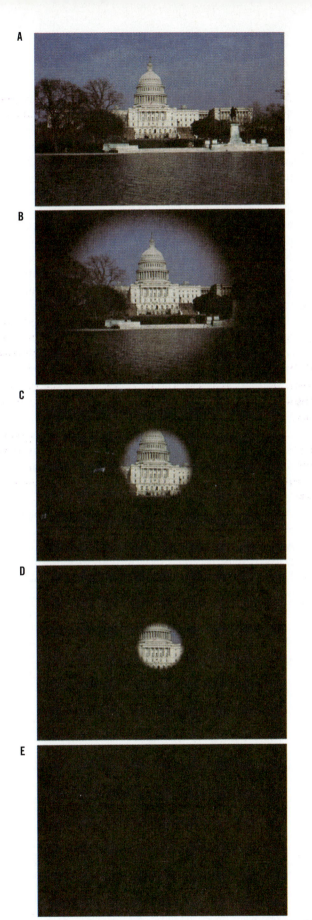

FIGURE 23-23 *A,* Normal vision. *B,* Tunnel vision. *C, D, E,* Visual loss continues with eventual blindness.

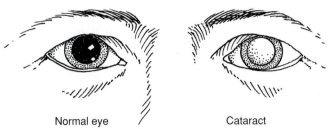

Normal eye   Cataract

FIGURE 23-24 *There is a cataract in the left eye.. (From Long, BC, et al: Medical-surgical nursing: a nursing process approach, ed 3, St. Louis, 1993, Mosby-Year Book.)*

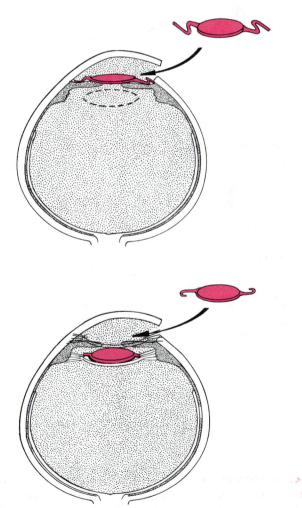

FIGURE 23-25 *Lens implant during cataract surgery. (From Long, BC, et al: Medical-surgical nursing: a nursing process approach, ed 3, St. Louis, 1993, Mosby-Year Book.)*

8. Remind the person not to rub the eye.
9. Report signs of constipation to the nurse. The resident should not strain to have a bowel movement.
10. Report coughing to the nurse. Forceful coughing can increase eye pressure.

Some residents are fitted with corrective lenses after surgery. Even with corrective lenses or implants, there will be some degree of impaired vision.

Corrective lenses. Eyeglasses and contact lenses are prescribed to correct vision problems. Eyeglasses may be worn only for certain activities, such as reading or seeing at a distance. Or they may be worn whenever the person is awake. Contact lenses are usually always worn while the person is awake.

Eyeglasses. People often are upset when told that glasses are necessary. However, adjustment usually is rapid. Most persons know that glasses will be needed sooner or later. Appearance often is a concern. Glasses come in many styles and shapes. Frames can be chosen that fit face shape, personality, and life-style.

Lenses are made of hardened glass or plastic. They are impact-resistant to prevent shattering. Glass lenses are washed with warm water and dried with soft tissue. Plastic lenses scratch easily. A special cleaning solution and special tissues and cloths are needed for cleaning and drying. Some of newer plastic lenses have a special hardened surface. They can be washed with soap and water. Check with the resident or the nurse for the proper cleaning method.

Glasses are costly. They must be protected from loss or damage. When not being worn, glasses are put in their case. The case is put in the drawer of the bedside stand. It is wise to label glasses with the resident's name.

Contact lenses. Contact lenses fit directly on the eye. Hard and soft contacts are available. Many people prefer contacts because they cannot be seen. Contacts do not break easily. However, they are more expensive than eyeglasses and are easily lost. Contacts are removed for activities such as swimming, showering, and sleeping.

People with contact lenses are taught to insert, remove, and clean them. If they are able, residents can perform these activities themselves. The eye can easily be damaged during insertion or removal of contact lenses. The nurse assists the resident who cannot insert or remove the lenses. Therefore you should not perform these measures.

Some elderly residents may have had cataract surgery. They may have extended-wear contact lenses. These lenses are in place 24 hours a day for weeks. They are removed and cleansed by the eye doctor or the nurse. Report any redness or drainage from the eyes to the nurse right away. Also report resident complaints of eye pain or blurred vision.

Special needs of the blind resident. Blindness has many causes—for example, birth defects, accidents, and eye disease. Blindness also can be a complication of diseases that affect other organs and body systems. Blindness usually occurs later in life. A blind person's life is seriously affected by the loss of sight. Physical and psychological adjustments can be long and hard. Special education and training are required. Moving about, activities of daily living, reading braille, and using a Seeing Eye dog require training. Some very elderly residents with recent loss of sight never master these special skills.

Braille is a method of writing for the blind that uses raised dots. Dots are arranged to represent each letter of the alphabet. The first 10 letters also represent the numbers 0 through 9 (Fig. 23-26). The person feels the arrangement of the dots with the fingers (Fig. 23-27). Many books, magazines, and newspapers are available in braille. There are also braille typewriters.

Braille is hard to learn, especially for many elderly persons. Entire books and articles are available on audio tapes. These are often called "talking books." They can be bought or borrowed from libraries. The activities director or family can obtain these "books" for residents.

The blind person can be taught to move about with a white cane or a Seeing Eye or guide dog. Both are recognized worldwide as signs that the person is blind. The dog serves as the eyes of the blind person. The dog recognizes danger and guides the person through traffic.

You must treat the blind person with respect and dignity—not with pity. Most blind people have adjusted to their blindness. They lead rather independent lives. Some have been blind for a long time, others for only a short time. Certain practices are necessary in dealing with blind persons. These following practices are necessary no matter how long the person has been blind:

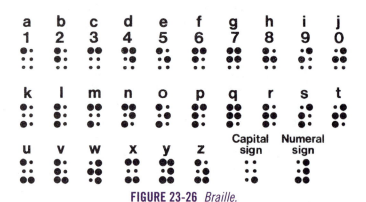

FIGURE 23-26 *Braille.*

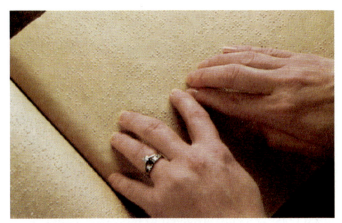

FIGURE 23-27 *Braille is "read" with the fingertips.*

1. Identify yourself promptly when you enter the room. Give your name, title, and reason for being there. Do not touch the person until you have indicated your presence in the room.
2. Orient the person to the room. Identify the location and purpose of furniture and equipment.
3. Let the person move about and touch and locate furniture and equipment if able.
4. Do not rearrange furniture and equipment.
5. Give step-by-step explanations of procedures as you perform them. Indicate when the procedure is over.
6. Tell the person when you are leaving the room.
7. Keep doors open or shut, never partially open.
8. Assist the person in walking by staying slightly ahead of him or her (Fig. 23-28). The person should touch your arm lightly. If the resident is weak or ill, provide the support needed. Never push or guide the blind person in front of you.
9. Inform the person of steps, doors, turns, furniture, curbs, and other obstructions when you are assisting with ambulation.
10. Assist in food selection by reading the menu to the person.
11. Explain the location of food and beverages on the tray. Use the face of a clock (see Chapter 15, p. 349), or guide the person's hand to the items on the tray.
12. Ask the person if assistance is needed in cutting meat, opening containers, buttering bread, and other similar activities. Assist only if needed.
13. Keep the signal light within reach.
14. Provide a radio, "talking books," television, and braille books for the person's entertainment.
15. Do not shout or speak in a loud voice. Just because a person is blind does not mean that hearing is impaired.
16. Let the person, if able, perform self-care activities.

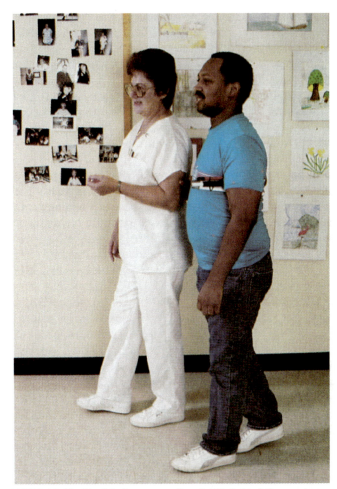

FIGURE 23-28 *The blind person walks slightly behind the nursing assistant and lightly touches the assistant's arm.*

RESPIRATORY DISORDERS

Residents with respiratory disorders are commonly seen in nursing facilities. The respiratory system brings oxygen into the lungs and removes carbon dioxide from the body. Respiratory disorders interfere with this function and threaten life.

Chronic Obstructive Pulmonary Disease

Four disorders are grouped under chronic obstructive pulmonary disease (COPD). They are chronic bronchitis, asthma, bronchiectasis, and emphysema. These disorders interfere with the normal exchange of oxygen and carbon dioxide in the lungs. They obstruct airflow.

Chronic bronchitis. Chronic bronchitis occurs after repeated episodes of bronchitis (inflammation of the bronchi). Common causes are cigarette smoking and air pollution. "Smoker's cough" in the morning usually is the first symptom. At first the cough is dry. Eventually the resident coughs up mucus that may contain pus and blood. The cough becomes more frequent as the disease progresses. The person also may have difficulty breathing and may tire easily. The mucus and inflammation of breathing passages "obstruct" airflow into the lungs. Therefore the body cannot get normal amounts of oxygen.

Asthma. Air passages narrow with asthma. Difficulty breathing results. Allergies and emotional stress are common causes. Episodes occur suddenly and are called *asthma attacks*. In addition to dyspnea, there is shortness of breath, wheezing, coughing, rapid pulse, perspiration, and cyanosis. The person usually is very frightened during the attack. Fear usually causes the attack to become worse.

Drugs are used to treat asthma. Emergency room treatment may be necessary for severe attacks. The person and family are taught how to prevent asthma attacks. Repeated attacks can damage the respiratory system.

Bronchiectasis. Bronchiectasis is a disorder in which the bronchi dilate (enlarge). Pus collects in the dilated bronchi. There are many causes, including respiratory infections and aspiration. The person has a chronic, productive cough. Large amounts of sputum are coughed up. The sputum contains pus and usually has a foul smell. The amount increases as the disease progresses. Eventually blood may be present in sputum. Weight loss, fatigue, and loss of appetite can occur. The doctor may order drugs, respiratory therapy, rest, and measures to improve nutrition. The person must be protected from others with respiratory infections. Smoking is not allowed. Removal of the diseased part of the lung may be necessary.

Emphysema. Emphysema is a disorder in which the alveoli become enlarged. Walls of the alveoli become less elastic. They do not expand and shrink normally with inspiration and expiration. As a result, some air remains trapped in the alveoli during expiration. The trapped air is not exhaled. As the disease progresses, more alveoli become involved. The normal exchange of oxygen and carbon dioxide cannot occur in the affected alveoli.

Smoking is the most common cause of emphysema. Signs and symptoms include shortness of breath and "smoker's cough." At first the shortness of breath occurs with exertion. You need to allow extra time for the resident to complete ADLs and other activities. Five minute rest periods between activities are helpful. For example, the person rests 5 minutes between dressing and putting on socks and shoes. As the disease progresses, shortness of breath may occur at rest. Sputum may contain pus. As more air is trapped in the lungs, the person develops a

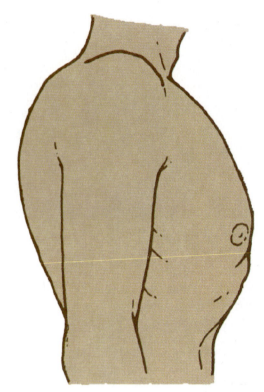

FIGURE 23-29 *Barrel chest resulting from emphysema.*

"barrel chest" (Fig. 23-29). Residents usually prefer to sit upright and slightly forward. Breathing is easier in this position. The nurse may ask you to assist the person in assuming such a position. To do so, place the overbed table at chest height in front of the resident. Then place a pillow on the table. Have the resident lean forward slightly and rest the arms and head on the pillow.

The person must stop smoking. Respiratory therapy, breathing exercises, oxygen, and drug therapy are ordered.

Pneumonia

Pneumonia is an inflammation of lung tissue. Alveoli in the affected area fill with fluid. Therefore oxygen and carbon dioxide cannot be exchanged normally.

Pneumonia is caused by bacteria, viruses, aspiration, or immobility. The person is very ill. Pneumonia is very serious in the elderly, the chronically ill, or the quadriplegic resident. It can be fatal. Signs and symptoms include fever, chills, painful cough, pain on breathing, and rapid pulse. Cyanosis may be present. Sputum color depends on the cause. It may be clear, green, yellowish, or rust colored.

Drugs are ordered for infection and pain relief. "Force fluids" often is ordered because of fever. Fluids also help thin mucous secretions. Thin secretions are easier to cough up. Oxygen may be necessary. A semi-Fowler's position usually is preferred for breathing. Mouth care is important. Frequent linen changes may be necessary because of fever. Transfer to a hospital may be required.

CARDIOVASCULAR DISORDERS

Cardiovascular disorders are leading causes of death in the United States. Problems may occur in the heart or in the blood vessels.

Hypertension

Hypertension is a condition in which the blood pressure is abnormally high. Narrowed blood vessels are a common cause. When vessels narrow, the heart has to pump with more force to move blood through them. Other disorders can cause high blood pressure. They include kidney disorders, head injuries, certain complications of pregnancy, and tumors of the adrenal gland.

Hypertension can damage other body organs. The heart may enlarge so that it can pump with more force. Blood vessels in the brain may burst and cause a stroke. Blood vessels in the eyes and kidneys may be damaged.

At first, hypertension may not cause signs or symptoms. Usually it is discovered when the blood pressure is measured. Signs and symptoms develop as the disorder progresses. Headache, blurred vision, and dizziness may be reported. Complications of hypertension include stroke, heart attack, kidney failure, and blindness.

Medications to lower blood pressure may be ordered. The person will be advised to quit smoking, exercise regularly if able, and get enough rest. A sodium-restricted diet may be ordered. If the person is overweight, a low-calorie diet is ordered.

Coronary Artery Disease

Coronary artery disease (CAD) is a disorder in which the coronary arteries become narrowed. One or all of the arteries may be affected. Because of narrowed vessels, blood supply to the heart muscle is reduced. Atherosclerosis is the most common cause of narrowed coronary arteries. In atherosclerosis, fatty material collects on the arterial walls (Fig. 23-30). This causes arteries to narrow and obstruct blood flow. Blood flow through an artery may be completely blocked. Permanent heart damage occurs in the part of the heart receiving its blood supply from that artery.

Risk factors for CAD have been identified. They include obesity, cigarette smoking, lack of exercise, a diet high in fat and cholesterol, and hypertension. Age and sex (male or female) are other risk factors. CAD is more likely to occur in older persons and in men. The type A personality also is a risk factor. The person with a type A personality is aggressive, competitive, and works very

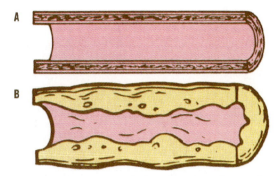

FIGURE 23-30 *A, Normal artery. B, Fatty deposits collect on the walls of the arteries in atherosclerosis.*

hard. The person has difficulty relaxing, has a sense of urgency, and does things at a rapid pace.

There are two major complications of coronary artery disease. They are angina pectoris and myocardial infarction (heart attack).

Angina pectoris. Angina *(pain)* pectoris *(chest)* means chest pain. The chest pain is due to reduced blood flow to part of the heart muscle (myocardium). Angina pectoris occurs when the heart needs more oxygen. Normally, blood flow to the heart increases when the heart's need for oxygen increases. Physical exertion, a heavy meal, emotional stress, and excitement increase the heart's need for oxygen. In CAD, the narrowed vessels prevent increased blood flow.

Signs and symptoms include chest pain. The pain may be described as a tightness, heaviness, or discomfort in the left side of the chest or across the chest. The pain may radiate to the left jaw and down the inner aspect of the left arm (Fig. 23-31, p. 506). Some have pain in both arms or elbows. The person may be pale, feel faint, and perspire. Dyspnea may be present. These signs and symptoms cause the person to stop activity and rest. Rest often relieves the symptoms in 3 to 15 minutes. Rest reduces the heart's need for oxygen. Therefore normal blood flow is achieved and heart damage is prevented.

In addition to rest, angina pectoris is treated with a medication called *nitroglycerin.* A nitroglycerin tablet is taken when an angina attack occurs. The tablet is put under the tongue. It dissolves under the tongue and is rapidly absorbed into the bloodstream. Some residents are allowed to keep the nitroglycerin with them. The resident takes a tablet when one is needed and then tells the nurse. The person does not have to wait for a nurse to answer the call light and then go get the tablet. The resident should have nitroglycerin tablets available at all times. This includes the times when the resident goes to physical therapy, occupational therapy, the dining room, the lounge, or other parts of the facility. The resident also should carry it on outings.

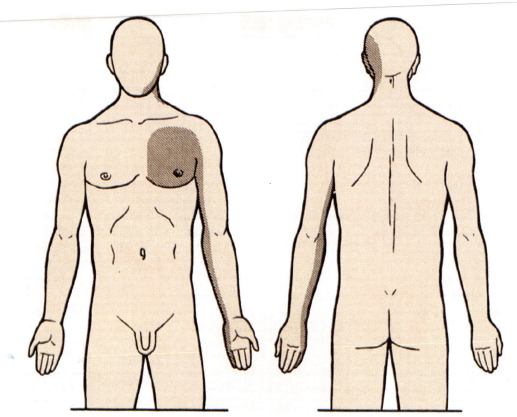

FIGURE 23-31 *The shaded area indicates where the pain of angina pectoris is located.*

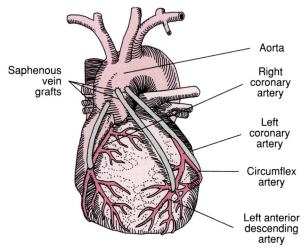

FIGURE 23-32 *Coronary artery bypass surgery. The diseased part of the artery is bypassed with a vein graft.*

Residents are taught to avoid situations likely to cause angina pectoris. These include overexertion, heavy meals and overeating, and emotional situations. Residents are advised to stay indoors during cold weather or during hot, humid weather. Some people have coronary artery bypass surgery. The surgery bypasses the diseased part of the artery (Fig. 23-32) and increases blood flow to the heart.

Many people with angina pectoris eventually have heart attacks. Chest pain that is not relieved by rest and nitroglycerin may have a more serious cause.

Myocardial infarction. A myocardial infarction (MI) is due to lack of blood supply to the heart muscle (myocardium). Tissue death occurs (infarction). Common terms for MI are *heart attack, coronary thrombosis,* and *coronary occlusion.* Blood flow to the myocardium is suddenly interrupted. Usually a thrombus obstructs the blood flow through an artery. The area of damage may be small or large. Cardiac arrest can occur (see Chapter 26).

Signs and symptoms include sudden, severe chest pain. The pain often is on the left side. It may be described as crushing, stabbing, or squeezing. Some have described the pain in terms of someone sitting on their

506

chest. Pain may radiate to the neck, jaw, and down the arms. The pain is more severe and lasts longer than angina pectoris. It is not relieved by rest and nitroglycerin. Other signs and symptoms include indigestion, dyspnea, nausea, dizziness, perspiration, pallor, cyanosis, cold and clammy skin, low blood pressure, and a weak and irregular pulse. The person is very fearful and apprehensive. Some have described a feeling of doom. All or some of these signs and symptoms may be present.

Myocardial infarction is an emergency. Hospital care is required. Efforts are directed at relieving the pain, stabilizing vital signs, giving oxygen, and calming the person. Many medications are given. Measures are taken to prevent life-threatening complications.

Congestive Heart Failure

Congestive heart failure (CHF) occurs when the heart cannot pump blood normally. Blood backs up and causes congestion of tissues. Left-sided heart failure or right-sided heart failure, or both, can occur.

When the left side of the heart fails to pump efficiently, blood backs up into the lungs. Signs and symptoms of respiratory congestion occur. These include dyspnea, increased sputum production, cough, and gurgling sounds in the lungs. In addition, blood is not pumped out of the heart to the rest of the body in adequate amounts. Organs do not receive enough blood. Signs and symptoms occur from the body's organs. For example, inadequate blood flow to the brain causes confusion, dizziness, and fainting. Inadequate blood flow to the kidneys causes reduced kidney function and decreased urinary output. The skin becomes pale or cyanotic. Blood pressure falls. A very severe form of left-sided failure is pulmonary edema (fluid in the lungs). Pulmonary edema is an emergency. Death can occur.

The right side of the heart may fail. Blood backs up into the venae cavae and into the venous system. The feet and ankles swell. Neck veins bulge. Congestion occurs in the liver, and liver function decreases. The abdomen may become congested with fluid. The right side of the heart cannot pump blood to the lungs efficiently. Therefore normal blood flow does not occur from the lungs to the left side of the heart. Less blood than normal is pumped from the left side of the heart to the rest of the body. Like left-sided failure, the body's organs have a reduced blood supply. Signs and symptoms described in the previous paragraph eventually occur.

Congestive heart failure usually is caused by a weakened heart. Myocardial infarction and hypertension are common causes. Damaged heart valves also can cause CHF. If a resident becomes acutely ill, he or she is transferred to a hospital for treatment.

Congestive heart failure can be treated and controlled. Drugs are given to strengthen the heart and to reduce the amount of fluid in the body. A sodium-restricted diet is ordered. Supplemental oxygen is given. Most residents prefer the semi-Fowler's or Fowler's position for breathing. Many elderly residents have CHF. You may be involved in the following aspects of the resident's care:

1. Maintaining prescribed activity limits
2. Measuring intake and output
3. Measuring weight daily
4. Restricting fluids as ordered by the doctor
5. Giving good skin care to prevent skin breakdown
6. Performing range-of-motion exercises
7. Assisting with transfers or ambulation
8. Assisting with self-care activities
9. Maintaining good body alignment
10. Applying elastic stockings, if ordered

THE ENDOCRINE SYSTEM

The most common endocrine disorder is diabetes mellitus. In this disorder the body cannot use sugar properly. For proper use of sugar, there must be enough insulin. Insulin is secreted by the pancreas. In diabetes mellitus, the pancreas fails to secrete enough insulin. Sugar builds up in the blood. Cells do not have enough sugar for energy. Therefore cells cannot perform their specific functions.

Diabetes mellitus can occur in children and adults. Persons at risk are those with a family history of diabetes. Aging and obesity increase the risk.

Signs and symptoms include increased urine production, increased thirst, hunger, and weight loss. A blood test shows sugar levels above normal. If diabetes is not controlled, complications occur. These include changes in the retina that lead to blindness, kidney damage, nerve damage, and circulatory disorders. Circulatory disorders can lead to stroke, heart attack, and slow wound healing. Foot and leg wounds are especially serious. Infection and gangrene often occur and may require amputation of the part.

Diabetes mellitus is treated with exercise, diet, oral hypoglycemic agents, and insulin therapy. Oral hypoglycemic agents are tablets that increase the production of insulin in the pancreas. Meals must be served on time. The resident must eat all foods served. Good foot care is especially important.

A hypoglycemic reaction (insulin shock) may occur if a resident gets too much medication or too little food. Hypoglycemic means low *(hypo)* blood *(emia)* sugar *(glyc)*. Diabetic coma develops if the person does not have enough insulin. Table 23-1 on p. 508 summarizes the causes, signs, and symptoms of hypoglycemic reactions and diabetic coma. Both can lead to death if not corrected.

Table 23-1

Hypoglycemic Reaction and Diabetic Coma

	Hypoglycemic Reaction	Diabetic Coma
Causes	Too much medication	Undiagnosed diabetes
	Omitting a meal	Not enough medication
	Eating too little food	
	Increased exercise	Eating too much food
	Vomiting	Too little exercise
		Stress from illness, surgery, emotional upset, etc.
Signs and Symptoms	Hunger	Weakness
	Weakness	Drowsiness
	Trembling	Thirst
	Perspiration	Hunger
	Headache	Frequent urination
	Dizziness	Flushed face
	Rapid pulse	Sweet breath odor
	Low blood pressure	Slow, deep, labored respirations
	Confusion	Dry skin
	Cold, clammy skin	Rapid, weak pulse
	Convulsions	Low blood pressure
	Unconsciousness	Headache
		Nausea and vomiting
		Coma

COMMUNICABLE DISEASES

Communicable diseases (contagious or infectious diseases) can be transmitted from one person to another. They can be transmitted in the following ways:

- Direct—from the infected person
- Indirect—from dressings, linens, or surfaces
- Airborne—from a person through sneezing or coughing
- Vehicle—through ingestion of contaminated food, water, drugs, blood, or fluids
- Vector—from animals, fleas, and ticks

This section discusses hepatitis and AIDS. Table 23-2 outlines common adult communicable diseases. A review of Chapter 8 may be helpful in studying this section.

Hepatitis

Hepatitis is an inflammatory disease of the liver. There are different types of hepatitis.

Type A (infectious hepatitis) usually is spread by the fecal-oral route. Food, water, or drinking or eating utensils or containers can be contaminated with feces. The virus is ingested when the person eats or drinks contaminated food or water. It also can be ingested when a person eats or drinks from a vessel contaminated with the virus. Causes include poor sanitation, crowded living conditions, poor nutrition, and poor hygiene practices. The disease is more common in children. You must be careful when handling bedpans, feces, and rectal thermometers. Good handwashing is essential for you and the residents.

Table 23-2

Common Communicable Diseases Seen in Adults

Disease	Signs and Symptoms	Mode of Transmission	Infective Material
AIDS	Fever, night sweats, weight loss, cough	Sexual contact, blood, needles	Blood, semen
Gonorrhea	Urethral or vaginal discharge, fever, lower abdominal pain	Sexual contact	Genital-urinary secretions
Hepatitis A	Fever, loss of appetite, jaundice, fatigue	Direct contact, oral ingestion of virus	Urine, stool
Hepatitis B	Fever, fatigue, loss of appetite, nausea, headache	Blood, oral secretions, sexual contact	Blood, saliva, semen
Hepatitis C	Fever, headache, fatigue, jaundice	Blood	Blood
Syphilis	Genital and cutaneous lesions	Sexual contact, blood	Drainage from lesions, blood
Pneumonia	Fever, cough	Airborne	Sputum
Tuberculosis	Fever, night sweats, cough, weight loss	Airborne	Sputum

PROTECTIVE MEASURES: Universal precautions are practiced with all residents. The bloodborne pathogen standard is also followed. Respiratory isolation is practiced for active tuberculosis and some types of pneumonia.

Type B (serum hepatitis) usually is transmitted by blood and sexual contact. The type B virus is present in blood, saliva, semen, and urine of infected persons. The virus is spread by contaminated blood or blood products and by sharing needles and syringes among injection drug users. Hepatitis B can be prevented by vaccination. (See Chapter 8 for review of Occupational Safety and Health Administration [OSHA] standard for occupational exposure to bloodborne pathogens.)

Hepatitis can be mild or can cause death. Signs and symptoms of hepatitis include the following:

- Loss of appetite
- Weakness, fatigue, exhaustion
- Nausea and vomiting
- Fever
- Skin rash
- Dark urine
- Jaundice (yellowish skin color)
- Light-colored stools
- Headache
- Chills
- Abdominal pain

You must protect yourself and others from the hepatitis virus. Universal precautions and OSHA's bloodborne pathogen standard are necessary to prevent the spread of this disease.

Acquired Immunodeficiency Syndrome

Acquired immunodeficiency syndrome (AIDS) is caused by a virus. The virus is known as the human immunodeficiency virus (HIV). The virus attacks the body's immune system. It affects the person's ability to fight other diseases.

At this time there is neither a cure for AIDS nor a vaccine to prevent the disease. AIDS eventually causes death.

The following persons are at risk for AIDS:

- Homosexual or bisexual men with multiple sex partners
- Heterosexual men and women who engage in unsafe sex with multiple partners
- Users of intravenous and other injected drugs who share needles
- Persons who received blood or blood products before 1985
- Sex partners of infected persons
- Children born to infected mothers

AIDS is transmitted mainly by blood or sexual contact. According to the Centers for Disease Control and Prevention (CDC), the AIDS virus has been found in blood, semen, saliva, tears, breast milk, vaginal secretions, and urine. However, the virus is known to be transmitted by contact with infected blood, semen, vaginal secretions, or breast milk.

The virus enters the blood stream through the rectum, vagina, penis, or mouth. Small breaks in the mucous membrane of the vagina or rectum may occur when the penis, finger, or other objects are inserted. Gum disease can cause breaks in the mucous membrane of the gums. The breaks in the mucous membrane of the mouth, vagina, or rectum provide a route for the virus to enter the blood stream.

Drug users transmit the virus through the use of contaminated needles and syringes. The virus is carried in the contaminated blood left by the users in the needles or syringes. When needles and syringes are used by others, the contaminated blood enters their blood streams.

Infection also can occur when infected body fluids come in contact with open skin areas. Babies can become infected during pregnancy or shortly after birth.

Some persons show positive HIV test reactions. They carry the AIDS virus but have no signs or symptoms. They may not develop symptoms of the disease for many years. However, they can spread the virus. The signs and symptoms of AIDS include the following:

- Loss of appetite
- Weight loss
- Chills and fever
- Night sweats
- Difficulty breathing
- Headache
- Diarrhea
- Fatigue, extreme or constant
- Skin rashes
- Swollen glands in the neck, underarms, and groin
- Dry cough
- White blotches in the mouth or on the tongue
- Purple blotches or bumps on the skin that look like bruises, but do not go away (Kaposi's sarcoma)
- Confusion

Persons with AIDS develop other diseases. Their bodies do not have the ability to fight disease. The AIDS virus has damaged the immune system, which fights disease. Affected persons are at risk for pneumonia, tuberculosis, and other communicable diseases. They also are at risk for central nervous system damage. Those with central nervous system damage may have memory loss, loss of coordination, paralysis, and mental disorders.

You may care for residents with AIDS. These persons are so ill that they can no longer care for themselves. They usually require nursing care until death occurs. They need the same care and compassion as other dying residents.

OSHA's bloodborne pathogen standard and universal precautions are important for all residents. You may care for residents who are HIV-positive but show no symptoms.

Quality OF LIFE

Quality of life is important for persons with the health problems described in this chapter. The care you give them has been presented in previous chapters. Safety, good alignment, turning and repositioning, preventing infection, skin care, urinary and bowel elimination, and nutrition are some examples. Quality of life issues discussed for such care also apply to the care of persons with these common health problems.

The right to privacy and confidentiality is very important. Remember, discuss the person's problems only with the nurse and health care team members involved in the person's care. You are not responsible for giving information to families and visitors. You must not discuss your residents outside the facility. Your own family and friends should not hear about the residents.

The right to personal choice must be protected. Be sure to explain what you are going to do. The resident's consent is necessary. Also involve the person in deciding when to begin care or procedures.

Be sure to protect the resident's right to be free from abuse, mistreatment, and neglect. This is very important for residents with communicable diseases. Health care team members may tend to avoid the person because they fear getting the disease themselves. However, the use of universal precautions protect others from contamination.

SUMMARY

A resident may have one or many disorders described in this chapter. For example, a resident may have arthritis, diabetes, heart disease, and osteoporosis. Problems increase if a fracture occurs. The resident is then at risk for infection, pneumonia, and the complications of bed rest. The amount of care required depends on the nature of the problem and the number of problems a resident has.

Only very basic information was given about each disorder. Entire textbooks have been written on many of these disorders. You are not expected to have an in-depth understanding of your residents' diagnoses. However, the information in this chapter will help you better understand your resident's physical, psychological, and social needs.

Review QUESTIONS

Circle the *best* answer.

1. The spread of cancer to other body parts is called
    a. Malignant tumor
    b. Metastasis
    c. Gangrene
    d. Benign tumor

2. Which is not a warning sign of cancer?
    a. Painful, swollen joints
    b. A sore that does not heal
    c. Unusual bleeding or discharge from a body opening
    d. Nagging cough or hoarseness

3. A resident has arthritis. Care does *not* include
    a. Measures to prevent contractures
    b. Range-of-motion exercises
    c. Local cold applications
    d. Assistance with activities of daily living

4. Mr. Day has a cast because of a fracture. The cast needs to dry. Which is *false?*
    a. The cast should be covered with blankets or plastic.
    b. He is turned as directed so the cast dries evenly.
    c. The entire length of the cast is supported with pillows.
    d. The cast is supported with the palms when lifted.

5. A resident has a cast. Which are reported immediately?
    a. Pain, numbness, or inability to move the fingers or toes
    b. Chills, fever, or nausea and vomiting
    c. Odor, cyanosis, or temperature changes of the skin
    d. All of the above

6. A resident has had a fractured hip repaired. The operated leg should be
    a. Abducted at all times
    b. Adducted at all times
    c. Externally rotated at all times
    d. Flexed at all times

7. The resident with osteoporosis is at risk of
    a. Fractures
    b. An amputation
    c. Phantom limb pain
    d. All of the above

8. Mr. Doe has had an amputation. Why will he have a psychological adjustment?
    a. Activities of daily living are affected.
    b. Appearance is affected.
    c. His life-style is affected.
    d. All of the above

9. Mr. Smith has had a CVA. Which is *false?*
    a. Blood supply to part of his brain was interrupted.
    b. Hemiplegia may occur.
    c. Aphasia may occur.
    d. Changes in brain tissue are progressive.

10. A resident has had a stroke. The nurse tells you to do the following. Which one should you question?
    a. Elevate the head of the bed to a semi-Fowler's position.
    b. Do range-of-motion exercises every 2 hours.
    c. Turn, reposition, and give skin care every 2 hours.
    d. Keep the bed in the highest horizontal position.

11. A resident has Parkinson's disease. Which is *false?*
    a. The disease affects part of the brain.
    b. Mental function is affected first.
    c. Signs and symptoms include stiff muscles, slow movements, and a shuffling gait.
    d. The person needs to be protected from injury.

12. A resident has multiple sclerosis. Which is *false?*
    a. Nerve impulses are sent to and from the brain in a normal manner.
    b. Symptoms begin in young adulthood.
    c. There is no cure.
    d. The resident eventually will be paralyzed and totally dependent on others for care.

13. Residents with head or spinal cord injuries require
    a. Rehabilitation
    b. Speech therapy
    c. Care in a nursing facility
    d. Psychiatric care

14. A resident is a quadriplegic from a spinal cord injury. The resident has paralysis
    a. Of the legs, arms, and trunk
    b. On one side of the body
    c. Of the legs
    d. Of the legs and trunk

15. You are talking to a person with a hearing loss. You should do the following *except*
    a. Speak clearly, distinctly, and slowly
    b. Sit or stand where there is a good light
    c. Shout
    d. Stand or sit on the side of the better ear

16. You are talking with a hearing-impaired person. You can do the following *except*
    a. State the topic of discussion
    b. Cover your mouth, smoke, or chew gum while talking
    c. Use short sentences and simple words
    d. Write out important names and words

17. When eyeglasses are not being worn, they should be
    a. Soaked in a cleansing solution
    b. Kept within the person's reach
    c. Put in the case and in the top drawer of the bedside stand
    d. Placed on the overbed table

18. Mrs. Smith is blind. You should
    a. Touch her to get her attention
    b. Move equipment and furniture to provide for variety
    c. Provide step-by-step explanations of procedures
    d. Have her walk in front of you as you guide from behind

19. Glaucoma and cataract result in
    a. Decreased mental function
    b. Paralysis
    c. Loss of vision
    d. Breathing difficulties

20. A resident has emphysema. Which is *false?*
    a. The resident will have dyspnea only with activity.
    b. Smoking is the most common cause.
    c. The resident probably will breathe more easily sitting upright and slightly forward.
    d. Sputum may contain pus.

21. A resident has pneumonia. Universal precautions are needed.
    a. True
    b. False

22. A resident has hypertension. Which complication can occur?
    a. Stroke
    b. Heart attack
    c. Kidney failure
    d. All of the above

23. A resident has hypertension. Treatment will probably include the following *except*
    a. No smoking and regular exercise
    b. A high-sodium diet
    c. A low-calorie diet if the resident is obese
    d. Medications to lower the blood pressure

24. A resident has angina pectoris. Which statement is *true?*
    a. Damage to the heart muscle occurs.
    b. The pain is described as crushing, stabbing, or squeezing.
    c. The pain is relieved with rest and nitroglycerin.
    d. All of the above

25. A resident is having a myocardial infarction. You know that
    a. The resident is having a heart attack
    b. This is an emergency situation
    c. The resident may have a cardiac arrest
    d. All of the above

26. A resident has congestive heart failure. The following measures have been ordered. Which should you question?
    a. Force fluids
    b. Measure intake and output
    c. Measure weight daily
    d. Perform range-of-motion exercises

27. Which is not a sign of diabetes mellitus?
    a. Increased urine production
    b. Weight gain
    c. Hunger
    d. Increased thirst

28. AIDS and hepatitis require
    a. Respiratory precautions
    b. Enteric precautions
    c. Universal precautions
    d. Drainage/secretion precautions

Review QUESTIONS

29. Hepatitis B usually is spread by contact with in-fected
    a. Blood
    b. Feces
    c. Wound drainage
    d. All of the above
30. AIDS usually is spread by contact with infected
    a. Blood
    b. Urine
    c. Tears
    d. Saliva

Answers

1. b	9. d	17. c	25. d
2. a	10. d	18. c	26. a
3. c	11. b	19. c	27. b
4. a	12. a	20. a	28. c
5. d	13. a	21. a	29. a
6. a	14. a	22. d	30. a
7. a	15. c	23. b	
8. d	16. b	24. c	

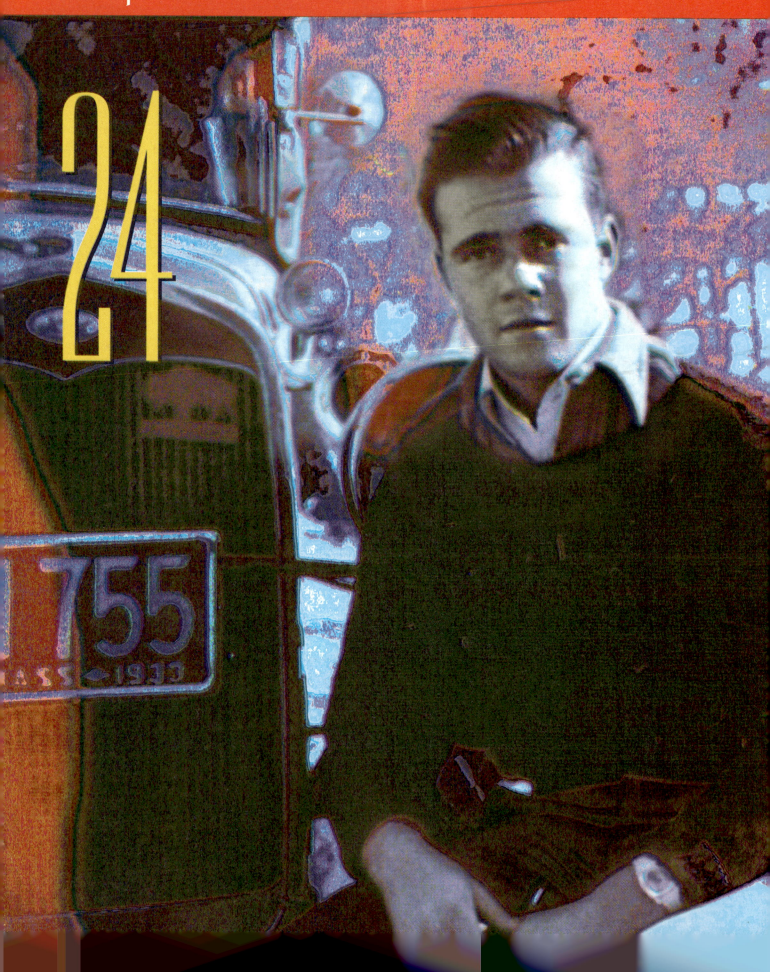

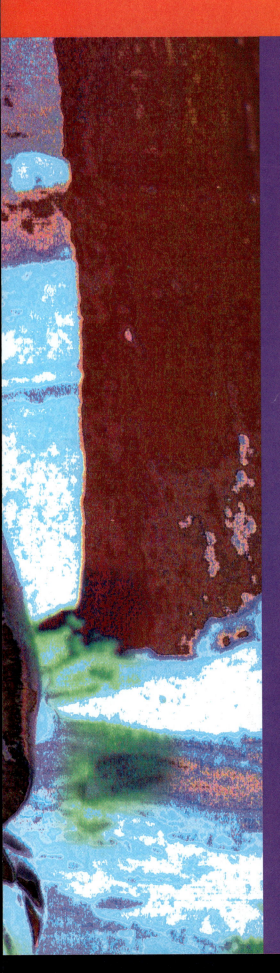

What You Will

LEARN

- The key terms listed in this chapter

- How to describe acute confusion

- The causes of acute confusion

- How to describe Alzheimer's disease

- Signs, symptoms, and behaviors associated with acute confusion and Alzheimer's disease

- The difference between acute confusion and dementia

- The effects of Alzheimer's disease on the family

- The care required by a person with Alzheimer's disease

- How to provide quality of life for confused and demented residents

cognitive impairment
A decrease in intellectual functioning

delusion
A false belief

dementia
The term used to describe mental disorders caused by changes in the brain

hallucination
Seeing, hearing, or feeling something that is not real

illusion
Misunderstanding sights and sounds in the environment

sundowning
Increased signs, symptoms, and behaviors of Alzheimer's disease during hours of darkness

My dad could grow and fix anything. He was very intelligent. Now he doesn't remember my name. 🙿

Intellectual functioning refers to memory, thinking, reasoning, understanding, judgment, and behavior. A decrease in intellectual functioning is known as **cognitive impairment.**

Many people believe that cognitive impairment is a part of aging. Actually, most elderly persons can function intellectually. They may be slower in reacting and more cautious. Some may have poor grammar or limited vocabularies. You must remember that many of today's elderly did not have a lot of schooling. They grew up when times were hard. Many had to work to support the family. Others went off to war. None of these factors, however, means slow reactions or a lack of intelligence. Nor do they mean that person is confused or disoriented.

Some elderly persons do develop acute confusion or dementia. Acute confusion usually can be reversed. Dementia cannot. Dementia is a chronic condition that eventually leads to death.

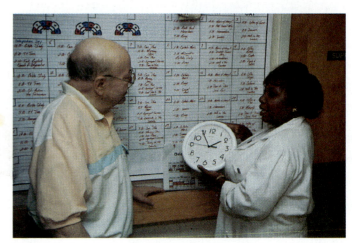

FIGURE 24-1 *A clock and calendar are used to orient a resident.*

ACUTE CONFUSION

Acute confusion (delirium) comes on suddenly. Disorientation occurs. Persons may not know the time, the date, or where they are. They may be lethargic. Lethargic people are drowsy, lack energy, and are sluggish. They may be very active at other times. They may sleep all day and be up all night. They cannot think clearly. There may be behavior shifts. A person may be alert, oriented, and active; and then disoriented and lethargic.

Hallucinations may occur. A **hallucination** is seeing, hearing, or feeling something that is not real. Affected persons may see animals, insects, or people that are not present. Some hear voices. They may feel bugs crawling on their bodies or feel that they are being touched.

Some have **illusions.** An illusion is misunderstanding the sights and sounds in the environment. Clothes hanging in the closet may be seen as people. The sound of a food cart may be heard as a car in the hallway.

Persons with acute confusion are easily distracted. Their speech may be rambling and may not make sense. Dressing, personal hygiene, and eating may be difficult. Memory is poor. They may not remember what they did just moments before. Judgment is poor. Therefore they are at risk for injury to themselves.

Acute confusion often is an early sign of illness in elderly persons. The confusion is caused by illnesses and disorders that affect brain function. The person often is physically ill. Chronic obstructive pulmonary disease, heart failure, diabetes, infection, and brain tumors can all cause acute confusion. Other causes include accidents, head injuries, surgery, medications, and immobility. A strange environment (hospital, nursing facility) can make the confusion worse.

Acute confusion may be an early sign of a medical emergency. You must report changes in behavior to the nurse immediately. You can help residents with acute confusion by following these practices:

1. Reorient the person. Give the time and location. Be sure to indicate if it is day or night. The use of calendars and clocks may be helpful (Fig. 24-1).
2. Provide a safe environment. Active and lethargic residents must be protected from falls and other accidents. Prevent burns from hot food. Cut food into small pieces for easier chewing and swallowing.
3. Keep care and activities simple. Assist with dressing, hygiene, and other personal care activities as needed.
4. Keep the person's stress level low.
   a. Give simple, step-by-step directions.
   b. Keep choices to a minimum.
   c. Have the person do one task at a time.
   d. Ask simple questions.
   e. Speak in simple sentences.
   f. Do not expose the person to excessive noise or activity.
   g. Do not rearrange furniture or the resident's personal possessions.

5. Sit with the person during meals so that he or she remembers to eat. Feed the person if necessary.
6. Walk with the agitated resident. This helps to distract the person.
7. Provide for the person's elimination needs. Confusion often increases when the person needs to urinate or have a bowel movement.
8. Use touch to calm and reassure the resident.
9. Do not restrain the person. The person may become more confused.
10. Show that illusions are not real. For example, let the person feel clothes in the closet or see the food on the cart.
11. Let the person who is up at night sit at the nurses' station. Offer milk, juice, or a snack, if these are allowed.
12. Control your nonverbal communication. The confused person often can tell when you are upset, angry, or frustrated.

DEMENTIA

Certain diseases cause changes in the brain. **Dementia** is the term used to describe the mental disorder caused by these changes. There are many causes of dementia. It is seen in the advanced stages of AIDS, multiple sclerosis, and Parkinson's disease. Multi-infarct dementia is due to multiple (many) small strokes. Signs and symptoms of dementia develop slowly. They may go unnoticed for a long time. Dementias are chronic. There is no cure, and they become progressively worse. Alzheimer's disease is the most common cause of dementia.

Alzheimer's Disease

Alzheimer's disease occurs in both men and women. Although it is more common in elderly persons, it also occurs in younger persons. Some people in their 40s and 50s have Alzheimer's disease. The cause is unknown.

Stages of Alzheimer's disease. Three stages of Alzheimer's disease have been described (List 24-1). Signs and symptoms become more severe with each stage. The disease ends in death.

Wandering, sundowning, hallucinations, delusions, and catastrophic reactions also occur. Persons with Alzheimer's disease are disoriented to person, time, and place. They may wander from the nursing facility and not be able to find their way back. They may be with a staff member one minute and be gone the next. Persons with Alzheimer's disease have poor judgment and cannot tell what is safe or dangerous. They are in danger of accidents. A person may walk into traffic or into a nearby river or lake. If not properly dressed, they risk exposure in cold climates.

Sundowning occurs in the late afternoon and evening. As daylight ends and darkness occurs, confu-

---

List 24-1

Stages of Alzheimer's Disease

Stage 1
Memory loss—forgetfulness; forgets recent events
Poor judgment; bad decisions
Disoriented to time
Lack of spontaneity—less outgoing or interested in things
Blames others for mistakes, forgetfulness, and other problems
Moodiness

Stage 2
Restlessness; increases during the evening hours
Sleep disturbances
Memory loss increases—may not recognize family and friends
Dulled senses—cannot tell the difference between hot and cold; cannot recognize dangers
Bowel and bladder incontinence
Needs assistance with activities of daily living—problems bathing, feeding, and dressing self; afraid of bathing; will not change clothes
Loses impulse control—may use foul language, have poor table manners, be sexually aggressive, or be rude
Movement and gait disturbances—walks slowly, has a shuffling gait
Communication problems—cannot follow directions; has problems with reading, writing, and math; speaks in short sentences or single words; statements may not make sense
Repeats motions and statements—may move things back and forth constantly; may say the same thing over and over again
Agitation—behavior may become violent

Stage 3
Seizures (see Chapter 26)
Cannot communicate—may groan, grunt, or scream
Does not recognize self or family members
Totally dependent on others for all ADL
Disoriented to person, time, and place
Totally incontinent of urine and feces
Cannot swallow—choking and aspiration are risks
Sleep disturbances increase
Becomes bed bound—cannot sit or walk
Coma
Death

sion, restlessness, and other symptoms increase. The person's behavior is worse after the sun goes down. Sundowning may relate to being tired or hungry. Inadequate light may cause the person to see things that are not there. Like children, persons with Alzheimer's disease may be afraid of the dark.

Senses are dulled. The person may have hallucinations as described on p. 516. Delusions may occur. **Delusions** are false beliefs. Persons with Alzheimer's disease have thought that they were God, movie stars, or some other person. Some believe they are in jail, are going to be murdered, or are being attacked. A person may believe that a family member is actually someone else. Many other false beliefs can occur.

Care of the person with Alzheimer's disease.
Alzheimer's disease is frustrating to the victim, family, and caregivers. Usually the person is cared for at home until symptoms become severe. Care in a nursing facility often is required. Thus you may care for residents with Alzheimer's disease. The resident and family need your support and understanding.

Remember, persons with Alzheimer's disease do not choose to be forgetful, incontinent, agitated, or rude. Nor do they choose to have all the other behaviors, signs, and symptoms of the disease. They have no control over what is happening to them. The disease causes the behaviors. Thus when a resident does something that a healthy person would not do, remember that the *disease* is responsible, not the *person*.

Care of persons with Alzheimer's disease is described in List 24-2. Such measures probably will be part of the person's comprehensive care plan.

The family.
The family of the person with Alzheimer's disease has special needs. Caring for the loved one can be exhausting. Family members may feel guilty because they can no longer care for the person at home and care in a nursing facility is now required. They need much support and encouragement. Many join Alzheimer's disease support groups. These groups are sponsored by hospitals, nursing facilities, and the Alzheimer's Association. The Alzheimer's Association has chapters in cities and towns throughout the country. Support groups offer encouragement, advice, and ideas about care. People in similar situations share feelings, anger, frustration, guilt, and other emotions.

Families often feel helpless. No matter what is done for the loved one, the person only gets worse. Much time, money, energy, and emotions are required to care for the person. Anger and resentment may result. The family may then feel guilty because of their anger and resentment. They know that the person did not choose to have the disease. The family also knows that the person cannot control behavior. They may be frustrated and hurt that the person no longer knows them or is unable to show love and affection.

The family has probably cared for the loved one at home. They have learned special care measures and procedures. They may want to help give some of that person's care in the nursing facility. Letting them participate helps them deal with guilt feelings. The health care team may meet with the family to plan their part in the person's care. The nurse and the support groups will help the family understand the disease. They also help the family understand the person's changing needs for care.

List 24-2

Care of the Person with Alzheimer's Disease

1. Safety
   a. Remove sharp and breakable objects from the environment. This includes knives, scissors, glass, dishes, and razors.
   b. Provide plastic eating and drinking utensils. This helps prevent breakage and cuts.
   c. Place safety plugs in electrical outlets.
   d. Keep cords and electrical equipment out of reach.
   e. Childproof caps should be on medicine containers and household cleaners.
   f. Store household cleaners and medicines in locked storage areas.
   g. Practice safety measures to prevent falls (see Chapter 7, p. 114).
   h. Practice safety measures to prevent burns (see Chapter 7, p. 114).

i. Practice safety measures to prevent poisoning (see Chapter 7, p. 113).

2. Wandering
    a. Make sure doors and windows are securely locked. Locks are often placed at the top and bottom of doors (Fig. 24-2, p. 520).
    b. Make sure door alarms are turned on. The alarm goes off when the door is opened. These are common in nursing facilities.
    c. Make sure the person wears an ID bracelet at all times.
    d. Exercise the person as ordered. Adequate exercise often reduces wandering.
    e. Do not restrain the person. Restraints require a doctor's order. They also tend to increase confusion and disorientation.
    f. Do not argue with the person who wants to leave. Remember, the person does not understand what you are saying.
    g. Go with the person who insists on going outside. Make sure he or she is properly dressed. Guide the person inside after a few minutes (Fig. 24-3, p. 520).
    h. Let the person wander in enclosed areas if provided. Many nursing facilities have enclosed areas where residents can walk about (Fig. 24-4, p. 520). These areas provide a safe place for the person to wander.

3. Sundowning
    a. Provide a calm, quiet environment late in the day. Treatments and activities should be done early in the day.
    b. Do not restrain the person.
    c. Encourage exercise and activity early in the day.
    d. Make sure the person has eaten. Hunger can increase restlessness.
    e. Promote urinary and bowel elimination. A full bladder or constipation can increase restlessness.
    f. Do not try to reason with the person. Remember, he or she cannot understand what you are saying.

g. Do not ask the person to tell you what is bothering him or her. The ability to communicate is impaired. He or she does not understand what you are asking. The person cannot think or speak clearly.

4. Hallucinations and delusions
    a. Do not argue with the person. He or she does not understand what you are saying.
    b. Reassure the person. Tell him or her that you will provide protection from harm.
    c. Distract the person with some item or activity.
    d. Use touch to calm and reassure the person (Fig. 24-5, p. 520).

5. Comfort, rest, and sleep
    a. Provide good skin care. Make sure the person's skin is free of urine and feces.
    b. Promote urinary and bowel elimination (see Chapters 13 and 14).
    c. Promote exercise and activity during the day. This helps reduce wandering and sundowning behaviors. The person may also sleep better.
    d. Reduce the person's intake of coffee, tea, and cola drinks. They contain caffeine. Caffeine is a stimulant. The person's restlessness, confusion, and agitation can increase because of caffeine.
    e. Provide a quiet, restful environment. Soft music is better in the evening than loud television programs.
    f. Promote personal hygiene. Do not force the person into a shower or tub. People with Alzheimer's disease are often afraid of bathing. Try bathing the person when he or she is calm.
    g. Provide oral hygiene.
    h. Have equipment ready for any procedure ahead of time. This reduces the amount of time the person has to be involved in care measures.

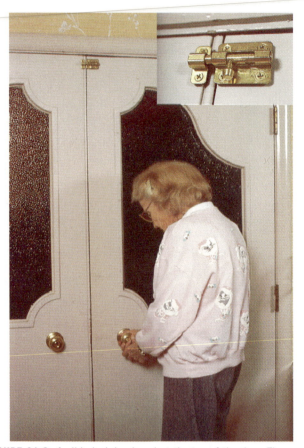

FIGURE 24-2 *A slide lock is placed at the top of the door. The person tries to open the lock on the knob.*

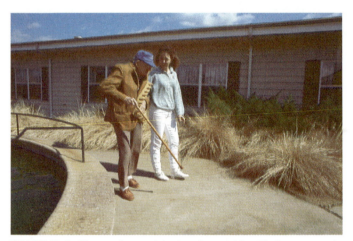

FIGURE 24-3 *The nursing assistant walks outside with the person who wanders. He is guided back into the facility.*

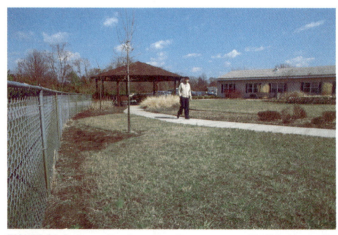

FIGURE 24-4 *An enclosed garden allows persons with Alzheimer's disease to wander in a safe environment.*

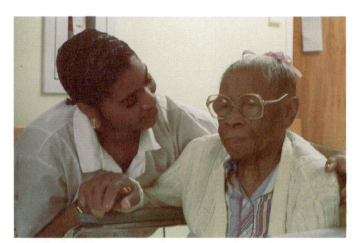

FIGURE 24-5 *The nursing assistant uses touch to calm a person with Alzheimer's disease.*

Quality OF LIFE

Quality of life is important for residents with acute confusion and dementia. They have the same rights under OBRA as do other residents. Confused and demented residents may not know or be able to exercise their rights. However, the family is aware of the resident's rights. They need to know that their loved one's rights are being protected. The family also needs to know that the loved one is being treated with respect and dignity.

Confused and demented residents have the right to privacy and confidentiality. You must still protect the person from exposure. Only those involved in the person's care should be present for care and procedures. The resident should still visit with others in private. When family and friends visit, they should be a given a space where they can visit privately. Confidentiality also is important. The resident's care and condition are not shared with others.

Even confused and demented residents have the right to personal choice. Some can still make simple choices. For example, a person may be able to choose between wearing a dress or slacks. Choosing to watch or not watch television may be a simple choice. Others cannot make choices themselves. The family may do so. Bath times, menus, clothing, activities, and other aspects of care may be chosen by the family.

The resident has the right to keep and use personal possessions. Some items may be a source of comfort for the resident. A pillow, blanket, afghan, or sweater may be important to the resident. The resident may not be able to tell you why or even recognize the item. Still, it is important. Personal items kept by the resident need to be safe (see List 24-2). You also must protect the person's property from loss or damage.

Confused and demented residents must be kept free from abuse, mistreatment, and neglect. Their care can be very frustrating. The person's behaviors may be difficult to deal with. Family and staff members can become short-tempered and angry. The resident must be protected from abuse (see Chapter 6, p. 106). Be sure to report any signs of abuse to the nurse right away. You need to be patient and calm when caring for these residents. Talk with the nurse if you find yourself becoming frustrated. Sometimes a change in assignment is needed for a while.

All residents have the right to be free from restraints. Remember, restraints require a doctor's order. They must be used only when it is the best method of protecting the resident. They are not used for staff convenience. Restraints can make confusion and demented behaviors worse. The nurse will tell you when restraints are to be used.

Activity and a safe environment promote quality of life. List 24-2 identifies safety measures for confused and demented residents. These residents also need activities that are safe, calm, and quiet. The recreation therapist and other health care team members will find activities that are best for each confused or demented resident. These will be part of the person's comprehensive care plan.

SUMMARY

Acute confusion and dementia affect a person's ability to think, reason and understand. Memory, judgment, and behavior also are affected. Therefore the person's ability to meet basic needs is affected. Physical, safety, love and belonging, esteem, and self-actualization needs are all affected.

Acute confusion is a temporary condition. The person needs reassurance that the condition will pass. Remember, acute confusion may signal a physical illness or medical emergency. A sudden change in a resident's behavior must be reported to the nurse immediately.

Dementia is a chronic condition. Persons with dementia do not choose to be forgetful, to wander, or to have poor manners. The disease is responsible for their behaviors. As frustrating as their behaviors may be, you must remember that they have no control over their actions.

The demented resident and family need much encouragement and emotional support. Required care can be physically, emotionally, and financially draining. There are no cures. However, a kind, caring nursing assistant can be a comfort.

Review QUESTIONS

Circle the *best* answer.

1. Cognitive impairment
   a. Is expected in elderly people
   b. Refers to a decrease in intellectual functioning
   c. Refers only to memory loss
   d. Is a permanent condition

2. Acute confusion is
   a. Caused by changes in the brain
   b. An illusion
   c. Caused by factors that affect brain function
   d. A chronic condition

3. An illusion is
   a. Misunderstanding sights and sounds in the environment
   b. Alzheimer's disease
   c. Dementia
   d. Seeing, hearing, and feeling things that are not real

4. Persons with acute confusion
   a. Should be restrained in bed at night
   b. Should be given many tasks to keep them busy
   c. Are easily distracted
   d. Are never a danger to themselves or others

5. Dementia describes
   a. A false belief
   b. Mental disorders caused by changes in the brain
   c. Sundowning
   d. Acute confusion

6. These statements are about Alzheimer's disease. Which is *true?*
   a. It occurs only in elderly persons.
   b. Diet and medications can control the disease.
   c. It is the same as cognitive impairment.
   d. The disease ends in death.

7. Persons with Alzheimer's disease
   a. Have memory loss, poor judgment, and sleep disturbances
   b. Lose impulse control and the ability to communicate
   c. May wander or have delusions and hallucinations
   d. All of the above

8. Sundowning means that
   a. The person becomes sleepy when the sun sets
   b. Behaviors become worse in the late afternoon and evening

   c. Behavior improves at night
   d. The person is in the third stage of the disease

9. Alzheimer's disease support groups do the following *except*
   a. Provide care
   b. Offer encouragement and care ideas
   c. Provide support for the family
   d. Promote the sharing of feelings and frustrations

10. A person with Alzheimer's disease tends to wander. You should
    a. Make sure doors and windows are locked
    b. Make sure the person wears an ID bracelet
    c. Exercise the person as ordered
    d. All of the above

11. A person has Alzheimer's disease. Which is *false?*
    a. Safety plugs should be placed in electrical outlets.
    b. Cleaners and medications should be out of the person's reach.
    c. The person can keep smoking materials.
    d. Sharp and breakable objects are removed from the person's environment.

12. A person has Alzheimer's disease. Which is *false?*
    a. It is possible to reason with the person.
    b. Touch can calm and reassure the person.
    c. A calm, quiet environment is important.
    d. Assistance is needed with ADLs.

13. The person with Alzheimer's disease cannot make choices. Therefore the person's right to personal choice does not have to be protected.
    a. True
    b. False

14. Confused and demented residents have the right to
    a. Privacy and confidentiality
    b. Be free from abuse, mistreatment, and neglect
    c. Keep and use personal possessions
    d. All of the above

Answers

1. b	5. b	9. a	13. b
2. c	6. d	10. d	14. d
3. a	7. d	11. c	
4. c	8. b	12. a	

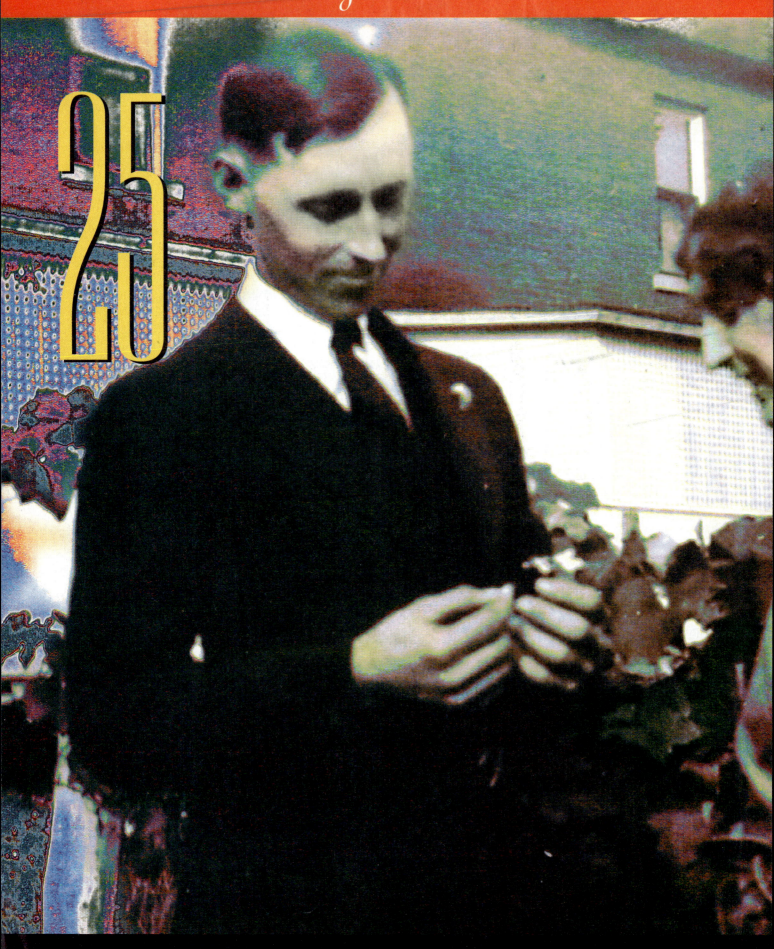

25

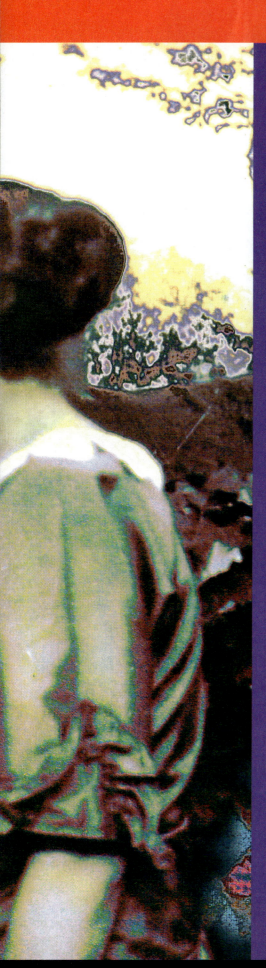

What You Will

LEARN

- The key terms listed in this chapter

- Differences between sex and sexuality

- Why sexuality is important throughout life

- Five types of sexual relationships

- How injury and illness can affect a person's sexuality

- The illnesses, injuries, and surgeries that affect sexuality

- How aging affects sexuality

- How the nursing team can promote a resident's sexuality and quality of life

- Why residents may become sexually aggressive

- Ways to deal with a sexually aggressive resident

- How sexually transmitted diseases are spread

- The common sexually transmitted diseases

bisexual
An individual who is attracted to persons of both sexes

heterosexual
A person who is attracted to individuals of the opposite sex

homosexual
A person who has a strong attraction to members of the same sex

impotence
The inability of the male to have an erection

menopause
The time when menstruation stops; it marks the end of the woman's reproductive years

sex
The physical activities that involve the organs of reproduction; the activities are done for pleasure or to have children

sexuality
That which relates to one's sex; those physical, psychological, social, cultural, and spiritual factors that affect a person's feelings and attitudes about his or her sex

transsexual
A person who believes that he or she is really a member of the opposite sex

transvestite
A person who becomes sexually excited by dressing in the clothes of the opposite sex

My husband died 7 years ago. I still miss him. We were together 57 years. I guess what I really miss is just feeling close to someone. ❧

Residents in nursing facilities were once viewed as having only physical problems. The person's physical needs were the first and often the only concern. Little attention was given to the psychological or social effects of the resident's disorder. The needs of love and belonging, esteem, and self-actualization were overlooked. Now attention is given to the total person. Physical, psychological, social, and spiritual needs of the person are considered.

Sexuality is one aspect of the person that involves the physical, psychological, social, and spiritual. This chapter describes the effects of aging, illness, and injury on sexuality. A review of the reproductive system in Chapter 5 will be helpful before studying this chapter.

SEX AND SEXUALITY

Sex and sexuality are different. **Sex** refers to the physical activities involving the reproductive organs. The activities are done for pleasure or to produce children. **Sexuality** involves the whole personality as well as the body. Attitudes and feelings are involved. In addition to physical and psychological factors, sexuality is influenced by social, cultural, and spiritual factors. The way a person behaves, thinks, dresses, and responds to others is related to that person's sexuality.

Sexuality is present from birth. When the infant's sex is known, a boy or girl name is given. Blue often is used for boys and pink for girls. Toys reflect sexuality. Dolls traditionally are given to girls. Trains and baseball bats are for boys. By 2 years of age, children know their own sex. By 3, they know the sex of other children. Children learn male and female roles from their parents (Fig. 25-1). Early on they learn that there are certain behaviors for boys and certain behaviors for girls.

As children grow older, interest increases about the human body and how it works. Body changes during adolescence bring a greater interest and curiosity about sex and the body.

Sexual activity is common in young adulthood. Sex takes on more meaning as young adults mature. Attitudes and feelings are important. Decisions about sexuality become more important. Some of the decisions relate to selecting a sexual partner, sex before marriage, and birth control.

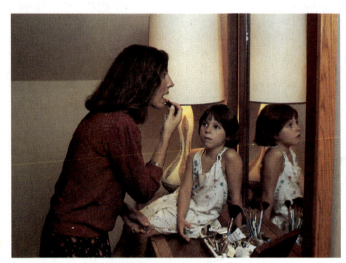

FIGURE 25-1 *This little girl is learning a female role from her mother.*

Sexuality continues to be important into adulthood and old age. Attitudes and the need for sex change as a person grows older. Life circumstances change. These changes may include divorce, death of a spouse, injury, or illness.

SEXUAL RELATIONSHIPS

Sex and sexuality imply a male partner and a female partner. Most people are heterosexuals. A **heterosexual** person is attracted to the opposite sex. Sexual activities involve a member of the opposite sex. However, you may meet or care for people who are not heterosexual.

A **homosexual** person is attracted to members of the same sex. The person has sexual relationships and is aroused by someone of the same sex. Men are attracted to men, and women are attracted to women. The word "gay" often is used in reference to a homosexual. A homosexual woman is called a *lesbian*.

Homosexuality is as old as humankind. For centuries, however, homosexual behavior was condemned in most societies. In our culture it has become more accepted since the 1960s and 1970s. Before, it was hidden. Now many homosexual persons are more open about their sexuality and sexual preferences and relationships.

Bisexual persons are attracted to both sexes. They can be aroused and excited by either men or women. Their pattern of sexual activity varies. Sometimes it is strictly heterosexual; at other times it is homosexual. Some persons move between homosexual and heterosexual relationships. Bisexual persons often are married and have children. Some seek a homosexual relationship or experience outside of marriage.

Some persons believe they really are members of the opposite sex. That is, a male born with male sex organs believes he is really a woman in a man's body. A woman born with female sex organs believes she really is a man in a woman's body. These individuals are called **transsexuals.** They often describe feelings of being "trapped" in the wrong body. Most transsexual persons have had these feelings for as long as they can remember. Some undergo psychiatric treatment. Some have had sex-change operations.

A **transvestite** enjoys dressing in clothing of the opposite sex. Most are male. Transvestites usually are married and heterosexual. They dress as men most of the time. Dressing as a woman usually occurs in private. Some men dress completely as women. Others focus on bras, panties, and other undergarments. The wife may not know about the practice. Some wives know their husbands are transvestites. If the wife agrees, she may be included in the transvestite's activities. Some transvestites have same-sex friends with similar interests.

INJURY AND ILLNESS

Sexuality and sex involve the mind and the body. Injury and illness can affect the way the body works. The mind also can be affected. A person may feel unclean, unwhole, unattractive, or mutilated after disfiguring surgery. Attitudes about sex may change. The person may feel unattractive and incapable of being loved. These feelings affect the person's ability to be close and intimate. Therefore the person may develop sexual problems that are psychological in nature. The individual can be helped to overcome these feelings. Time, understanding, and a caring partner are very helpful. Some may need counseling or psychiatric assistance.

Many illnesses, injuries, and surgeries cause changes in the nervous, circulatory, and reproductive systems. If any of these systems are affected, the person may experience changes in sexual ability. Most chronic illnesses also affect sexual functioning.

Impotence may occur. Impotence is the inability of the male to have an erection. Diabetes mellitus, spinal cord injuries, multiple sclerosis, and alcoholism are common causes. Circulatory disorders and medications can affect the man's ability to have an erection. Medications to control blood pressure often have impotence as a side effect.

Heart disease, stroke, chronic obstructive pulmonary disease, and nervous system disorders also may affect sexual ability. Surgery that affects the reproductive organs may have physical and psychological effects. Removal of the prostate or the testes affects a man's ability to achieve an erection. Removal of the uterus, ovaries, or a breast may affect a woman psychologically. A colostomy or ileostomy may psychologically affect both men and women.

You will care for residents with disorders that can affect sexual functioning. Changes in sexual functioning have a great impact on the resident. Fear, anger, worry, and depression often occur. These are evident in the resident's behavior and comments. You need to understand that the resident's feelings are normal and expected.

SEXUALITY AND ELDERLY PERSONS

Many people think that sex, love, and intimacy are for the young. Young people fall in love, hold hands, embrace, and have sex. A common attitude is that older people are not supposed to need sex, love, and affection. There is also the idea that older people are not capable of sexual activities. Fortunately these ideas are untrue. Sexual relationships are psychologically and physically important to elderly persons (Fig. 25-2).

Love, affection, and intimacy are needed throughout life. As the elderly person experiences other losses, feeling close to another human being becomes even more important. Children leave home. Friends and relatives

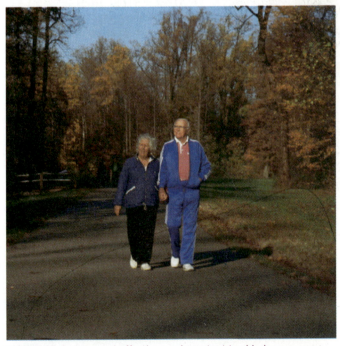

FIGURE 25-2 *Love and affection are important to elderly persons.*

die. Retirement means job loss. Health problems may develop. These losses may be compounded by decreasing physical strength and changes in appearance.

Reproductive organs change with age. These changes, however, do not eliminate sexual needs or abilities. Changes in men are related to decreases in the male hormone testosterone. The hormone affects strength, sperm production, and reproductive tissues. These changes affect sexual activity. It takes longer for an erection to occur. The phase between erection and orgasm also is longer. Orgasm is less forceful than in the younger years. After orgasm the erection is lost quickly. The time between erections also is longer. Older men may need stimulation of the penis to become sexually excited. Younger men can become sexually excited by just thinking about sex or a sexual partner.

Elderly men usually experience decreased frequency in sexual activity. Decreased frequency can result from the physical changes just described. Other reasons include boredom with his sexual partner, mental and physical fatigue, overeating, and excessive drinking. The man may fear that he cannot perform. Therefore he avoids sexual activity. Pain and reduced mobility from illness and aging can affect frequency. One or both partners may have a chronic illness. The illness may result in decreased frequency or the complete absence of sex.

Physical changes also occur in women. **Menopause** occurs around 50 years of age. Menopause is the time when a woman stops menstruating. It marks the end of her reproductive years. A related change is the decreased secretion of female hormones (estrogen and progesterone). Reduced hormone levels affect reproductive tissues. The uterus, vagina, and external genitalia atrophy. The vagina can still receive the penis during intercourse. However, intercourse may be uncomfortable or painful. Pain and discomfort are due to thinning of the vaginal walls and vaginal dryness. This condition can be relieved by hormones taken orally or used vaginally. Like elderly men, older women have changes in sexual excitement. It takes longer to become sexually excited. The time between excitement and orgasm is longer. Orgasm is less intense, and the woman returns to a pre-excitement state more quickly.

Most elderly women experience decreased frequency of sexual activity. Reasons relate to weakness, mental and physical fatigue, pain, and reduced mobility. These may be due to chronic illness.

Some elderly persons do not have sexual intercourse. This does not mean they lack sexual needs and desires. Their needs may be expressed in other ways. Handholding, touching, caressing, and embracing are ways of expressing closeness and intimacy.

Having a sexual partner also is important. Divorce results in the loss of a sexual partner. So does death. This is a greater problem for women. Women live longer than men. Therefore there are more widows than single elderly men. The partner may be in a hospital or a nursing facility. Or the partner may have a condition that makes sexual intercourse impossible. These situations are seen in adults of all ages.

THE SEXUALLY AGGRESSIVE RESIDENT

Some residents try to have their sexual needs met by health care workers. Residents may flirt, make sexual advances or comments, expose themselves, masturbate, or touch the worker. Health care workers usually are angry or embarrassed. Such reactions are normal. Often there are reasons for the resident's behavior. Understanding the behavior may help you deal with the situation.

Illness, injury, surgery, or aging may threaten the male's sense of manhood. He may try to reassure or prove to himself that he is still attractive and able to perform sexually. He may do so by behaving sexually behavior toward health care workers.

Sometimes sexually aggressive behaviors are due to confusion or disorientation. Nervous system disorders, medications, fever, dementia, and poor vision are common causes of confusion and disorientation. The resident may confuse a health care worker with his or her sexual partner. Or the resident cannot control behavior because of changes in mental function. Normally the person would be able to control any urges toward a worker. Changes in the brain, however, may make control difficult. The resident's sexual behavior in these situations usually is innocent.

Sometimes residents touch workers inappropriately. Their purpose is sexual. Sometimes, however, touch is the only way the resident can get the health care worker's attention. Consider the following situation. Mr. Green has had a stroke. He is paralyzed on one side of his body and cannot speak. You have your back to him and are bending over. Your buttocks are the closest part of your body to him. To get your attention he touches your buttocks. You should not consider the behavior to be sexual in this situation.

Sexual advances may be intentional. You need to deal with the situation in a professional manner. There is no ideal way to deal with the advances. The following suggestions may be helpful:

1. Look at your own behavior toward the resident. In nursing facilities it is common to view residents as "family" rather than "patients." They are treated respectfully, but with affection. A resident may view this affection as a sexual advance and respond in a sexual manner. If this occurs, you may want to change your behavior toward that resident.

2. Discuss the situation with the nurse. The nurse can help you deal with or understand the resident's behavior.
3. Ask the resident not to touch you in places where you were touched.
4. Explain to the resident that you will not do what he or she suggests.
5. Explain to the resident that his or her behavior makes you uncomfortable. Then politely ask the resident not to act in that way.
6. Allow privacy if the resident is becoming sexually aroused or is masturbating. Provide for safety (e.g., raise side rails, place the signal light within reach), and tell the resident when you will return.

SEXUALLY TRANSMITTED DISEASES

Some diseases are spread by sexual contact. They are called sexually transmitted diseases (STDs) (see Table 25-1 on p. 530 and Figs. 25-3 and 25-4). Residents may have STDs. Some are not aware that they have been infected.

The genital area usually is associated with STDs. Other body areas, however, may be involved. These areas include the rectum, ears, mouth, nipples, throat, tongue, eyes, and nose. Most STDs are spread by sexual contact. The use of condoms helps prevent their spread. Some are spread through a break in the skin, by contact with the infected person's body fluids (blood, semen, saliva), or by contaminated blood or needles.

Universal precautions are necessary for your protection and the protection of others. Handwashing before and after resident contact is essential. The bloodborne pathogen standard is also followed.

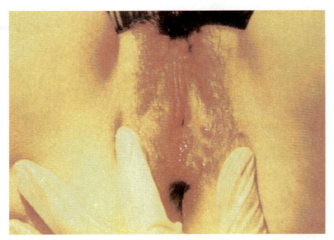

FIGURE 25-3 *Genital herpes sore.*

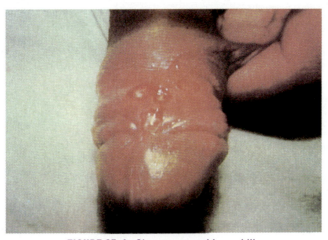

FIGURE 25-4 *Chancre caused by syphilis.*

Table 25-1

Sexually Transmitted Diseases

Disease	Signs and Symptoms	Treatment
Genital herpes	Painful, fluid-filled sores on or near the genitalia (Fig. 25-5) The sores may have a watery discharge Itching, burning, and tingling in the genital area Fever Swollen glands	No known cure Medications can be given to control discomfort
Venereal warts	Male—Warts appear on the penis, anus, or genitalia Female—Warts appear near the vagina, cervix, and labia	Application of special ointment that causes the warts to dry up and fall off Surgical removal may be necessary if the ointment is not effective
AIDS (Acquired Immunodeficiency Syndrome)	Fever, night sweats, weight loss, cough (see Chapter 23, p. 509)	No known treatment at this time
Gonorrhea	Burning on urination Urinary frequency and urgency Vaginal discharge in the female Urethral discharge in the male	Antibiotic medications
Syphilis	*Stage 1:* 10-90 days after exposure Painless chancre on the penis, in the vagina, or on genitalia (Fig. 25-4); the chancre may also be on the lips or inside of the mouth, or anywhere else on the body *Stage 2:* about two months after the chancre General fatigue, loss of appetite, nausea, fever, headache, rash, sore throat, bone and joint pain, hair loss, lesions on the lips and genitalia *Stage 3:* 3 to 15 years after infection Damage to the cardiovascular system and central nervous system, blindness	Antibiotic medications

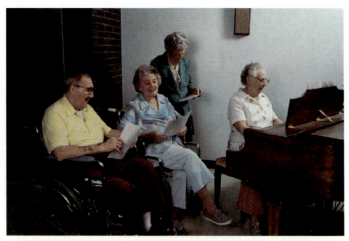

FIGURE 25-5 *Intimate relationships occur in nursing facilities.*

Quality OF LIFE

Sexuality is part of the total person. Illness or injury does not mean that sexuality is unimportant. Some residents are so ill that sexual activity is impossible. Others, however, want to be and can be sexually active. Sexual activity does not always mean intercourse. It may be expressed in other ways. Nursing staff members used to discourage any form of sexual expression, particularly among the elderly. Hand holding was okay. But two people were not to get any closer! There is now increased awareness of the importance of sexuality in health and in illness. The nursing team plays an important role in allowing residents to meet their sexual needs. The following measures are appreciated by residents. They are carried out in cooperation with the nurse supervising your work.

1. Let the person practice grooming routines. This includes applying make-up, nail polish, body lotion, and cologne. Hair care and shaving also are important. Men may wish to use after-shave lotion or cologne. The resident may need assistance in performing these activities.
2. Let the person choose what to wear. Remember, the resident has the right to personal choice.
3. Protect the right to privacy. Do not expose the resident. Care and procedures are performed so the resident is not exposed unnecessarily. The resident must be draped and screened appropriately.
4. Accept the person's sexual relationships. The resident may not share your sexual attitudes, values, or practices. You cannot expect the resident to act according to your standards. The resident may have a homosexual, a premarital, or an extramarital relationship. There may be more than one sexual partner. Do not make judgments or gossip about the resident's relationships. You must protect the resident's right to confidentiality.

5. The right to privacy includes the right to visit with the resident in private. You usually can tell when people want to be alone. If the resident has a private room, you can close the door for privacy. Some facilities have "Do not disturb" signs for doors. Let the resident and partner know how much time they can expect to have alone. For example, you can remind them when to expect a meal tray, medications, or a treatment. This tells them when to expect someone. Knocking before you enter any room is a common courtesy. It shows respect for privacy. Other staff members should be told that the resident wants some time alone. Other measures are necessary if there is a roommate. Consideration must be given to the roommate. The curtain between the two beds provides little privacy. Privacy can be arranged when the roommate is out of the room. Sometimes roommates volunteer to leave for a while when they sense that couples need time alone. If the roommate cannot leave, other areas can be found for privacy.
6. Allow married couples to share the same room. This is an OBRA requirement. They have lived together for years. Being in a nursing facility is no reason to separate them. Allow them to share the same bed if their conditions permit. A double, queen, or king-size bed may be provided by the facility or by the couple.
7. Let single elderly people develop new relationships. Death and divorce result in loss of a sexual partner. A widowed or divorced resident may develop a relationship with another resident. Instead of keeping them apart, measures should be taken to give them time together (Fig. 25-5). Both persons, however, must want the relationship. A confused, disoriented person must be protected from others. You may feel that a disoriented resident does not understand the behavior of the other resident. In this case, you should separate the two persons and report the situation to the nurse.

SUMMARY

Sexuality is part of the total person. Ill or injured people still need love, affection, and closeness to other persons. Health care workers should promote, rather than discourage, a resident's sexual expression. This is especially true for elderly persons.

Illness, injury, and surgery may affect a person's sexuality. The problem may be temporary or permanent. Reproductive organs, the circulatory system, or the nervous system may be affected. Consequently the resident may have problems in sexual performance. Some injuries and surgeries are disfiguring. These persons may feel unclean and unattractive. Their sexuality and sexual performance may be affected psychologically. Those who have physical or psychological changes in sexuality need understanding and caring. Try to understand the resident's situation. How you would feel if you had the resident's problem?

Review QUESTIONS

Circle the *best* answer.

1. Sex involves
   a. The organs of reproduction
   b. Attitudes and feelings
   c. Culture and spiritual factors
   d. All of the above

2. Sexuality is important to
   a. Small children
   b. Teenagers and young adults
   c. Middle-aged adults
   d. Persons of all ages

3. A person is attracted to a member of the opposite sex. This person is a
   a. Heterosexual
   b. Homosexual
   c. Bisexual
   d. Transsexual

4. Illness and injury can result in impotence. Impotence is
   a. When menstruation stops
   b. A psychological reaction to disfigurement
   c. The inability of the male to achieve an erection
   d. The complete absence of sexual activity

5. Changes in reproductive organs occur with aging. These changes can make sexual activity difficult or impossible.
   a. True
   b. False

6. Which will *not* promote sexuality?
   a. Allowing normal grooming routines.
   b. Having the resident wear a hospital gown.
   c. Allowing the resident and his or her partner privacy.
   d. Accepting the resident's relationship.

7. An oriented elderly lady and an oriented elderly gentleman seem to be developing a relationship. They live in a nursing facility. Nursing personnel should keep them separated.
   a. True
   b. False

8. Mr. Gibson wants some time alone with his wife. The nurse tells you this is okay. You should
   a. Close the door to the room
   b. Put a "Do not disturb" sign on the door
   c. Tell them how long they can expect to be undisturbed
   d. All of the above

9. A husband and wife are both admitted to a nursing facility. They should be assigned to separate rooms. Men and women should not share rooms in nursing facilities.
   a. True
   b. False

10. Mr. Robinson is showing sexually aggressive behavior. The behavior may be
    a. An attempt to prove he is still attractive and able to perform sexually
    b. Due to confusion or disorientation
    c. Done on purpose
    d. All of the above

11. Mr. Robinson has made sexual advances to you. You should do the following *except*
    a. Discuss the situation with the nurse
    b. Do what the resident asks
    c. Explain to the resident that his behavior makes you uncomfortable
    d. Examine your own behavior toward the resident

12. These statements are about sexually transmitted diseases (STDs). Which is *false?*
    a. STDs usually are spread by sexual contact.
    b. STDs can affect the genital area and other body parts.
    c. Signs and symptoms of STDs always are obvious.
    d. Universal precautions are required.

Answers

1. a	4. c	7. b	10. d
2. d	5. b	8. d	11. b
3. a	6. b	9. b	12. c

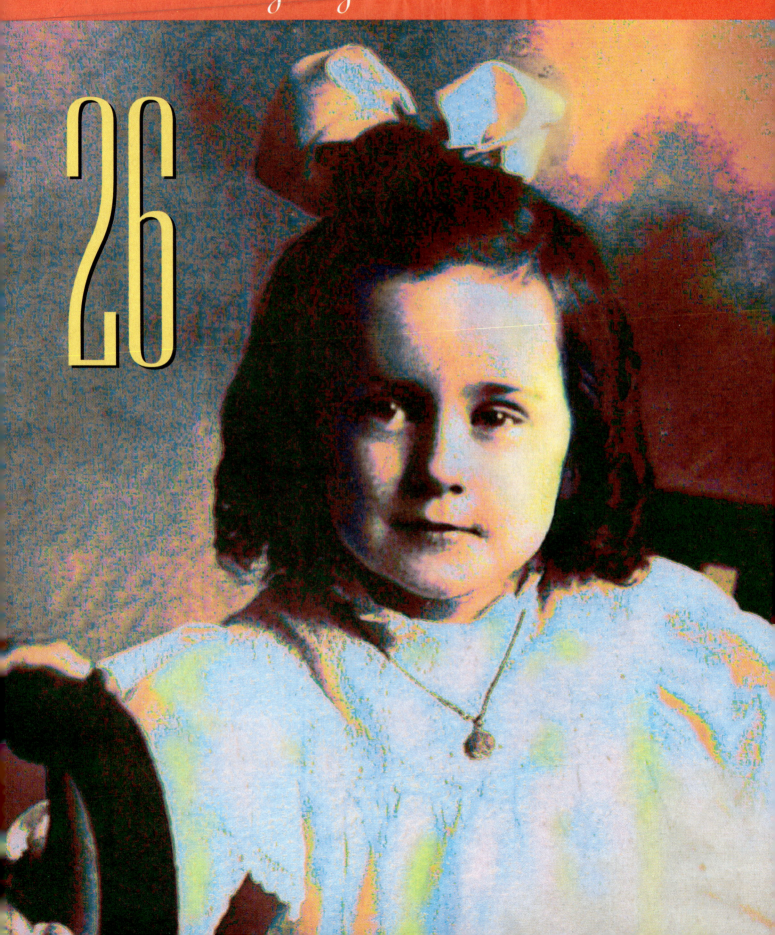

26

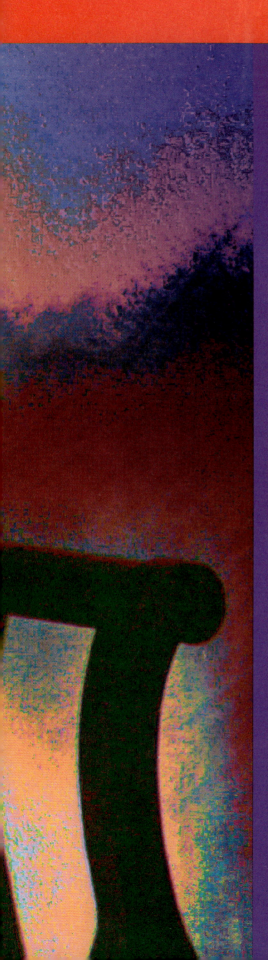

What You Will LEARN

- The key terms listed in this chapter

- Signs of an obstructed airway

- How to relieve an obstructed airway

- The difference between internal and external hemorrhage

- The difference between arterial and venous bleeding

- How to control hemorrhage

- The different types of seizures and how to care for a person during a seizure

- Common causes of and emergency care for fainting

- Signs of stroke and emergency care for stroke victims

- How to help a person who is vomiting

- How to promote quality of life in emergency situations

cardiac arrest
The sudden stoppage of breathing and heart action

convulsion
Violent and sudden contractions or tremors of muscles; seizure

first aid
Emergency care given to an ill or injured person before medical help arrives

hemorrhage
The excessive loss of blood from a blood vessel

respiratory arrest
Breathing stops but the heart continues to pump for several minutes

seizure
A convulsion

shock
A condition that results when there is an inadequate blood supply to organs and tissues

They said I had a stroke. I had to go to the hospital by ambulance. The staff made sure I had my glasses and rosary. I was so afraid they would get lost or broken.

Emergency situations can occur in nursing facilities, homes, public places, or on the highway. Knowing what to do may mean the difference between life or death. This chapter describes some common emergencies and the basic care that should be given. You are encouraged to take a first aid course offered by the American Red Cross and a basic life support course offered by the American Heart Association or the Red Cross. These courses will prepare you to give care in emergency situations.

GENERAL RULES OF EMERGENCY CARE

First aid is the emergency care given to an ill or injured person before medical help arrives. The goals of first aid are to prevent death and to prevent injuries from becoming worse.

When an emergency occurs, the local Emergency Medical Service (EMS) system is activated. The system involves emergency personnel (paramedics, emergency medical technicians) who have had education and training in emergency care. They have learned how to treat, stabilize, and transport persons who are experiencing life-threatening conditions. Their emergency vehicles have the equipment, supplies, and drugs used in emergencies. Emergency personnel communicate by two-way radio with doctors based in hospital emergency rooms. The doctors tell them what to do. In many areas the EMS system can be activated by dialing 911. The system also can be activated by calling the local fire or police department or the telephone operator.

In nursing facilities a nurse decides when to activate the EMS system. The nurse will tell you what to do to help in the situation. If the resident has stopped breathing or is having a cardiac arrest, the nurse may start cardiopulmonary resuscitation (CPR) (see p. 537-542). Facility policies vary about nursing assistants starting CPR. Some allow nursing assistants to start CPR and others do not. You need to know your facility's policy about CPR.

Some residents are not resuscitated. The family and doctor have decided that the person should be allowed to die with peace and dignity. If so, the doctor writes a "Do not resuscitate" (DNR) order. You need to know your facility's policy about DNR orders. The nurse will tell you which residents have DNR orders.

Each emergency is different. However, the following rules apply to any emergency:

1. Know your limitations. Do not try to do more than you are able. Do not perform a procedure with which you are unfamiliar. Do what you can under the circumstances.
2. Stay calm. Calm and efficient functioning will help the victim feel more secure.
3. Make quick observations for life-threatening problems. Check for breathing, pulse, and bleeding.
4. Keep the victim lying down or in the position in which he or she was found. You could make an injury worse by moving the victim.
5. Perform necessary emergency measures.
6. Call for help or have someone activate the EMS system. An operator will send emergency vehicles and personnel to the scene. Do not hang up until the operator has hung up. Give the operator the following information.
   a. Your location—include the street address and the city or town you are in. Give names of cross streets or roads and landmarks if possible. Also give the telephone number you are calling from.
   b. What has happened (e.g., heart attack, accident)—police, fire equipment, and ambulances may be needed.
   c. How many people need help.
   d. The condition of the victims, any obvious injuries, and if there are life-threatening situations.
   e. What aid is being given.
7. Do not remove clothes unless you have to. If clothing must be removed, tear the garment along the seams.
8. Keep the victim warm. Cover the victim with a blanket. Use coats and sweaters if there is no blanket.
9. Reassure the conscious victim. Explain what is happening and that help has been called.
10. Do not give the victim any food or fluids.
11. Do not move the victim. Emergency personnel have been trained to do so.

12. Keep bystanders away from the victim. They tend to stare, offer advice, and make comments about the victim's condition. The victim may think the situation is worse than it really is. Also, privacy is invaded by onlookers.

BASIC LIFE SUPPORT

When the heart and breathing stop, the person is clinically dead. Blood and oxygen are not circulated through the body. Permanent brain damage and other organ damage occur within 4 to 6 minutes. Death may be expected. Death is expected in persons suffering from long illnesses for which there is no hope of recovery. However, the heart and breathing can stop suddenly and without warning. This is a state of **cardiac arrest.**

Cardiac arrest is a sudden, unexpected, and dramatic event. People have had cardiac arrests while driving, shoveling snow, playing golf or tennis, watching television, eating, and sleeping. Cardiac arrest can occur anywhere and at any time. Common causes include heart disease, drowning, electrical shock, severe injury, obstruction of the air passages, and drug overdose. The victim suffers permanent brain damage unless breathing and circulation are restored.

Respiratory arrest is when breathing stops but the heart continues to pump blood for several minutes. If breathing is not restored, cardiac arrest occurs. Causes of respiratory arrest include drowning, stroke, obstructed airway, drug overdose, electrocution, smoke inhalation, suffocation, injury from lightening, myocardial infarction, coma, and other injuries.

Basic life support involves preventing or promptly recognizing cardiac arrest or respiratory arrest. Basic life support procedures support breathing and circulation. These life-saving measures require speed, skill, and efficiency. Again, you are advised to take a course to become certified in basic life support.

Cardiopulmonary Resuscitation

There are three major signs of cardiac arrest—no pulse, no breathing, and unconsciousness. The person's skin is cool, pale, and gray. The person has no blood pressure.

Cardiopulmonary resuscitation (CPR) must be started as soon as cardiac arrest occurs. CPR provides oxygen to the brain, heart, kidneys, and other organs until more advanced emergency care can be given. CPR has three basic parts (the ABCs of CPR): airway, breathing, and circulation.

Airway. The respiratory passages (airway) must be open if breathing is to be restored. The airway often is blocked or obstructed during cardiac arrest. The victim's tongue falls toward the back of the throat and blocks the airway. The head-tilt/chin-lift maneuver is used to open the airway (Fig. 26-1). One hand is placed on the vic-

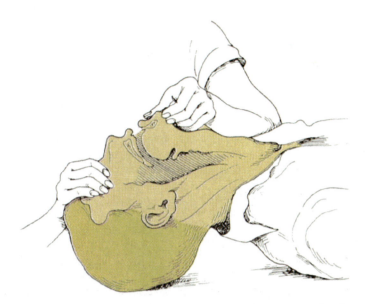

FIGURE 26-1 *The head-tilt/chin-lift maneuver is used to open the airway. One hand is on the victim's forehead, and pressure is applied to tilt the head back. The fingers of the other hand are placed under the chin. The chin is lifted forward with the fingers.*

tim's forehead. Pressure is applied on the forehead with the palm to tilt the head back. The fingers of the other hand are placed under the bony part of the chin. The chin is lifted forward as the head is tilted backward with the other hand.

Breathing. Oxygen is not inhaled when breathing stops. The victim must get oxygen. Otherwise, permanent brain and organ damage will occur. Because the victim cannot breathe, breathing is done for the victim. This is accomplished during CPR by *mouth-to-mouth* resuscitation (Fig. 26-2, p. 538).

The airway is kept open to give mouth-to-mouth resuscitation. The victim's nostrils are pinched shut with the thumb and index finger of the hand on the forehead. Shutting the nostrils prevents air from escaping through the nose. After taking a deep breath, place your mouth tightly over the victim's mouth. Blow air into the victim's mouth as you exhale. You should see the victim's chest rise as the lungs fill with air. After you give a ventilation, remove your mouth from the victim's mouth. Then take in a quick, deep breath.

Mouth-to-mouth resuscitation is not always indicated or possible. The *mouth-to-nose* technique may be necessary. The mouth-to-nose technique is suggested when:

1. You cannot ventilate the victim's mouth
2. You cannot open the mouth
3. You cannot make a tight seal for mouth-to-mouth resuscitation
4. The mouth is severely injured

The mouth must be closed for mouth-to-nose resuscitation. The head-tilt/chin-lift method is used to open the airway. Pressure is placed on the chin to close the mouth. To give the ventilation, place your mouth over the victim's nose and blow air into the nose (Fig. 26-3).

Some people breathe through openings *(stomas)* in their necks (Fig. 26-4). They need *mouth-to-stoma* ventilation during cardiac or respiratory arrest. You will seal your mouth around the stoma and blow air into the stoma (Fig. 26-5). To see if the person is a "neck-breather," check for an opening at the front of the neck.

You will have contact with the victim's body fluids or body substances when giving artificial ventilation. If available, a pocket mask with a one-way valve is used for mouth-to-mouth resuscitation (Fig. 26-6). This provides a barrier between you and the victim's fluids or body substances.

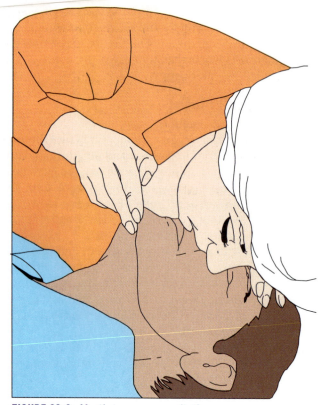

FIGURE 26-3 *Mouth-to-nose resuscitation.*

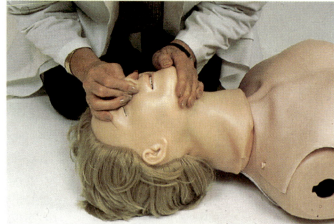

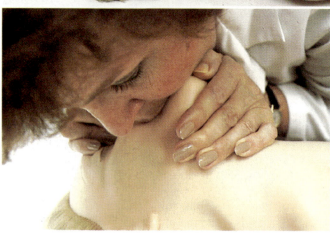

FIGURE 26-2 *Mouth-to-mouth resuscitation.* **A,** *The victim's airway is opened, and the nostrils are pinched shut.* **B,** *The victim's mouth is sealed by the rescuer's mouth.*

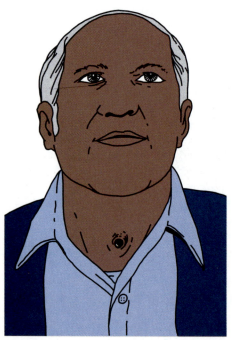

FIGURE 26-4 *A stoma in the neck. The person breathes air in and out of the stoma.*

Circulation. Blood flow to the brain and other organs must be maintained. Otherwise permanent damage results. In cardiac arrest the heart has stopped beating. Therefore blood must be pumped through the body in some other way. Artificial circulation is accomplished by external chest compression. This also is called *external cardiac massage.* Each chest compression forces blood through the circulatory system.

The heart lies between the sternum (breastbone) and the spinal column. When pressure is applied to the sternum, the sternum is depressed. This compresses the heart between the sternum and spinal column (Fig. 26-7). For effective chest compressions, the victim must be supine and on a hard, flat surface.

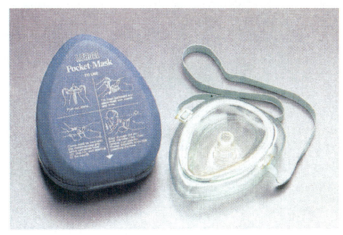

FIGURE 26-6 *A pocket mask with a one-way valve.*

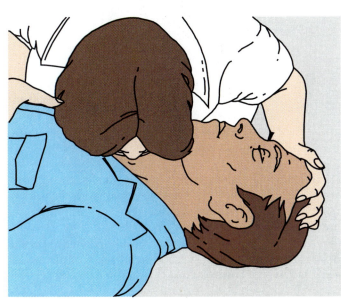

FIGURE 26-5 *Mouth-to-stoma resuscitation.*

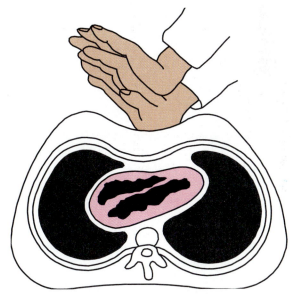

FIGURE 26-7 *The heart lies between the sternum and spinal cord. The heart is compressed when pressure is applied to the sternum. (From Rosen P et al: Emergency medicine: concepts and clinical practice, ed 3, St Louis, 1992, Mosby–Year Book.)*

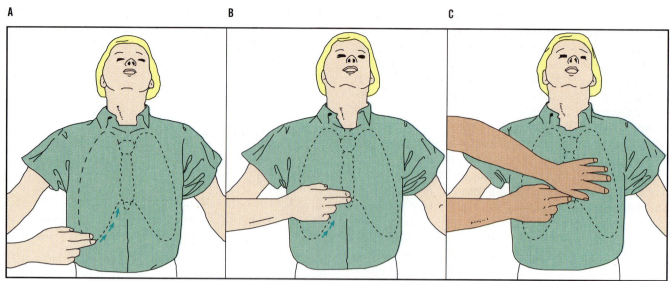

FIGURE 26-8 *Proper hand position for CPR.* **A,** *Locate the rib cage.* **B,** *Run the fingers along the rib cage to the notch.* **C,** *The heel of the hand is placed next to the index finger.*

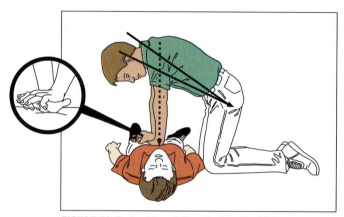

FIGURE 26-9 *Position of the shoulder for CPR.*

Proper hand position is important for external chest compressions. The process of locating hand position for adults is shown in Fig. 26-8 on p. 540.

1. Use your index and middle fingers to locate the lower part of the victim's rib cage on the side nearest you.
2. Then run your fingers up along the rib cage to the notch at the center of the chest. The notch is where the ribs and sternum meet.
3. Use your middle finger to mark the notch.
4. Place your index finger next to your middle finger on the lower end of the sternum.
5. Place the heel of your other hand on the lower half of the sternum next to your index finger.
6. Remove your index finger and middle finger from the notch.
7. Place that hand on the hand already on the sternum.
8. Extend or interlace your fingers to keep them off the chest.

You must be positioned properly for chest compressions. Your elbows must be straight. Your shoulders must be directly over the victim's chest (Fig. 26-9). Firm downward pressure is exerted to depress the sternum about 1½ to 2 inches. Then the pressure is released without removing your hands from the chest. Compressions are given in a regular, rhythmic fashion.

Performing CPR. CPR is performed only for cardiac arrest. You must determine if cardiac arrest or fainting has occurred. CPR is done when there is unresponsiveness, breathlessness, and pulselessness. Determine unresponsiveness by tapping or gently shaking the victim and shouting "Are you OK?" If there is no response, the victim is unconscious.

Establishing breathlessness involves three steps. *Look* at the victim's chest to see if it rises and falls. *Listen* for the escape of air during expiration. Place your ear near the victim's nose and mouth to listen for the escape of air. *Feel* for the flow of air. To feel for air, place your cheek near the victim's nose.

The carotid artery is used to check for pulselessness. To find the carotid pulse, place the tips of your index and middle fingers on the victim's trachea (windpipe). Then slide your fingertips down off the trachea to the groove of the neck on the side near you (Fig. 26-10).

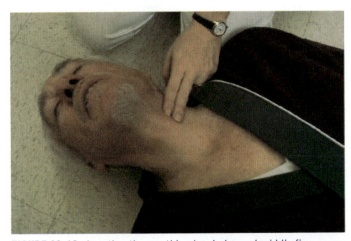

FIGURE 26-10 *Locating the carotid pulse. Index and middle fingers are placed on the trachea. The fingers are moved down into the groove of the neck where the carotid pulse is located.*

PROCEDURE

Adult CPR—One Rescuer

1. Check for unresponsiveness.

2. Call for help. Activate the EMS system.

3. Position the victim supine. Logroll the victim so there is no twisting of the spine. The victim must be on a hard, flat surface. Place the victim's arms alongside the body.

4. Open the airway. Use the head-tilt/chin-lift maneuver.

5. Check for breathlessness.

6. Give 2 ventilations. Each should be 1½ seconds long. Let the victim's chest deflate between ventilations.

7. Check for pulselessness. Check the pulse for 5 to 10 seconds. Use your other hand to keep the airway open with the head-tilt maneuver.

8. Give chest compressions at a rate of 80 to 100 per minute. Give 15 compressions and then 2 ventilations.
   a. Establish a rhythm and count out loud (try: "1 and, 2 and, 3 and, 4 and, 5 and, 6 and, 7 and, 8 and, 9 and, 10 and, 11 and, 12 and, 13 and, 14 and, 15").
   b. Open the airway and give 2 ventilations.
   c. Repeat this step until 4 cycles of 15 compressions and 2 ventilations have been given.

9. Check for a carotid pulse (5 seconds).

10. Resume cycle of 15 compressions and 2 ventilations.

11. Repeat step 8. Check for a pulse every 4 to 5 minutes. Do not interrupt CPR for more than 7 seconds.

PROCEDURE

Adult CPR—Two Rescuers

1. Perform one-person CPR until a helper arrives.

2. Continue chest compressions. The helper says, "I know CPR. Can I help?"

3. Indicate that you want help. Ask that the EMS system be activated, if not already done.

4. Do not stop the chest compressions. The helper kneels on the other side of the victim. The two-rescuer procedure begins after you complete a cycle of 15 compressions and 2 ventilations.

5. Stop compressions for 5 seconds. The helper checks for a carotid pulse. The helper states "No pulse."

6. Perform two-person CPR (Fig. 26-11) as follows:
   a. The helper gives 2 ventilations.
   b. Give chest compressions at a rate of 80 to 100 per minute. Count out loud in a rhythm (try: "1 and, 2 and, 3 and, 4 and, 5").
   c. The helper gives a ventilation immediately after the fifth compression. Pause 1 to 1½ seconds for the ventilation. Continue chest compressions after the ventilation.
   d. A ventilation is given after every fifth compression. Your helper checks for a pulse during the compressions.

7. Stop compressions after 1 minute. Your helper checks for breathing and a pulse. After the first minute, compressions are stopped every few minutes to check for breathing and circulation. Compressions are stopped for only 5 seconds.

8. Call for a switch in positions when you are tired.

9. Change positions quickly as follows:
   a. Helper gives a ventilation after you give the fifth compression.
   b. Helper moves down to kneel at the victim's shoulder and finds the proper hand position.
   c. You move to the victim's head after giving the fifth compression.
   d. Check for a pulse (5 seconds).
   e. Say "No pulse."
   f. Give 1 ventilation before your helper begins chest compressions.

10. Give 1 ventilation after every fifth compression.

11. Switch positions when the person giving the compressions is tired. Check for a pulse and breathing at every position change.

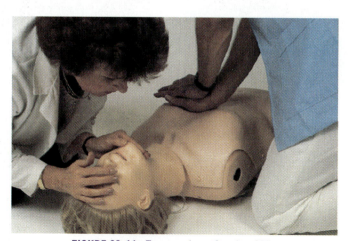

FIGURE 26-11 *Two people performing CPR.*

Obstructed Airway

Airway obstruction (*choking*) can lead to cardiac arrest. Air cannot pass through the air passages to the lungs. The entire body is deprived of oxygen. Airway obstruction often occurs during eating. Meat is the most common food to cause airway obstruction. Choking often occurs on large, poorly chewed pieces of meat. Laughing and talking while eating also are common causes. Elderly persons, especially those in nursing facilities, are at risk for choking. Weakness, poorly fitting dentures, poor swallowing reflexes, and chronic illnesses can lead to choking in these persons. Residents also can choke on hard candy, apples, or pieces of hot dog. Airway obstruction can occur in the unconscious person. Common causes are aspiration of vomitus and the tongue falling back into the airway.

When airway obstruction occurs, the conscious victim will clutch at the throat (Fig. 26-12). The person cannot breathe, speak, or cough and appears pale and cyanotic. The victim will be very apprehensive. The obstruction must be removed immediately before cardiac arrest occurs. The Heimlich maneuver is used to relieve an obstructed airway. It involves abdominal thrusts. The maneuver can be performed with the victim standing, sitting, or lying. The finger sweep is an another maneuver used when an adult victim is unconscious. Call for help when a victim has an obstructed airway. Have someone activate the EMS system.

The Heimlich maneuver is not effective in extremely obese persons or pregnant women. Chest thrusts are used. They are performed as follows:

1. The victim is sitting or standing (Fig. 26-13).
   a. Stand behind the victim.
   b. Place your arms under the victim's arms. Wrap your arms around the victim's chest.
   c. Make a fist. Place the thumb side of the fist on the middle of the sternum.
   d. Grasp the fist with your other hand.
   e. Give backward chest thrusts until the object is expelled or the victim becomes unconscious.
2. The victim is lying down or unconscious.
   a. Position the victim supine.
   b. Kneel next to the victim's body.
   c. Position your hands as for external chest compression.
   d. Give chest thrusts until the object is expelled or the victim becomes unconscious.

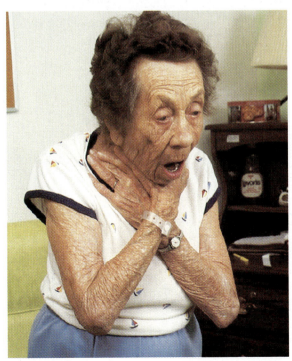

FIGURE 26-12 *A choking person usually will clutch the throat.*

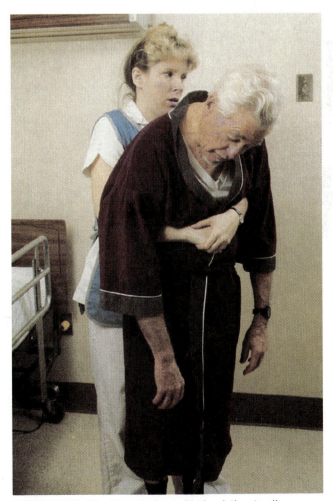

FIGURE 26-13 *Chest thrusts done with the victim standing.*

PROCEDURE

Clearing the Obstructed Airway—The Conscious Adult

1. Ask the victim if he or she is choking.

2. Determine if the victim can cough or speak.

3. Perform the Heimlich maneuver (abdominal thrusts) if the victim is standing or sitting (Fig. 26-14).
   a. Stand behind the victim.
   b. Wrap your arms around the victim's waist.
   c. Make a fist with one hand. Place the thumb side of the fist against the abdomen. The fist is in the middle above the navel and below the end of the sternum.

   d. Grasp your fist with your other hand.
   e. Press your fist and hand into the victim's abdomen with a quick, upward thrust.
   f. Repeat the abdominal thrust until the object has been expelled or the victim loses consciousness.

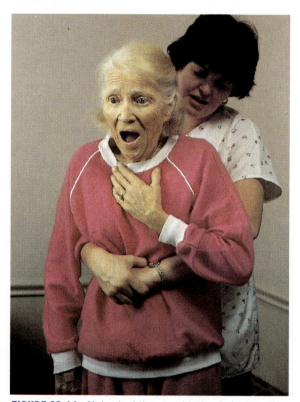

FIGURE 26-14 *Abdominal thrusts with the victim standing.*

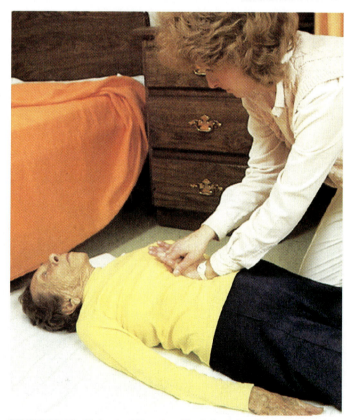

FIGURE 26-15 *Abdominal thrusts with victim lying down.*

PROCEDURE

Clearing the Obstructed Airway—The Unconscious Adult

1. Check for unresponsiveness.

2. Call for help.

3. Logroll the victim to the supine position with his or her face up. The victim's arms should be at the sides.

4. Open the airway. Use the head-tilt/chin-lift maneuver.

5. Check for breathlessness.

6. Give 1 ventilation. Reposition the victim's head, and open the airway if you could not ventilate. Give 1 ventilation.

7. Have someone activate the EMS system.

8. Do the Heimlich maneuver.
   a. Kneel next to the victim's thighs.
   b. Place the heel of one hand against the middle of the victim's abdomen. It should be in the middle of the abdomen between the lower end of the sternum and the navel.
   c. Place your other hand on top of the hand on the victim's abdomen (Fig. 26-15).
   d. Give an abdominal thrust. Press inward and upward.
   e. Give 5 abdominal thrusts.

9. Do the finger sweep maneuver to check for a foreign object.
   a. Open the victim's mouth. Use the tongue-jaw lift maneuver (Fig. 26-16).
      (1) Grasp the tongue and lower jaw with your thumb and fingers.
      (2) Lift the lower jaw upward.
   b. Insert your other index finger into the mouth along the side of the cheek and deep into the throat. Your finger should be at the base of the tongue.
   c. Form a hook with your index finger.
   d. Try to dislodge and remove the foreign object. Do not push it deeper into the throat.
   e. Grasp and remove the object if it is within reach.

10. Open the airway with the head-tilt/chin-lift method.

11. Give 1 ventilation. Repeat steps 8 through 10, and give 1 ventilation.

12. Repeat step 8 through 11 for as long as necessary.

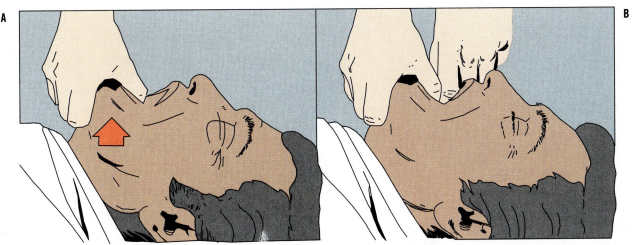

FIGURE 26-16 *Tongue-jaw lift maneuver. **A,** The victim's tongue is grasped, and the jaw is lifted forward with one hand. **B,** The index finger of the other hand is used to check for a foreign object.*

HEMORRHAGE

Life and body functions require an adequate blood supply. Circulation of blood through the body also is required. If a blood vessel is torn or cut, bleeding and blood loss occur. The larger the blood vessel, the greater the bleeding and blood loss. **Hemorrhage** is the excessive loss of blood from a blood vessel. If bleeding is not stopped, death will result.

Hemorrhage may be internal or external. Internal hemorrhage cannot be seen. Bleeding occurs inside the body into tissues and body cavities. Pain, shock (see p. 548), vomiting blood, coughing up blood, and loss of consciousness are signs of internal hemorrhage. There is little you can do for internal bleeding. Keep the person warm, flat, and quiet until medical help arrives. Fluids are not given.

External bleeding usually is seen. However, it may be hidden by clothing. Bleeding may be from an injured artery or a vein. Bleeding from an artery is bright red and occurs in spurts. There is a steady flow of blood when bleeding is from a vein. Basic emergency care for external hemorrhage involves stopping the bleeding. The treatment of choice is to apply direct pressure to the bleeding site. If direct pressure does not control bleeding, pressure is applied to the artery above the bleeding site. You can do the following to control external hemorrhage:

1. Call for help. Have someone activate the EMS system if possible.
2. Use universal precautions and follow the blood-borne pathogen standard. Wear gloves if possible.
3. Place a sterile dressing directly over the wound. Any clean material (handkerchief, towel, cloth, or sanitary napkin) can be used if there is no sterile dressing.
4. Apply pressure with your hand directly over the bleeding site (Fig. 26-17). Do not release the pressure until the bleeding is controlled.
5. If direct pressure does control bleeding, apply pressure over the artery above the bleeding site (Fig. 26-18). Use your first three fingers. For example, if bleeding is from the lower arm, apply pressure over the brachial artery. The brachial artery supplies blood to the lower arm.

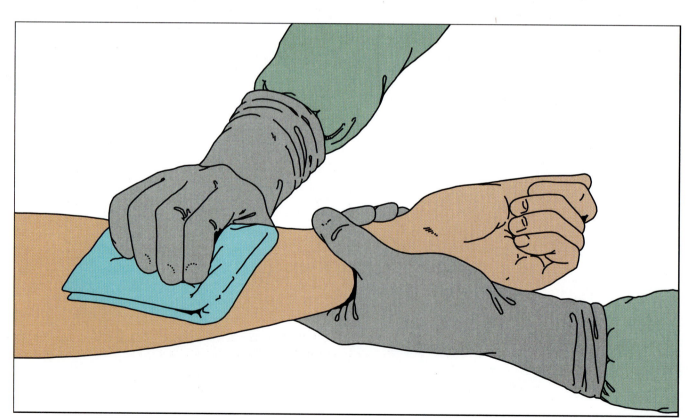

FIGURE 26-17 *Direct pressure is applied to the wound to stop bleeding. The hand is placed over the wound.*

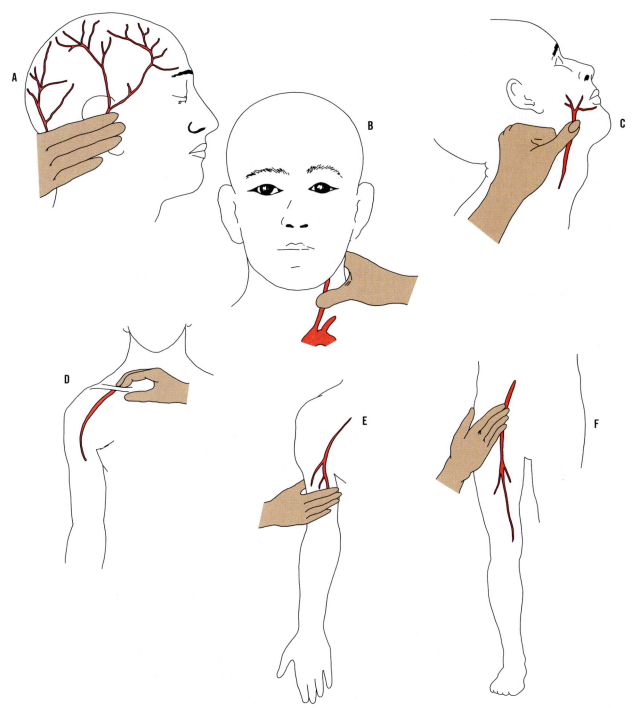

FIGURE 26-18 *Pressure points to control bleeding.* **A,** *Temporal artery.* **B,** *Carotid artery.* **C,** *External maxillary artery.* **D,** *Subclavian artery.* **E,** *Brachial artery.* **F,** *Femoral artery. (Modified from Billings DM, Stokes LG:* Medical-surgical nursing: common health problems of adults and children across the life span, *St Louis, 1982, Mosby–Year Book.)*

SHOCK

Shock occurs when there is an inadequate blood supply to organs and tissues. Blood loss, heart disease, and severe infection can cause shock. Signs and symptoms include low or falling blood pressure; a rapid and weak pulse; cold, moist, and pale skin; rapid respirations; thirst; and restlessness. Confusion and loss of consciousness occur as shock becomes worse.

Shock is possible in any person who is acutely ill or injured. Do the following to prevent or to treat shock:

1. Keep the victim lying down.
2. Control hemorrhage.
3. Keep the victim warm. Place a blanket over and under the victim if possible.
4. Reassure the victim.
5. Summon medical assistance.

SEIZURES

Seizures (convulsions) are violent and sudden contractions or tremors of muscles. They are due to an abnormality within the brain. The abnormality may be caused by head injury during birth, high fever, brain tumors, poisoning, or central nervous system infections. Head trauma and lack of blood flow to the brain also can cause seizures. The terms "attack" and "fits" have been used by people outside the health profession in referring to seizures. Do not use these terms. They have unpleasant and disturbing meanings.

There are many types of seizures. You need to be aware of two types. The *tonic-clonic* type *(grand mal seizure)* has two phases. The tonic phase is first. The person loses consciousness. The person, if standing or sitting, falls to the floor. The body is rigid. This occurs because all muscles contract at once. The clonic phase is next. Muscle groups contract and relax. This causes jerking and twitching movements of the body. Urinary and fecal incontinence may occur during this phase. After the seizure the person usually falls into a deep sleep. On awakening, the person may experience confusion and headache.

The *generalized absence* type *(petit mal seizure)* usually lasts 5 to 15 seconds. There is loss of consciousness, twitching of arm and face muscles, and rolling of the eyes. The person appears to be staring.

The person must to be protected from injury during a seizure. The following measures are performed:

1. Call for help.
2. Lower the person to the floor.
3. Place a folded bath blanket or towel under the person's head. Or cradle the persons's head in your lap or on a pillow (Fig. 26-19). This prevents the persons's head from striking the floor.
4. Turn the head to one side.
5. Loosen tight clothing.
6. Move furniture and equipment away from the person. The person may strike these objects during the uncontrolled body movements.
7. Do not try to restrain body movements during the seizure.
8. Position the person on one side if possible.
9. Summon medical help. Do not leave the resident during the seizure.

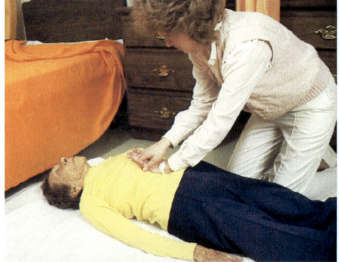

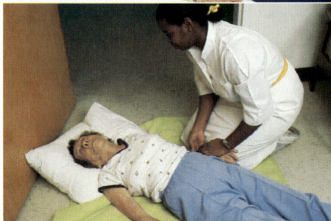

FIGURE 26-19 *Resident's head is protected during a seizure.*

4. Do not let the person get up until symptoms have subsided for about 5 minutes.
5. Help the person to a sitting position after recovery from fainting. Observe for symptoms of fainting.

STROKE

Stroke (cerebrovascular accident) was described in Chapter 23. A stroke occurs when the brain is suddenly deprived of its blood supply. Usually only a part of the brain is affected. A stroke may be caused by a thrombus, an embolus, or cerebral hemorrhage. Cerebral hemorrhage is due to the rupture of a blood vessel in the brain.

The signs of stroke vary. They depend on the size and location of brain injury. Loss of consciousness or semi-consciousness, rapid pulse, labored respirations, elevated blood pressure, vomiting, and hemiplegia are signs of stroke. The person may have aphasia (the inability to speak). Seizures may occur.

Emergency care includes the following:

1. Turn the person onto the affected side. The affected side is limp and the cheek appears puffy.
2. Elevate the head without flexing the neck.
3. Loosen tight clothing.
4. Keep the person quiet and warm.
5. Reassure the person.
6. Summon medical help

VOMITING

Vomiting is the act of expelling stomach contents through the mouth. Although not a true emergency, vomiting is a sign of illness or injury. It can be life-threatening. The vomitus (material vomited) can be aspirated and obstruct the airway. Shock also can occur if large amounts of blood are vomited.

The following measures will help the vomiting resident:

1. Use universal precautions. Wear gloves if possible. Also follow the bloodborne pathogen standard
2. Turn the person's head well to one side. This prevents aspiration.
3. Place an emesis basin under the person's chin.
4. Remove the vomitus from the resident's immediate environment.
5. Let the person use mouthwash and perform oral hygiene. This helps eliminate the taste of vomitus.
6. Eliminate odors.
7. Change linens as necessary.

Observe the vomitus for color, odor, and undigested food. Vomitus that looks like coffee grounds contains digested blood. This indicates bleeding. The amount of vomitus is measured. The amount is reported to the nurse and recorded on the I&O record. A specimen may be saved for laboratory study. Do not discard vomitus until it has been observed by the nurse.

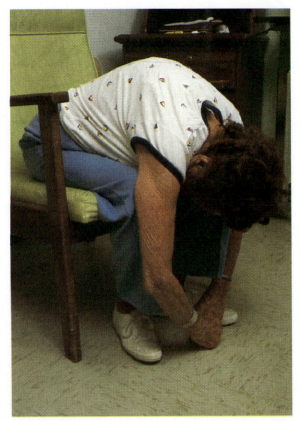

FIGURE 26-20 *A person bends forward and places the head between the knees to prevent fainting.*

FAINTING

Fainting is the sudden loss of consciousness as a result of an inadequate blood supply to the brain. Hunger, fatigue, fear, and pain are common causes. Some people faint at the sight of blood or injury. Fainting also can be caused by standing in one position for a long time or being in a warm, crowded room. Dizziness, perspiration, and blackness before the eyes may occur before the person faints. The person looks pale. The pulse is weak. Respirations are shallow if the person loses consciousness. Emergency care for fainting includes the following:

1. Have the person sit or lie down before fainting occurs.
   a. If the person is in the sitting position, have him or her bend forward and place the head between the knees if this position is possible (Fig. 26-20).
   b. If the person is lying down, elevate his or her legs.
2. Loosen tight clothing.
3. Keep the person lying down if fainting has occurred.

Quality OF LIFE

Quality of life must be protected in emergency situations. The victim is a person. He or she must be treated with dignity and respect.

The right to privacy and confidentiality must be protected. The person should not be exposed unnecessarily. You may be in a place where you cannot close doors, shades, and curtains. The victim may be in a lounge, dining area, or public place. Do what you can to protect the person's privacy.

Onlookers are major threats to privacy and confidentiality. If you are giving emergency care, your main concern is the victim's illness or injuries. It is hard to give care and manage onlookers at the same time. You can ask someone else to deal with the onlookers. If someone else is giving care, you can help by keeping onlookers away from the victim.

People are naturally curious. They want to know what happened, the extent of injuries or illness, and if the person will be okay. You must be careful not to discuss the situation. Remember, information about the person's care, treatment, and condition are confidential. Also remember that only doctors can make diagnoses. You can make observations about signs and symptoms. Only the doctor can determine what is wrong with the person.

The right to personal choice also must be protected. It is often hard to give the choices in emergencies. However, they should be given when possible. Hospital care may be required. The person has the right to choose which hospital to be taken to.

Personal possessions must be protected from loss and damage. Dentures and eyeglasses often are lost or broken in emergencies. Watches and other jewelry are easily lost. Clothing may be torn or cut. You must be very careful to protect the person's property. In public places the victim's personal items are given to family members, police, or EMS personnel.

The resident has a right to a safe environment. Physical and psychological safety are important. The person needs to be protected from further injury. For example, the stroke victim must be protected from falls. The person having a seizure must be protected from head injuries. All emergency victims need to feel safe and secure. Reassurance, explanations about care, and a calm approach are important. They help the person feel safe and secure.

SUMMARY

Emergencies are sudden and unexpected. They are frightening to the victim and others nearby. Quick action may be needed to save the victim's life and to prevent injuries from becoming worse. Emergencies can occur anywhere. You may be with the victim when an emergency occurs. Staying calm, knowing what to do, and calling for help are important for the person's physical and psychological well-being.

Cardiac arrest and airway obstruction are deadly and frightening emergencies. You are advised to take a basic life support course. You may be able to save a person's life with the basic life support procedures.

A first aid course also is beneficial. A first aid course will prepare you to function if injuries occur. These include insect stings, fractures, frostbite, poisoning, and eye injuries. The general rules of emergency care apply to any emergency situation. You may not know how to care for the specific injury. However, you can help the victim by following the general rules of emergency care.

Review QUESTIONS

Circle the *best* answer.

1. The goals of first aid are to
   a. Call for help and keep the victim warm
   b. Prevent death and prevent injuries from becoming worse
   c. Stay calm and perform emergency measures
   d. Reassure the victim and keep bystanders away

2. When giving first aid you should
   a. Be aware of your own limitations
   b. Move the victim
   c. Give the victim fluids
   d. Perform any necessary emergency measures

3. Cardiac arrest is
   a. The same as stroke
   b. The sudden stopping of heart action and breathing
   c. The sudden loss of consciousness
   d. The condition that results when there is inadequate blood supply to the organs and tissues of the body

4. Which is *not* a sign of cardiac arrest?
   a. No pulse
   b. No breathing
   c. A sudden drop in blood pressure
   d. Unconsciousness

5. You are going to give mouth-to-mouth resuscitation. You should do the following *except*
   a. Pinch the victim's nostrils shut
   b. Place your mouth tightly over the victim's mouth
   c. Blow air into the victim's mouth as you exhale
   d. Cover the victim's nose and mouth

6. External chest compressions are to be performed. The chest is compressed
   a. ½ to 1 inch
   b. 1 to 1½ inches
   c. 1½ to 2 inches
   d. 2 to 2½ inches

7. Which does *not* determine breathlessness?
   a. Looking to see if the chest rises and falls
   b. Counting respirations for 30 seconds
   c. Listening for the escape of air
   d. Feeling for the flow of air

8. Which is used to feel for a pulse during CPR?
   a. The apical pulse
   b. The brachial pulse
   c. The carotid pulse
   d. The dorsalis pedis pulse

9. CPR is being given by two persons. Ventilations are given
   a. After every fifth compression
   b. After every fifteenth compression
   c. After every compression
   d. Only when positions are changed

10. If airway obstruction occurs, the victim usually will
    a. Clutch at the throat
    b. Be able to speak, cough, and breathe
    c. Be calm
    d. Have a seizure

11. The Heimlich maneuver is used to relieve an obstructed airway. Which statement is *false?*
    a. The victim can be standing, sitting, or lying down.
    b. A fist is made with one hand.
    c. The thrusts are given inward and upward at the lower end of the sternum.
    d. The hands are positioned in the person's midsection, between the waist and lower end of the sternum.

12. A victim has an obstructed airway. You should use poking motions to sweep the victim's mouth out with your index finger.
    a. True
    b. False

13. Arterial bleeding
    a. Cannot be seen
    b. Occurs in spurts
    c. Is dark red
    d. Oozes from the wound

14. A victim is hemorrhaging from the left forearm. Your first action should be to
    a. Lower the body part
    b. Apply pressure to the brachial artery
    c. Apply direct pressure to the wound
    d. Cover the victim

15. The following statements relate to tonic-clonic seizures. Which statement is *false?*
    a. There is contraction of all muscles at once.
    b. The person may stop breathing.
    c. The seizure usually lasts about 10 to 20 seconds.
    d. There is loss of consciousness during the seizure.

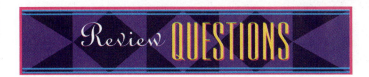

Review QUESTIONS

16. A victim is in shock. You should
    a. Open the airway
    b. Remove the victim's clothing
    c. Keep the victim lying down
    d. Elevate the person's head

17. A person is about to faint. Which statement is *false?*
    a. Take the person outside for some fresh air.
    b. Have the person sit or lie down.
    c. Loosen tight clothing.
    d. Elevate the legs if the person is lying down.

18. Emergency care of the stroke victim includes all of the following *except*
    a. Positioning the resident on the affected side
    b. Giving the person sips of water
    c. Loosening tight clothing
    d. Keeping the person quiet and warm

19. Vomiting is dangerous because of
    a. Aspiration
    b. Cardiac arrest
    c. Fluid loss
    d. Stroke

20. You can promote quality of life in emergency situations by
    a. Providing privacy
    b. Protecting personal possessions from loss or breakage
    c. Protecting the person from further injury
    d. All of the above

Answers

1. b	6. c	11. c	16. c
2. a	7. b	12. b	17. a
3. b	8. c	13. b	18. b
4. c	9. a	14. c	19. a
5. d	10. a	15. c	20. d

27

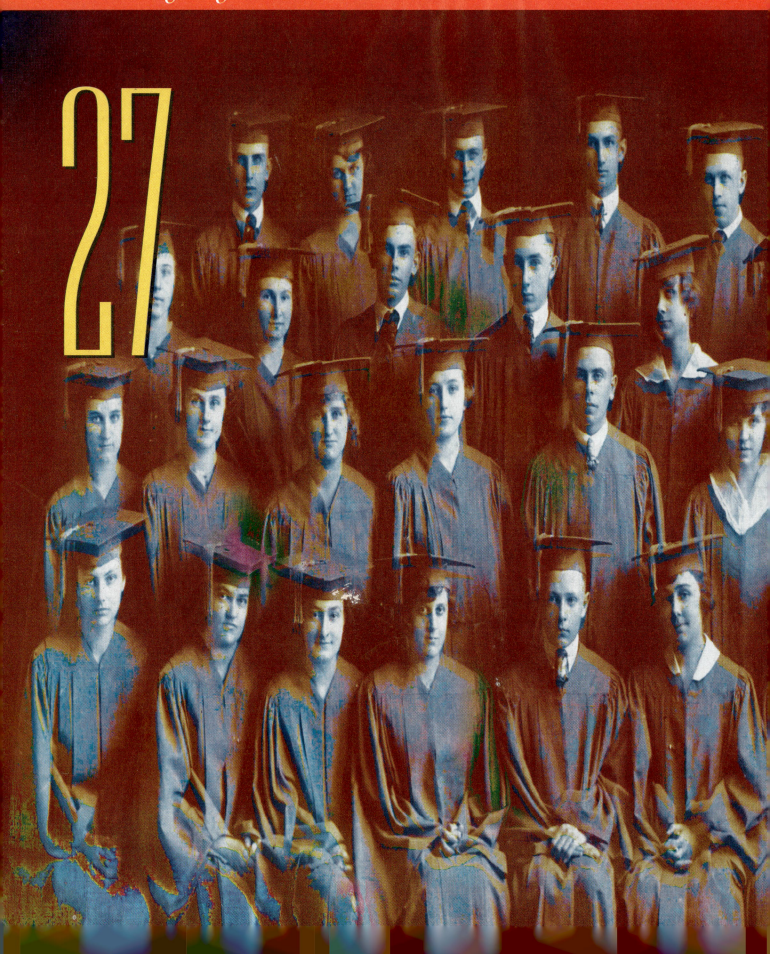

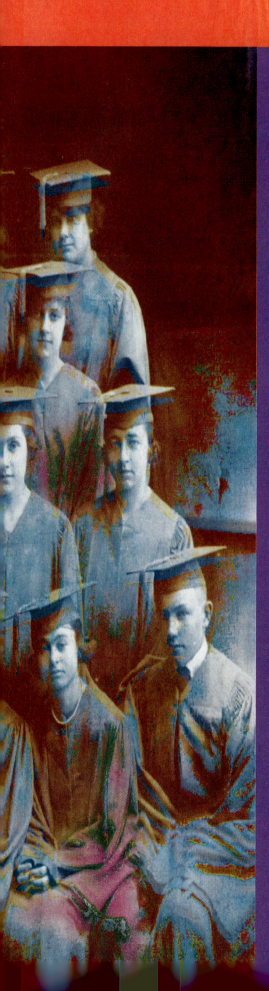

What You Will LEARN

- The key terms listed in this chapter

- Two psychological forces that affect living and dying

- How religion affect attitudes about death

- Beliefs about death held by different age groups

- The five stages of dying

- How to meet the dying resident's psychological, social, and spiritual needs

- How to meet the physical needs of the dying resident

- The needs of the family during the dying process

- The goals of hospice care

- What is meant by a "do not resuscitate" order

- The purpose of living wills

- The signs of approaching death

- The signs of death

- How to assist in giving postmortem care

postmortem
After (post) death (mortem)

reincarnation
The belief that the spirit or soul is reborn in another human body or in another form of life

rigor mortis
The stiffness or rigidity (rigor) of skeletal muscles that occurs after death (mortis)

terminal illness
An illness or injury for which there is no reasonable expectation of recovery

I know I'm not going to get any better. I just hope that my family is with me those final days. ✎

Dying residents often are cared for in nursing facilities. Some are in hospice programs (see Chapter 1). Death can occur suddenly and without warning. Often it is expected.

Health care workers see death often. Many, however, are unsure of their feelings about death. They are uncomfortable with dying people and the subject of death. Dying persons remind them of their own eventual death or the death of a loved one. Dying persons represent helplessness and the failure to cure.

You must examine your own feelings about death. Your attitude about death and dying affects the care you give. Your role is to help meet the person's physical, psychological, social, and spiritual needs. To do so, you need to understand the dying process. Then you can approach the dying resident with caring, kindness, and respect.

TERMINAL ILLNESS

Many illnesses and diseases can be cured or controlled. Others have no cure. Many injuries can be repaired. Others are so serious that the body cannot continue to function. Recovery is not expected. The disease or injury will result in death. An illness or injury for which there is no reasonable expectation of recovery is a **terminal illness.**

Doctors cannot tell exactly when a terminal illness will result in death. A person may be given days, months, weeks, or years to live. Predictions can be wrong. Individuals expected to live for only a short time have lived for years. Others have been given longer to live and have died much sooner.

Modern medicine has brought cures or has prolonged life in many cases. Future research is likely to bring new cures. Living and dying, however, are influenced by two very powerful psychological forces. They are hope and the will to live. Individuals have died sooner than expected or for no apparent reason when they have given up hope or lost the will to live.

ATTITUDES ABOUT DEATH

Experiences, culture, religion, and age influence a person's attitude about death. Many people fear death. Others refuse to believe they will die. Some look forward to and accept death. Attitudes and beliefs about death often change as a person grows older. They also are affected by changing circumstances.

Dying persons often are cared for in health care facilities. As death nears, the family may gather at the bedside to comfort the dying person and each other. In some cultures the dying person is cared for at home by the family. Care for the body after death and preparing it for burial may also be a cultural practice. More commonly, this is done by a funeral director.

People are living longer. Adult children often live far away from elderly parents and grandparents. Therefore many adults and children have never had contact with a dying person. Nor have they been present when death occurred. The process of dying is not seen. Therefore it is viewed as frightening, morbid, and mysterious.

Attitudes about death are closely related to religion. Some persons believe that life after death is free of suffering and hardship. They believe there will be reunion with family and loved ones. Some believe there is punishment and suffering for sins and misdeeds in the afterlife. Others do not believe in an afterlife. They believe that death is the end of life. There also are religious beliefs about the form of the body after death. Some believe the body keeps its physical form. Others believe that only the spirit or soul is present in the afterlife. Still others believe in reincarnation. **Reincarnation** is the belief that the spirit or soul is reborn into another human body or into another form of life. Many people strengthen their religious beliefs during the dying process. Religion often provides a source of comfort for the dying person and the family.

Ideas about death change as people grow older. Infants and toddlers have no concept of death. Children between the ages of 3 and 5 years start to be curious and have ideas about death. They recognize deaths of family members or pets and notice dead birds or bugs. They view death as temporary. Children often blame themselves when someone or something dies. They see the event as punishment for being bad. When children ask questions about death, answers from adults often cause fear and confusion. Children who are told "He is sleeping" may be afraid to go to sleep.

Between the ages of 5 and 7 years, children view death as final. They do not see death in relation to themselves. Death is something that happens to other people. They also think death can be avoided. Children associate death with punishment and mutilation of the body. It also is associated with witches, ghosts, goblins, and monsters.

These ideas come from fairy tales, cartoons, movies, and television.

Adults have more fears about death than do children. They fear pain and suffering, dying alone, and invasion of privacy. They also fear loneliness and being separated from family and loved ones. They worry about who will care for and support loved ones left behind. Adults often resent death. This is particularly true when it interferes with plans, hopes, dreams, and ambitions.

Elderly persons usually have fewer fears about death than do younger adults. They are more accepting that death will occur. They have had more experiences with dying and death. Many have lost family members and friends. Some welcome death as freedom from pain, suffering, and disability. Like younger adults, elderly persons often fear dying alone.

THE STAGES OF DYING

Dr. Elisabeth Kübler-Ross has identified five stages of dying. They are denial, anger, bargaining, depression, and acceptance. During *denial,* persons refuse to believe they are dying. "No, not me" is a common response. The person believes a mistake has been made. Information about the illness or injury is not heard. The person cannot deal with any problem or decision related to the illness or injury. This stage can last for a few hours, days, or much longer. Some people are still in the stage of denial at the time of death.

Anger is the second stage. The person thinks, "Why me?" People behave with anger and rage. They envy and resent those who have life and health. Family, friends, and the health care team usually are targets of their anger. They blame others. They find fault with those who are loved and needed the most. The health care team and family may have a hard time dealing with residents during this stage. Anger is a normal and healthy reaction. Do not take the person's anger personally. You must control any urges to attack back or to avoid the resident.

The third stage is *bargaining.* The person now says, "Yes, me. but. . . ." There is bargaining with God for more time. Promises are made in exchange for more time. The resident may want to see a child marry, see a grandchild, have one more Christmas, or live to see an important event. Usually more promises are made as the resident makes "just one more" request. This stage may not be obvious. Bargaining usually is private and on a spiritual level.

Depression is the fourth stage. The person thinks, "Yes, me." The person is very sad. There is mourning over things that have been lost and the loss of future life. The person may cry or say little. Sometimes the person talks about people and things that will be left behind.

The fifth and final stage of dying is *acceptance* of death. The person is calm and at peace. The person has said what needs to be said. Unfinished business is completed. The person is ready to accept death. A person may be in this stage for many months or years. Reaching acceptance does not mean that death is near.

Dying persons do not always go through all five stages. A person may never get beyond a certain stage. Some move back and forth between stages. For example, a person who has reached acceptance may move back to bargaining. Then the person may move forward to acceptance. Some people are in one stage until death.

PSYCHOLOGICAL, SOCIAL, AND SPIRITUAL NEEDS

Dying persons continue to have psychological, social, and spiritual needs. They may want family and friends present. They may want to talk about the fears, worries, and anxieties of dying. Some want to be alone. Often they want to talk to a member of the nursing team. Residents often need to talk at night. Things are quiet and there are few distractions at this time.

There are two very important aspects of communication in dealing with the dying person. These are listening and touch. The person needs to talk, express feelings, and share worries and concerns. Let the person express feelings and emotions in his or her own way. Just being there and listening helps meet the person's psychological and social needs. Do not worry about saying the wrong thing. Do not worry about finding the right words to comfort the person. Nothing really must be said. Being there for the person is what counts. Touch conveys caring and concern when words cannot. Sometimes the person does not want to talk but needs to have you nearby. Do not feel that you need to talk. Silence, along with touch, is a powerful and meaningful way to communicate.

Spiritual needs are important. The person may wish to see a priest, rabbi, or minister. The person also may want to take part in religious practices. Privacy is provided during spiritual moments. Courtesy is given to the clergy. The resident has the right to have religious objects nearby (medals, pictures, statues, or Bibles). Handle these items like any other valuable.

PHYSICAL NEEDS

Dying may take a few minutes, hours, days, or weeks. There is a general slowing of body processes, weakness, and changes in the level of consciousness. The person is given as much independence as possible. As the person weakens, the nursing team helps meet basic needs. The person may totally depend on others for basic needs and activities of daily living. Every effort is made to promote physical and psychological comfort. The person is allowed to die in peace and dignity.

Vision, Hearing, and Speech

Vision becomes blurred and gradually fails during the dying process. The person naturally turns toward light. A darkened room may be frightening. The eyes may be half open. Secretions may collect in the corners of the eyes. Because of failing vision, you need to explain what is being done to the person or in the room. The room should be well lit. Bright lights and glares, however, are avoided. Good eye care is essential (see Chapter 12). If the eyes stay open, a nurse may apply a protective ointment. Then the eyes are covered with moistened pads to protect them from injury.

Speech becomes difficult and may be hard to understand. Sometimes the person cannot speak. The nursing team needs to anticipate the resident's needs. You should not ask questions that need long answers. "Yes" or "no" questions can be asked but should be kept to a minimum. Although speech may be difficult or impossible for the person, you must still talk to him or her.

Hearing is one of the last functions to be lost during the dying process. Many people hear until the moment of death. Even if unconscious, the person may hear. Always assume that the dying, or any unconscious person, can hear. Speak in a normal voice, and provide reassurance and explanations about care. Offer words of comfort. Topics that could upset the resident are avoided.

Mouth, Nose, and Skin

Oral hygiene is very important for comfort. Routine mouth care usually is enough if the resident can eat and drink. Frequent oral care is given as death nears and when the person has difficulty taking oral fluids. Oral hygiene also is important if mucus collects in the mouth and the person cannot swallow.

Crusting and irritation of the nostrils can occur. Common causes are increased nasal secretions, an oxygen cannula, or an NG tube. Careful cleansing of the nose is important. The nurse may have you apply a lubricant to the nostrils.

Circulation fails and body temperature rises as death approaches. The skin is cool and pale. Perspiration increases. Good skin care, bathing, and the prevention of pressure sores are necessary. Linens and gowns are changed whenever needed because of perspiration. Although the skin feels cool, only light bed coverings may be needed. Blankets may make the person feel warm and cause restlessness.

Elimination

Dying persons may have urinary and anal incontinence. Bed protectors are used. Perineal care is given as necessary. Some residents have constipation and urinary retention. Doctors may order enemas. Foley catheters may be ordered. You may be asked to give enemas and perform catheter care.

Comfort and Positioning

Measures are taken to promote comfort. Good skin care, personal hygiene, back massages, and oral hygiene help to increase comfort. Some people have severe pain. They need strong pain medications, which are given by nurses. You can promote comfort by frequent position changes. Good alignment and supportive devices also promote comfort. Take care when turning the person. You may need help to turn the resident slowly and gently. Residents with breathing difficulties usually prefer the semi-Fowler's position.

The Resident's Room

The person's room should be as pleasant as possible. In addition to being well-lit, it should be well-ventilated. Unnecessary equipment is removed. Some equipment is upsetting to look at (suction machines, drainage containers). If possible, this equipment is kept out of the person's sight.

Mementos, pictures, cards, flowers, religious items, and other significant items comfort and reassure the person. Arranging them within the person's view is appreciated. The resident and family are allowed to arrange the room as they wish. This helps meet the needs of love, belonging, and esteem. The room should be comfortable, pleasant, and reflect the person's choices. This promotes physical and psychological comfort.

THE RESIDENT'S FAMILY

The family is going through a hard time. It may be very hard to find words to comfort them. You can show your feelings to the family by being available, courteous, and considerate. Use touch to show your concern.

The family usually is allowed to spend a lot of time with their loved one. Normal visiting hours usually do not apply if the resident is dying. You must respect the resident's and family's right to privacy. They need as much time together as possible. The resident's care, however, cannot be neglected just because the family is present. Let family members help give care if they wish. If they do not want to help, you can suggest that they take a break. They can use the time to have a beverage or meal.

The family may be very tired, sad, and tearful. They need support and understanding. Watching a loved one die is very painful. So is dealing with the eventual loss of that person. In their grief the family goes through stages like the dying person. They may be very angry. Do not take the anger personally. Try to be understanding. Treat the family with courtesy and respect. Visiting with a member of the clergy may be comforting to the family. You need to communicate this request to the nurse immediately.

HOSPICE CARE

Many residents seek hospice care when they are dying (see Chapter 1). Hospices focus on the physical, emotional, social, and spiritual needs of dying residents and their families. Hospices are not concerned with cure or with life-saving procedures. They emphasize pain relief and comfort measures. Care is designed to improve the dying person's quality of life.

A hospice may be part of a health care facility or a separate facility. Many hospices offer home care. Follow-up care and support groups for survivors also are part of hospice services.

"DO NOT RESUSCITATE" ORDERS

When death is sudden and unexpected, every effort is made to save the person's life. CPR is started. Nurses, doctors, and other emergency staff members rush to the person's bedside. They bring emergency and life-saving equipment. CPR and other life-support measures are continued until the person is resuscitated or until declared dead by the doctor.

Doctors often write "do not resuscitate" (DNR) orders for terminally ill residents. This means that no attempts will be made to resuscitate the person. The person will be allowed to die with peace and dignity. The orders are written after the resident and family have been consulted. The family makes the decision if the resident is not mentally able.

LIVING WILLS

Some persons, especially the terminally ill or elderly, choose not to be resuscitated. They have the right to refuse treatment. Some have written instructions about acceptable treatments and life-prolonging measures. These are called "living wills." A living will states that the person does not want life prolonged by extraordinary means if there is no reasonable expectation of recovery.

Currently, 41 states allow living wills. State laws vary. Most require that the person making the will be 18 years of age or older. Some states require new living wills every 5 or 7 years.

Living wills have been a focus of financial abuse of elderly persons. Some have been charged excessive legal fees—as much as $7,000. Be aware that living wills can be drawn up free or for a very small charge. A local Legal Aid office will give assistance in making living wills.

You may not agree with decisions made about treatment and resuscitation. However, you must follow the resident's or family's wishes and the doctor's orders. These may be against your personal, religious, and cultural values. If so, discuss the situation with the nurse. It may be necessary to change your assignments.

SIGNS OF DEATH

You need to know the signs of approaching death. The following signs may occur rapidly or gradually:

1. Movement, muscle tone, and sensation are lost. This usually begins in the feet and legs and eventually spreads to the rest of the body. When mouth muscles relax, the jaw drops. The mouth may stay open. There is often a peaceful facial expression.
2. Peristalsis and other gastrointestinal functions slow down. There may be abdominal distention, anal incontinence, fecal impaction, nausea, and vomiting.
3. Circulation fails and body temperature rises. The resident feels cool or cold, looks pale, and perspires heavily. The pulse is fast, weak, and irregular. Blood pressure begins to fall.
4. The respiratory system fails. Cheyne-Stokes, slow, or rapid and shallow respirations may be observed. Mucus collects in the respiratory tract. This causes the "death rattle" to be heard.
5. Pain decreases as the resident loses consciousness. Some persons, however, are conscious until the moment of death.

The signs of death include the absence of pulse, respirations, and blood pressure. The pupils are fixed and dilated. A doctor determines that death has occurred and pronounces the person dead.

CARE OF THE BODY AFTER DEATH

Care of the body after (*post*) death (*mortem*) is called **postmortem** care. A nurse is responsible for postmortem care. You may be asked to assist. Care begins as soon as the doctor pronounces the resident dead. Universal precautions and the bloodborne pathogen standard are followed. You may have contact with infected body fluids or body substances.

Postmortem care is done to maintain good appearance of the body. Discoloration and skin damage are prevented. Postmortem care also includes gathering valuables and personal items for the family. The right to privacy and the right to be treated with dignity and respect apply.

Within 2 to 4 hours after death, rigor mortis develops. **Rigor mortis** is the stiffness or rigidity (*rigor*) of skeletal muscles that occurs after death (*mortis*). Postmortem care involves positioning the body in normal alignment before rigor mortis sets in. Also, the family may wish to view the body before it is taken to the funeral home. The body should appear in a comfortable and natural position for viewing by the family.

In some facilities the body is prepared only for viewing. Postmortem care is completed later by the funeral director.

Assisting With Postmortem Care

1. Wash your hands.

2. Collect the following:
   a. Postmortem kit if used in your facility (shroud, gown, two tags, gauze squares, and safety pins)
   b. Valuables list
   c. Waterproof bed protectors
   d. Wash basin
   e. Bath towels
   f. Washcloth
   g. Tape
   h. Dressing
   i. Disposable gloves

3. Provide for privacy.

4. Raise the bed to the best level for good body mechanics.

5. Make sure the bed is flat.

6. Put on gloves.

7. Position the body supine. Arms and legs are straight. Place a pillow under the head and shoulders (Fig. 27-1).

8. Close the eyes. Gently pull the eyelids over the eyes. Apply moistened cotton balls gently over the eyelids if the eyes will not stay closed.

9. Insert dentures if it is facility policy. If not, put them in a labeled denture container.

10. Close the mouth. Place a rolled towel under the chin to support the mouth in the closed position if necessary.

11. Remove all jewelry except for wedding rings. List jewelry that has been removed. Place the jewelry and the list in an envelope to be given to the family.

12. Place a cotton ball over the ring and secure it in place with tape.

13. Remove drainage bottles, bags, and containers. Leave tubes and catheters in place if an autopsy is to be performed. Ask the nurse about the removal of tubes.

14. Bathe soiled areas with plain water. Dry thoroughly.

15. Place a bed protector under the buttocks.

16. Remove soiled dressings and replace them with clean ones.

17. Put a clean gown on the body. Make sure the body is positioned as in Step 7.

18. Brush and comb the hair if necessary.

19. Fill out the ID tags. Tie one to an ankle or to the right big toe.

20. Cover the body to the shoulders with a sheet if the family is to view the body.

21. Collect the resident's belongings. Put them in a bag marked with the resident's name.

22. Remove all used supplies, equipment, and linens except the shroud and the other ID tag. Make sure the room is neat. Adjust the lighting so it is soft.

23. Let the family view the body. Provide for privacy. Give the resident's belongings to the family.

24. Place the body on the shroud or cover the body with a sheet after the family has left the room. Apply the shroud (Fig. 27-2).
    a. Bring the top down over the head.
    b. Fold the bottom up over the feet.
    c. Fold the sides over the body.

25. Secure the shroud in place with safety pins or tape.

26. Attach the second ID tag to the shroud.

27. Leave the body on the bed for the funeral director. Leave the denture cup with the body.

28. Remove the gloves.

29. Strip the resident's unit after the body has been removed. Wear gloves for this step.

30. Wash your hands.

31. Report the following to the nurse:
    a. The time the body was taken by the funeral director
    b. What was done with jewelry and personal belongings
    c. What was done with dentures

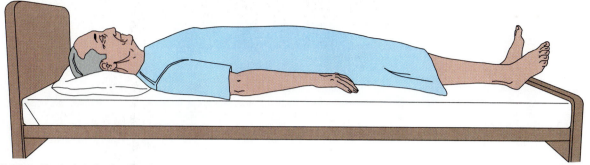

FIGURE 27-1 *The body is in the dorsal recumbent position. Arms are straight at the sides. There is a pillow under the head and shoulders.*

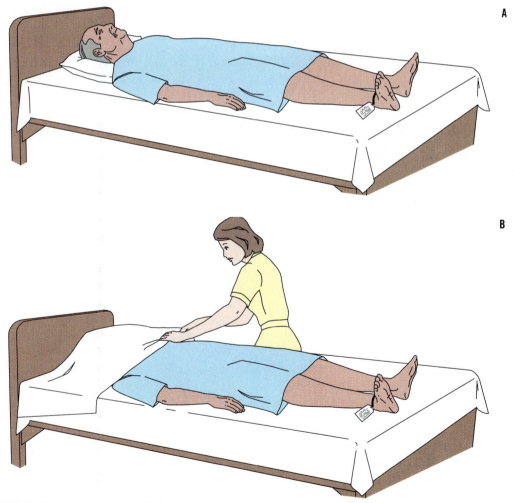

A

B

FIGURE 27-2 *Applying a shroud. **A,** Place the body on the shroud. **B,** Bring the top of the shroud down over the head.*

Continued.

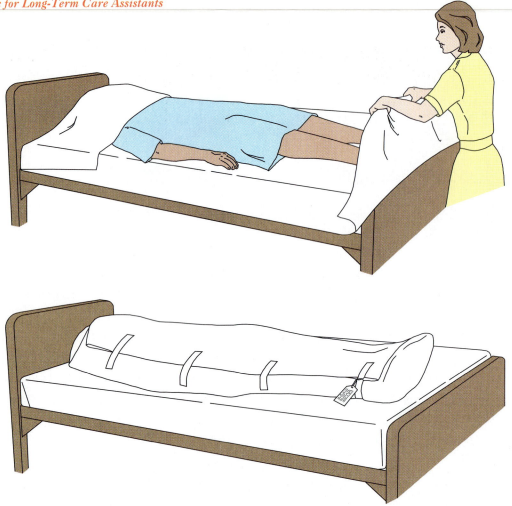

FIGURE 27-2 *C, Fold the bottom over the feet.* **D,** *Fold the sides over the body, tape or pin the sides together, and attach the identification tag.*

List 27 -1

The Dying Person's Bill of Rights

I have the right to be treated as a living human being until I die.

I have the right to maintain a sense of hopefulness, however changing its focus may be.

I have the right to be cared for by those who can maintain a sense of hopefulness, however changing this might be.

I have the right to express my feelings and emotions about my approaching death, in my own way.

I have the right to participate in decisions concerning my care.

I have the right to expect continuing medical and nursing attention even though "cure" goals must be changed to "comfort" goals.

I have the right not to die alone.

I have the right to be free from pain.

I have the right to have my questions answered honestly.

I have the right not to be deceived.

I have the right to have help from and for my family accepting my death.

I have the right to die in peace and dignity.

I have the right to retain my individuality and not be judged for my decisions, which may be contrary to the beliefs of others.

I have the right to discuss and enlarge my religious and/or spiritual experiences, regardless of what they may mean to others.

I have the right to expect that the sanctity of the human body will be respected after death.

I have the right to be cared for by caring, sensitive, knowledgeable people who will attempt to understand my needs and will be able to gain some satisfaction in helping me face my death.

From Barbus AJ: *Am J Nurs* 75(1):99, 1975.

562

Quality OF LIFE

Quality of life is important to residents and their families. A person has the right to die in peace and with dignity. See List 27-1 for the Dying Person's Bill of Rights. The dying person also has rights under OBRA.

You must protect the resident's right to privacy and confidentiality. Remember, the person must not be exposed unnecessarily. The person has the right not to have his or her body seen by others. Proper draping and screening procedures are important.

The resident and family or other visitors have the right to visit in private. The dying person is likely to be too weak to leave the bed or room. Therefore the roommate may have to leave the room. The nurse will try to work out an arrangement that is satisfactory to both roommates. The dying resident may be moved to a private room. This gives the resident and family privacy. The family also can stay as long as they like. In addition, a roommate's right to privacy is protected.

The right to confidentiality is important. This right must be protected before and after death. The resident's condition and diagnoses are shared only with those involved with the person's care. The resident's final moments and cause of death also are kept confidential. So are statements, conversations, and reactions of the family.

The dying resident has the right to be free from abuse, mistreatment, and neglect. Some health care workers avoid the dying person. They are uncomfortable with death and dying. Others have superstitions or religious beliefs about being near dying people. Abuse and mistreatment may occur. Family members or health care workers may be the sources of such actions. The dying person may be too weak to report the abuse or mistreatment. Or the person may feel that punishment is deserved for needing so much care. The person has the right to receive kind and respectful care before and after death. Be sure to report signs of abuse, mistreatment, or neglect to the nurse.

Freedom from restraint applies to the dying resident. Restraints are used only if ordered by the doctor. Dying residents often are too weak to be dangerous to themselves or others.

You must be careful to protect the resident's personal possessions. Dying residents may want certain photos and religious items nearby. Such religious items may include medals, a rosary, a Bible, a crucifix, and candles. It is important that such items be provided if possible. The resident's possessions must be protected from loss or damage before and after death. They may be passed on as family treasures or momentos.

The resident has a right to a safe and homelike environment. Dying residents usually depend on others for safety. All health care workers are responsible for keeping the environment safe and homelike. Remember, the facility is the resident's home. Try to keep equipment and supplies out of the view. The room also should be free of unpleasant odors and noises. Do your best to keep the room neat and clean.

Continued.

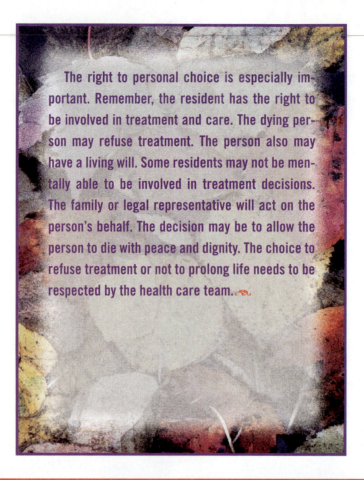

The right to personal choice is especially important. Remember, the resident has the right to be involved in treatment and care. The dying person may refuse treatment. The person also may have a living will. Some residents may not be mentally able to be involved in treatment decisions. The family or legal representative will act on the person's behalf. The decision may be to allow the person to die with peace and dignity. The choice to refuse treatment or not to prolong life needs to be respected by the health care team.

SUMMARY

American society values youth, beauty, and life. The topic of death usually is avoided. Many people die in health care facilities. Therefore health care workers see death often.

You may be uncomfortable with the subject of death. If so, you will be uncomfortable with dying residents. Some people feel medicine should keep people alive. They will be angry and frustrated with the dying resident. Certain behaviors are seen when health care workers are not comfortable with death and dying. They include avoiding the resident, nervous conversation, hurried care, rough handling, and minimizing the resident's needs. You may need to discuss your feelings about death with a nurse, other health care workers, or a member of the clergy. This will help you develop a more positive attitude about death.

The terminally ill resident must be allowed to die with peace and dignity. The person is encouraged to be independent for as long as possible. As the person weakens and death approaches, the nursing team will assist with basic needs. The resident will rely more and more on the nursing team for care and comfort. Even though the person is dying, basic needs continue.

The health care team is concerned with the dying person's psychological, social, and spiritual comfort. Visits from the clergy often are appreciated. The dying person also likes staff members to visit, sit quietly at the bedside, and use touch. Remember that silence and touch are very effective ways to communicate with the resident and family. Respect and protect the resident's rights. They must be protected both before and after death.

Postmortem care is given after death. Each facility has its own policies and procedures about care of the body after death. Postmortem care always includes treating the body with dignity and respect and respecting the right to privacy.

Circle the *best* answer.

1. Which is *true?*
   a. Death from terminal illness is sudden and unexpected.
   b. Doctors know when death will occur.
   c. An illness is terminal when there is no reasonable hope of recovery.
   d. All severe injuries result in death.

2. Two psychological forces that influence living and dying are
   a. Hope and the will to live
   b. Reincarnation and belief in the afterlife
   c. Denial and anger
   d. Bargaining and depression

3. These statements relate to attitudes about death. Which is *false?*
   a. Dying people often are cared for in health care facilities.
   b. Attitudes about death are influenced by religion.
   c. Infants and toddlers understand death.
   d. Families often gather around the bed of the dying person.

4. Reincarnation is the belief that
   a. There is no afterlife
   b. The spirit or soul is reborn into another human body or another form of life
   c. The body keeps its physical form in the afterlife
   d. Only the spirit or soul is present in the afterlife

5. Infants and toddlers view death
   a. As temporary
   b. Have no concept of death
   c. As adults do
   d. As going to sleep

6. Adults and elderly persons usually fear
   a. Dying alone
   b. Punishment for sins
   c. Reincarnation
   d. The five stages of dying

7. Persons in the stage of denial
   a. Are angry
   b. Make "deals" with God
   c. Are sad and quiet
   d. Refuse to believe they are dying

8. The dying person tries to gain more time during
   a. Anger
   b. Bargaining
   c. Depression
   d. Acceptance

9. When caring for the dying resident, you should
   a. Use touch and listening
   b. Do most of the talking
   c. Keep the room darkened
   d. Speak in a loud voice

10. As death approaches, the last sense to be lost is
    a. Sight
    b. Taste
    c. Smell
    d. Hearing

11. Care of the dying resident includes the following *except*
    a. Eye care
    b. Mouth care
    c. Active range-of-motion exercises
    d. Position changes

12. The dying resident should be positioned in
    a. The supine position
    b. The Fowler's position
    c. Good body alignment
    d. The dorsal recumbent position

13. A "do not resuscitate" order has been written. This means that
    a. CPR will not be done
    b. The person has a living will
    c. Life-prolonging measures will be carried out
    d. The person will be kept alive as long as possible

14. Which are *not* signs of approaching death?
    a. Increased body temperature and rapid pulse
    b. Loss of movement and muscle tone
    c. Increased pain and blood pressure
    d. Cheyne-Stokes respirations and the "death rattle"

15. The signs of death are
    a. Convulsions and incontinence
    b. No pulse, respirations, or blood pressure
    c. Loss of consciousness and convulsions
    d. The eyes stay open, there are no muscle movements, and the body is rigid

16. Postmortem care is done
    a. After rigor mortis sets in
    b. After the doctor pronounces the person dead
    c. When the funeral director arrives for the body
    d. After the family has viewed the body

Answers

1. c	5. b	9. a	13. a
2. a	6. a	10. d	14. c
3. c	7. d	11. c	15. b
4. b	8. b	12. c	16. b

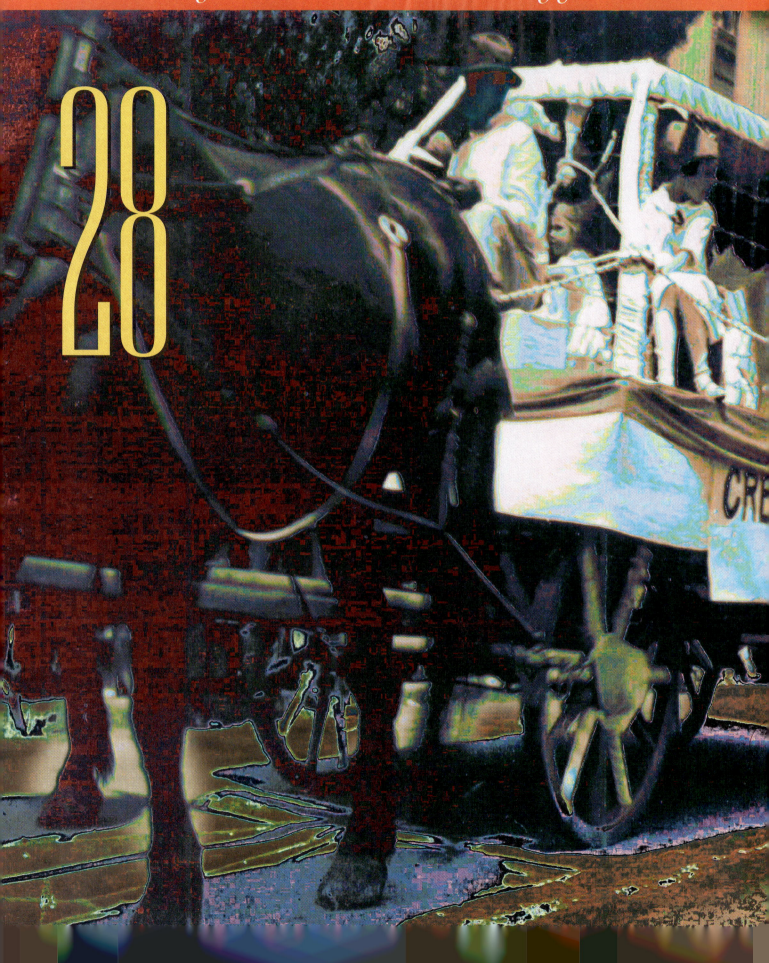

28

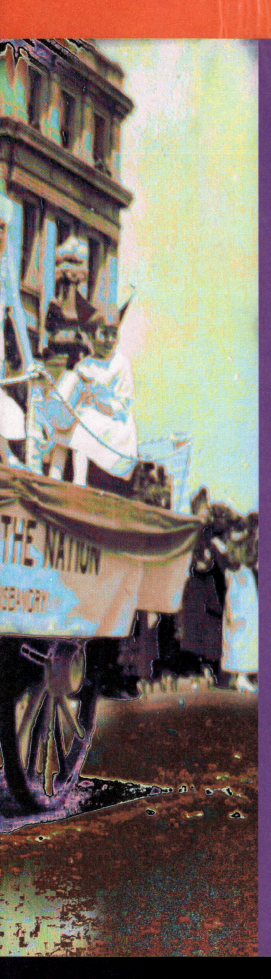

What You Will LEARN

- The key terms listed in this chapter

- Three word elements used in medical terms

- How to translate Greek and Latin prefixes and suffixes into the English language

- How to combine word elements into medical terms

- How to translate medical terms into English

- The four abdominal regions

- The directional terms used to describe the positions of the body in relation to other body parts

- The abbreviations used in health care and their meanings

abbreviation
A shortened form of a word or phrase

combining vowel
A vowel added between two roots or a root and a suffix to make pronunciation easier

prefix
A word element placed at the beginning of a word to change the meaning of the word

root
A word element that contains the basic meaning of the word

suffix
A word element placed at the end of a root to change the meaning of the word

word element
A part of a word

Some of those medical words sound awfully scary. The staff doesn't use many of those words. They tell me the meaning when they do.

Many people think there are secrets and mysteries to the language of medicine—the private language of doctors and nurses. Yet people use medical terms every day. You probably know the terms "flu," "cancer," "appendectomy," and "pneumonia." Health and medicine get a lot of attention on television and in newspapers and magazines. Because of greater news coverage, medical terms are used and understood more now than in the past.

Learning medical terminology is important for nursing assistants. As you gain more knowledge and experience, you will understand and use medical terms with ease and frequency. Learning medical terms for illnesses, diseases, and such common things as bruises, baldness, and a "runny nose" can be fun and educational. This chapter introduces medical terminology and the common abbreviations used in health care.

WORD ELEMENTS OF MEDICAL TERMS

Like all words, medical terms are made up of parts or **word elements.** These elements are combined in various ways to form the medical term. The term can be translated by separating the word into its elements. The word elements important to medical terminology are prefixes, roots, and suffixes.

Prefixes

A **prefix** is a word element placed at the beginning of a word. A prefix changes the meaning of the word. The prefix *olig* (scant, small amount) can be placed before the word *uria* (urine). The word *oliguria* is made. It means a scant amount of urine. Prefixes always are combined with other words. They are never used alone. Most prefixes are Greek or Latin. You need to learn the following prefixes to begin understanding medical terminology.

Prefix	Meaning
a-, an-	without or not
ab-	away from
ad-	toward
ante-	before, forward
anti-	against
auto-	self
bi-	double, two

Prefix	Meaning
brady-	slow
circum-	around
contra-	against, opposite
de-	down, from, away from, not
dia-	across, through, apart
dis-	separation, away from
dys-	bad, difficult, abnormal
ecto-	outer, outside
en-	in, into, within
endo-	inner, inside
epi-	over, on, upon
eryth-	red
ex-	out, out of, from, away from
hemi-	half
hyper-	excessive, too much, high
hypo-	under, decreased, less than normal
in-	in, into, within, not
inter-	between
intra-	within
intro-	into, within
leuk-	white
macro-	large
mal-	bad, illness, disease
mega-	large
micro-	small
mono-	one, single
neo-	new
non-	not
olig-	small, scant
para-	similar, beside
per-	by, through
peri-	around
poly-	many, much
post-	after, behind
pre-	before, in front of, prior to
pro-	before, in front of
re-	again
retro-	backward
semi-	half
sub-	under
super-	above, over, excess
supra-	above, over
tachy-	fast, rapid
trans-	across
uni-	one

ROOTS

The **root** contains the basic meaning of the word. It can be combined with another root, with prefixes, and with suffixes in various combinations to form a medical term. Like prefixes, roots are mainly from the Greek and Latin languages.

A vowel may be added when two roots are combined or when a suffix is added to a root. The vowel is called a **combining vowel.** It usually is an "o." An "i" sometimes is used when there is no vowel between the two combined roots or between the root and the suffix. A combining vowel makes pronunciation easier.

The most common roots and their combining vowels are listed here.

Root (combining vowel)	Meaning
abdomin(o)	abdomen
aden(o)	gland
adren(o)	adrenal gland
angi(o)	vessel
arterio	artery
arthr(o)	joint
broncho	bronchus, bronchi
card, cardi(o)	heart
cephal(o)	head
chole, chol(o)	bile
chondr(o)	cartilage
colo	colon, large intestine
cost(o)	rib
crani(o)	skull
cyan(o)	blue
cysto(o)	bladder, cyst
cyt(o)	cell
dent(o)	tooth
derma	skin
duoden(o)	duodenum
encephal(o)	brain
enter(o)	intestines
fibr(o)	fiber, fibrous
gastr(o)	stomach
gloss(o)	tongue
gluc(o)	sweetness, glucose
glyc(o)	sugar
gyn, gyne, gyneco-	woman
hem, hema, hemo, hemat(o)	blood
hepat(o)	liver
hydr(o)	water
hyster(o)	uterus
ile(o), ili(o)	ileum
laparo	abdomen, loin, or flank
laryng(o)	larynx
lith(o)	stone
mamm(o)	breast, mammary gland
mast(o)	mammary gland, breast
meno	menstruation
my(o)	muscle
myel(o)	spinal cord, bone marrow

Root (combining vowel)	Meaning
necro	death
nephr(o)	kidney
neur(o)	nerve
ocul(o)	eye
oophor(o)	ovary
ophthalm(o)	eye
orth(o)	straight, normal, correct
oste(o)	bone
ot(o)	ear
ped(o)	child, foot
pharyng(o)	pharynx
phleb(o)	vein
pnea	breathing, respiration
pneum(o)	lung, air, gas
proct(o)	rectum
psych(o)	mind
pulmo	lung
py(o)	pus
rect(o)	rectum
rhin(o)	nose
salping(o)	eustachian tube, uterine tube
splen(o)	spleen
sten(o)	arrow, constriction
stern(o)	sternum
stomat(o)	mouth
therm(o)	heat
thoraco	chest
thromb(o)	clot, thrombus
thyr(o)	thyroid
toxic(o)	poison, poisonous
toxo	poison
trache(o)	trachea
urethr(o)	urethra
urin(o)	urine
uro	urine, urinary tract, urination
uter(o)	uterus
vas(o)	blood vessel, vas deferens
ven(o)	vein
vertebr(o)	spine, vertebrae

Suffixes

A **suffix** is placed at the end of a root to change the meaning of the word. Suffixes cannot be used alone. Like prefixes and roots, they are mainly from Greek and Latin. When translating medical terms, begin with the suffix.

A combining vowel is needed if the root ends with a consonant. If the root ends with a vowel and the suffix begins with a vowel, the vowel at the end of the root is dropped. For example, *nephritis,* means inflammation of the kidney. It was formed by combining *nephro* (kidney) and *itis* (inflammation). The "o" in nephro was dropped because the suffix began with a vowel.

You need to learn the suffixes listed in this chapter.

Suffix	Meaning
-algia	pain
-asis	condition, usually abnormal
-cele	hernia, herniation, pouching
-centesis	puncture and aspiration of
-cyte	cell
-ectasis	dilation, stretching
-ectomy	excision, removal of
-emia	blood condition
-genesis	development, production, creation
-genic	producing, causing
-gram	record
-graph	a diagram, a recording instrument
-graphy	making a recording
-iasis	condition of
-ism	a condition
-itis	inflammation
-logy	the study of
-lysis	destruction of, decomposition
-megaly	enlargement
-meter	measuring instrument
-metry	measurement
-oma	tumor
-osis	condition
-pathy	disease
-penia	lack, deficiency
-phasia	speaking
-phobia	an exaggerated fear
-plasty	surgical repair or reshaping
-plegia	paralysis
-ptosis	falling, sagging, dropping, down
-rrhage, -rrhagia	excessive flow
-rrhaphy	stitching, suturing
-rrhea	profuse flow, discharge
-scope	examination instrument
-scopy	examination using a scope
-stasis	maintenance, maintaining a constant level
-stomy, -ostomy	creation of an opening
-tomy, -otomy	incision, cutting into
-uria	condition of the urine

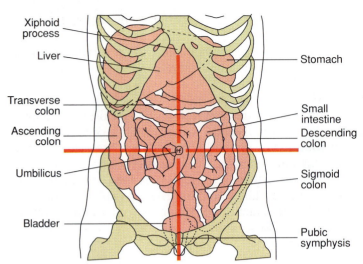

Fig 28-1 *The four regions of the abdomen.* **A,** *Right upper quadrant,* **B,** *Left upper quadrant.* **C,** *Right lower quadrant.* **D,** *Left lower quadrant.*

Combining Word Elements

Medical terms are formed by combining word elements. A root can be combined with prefixes, roots, or suffixes. The prefix *dys* (difficult) can be combined with the root *pnea* (breathing). This forms the term *dyspnea,* meaning difficulty in breathing.

Roots can be combined with suffixes. The root *mast* (breast) combined with the suffix *ectomy* (excision or removal) forms the term *mastectomy.* It means the removal of a breast.

Combining a prefix, root, and suffix is another way of forming medical terms. *Endocarditis* consists of the prefix *endo* (inner), the root *card* (heart), and suffix *itis* (inflammation). *Endocarditis* means inflammation of the inner part of the heart.

There are more complex combinations of prefixes, roots, and suffixes. There may be two prefixes, a root, and a suffix. Or there may be a prefix, two roots, and a suffix. Another pattern involves two roots and a suffix. The important things to remember are that prefixes always come before the root and suffixes always come after the root. You can practice forming medical terms by combining the word elements listed in this chapter.

ABDOMINAL REGIONS

To help describe the location of body structures, pain, or discomfort, the abdomen is divided into regions. The four regions (quadrants) are shown in Fig. 28-1. The regions are the right upper quadrant (RUQ), left upper quadrant (LUQ), right lower quadrant (RLQ), and left lower quadrant (LLQ).

DIRECTIONAL TERMS

Certain terms are used to describe the position of one body part in relation to another. These terms give the direction of the body part when a person is standing and facing forward. The directional terms that follow come from some of the prefixes listed in this chapter:

1. *Anterior (ventral)*—located at or toward the front of the body or body part
2. *Distal*—the part farthest from the center or from the point of attachment
3. *Lateral*—relating to or located at the side of the body or body part
4. *Medial*—relating to or located at or near the middle or midline of the body or body part

5. *Posterior* (dorsal)—located at or toward the back of the body or body part
6. *Proximal*—the part nearest to the center or to the point of origin

ABBREVIATIONS

Abbreviations are shortened forms of words or phrases. They often are used in written communication to save time and space. Some facilities use abbreviations other than the ones listed here. Most facilities have a list of the abbreviations they accept. You should obtain the list when you are hired and use only the abbreviations accepted by that facility. If you are not sure if an abbreviation is acceptable, write the term out in full to communicate accurately.

Abbreviation	Meaning
abd	Abdomen
ac	Before meals
ADL	Activities of daily living
ad lib	As desired

Abbreviation	Meaning
Adm (adm)	Admitted or admission
AM (am)	Morning
amb	Ambulatory
amt	Amount
ap	Apical
approx	Approximately
bid	Twice a day
BM (bm)	Bowel movement
BP	Blood pressure
BRP	Bathroom privileges
c̄	With
C	Centigrade
Ca	Cancer
Cath	Catheter
CBC	Complete blood count
CBR	Complete bed rest
cc	Cubic centimeter
CCU	Coronary care unit
c/o	Complains of
CPR	Cardiopulmonary resuscitation
CVA	Cerebrovascular accident, stroke
dc (d/c)	Discontinue
DOA	Dead on arrival
DON	Director of nursing
drsg	Dressing
Dx	Diagnosis
ECG (EKG)	Electrocardiogram
EEG	Electroencephalogram
ER	Emergency room
F	Fahrenheit
FBS	Fasting blood sugar
FF	Force fluids
fld	Fluid

ft	Foot or feet
gal	Gallon
GI	Gastrointestinal
h (hr)	Hour
H_2O	Water
HS (hs)	Hour of sleep
ht	Height
ICU	Intensive care unit
in	Inch
I&O	Intake and output
IV	Intravenous
L	Liter
Lab	Laboratory
lb	Pound
liq	Liquid
LLQ	Left lower quadrant
LMP	Last menstrual period
LPN	Licensed practical nurse
lt	Left
LVN	Licensed vocational nurse
LUQ	Left upper quadrant
meds	Medications
mid noc	Midnight

Abbreviation	Meaning
min	Minute
ml	Milliliter
NA	Nursing assistant
neg	Negative
nil	None
no	Number
noc	Night
NPO	Nothing by mouth
O_2	Oxygen
OB	Obstetrics
OJ	Orange juice
OOB	Out of bed
OR	Operating room
Ord	Orderly
OT	Occupational therapy
oz	Ounce
PAR	Postanesthesia room
pc	After meals
Peds	Pediatrics
per	By, through
PM (pm)	After noon
po (per os)	By mouth
postop (post op)	Postoperative
preop (pre op)	Preoperative
prep	Preparation
prn	When necessary
Pt (pt)	Patient
PT	Physical therapy
q	Every
qd	Every day
qh	Every hour
q2h, q3h, etc.	Every 2 hours, every 3 hours, etc.
qhs	Every night at bedtime

Abbreviation	Meaning
qid	Four times a day
qod	Every other day
R	Rectal temperature
RLQ	Right lower quadrant
RN	Registered nurse
ROM	Range of motion
RR	Recovery room
RUQ	Right upper quadrant
s̄	Without
Spec (spec)	Specimen
SSE	Soap suds enema
stat	At once, immediately
surg	Surgery
tbsp	Tablespoon
tid	Three times a day
TLC	Tender loving care
TPR	Temperature, pulse, and respiration
tsp	Teaspoon
U/a (U/A, u/a)	Urinalysis
VS (vs)	Vital signs
WBC	White blood count
w/c	Wheelchair
wt	Weight

SUMMARY

Medical terminology involves the use of word elements derived mainly from Greek and Latin. Word elements are prefixes, roots, and suffixes. They are combined in various ways to form medical words. Prefixes go before the root and suffixes go after the root. They are never used alone. You can practice forming and translating medical words by learning the word elements listed in this chapter. Use a nursing dictionary to check your accuracy.

Knowing commonly accepted abbreviations will help you to communicate with other health care workers. Abbreviations save time and space in making notes about assignments and observations. If you are allowed to chart in the resident's record, use abbreviations accepted by your facility whenever possible.

Review QUESTIONS

Fill in the blanks.

1. The three word elements used in medical terminology are
   a. _____
   b. _____
   c. _____

2. A _____ is a word element placed at the beginning of a word to change the meaning of the word.

3. A _____ is a word element placed at the end of a word to change the meaning of the word.

4. The four regions of the abdomen are
   a. _____
   b. _____
   c. _____
   d. _____

Match the item in column A with the item in column B.

Column A	Column B
5. Distal	A. The part nearest to the center or point of origin
6. Proximal	B. Relating to or located at the side of the body or body part
7. Anterior (ventral)	C. Located at or toward the front part of the body or body part
8. Medial	D. The part farthest from the center or point of attachment
9. Posterior (dorsal)	E. Located at or toward the back of the body or body part
10. Lateral	F. Relating to or located at or near the middle or the midline of the body or body part

Write the definition of the following prefixes.

11. a- _____
12. dys- _____
13. ab- _____
14. trans- _____
15. post- _____
16. olig- _____
17. hyper- _____
18. hypo- _____
19. ad- _____

Write the definition of the following suffixes.

20. -algia _____
21. -itis _____
22. -ostomy _____
23. -ectomy _____
24. -osis _____
25. -rrhage _____
26. -pathy _____
27. -otomy _____
28. -plasty _____

Write the definition of the following roots.

29. cranio _____
30. cardio _____
31. mammo _____
32. veno _____
33. urino _____
34. cyano _____
35. arterio _____
36. arthro _____
37. litho _____
38. gastro _____
39. encephalo _____
40. hemo _____
41. hystero _____
42. hepato _____
43. myo _____
44. phlebo _____
45. osteo _____
46. neuro _____
47. pneumo _____
48. toxo _____
49. psycho _____
50. thoraco _____

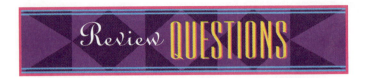

Match the item in *column A* with the item in *column B*.

Column A

		Column B
51.	Intravenous	A. Inflammation of a joint
52.	Apnea	B. Blood in the urine
53.	Hemiplegia	C. Excessive flow of blood
54.	Thoracotomy	D. Paralysis on one side
55.	Arthritis	E. Surgical removal of the uterus
56.	Bronchitis	F. No breathing
57.	Anuria	G. Inflammation of the bronchi
58.	Hematuria	H. Incision into the chest
59.	Hysterectomy	I. No urine
60.	Hemorrhage	J. Within a vein

Write the abbreviation for the following terms.

61. Bathroom privileges _____
62. As desired _____
63. Complains of _____
64. Twice a day _____
65. Hour of sleep _____
66. Nothing by mouth _____
67. When necessary _____
68. Postoperative _____
69. Every _____
70. At once, immediately _____

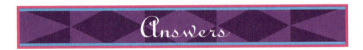

1. a. Prefix
   b. Root
   c. Suffix
2. Prefix
3. Suffix
4. a. Right upper quadrant
   b. Left upper quadrant
   c. Right lower quadrant
   d. Left lower quadrant

5. D
6. A
7. C
8. F
9. E
10. B
11. Without
12. Bad, difficult, abnormal
13. Away from
14. Across, over
15. After, behind
16. Scant, small
17. Excessive, too much
18. Decreased, less than normal
19. Toward
20. Pain
21. Inflammation
22. Creation of an opening
23. Removal of, excision
24. Condition
25. Excessive flow
26. Disease
27. Incision, cutting into
28. Surgical repair or reshaping
29. Skull
30. Heart
31. Breast
32. Vein
33. Urine
34. Blue
35. Artery
36. Joint
37. Stone
38. Stomach
39. Brain
40. Blood
41. Uterus
42. Liver
43. Muscle
44. Vein
45. Bone
46. Nerve
47. Lung
48. Poison

Answers

49. Mind
50. Chest
51. J
52. F
53. D
54. H
55. A
56. G
57. I
58. B
59. E
60. C
61. BRP
62. ad lib
63. c/o
64. bid
65. HS (hs)
66. NPO
67. prn
68. postop (post op)
69. q
70. stat

GLOSSARY

abbreviation   A shortened form of a word or phrase

abduction   Moving a body part away from the body

activities of daily living (ADL)   Those self-care activities a person performs daily to remain independent and to function in society

acute illness   A sudden illness from which the person is expected to recover

adduction   Moving a body part toward the body

admission   Official entry of a person into a facility or nursing unit

alimentary canal   The long tube extending from the mouth to the anus; the gastrointestinal tract

alopecia   Loss of hair

Alzheimer's disease   A disease that affects brain tissue; victims suffer increasing memory loss and confusion until they cannot meet their simplest personal needs; some even forget their own names

AM care   Care performed before breakfast; early morning care

ambulation   The act of walking

amputation   The removal of all or part of an extremity

anal incontinence   The inability to control the passage of feces and gas through the anus; fecal incontinence

anorexia   Loss of appetite

aphasia   The inability *(a)* to speak *(phasia)*

apical-radial pulse   Taking the apical and radial pulse at the same time; two workers are needed

apnea   The lack of or absence *(a)* of breathing *(pnea)*

artery   A blood vessel that carries blood away from the heart

arthritis   Joint *(arthr)* inflammation *(itis)*

arthroplasty   Joint *(arthro)* replacement *(plasty)*

asepsis   The absence of pathogens

aspiration   Breathing fluid or an object into the lungs

assault   Intentionally attempting or threatening to touch the body of another person without the person's consent

atelectasis   A collapse of a portion of the lung

atrophy   A decrease in size or a wasting away of tissue

autoclave   A pressure steam sterilizer

autonomic nervous system   A division of the peripheral nervous system; the system controls involuntary muscles and functions that occur without conscious effort

bacteria   Microscopic one-celled plant life that multiply rapidly; germs

base of support   The area on which an object rests

battery   The actual unauthorized touching of another person's body without the person's consent

bedsore   A decubitus ulcer; a pressure sore

benign tumor   A tumor that grows slowly and within a localized area; it usually does not cause death

bisexual   An individual who is attracted to persons of both sexes

blood pressure   The amount of force exerted against the walls of an artery by the blood

bloodborne pathogen   A pathogen found in the blood

board and care facility   A facility that provides custodial care to a few independent residents, often in a home setting; no licensed nurse is required

body alignment   The way in which body parts are aligned with one another; posture

body language   Facial expressions, gestures, posture, and other body movements that send messages to others

body mechanics   Using the body in an efficient and careful way

body temperature   The amount of heat in the body that is a balance between the amount of heat produced and the amount lost by the body

bone marrow   The substance within the hollow center of bones that manufactures blood cells

bowel movement   Defecation

bradypnea   Slow *(brady)* breathing *(pnea)*; the respiratory rate is less than 10 respirations per minute

braille   A method of writing for the blind; raised dots are arranged to represent each letter of the alphabet; the first 10 letters also represent the numbers 0 through 9

calorie   The amount of energy produced from the burning of food by the body

capillary   A tiny blood vessel; food, oxygen, and other substances pass from the capillaries to the cells

cardiac arrest   The sudden stoppage of breathing and heart action

carrier   A human being or animal that is a reservoir for microorganisms but that does not have the signs and symptoms of an infection

cartilage   Connective tissue at the end of long bones

caster   A small wheel made of rubber or plastic

catheter   A tube used to drain or inject fluid through a body opening

catheterization   The process of inserting a catheter

cell   The basic unit of body structure

cell membrane   The outer covering that encloses the cell and helps the cell hold its shape

central nervous system   One of two main divisions of the nervous system; made up of the brain and spinal cord

cerebrospinal fluid   The fluid that circulates around the brain and spinal cord

cerumen   The waxy substance secreted in the ear

chart   The resident's record

Cheyne-Stokes   A pattern of breathing in which respirations gradually increase in rate and depth and then become shallow and slow; breathing may stop (apnea) for 10 to 20 seconds

chromosomes   The threadlike structures in the cell nucleus; they contain genes

chronic illness   An illness, slow or gradual in onset, for which there is no known cure; the illness can be controlled and complications prevented

chyme   Partially digested food and fluid that pass from the stomach into the small intestine

civil law   Laws concerned with the relationships among people; private law

clean technique   Medical asepsis

closed fracture   The bone is broken but the skin is intact; a simple fracture

cognitive impairment   A decrease in intellectual functioning

colostomy   An artificial opening between the colon and abdomen

coma   The state of being completely unaware of one's surroundings and unable to react or respond

comatose   The inability to respond to verbal stimuli

combining vowel   A vowel added between two roots or a root and a suffix to make pronunciation easier

communicable disease   A disease caused by pathogens that are easily spread; an infectious disease; a disease that can be spread from one person to another

communication   The exchange of information; a message sent is received and interpreted by the intended person

complete bed bath   Washing the entire body of a resident who is in bed

compound fracture   The bone is broken and has come through the skin; open fracture

comprehensive care plan   A written guide that gives direction about the care a resident should receive from the health care team

constipation   The passage of a hard, dry stool

constrict   To narrow

contagious disease   A communicable disease

contamination   The process by which an object or area becomes unclean

contracture   The abnormal shortening of a muscle

convulsion   Violent and sudden contractions or tremors of muscles; seizure

crime   An act that is a violation of criminal law

criminal law   Laws concerned with offenses against the public and society in general; public law

culture   The values, beliefs, habits, likes, dislikes, customs, and characteristics of a group that are passed from one generation to the next

custodial care   Care provided on a 24-hour basis that meets a person's basic physical needs

cyanosis   Bluish discoloration of the skin

cytoplasm   The portion of the cell that surrounds the nucleus

dangling   Sitting on the side of the bed; sitting on the side of the bed and moving the legs back and forth and around in circles

deconditioning   The process of becoming weak from illness or lack of exercise; the loss of muscle strength due to inactivity

decubitus ulcer   A bedsore; a pressure sore

defamation   Injuring the name and reputation of another person by making false statements to a third person

defecation   The process of excreting feces from the rectum through the anus; a bowel movement

dehydration   A decrease in the amount of water in body tissues

delusion   A false belief

dementia   A set of chronic symptoms in which a person loses memory and the ability to think and reason; the term used to describe mental disorders caused by changes in the brain

dermis   The inner layer of the skin

diarrhea   The frequent passage of liquid stools

diastole   The period of heart muscle relaxation

diastolic pressure   The pressure in the arteries when the heart is at rest

digestion   The process of physically and chemically breaking down food so that it can be absorbed for use by the cells of the body

dilate   To expand or to open wider

disaster   A sudden, catastrophic event in which many people are injured and killed and property is destroyed; may be of natural or human origin

discharge   Official departure of a resident from a facility

disinfection   The process by which pathogens are destroyed

dorsal recumbent position   The back-lying or supine position; the supine or back-lying examination position; legs are together

dorsiflexion   Bending backward

drawsheet   A small sheet placed over the middle of the bottom sheet; it helps keep the mattress and bottom linens clean and dry; it can be used to turn and move residents in bed; the "cotton drawsheet"

dysphagia   Difficulty (*dys*) swallowing (*phagia*)

dyspnea   Difficult, labored, or painful (*dys*) breathing (*pnea*)

dysuria   Painful or difficult (*dys*) urination (*uria*)

early morning care   AM care

edema   The swelling of body tissues with water

embolus   A blood clot that travels through the vascular system until it lodges in a distant blood vessel

empathy   The ability to see things from another person's point of view

endometrium   The lining of the uterus

enema   The introduction of fluid into the rectum and lower colon

epidermis   The outer layer of the skin

esteem   The worth, value, or opinion one has of a person

ethics   What is right and wrong conduct

exhalation   The act of breathing out; expiration

extension   Straightening of a body part

external rotation   Turning the joint outward

face mask   A device used in the administration of oxygen; it covers the nose and mouth

fainting   The sudden loss of consciousness caused by an inadequate blood supply to the brain

false imprisonment   The unlawful restraint or restriction of another person's movement

fecal impaction   The prolonged retention and accumulation of fecal material in the rectum

fecal incontinence   The inability to control the passage of feces and gas through the anus, anal incontinence

feces   The semisolid mass of waste products in the colon

fertilization   The process whereby the male sex cell (sperm) unites with the female sex cell (ovum) to form one cell

first aid   Emergency care given to an ill or injured person before medical help arrives

flatulence   The excessive formation of gas in the stomach and intestines

flatus   Gas or air in the stomach or intestines

flexion   Bending a body part

Foley catheter   A catheter that is left in the urinary bladder so that urine drains continuously into a collection bag; an indwelling or retention catheter

footdrop   Permanent plantar flexion

Fowler's position   A semisitting position in which the head of the bed is elevated 45 to 60 degrees

fracture   A broken bone

fracture pan   A bedpan with a thinner rim that is shallower at one end than a regular bedpan

friction   The rubbing of one surface against another

functional nursing   A method of organizing nursing care; nursing staff members perform specific tasks for all assigned residents

fungi   Plants that live on other plants or animals

gait belt   A transfer belt

gangrene   A condition in which there is death of tissue; tissues become black, cold, and shriveled

gastrostomy   Surgically created opening in the stomach

gavage   Tube feeding

genes   The structures within the chromosomes that control the physical and chemical traits inherited by children from their parents

geriatrics   The care of aging people

germs   Bacteria

gerontology   The study of the aging process

glucosuria   Sugar *(glucose)* in the urine *(uria)*

gonad   The sex gland

graduate   A calibrated container used to measure fluid

ground   That which carries leaking electricity to the earth and away from the electrical appliance

hallucination   Seeing, hearing, or feeling something that is not real

health care team   A variety of health care workers who work together in providing health care for residents; interdisciplinary health care team

hearing aid   An instrument that amplifies sound

hemiplegia   Paralysis on one side of the body

hemoglobin   The substance in red blood cells that gives blood its color and carries oxygen in the blood

hemorrhage   The excessive loss of blood from a blood vessel

heterosexual   A person who is attracted to individuals of the opposite sex

homosexual   A person who has a strong attraction to members of the same sex

horizontal recumbent position   The dorsal recumbent position

hormone   A chemical substance secreted by the glands into the bloodstream

hospice   A health care facility or program for individuals dying of terminal illness

hospital   A health care facility where ill and injured persons are given health care, including medical and nursing care

host   The environment in which microorganisms live and grow; reservoir

HS care   Care given to the resident in the evening at bedtime

hyperextension   Excessive straightening of a body part

hypertension   Persistent blood pressure measurements above the normal systolic (140 mm Hg) or diastolic (90 mm Hg) pressures; in the elderly, persistent blood pressure measurements above 160 mm Hg systolic or 95 mm Hg diastolic

hyperventilation   Respirations that are rapid *(hyper)* and deeper than normal

hypotension   A condition in which the systolic blood pressure is below 90 mm Hg and the diastolic pressure is below 60 mm Hg

hypoventilation   Respirations that are slow *(hypo)*, shallow, and sometimes irregular

ileostomy   An artificial opening between the ileum (small intestine) and the abdomen

illusion   Misunderstanding sights and sounds in the environment

immunity   Having protection against a specific disease; the person does not get or become affected by the disease

impotence   The inability of the male to have an erection

indwelling catheter   A retention or Foley catheter

infection   A disease state that results from the invasion and growth of microorganisms in the body

infection precautions   Practices that limit the spread of pathogens; barriers are set up that prevent the escape of the pathogen

infectious disease   Communicable disease

inhalation   The act of breathing in; inspiration

integumentary system   The skin

interdisciplinary health care team   The health care team

internal rotation   Turning the joint inward

intravenous therapy   Fluid administered through a needle within a vein; IV and IV infusion

invasion of privacy   A violation of a person's right not to have his or her name, photograph, or private affairs exposed or made public without giving consent

involuntary muscles   The muscles that work automatically and that cannot be consciously controlled

iris   The part of the eye that gives the eye its color

isolation techniques   Practices that limit the spread of pathogens; barriers are set up that prevent the escape of the pathogen

joint   The point at which two or more bones meet

Kardex   Card file that summarizes information in the resident's record; it includes treatments, diagnosis, routine care measures, and special equipment used by the resident

knee-chest position   The resident kneels and rests the body on the knees and chest; the head is turned to one side, the arms are above the head or flexed at the elbows, the back is straight, and the body is flexed about 90 degrees at the hips

laryngeal mirror   Instrument used to examine the mouth, teeth, and throat

lateral position   The side-lying position

law   A rule of conduct made by a government body

legal   That which pertains to laws

liable   Being responsible for one's own action

libel   Defamation through written statements

licensed practical nurse (LPN)   An individual who has completed a 1-year nursing program and who has passed the licensing examination for practical nurses; called licensed vocational nurse (LVN) in some states

ligament   A strong band of connective tissue that holds bones together

lithotomy position   Resident is in a back-lying position, hips are at the edge of the examination table, knees are flexed, hips are externally rotated, and feet are in stirrups

logrolling   Turning the resident as a unit in alignment with one motion

malignant tumor   A tumor that grows rapidly and invades other tissues; it causes death if untreated

malpractice   Negligence by a professional person

meatus   The opening at the end of the urethra

Medicaid   A health insurance program sponsored by state and federal governments

medical asepsis   The techniques and practices used to prevent the spread of pathogens from one person or place to another person or place; clean technique

Medicare   A health insurance plan administered by the Social Security Administration of the federal government

menarche   The time when menstruation first begins

meninges   The connective tissue that covers and protects the brain and spinal cord; there are three layers: the outer layer called the dura mater, the middle layer called the arachnoid and the inner layer called the pia mater

menopause   The time when menstruation stops; it marks the end of the woman's reproductive years

menstruation   The process in which the endometrium of the uterus breaks up and is discharged from the body through the vagina

metabolism   The burning of food by the cells for heat and energy

metastasis   The spread of cancer to other body parts

microbe   A microorganism

microorganism   A small living plant or animal that cannot be seen without the aid of a microscope; a microbe

micturition   The process of emptying the bladder; urination or voiding

minimum data set (MDS)   A form used by nurses to assess a resident's mental, physical, and psychosocial function

mitosis   The process of cell division

morning care   Care given after breakfast; cleanliness and skin care measures are more thorough at this time

nasal cannula   A two-pronged device used in the administration of oxygen; the prongs are inserted a short distance into the nostrils

nasal catheter   A device used in the administration of oxygen; it is inserted into the nostril to the back of the throat

nasal speculum   Instrument used to examine the inside of the nose

need   That which is necessary or desirable for maintaining life and mental well-being

negligence   An unintentional wrong in which a person fails to act in a reasonable and careful manner and thereby causes harm to another person or to the person's property

nephron   The basic working unit of the kidney

neuron   The nerve cell; the basic unit of the nervous system

nonpathogen   A microorganism that does not usually cause an infection

nonverbal communication   Communication that does not involve the use of words

normal flora   Microorganisms that usually live and grow in a certain location

nucleus   The control center of the cell that directs the cell's activities

nurse practitioner (NP)   A registered nurse who has received advanced training in physical examination and assessment; in some states the NP can diagnose and prescribe under a doctor's supervision

nursing assistant   An individual who gives basic nursing care under the supervision of an RN or an LPN; also called nurse's aide, nursing attendant, health care assistant, and orderly

nursing facility (NF)   A facility that provides nursing care for many residents; a licensed nursing staff is required; commonly called a nursing home or convalescent hospital

nursing team   The individuals involved in providing nursing care: registered nurses, LPNs, and nursing assistants

nutrient   A substance that is ingested, digested, absorbed, and used by the body

nutrition   The many processes involved in the ingestion, digestion, absorption, and use of foods and fluids by the body

objective data   Information about a resident that can be seen, heard, felt, or smelled by another person; signs

OBRA   The Omnibus Budget Reconciliation Act of 1987; concerned with the quality of life, health, and safety of residents

observation   Using the senses of sight, hearing, touch, and smell to collect information about the resident

old   Those persons between the ages of 65 and 85

old-old   Those persons over the age of 85

open fracture   A fracture in which the bone is broken and has come through the skin; a compound fracture

ophthalmoscope   Lighted instrument used to examine the internal structures of the eye

optimal level of function   A person's highest potential for mental and physical performance

oral hygiene   Measures performed to keep the mouth and teeth clean; mouth care

orderly   A male nursing assistant

organ   Groups of tissues with the same function

ostomy   The surgical creation of an artificial opening

otoscope   Lighted instrument used to examine the external ear and the eardrum (tympanic membrane)

ovary   The female sex gland

ovulation   The process whereby an ovum is released by the ovary

ovum   The female sex cell

paraplegia   Paralysis from the waist down

parasympathetic nervous system   A division of the autonomic nervous system; the system tends to slow down functions

partial bed bath   Bathing the resident's face, hands, axillae, genital area, and buttocks

pathogen   A microorganism that is harmful and capable of causing an infection

percussion hammer   Instrument used to tap body parts to test reflexes

pericare   Perineal care

perineal care   Cleansing the genital and anal areas of the body; pericare

periosteum   The membrane that covers bone

peristalsis   Involuntary muscle contractions in the digestive system that move food through the alimentary canal; the alternating contraction and relaxation of intestinal muscles

personal protective equipment   Specialized clothing or equipment (gloves, goggles, gowns, masks) worn for protection against a hazard

phantom limb pain   A situation in which a resident complains of pain in an amputated part; it may feel as if the part is still there

plantar flexion   The foot is bent; footdrop

plasma   The fluid portion of the blood

plastic drawsheet   A drawsheet made of plastic; it is placed between the bottom sheet and the cotton drawsheet to keep the mattress and bottom linens clean and dry

pneumonia   An inflammation of the lung

postmortem   After *(post)* death *(mortem)*

posture   The way in which the body parts are aligned with one another; body alignment

prefix   A word element placed at the beginning of a word to change the meaning of the word

pressure sore   An area where the skin and underlying tissues are eroded as a result of a lack of blood flow; a bedsore or decubitus ulcer

primary nursing   A method of organizing nursing care; a nurse is responsible for the total care of specific residents on a 24-hour basis

pronation   Turning downward

prone   Lying on the abdomen with the head turned to one side

prosthesis   An artificial replacement for a body part

protoplasm   A term that refers to all of the structures, substances, and water within the cell

protozoa   Microscopic one-celled animals

pulse   The beat of the heart felt at an artery as a wave of blood passes through the artery

pulse deficit   The difference between the apical and radial pulse rates

pulse rate   The number of heartbeats or pulses felt in 1 minute

pupil   The opening in the middle of the eye

quadriplegia   Paralysis from the neck down

range of motion   The movement of a joint to the extent possible without causing pain

recording   Writing or charting resident care and observations

reflex   An involuntary movement

registered nurse (RN)   A person who has studied nursing for 2, 3, or 4 years and who has passed a licensing examination

rehabilitation   The process of restoring the disabled person to the highest possible level of physical, psychological, social, and economic functioning

reincarnation   The belief that the spirit or soul is reborn in another human body or in another form of life

religion   Spiritual beliefs, needs, and practices

reporting   An oral account of the resident's care and observations

reservoir   The environment in which microorganisms live and grow; the host

resident   A person living in a long-term care facility

resident assessment protocol summary (RAPS)   Guidelines used in developing the comprehensive care plan

resident's record   A written account of the resident's physical or mental status and his or her response to the treatment and care given by members of the health team; the chart

resident unit   The furniture and equipment provided for the individual by the facility

respiration   The process of supplying the cells with oxygen and removing carbon dioxide from them; the act of breathing air into (inhalation) and out of (exhalation) the lungs

respiratory arrest   Breathing stops but the heart continues to pump for several minutes

respite care   The admission of a person from home to a nursing facility for a short stay; the caregiver is given time for a vacation, business, or a short rest

responsibility   A duty; an obligation to perform some act or function; being able to answer for one's actions

restorative aide   A nursing assistant who has special training in rehabilitation skills

restraint   Devices or chemicals that limit freedom of movement or prevent access to one's body

retention catheter   A Foley or indwelling catheter

reverse Trendelenburg's position   The head of the bed is raised and the foot of the bed is lowered

rickettsiae   Microscopic forms of life found in the tissues of fleas, lice, ticks, and other insects

rigor mortis   The stiffness or rigidity (*rigor*) of skeletal muscles that occurs after death (*mortis*)

root   A word element that contains the basic meaning of the word

sclera   The white of the eye

seizure   A convulsion

self-actualization   Experiencing one's potential

semi-Fowler's position   The head of the bed is raised 45 degrees and the knee portion is raised 15 degrees; or the head of the bed is raised 30 degrees and the knee portion is not raised

sex   The physical activities involving the organs of reproduction; the activities are done for pleasure or to have children

sexuality   That which relates to one's sex; those physical, psychological, social, cultural, and spiritual factors that affect a person's feelings and attitudes about his or her sex

shear   That which occurs when skin sticks to a surface and the bones move forward or backward within the skin; blood supply to the skin is affected

shock   A condition that results when there is an inadequate blood supply to organs and tissues

side-lying position   The lateral position

signs   Objective data

simple fracture   A closed fracture; the bone is broken but the skin is intact

Sims' position   A side-lying position in which the upper leg is sharply flexed so that it does not rest on the lower leg and the lower arm is behind the resident

skilled nursing facility (SNF)   A facility that provides nursing care for residents who need complex care but do not require hospital services; it may be part of a nursing facility or a hospital

slander   Defamation through oral statements

sperm   The male sex cell

sphygmomanometer   The instrument used to measure blood pressure; it has a cuff (applied to the upper arm) and a measuring device

spore   A bacterium protected by a hard shell that forms around the microorganism

sputum   Mucus secreted by the lungs, bronchi, and trachea during respiratory illnesses or disorders

sterile   The absence of all microorganisms

sterilization   The process by which all microorganisms are destroyed

stethoscope   An instrument used to listen to the sounds produced by the heart, lungs, and other body organs

stoma   An opening; see **colostomy** and **ileostomy**

stomatitis   Inflammation (*itis*) of the mouth (*stomat*)

stool   Feces that have been excreted

stroke   A cerebral vascular accident (CVA); blood supply to a part of the brain is suddenly interrupted

subjective data   Information communicated by the resident that the health care worker cannot observe by using the senses; symptoms

suction   The process of withdrawing or sucking up fluids

suffix   A word element placed at the end of a root to change the meaning of the word

suffocation   The termination of breathing that results from lack of oxygen

sundowning   Increased signs, symptoms, and behaviors of Alzheimer's disease during hours of darkness

supination   Turning upward

supine position   The back-lying or dorsal recumbent position

suppository   A cone-shaped solid medication that is inserted into a body opening; it melts at body temperature

sympathetic nervous system   A division of the autonomic nervous system; the system tends to speed up functions

symptoms   Subjective data

synovial fluid   The fluid secreted by the synovial membrane that acts as a lubricant; the fluid allows the joint to move smoothly

system   Organs that work together to perform special functions

systole   The period of heart muscle contraction

systolic pressure   The amount of force it takes to pump blood out of the heart into the arterial circulation

tachypnea   Rapid *(tachy)* breathing *(pnea);* the respiratory rate is usually greater than 24 respirations per minute

team nursing   A method of organizing nursing care in which a nurse serves as a team leader; the team leader assigns other nurses and nursing assistants to care for certain residents

tendons   The tough connective tissue that connects muscles to bones

terminal illness   An illness or injury for which there is no reasonable expectation of recovery

testis   The male sex gland

thrombus   A blood clot

tissue   Groups of cells with the same function

tort   A wrong committed against another person or the person's property

transfer   Moving a resident from one room, nursing unit, or facility to another

transfer belt   A belt used to hold onto a resident during a transfer or when a worker is walking with the resident; a gait belt

transsexual   A person who believes that he or she is really a member of the opposite sex

transvestite   A person who becomes sexually excited by dressing in the clothes of the opposite sex

Trendelenburg's position   The head of the bed is lowered and the foot of the bed is raised

triggers   Clues that direct the caregiver to the appropriate resident assessment protocols (RAPS)

tumor   A new growth of abnormal cells; tumors can be benign or malignant

tuning fork   Instrument used to test hearing

urethra   The structure through which urine passes from the bladder and is eliminated from the body

urinary incontinence   The inability to control the passage of urine from the bladder

urination   The process of emptying the bladder; micturition or voiding

vaccination   The administration of a vaccine to produce immunity

vaccine   A preparation containing microorganisms

vaginal speculum   Instrument used to open the vagina so that it and the cervix can be examined

vein   A blood vessel that carries blood back to the heart

verbal communication   Communication that uses the written or spoken word

virus   A microscopic organism that grows in living cells

vital signs   Temperature, pulse, respirations, and blood pressure

voiding   Urination or micturition

voluntary muscles   The muscles that can be consciously controlled; skeletal muscles

vomiting   The act of expelling stomach contents through the mouth

will   A legal statement of how an individual wishes to have property distributed after death

word element   A part of a word

young-old   Those persons between the ages of 55 and 65

INDEX